MENTAL ILLNESSES AND TREATMENTS

MENTAL EPIDEMICS

FROM MOBBING TO TERRORISM HANDBOOK

Mental Illnesses and Treatments

Additional books in this series can be found on Nova's website under the Series tab.

Additional e-books in this series can be found on Nova's website under the e-books tab.

MENTAL ILLNESSES AND TREATMENTS

MENTAL EPIDEMICS

FROM MOBBING TO TERRORISM HANDBOOK

PAVEL IVANOVICH SIDOROV

NOVA BIOMEDICAL
New York

Library of Congress Cataloging-in-Publication Data

ISBN: 978-1-63484-809-1

Published by Nova Science Publishers, Inc. † New York

Contents

Preface vii

Acknowledgements ix

Introduction. Adaptive Engineering and Management of Mind and Health as the Mission of Mental Medicine xi

List of Abbreviations xvii

About the Author xix

Section I. Conceptual and Methodological Basis of Mental Medicine and Epidemiology 1

Chapter 1 Mental Ecology 3

Chapter 2 Synthesis of Mental Medicine 13

Chapter 3 From Nosocentric Psychiatry to Health-Oriented Mental Medicine 21

Chapter 4 Synergetic Methodology of Mental Medicine 27

Chapter 5 Mental Epidemiology 35

Chapter 6 Ethical Propaedeutics of Mental Epidemiology 51

Section II. Mental Epidemics of Psychosomatic Disorders 69

Chapter 7 Synergetic Biopsychosociospiritual Concept of Mental Epidemics of Psychosomatic Disorders 71

Chapter 8 Arterial Hypertension 83

Chapter 9 Coronary Heart Disease 97

Chapter 10 Peptic Ulcer 111

Chapter 11 Bronchial Asthma 123

Chapter 12 Diabetes Mellitus 135

Chapter 13 Oncological Diseases 147

Chapter 14 Overweight and Obesity 159

Chapter 15	Rheumatoid Arthritis	**169**
Section III. Mental Epidemics of Somatoform Disorders		**181**
Chapter 16	Somatoform Disorders	**183**
Chapter 17	Induced Neuropsychiatric Disorders: History and Hystero-Demonical Renaissance	**191**
Chapter 18	Destructive Professiogenesis	**205**
Section IV. Mental Epidemics of Dependent Personality Disorders		**219**
Chapter 19	Dependent Personality Disorders	**221**
Chapter 20	Mobbing Syndrome: Mental Terrorism of "Office Wars"	**233**
Chapter 21	Terrorism as a Polymodal Dependent Disorder	**243**
Chapter 22	Mental Terrorism of Hybrid Wars and Synergetics of Protection	**265**
Section V. Mental Epidemics of Endoecological Mental Disorders		**283**
Chapter 23	Schizophrenia	**285**
Chapter 24	Depressive Disorders	**305**
Section VI. Preventive-Correctional and Treatment-Rehabilitational Resources of Mental Medicine		**315**
Chapter 25	Biological Resources of Mental Medicine	**317**
Chapter 26	Psychological Resources of Mental Medicine	**337**
Chapter 27	Social Resources of Mental Medicine	**347**
Chapter 28	Spiritual and Moral Resources of Mental Medicine	**357**
Chapter 29	Religious Resources of Mental Medicine	**371**
Section VII. Synergetic Technological Platform of Mental Health Service		**385**
Chapter 30	Synergetic Integrativity and Health-Oriented Optimisticity of Mental Medicine	**387**
Chapter 31	Mental Health Service as an Interface of Public Conscience	**395**
Chapter 32	Mental Engineering of Public Conscience	**407**
Chapter 33	Mental Preventology as a System of Integration of Healthy Way and Moral Meaning of Life	**421**
Chapter 34	Mental Immunity as the Matrix of Identity and the Basis of Security	**441**
Conclusion	**Development Strategies for Mental Epidemiology and Medicine**	**455**
References		**461**
Index		**485**

Preface

The Handbook focuses on a new research area: mental medicine as a psychiatric paradigm of integrative medicine. The scientific basis of mental medicine is "synergetics." Synergetics is an interdisciplinary science of development and self-organization, which has allowed the successive and systematical combination of treatment and rehabilitation strategies of nosocentric clinical psychiatry with preventive and correctional methods of health-oriented mental preventology. Mental medicine strengthens mental health and treats mental illnesses. Its mission lies in enabling adaptive engineering and management of mind and health.

This book presents a synergetic biopsychosociospiritual concept of development of mental epidemics – that is, contagious polymodal and polymorphic mental diseases and states. The conceptual provisions of mental health services are proposed, and requirements for mental health system monitoring as an interface of the public conscience are included.

The features of anti-epidemic biopsychosociospiritual care are examined in this book. These features include somatotropic and psychotropic management, psychotherapeutic and sanogenetic management in multidisciplinary teams, as well as social, spiritual, and moral correction and rehabilitation. The principles and techniques of mental preventology are grounded. Mental preventology grows out of a synergetic rendering of mental hygiene and psychoprophylaxis, ethical and psychological support of adaptive professiogenesis and business communication, integration of healthy ways and the moral meaning of life. The system of biopsychosociospiritual protection of the personality and society is represented by the resources of mental immunity, which is behaviorally embodied in the profile registers of mental resilience.

This book is intended for general practitioners and psychotherapists, psychiatrists and narcologists, clinical psychologists and educators, specialists in social work and bioethics, churchmen and volunteers.

Acknowledgements

Reviewers: *I. L. Andreev*, Professor, Doctor of Philosophy, Chief Researcher, Institute of Philosophy of Russian Academy of Sciences; *V. V. Makarov*, Professor, Head of the Department of Psychotherapy and Sexual Pathology of the Russian Academy of Postgraduate Education; *M. M. Burkin*, Professor, Head of the Department of Psychiatry and Neurology, Petrozavodsk State University.

Translation into English – by *Maria A. Zakharova*, BA. Medical and science translation review – by *Evgeniya P. Sovershaeva*, MD.

Photo: *Igor Slobodyanyuk*, *Aleksey Sukhanovsky*.

Introduction. Adaptive Engineering and Management of Mind and Health as the Mission of Mental Medicine

Every age in the history of medicine left its mark by furthering the development of philosophy and natural science. During its whole history, humanity has pondered over the World Secret of orderliness and destruction, asking eternal questions about the nature of order and chaos, birth, and death, health and disease, the cycle of phenomena and the singularity of processes. These questions are still of great concern for modern science and the scientific community's mindset.

Mentality is the perception of reality that is, developed during the process of upbringing, education, and acquisition of life experience in a particular cultural environment. The word "mentality" comes from the Latin "mens, mentis," which means "mind."

The French ethnologist and socio-anthropologist Lucien Lévy-Bruhl was the first to introduce the term "mentality" to the scientific community. Gaston Bouthoul (1952) described mentality as "the sum of ideas and intellectual sets of a certain person connected with each other either logically or by religious beliefs," and the majority of researches have agreed with this definition.

Mental ecology is a sector of human ecology that studies the various relationships between the environment, -society, and -individuals.

According to the World Health Organization (WHO 1992), there are four groups of factors that form a person's general level of health. They include lifestyle, life environment, public health service, and genetics. In the present research, we single out *"mentality"* from "lifestyle," which is the behavioristic incarnation of mentality. By the method of «Health ecology estimation», we calculated the contribution of each factor in general health level: lifestyle-25%, life environment-21%, mentality-20%, public health service-18% and genetics-16%.

According to the WHO definition (2001), *mental health* is the mental well-being of a person that helps him to fulfill own potential, assists with managing stress, helps to work effectively and participate in the development of society. Mental health is not just the absence of psychiatric disorder.

It is crucially important to note that the definition consists of not merely G. L. Engel's (1977) classical biopsychosocial triad, but also of a moral part of "well-being," "self-actualization," "ability to handle stress" and "productivity," that are impossible without ethics of business communication. The civil, political part represented by the appeal to "contribute to the society development" looks even more pretentious.

The canons of all the world religions have a compulsory concern for people's moral and mental health, for the prevention of stress and addictions. In this context, mental health is the common, canonical religious priority.

According to WHO, there is none of "official" definition of the term "mental health" because of cultural differences, subjective judgments and competing professional theories. Meanwhile mental health is the crucial criteria of the state and society development. This fact is important to take into consideration given that the amount of people with mental disorders of nonpsychotic origin has increased by a factor of 60 for the last century.

That is why very disturbing tendencies characterize public conscience in Russia as an integral quality of mental health. The prevalence rate of mental and behavior disorders is about 20-30% of the population. 30-50% of those who have taken medical advice suffer from mental disorders. Mental disorders constitute more than 40% of exemptions from military service. 25% of schoolchildren and 45% of university students have experimented with drugs. 75% of men and 47% of women abuse alcohol. Official statistics differs significantly from epidemiological research data, according to which the prevalence rate of subclinical forms of mental disorders is higher by a factor of 5; neurotic disorders – by a factor of 19; personality disorders – by a factor of 17. According to all these facts, it can be stated that *public conscience in Russia is in critical condition.*

Thousands of extremist organizations make a profit of this situation, and the whole situation is getting even worse. There are more than 12 millions of people involved in almost 3000 destructive sects that manage to manipulate public conscience of the population. Besides, there are 300 thousands of magicians, wizards, sorcerers and shamans who influence up to 30 millions of people every year. All the mentioned above are engaged in mental, political or religious terrorism which means manipulative influence on a person's mind for the purpose of destruction his individuality and taking control of the individual's behavior, emotions and will (often for mercenary reasons). *Mental terrorism is a non-lethal weapon of mass destruction and a threat to national security.*

Destructive mental manipulation supports and extends *pessimistically-catastrophic mental paradigm*. A considerable part of the population anxiously sees their future and future of their kids as rather a depressive. Most of the TV-shows and news focus on negative and fearsome events as well. It results in the shaping of a catastrophic type of mind when people expect only grief and defeats. Such *self-destructive mentality* has already been formed and is continuing to root in the public conscience. Creating new means of resistance to *mental* terrorism and *building self-preservative optimistic-resourceful mental paradigm* is the crucially primary public aim.

Igor Guberman in his "garicks" (a kind of humorous limericks) expressed current dramatic and tragic-comic contradictions of Russian public conscience in a very amusing and laconical way, showing the essential impossibility of a dialog neither between orthodox and liberal mentality nor within those two paradigms. Here is one of his garicks illustrating the illness of "marginal mentality":

The sky above is full of promise
And life ahead is nice and sweet
It's not because the world is flawless
But it's because I am a twit.

The marginal mentality in its most purified form is very easy to find in a mental asylum. If we imagine for a moment our world as a madhouse, then it is not the doctors but the elite of acutely psychotic patients who will rule such a place. The world has not gone mad yet, but it is teetering on the edge hardly resisting attacks of social epidemics of reckless violence and terrorism. The government cannot fight these phenomena with crude force anymore. It is crucial to change the mental paradigm of the civilizational development, strengthening social-humanistic and spiritual and moral priorities.

The mental paradigm of Russian state national security includes mitigation of mental diseases consequences and reduction of prevalence of mental and social epidemics, self-destructive and antisocial behavior. Lowering high level of death rate and violence in the society, diminution of social differentiation, poverty and unemployment are also the elements of this paradigm. Liquidation of social vulnerability of the disabled and the ill, overcoming of the anomie and deformation of public and personal conscience, as well as avoidance of a person's isolation from society, and forming of the strategies of adaptive professiogenesis and effective self-management are also the aspects of this mental paradigm.

Mental medicine is a science that studies etiopathogenesis and diagnostics, clinical picture and treatment of mental diseases, biopsychosociospiritual resources of an individual and society development, strategies and mechanisms of adaptation and professiogenesis based on integrated and synergetic methodology. This formula includes the classical definition of psychiatry and all the modalities that were marked out by WHO (2001) in its description of mental health which is the target of mental preventology.

Mental preventology as a part of general preventology studies the means of forming and maintenance an optimal level of mental health, psycho-hygiene, and psycho-prevention basing on systematic and multi-disciplined synergetic approach. Defensive biopsychosociospiritual resources of the personality are accumulated in the *mental immunity*, behaviorally embodying in the profile registers of *mental resilience*.

Mental epidemiology studies the spread of mental health-related states and events (and their determinants) within certain populations, as well as the application of these studies to the adaptive defense of public health and conscience.

Mental epidemics are contagious polymodal and polymorphic mental diseases and states.

Organizational and manpower need of mental medicine manifests itself in multiple attempts to bring "The Psychotherapy" bill in the State Duma which would provide more legal substance to clinical psychologists and psychotherapists. According to expert evaluation, there are more than 100 thousand practicing psychologists and 40 thousand of psychotherapists in Russia nowadays. It is crucially important to note that even now these specialists attend to not only patients but the mentally healthy clients who experience certain problems and adaptation troubles. The therapists use the technology of health-centered mental medicine helping healthy people, improving their outlook on the world and self-perception in this world.

The mission of mental medicine lies in the adaptive engineering and management of individual and public conscience and health. It represents the new stage of development of personalized integrative medicine on the synergetic conceptually-methodological and instrumentally-technological platform.

The goal of mental medicine is to reinforce evolutionarily the health-centered potential of mental health protection (on the base of clinical psychiatry) which is of great importance for joint support of civilizational and modernization trends. The global crisis of modern world in the first instance demands reconsideration of the basic mental paradigm of the humanity development which means socio-humanistic principles that supplant selfish and exploitative attitude. Mental medicine is going to be the medicine of tomorrow's post-crisis society.

Substantial characteristics of mental medicine in a generalized sense can be defined within the following blocks:

1. *philosophic and gnoseological* block deals with paradigm evolution of mental medicine;
2. *a conceptually-methodological* block which is a synergetic biopsychosociospiritual methodology of mental medicine;
3. *the parametric block* is used to estimate the efficiency of prevention and correction, treatment and rehabilitation;
4. *instrumental and technological* block embraces multi-discipline resources of mental medicine;
5. *normative legal* block institutionalizes new integral grade of an inter-sectoral professional community.

Health-centered mental medicine extends the potential of psychiatry and narcology, psychotherapy and clinical psychology. Such medicine destigmatizes the psycho-narcological field and its professional communities, ensures inclusion of psycho- and socio-therapy in all the preventive, therapeutic, and rehabilitation programs and routes thus implementing new conceptual and technological methodology which aims ultimately at preservation and strengthening of mental health. Essentially mental medicine systematically tackles the challenges of the global crisis. It is not a mere coincidence that "crisis" in Chinese consists of two hieroglyphs – "*danger*" and "feasibility of *overcoming*." Mental medicine accumulates new resources and opportunities on a multi-discipline and synergetic basis.

Mental health service (MHS) is a new synergetic productive cluster which is being formed nowadays in Russia. This service solves mental medicine tasks on a target-oriented level, mobilizing federal, regional, corporative and private resources of the state-private and society-state partnerships. MHS is a synergetic biopsychosociospiritual Ψ-cluster of society and state. It provides the mentally-ill with preventive and correctional defense of the mental health along with medical and rehabilitation care.

The interface function of the public conscience of the MHS is performed by the system monitoring of mental health (SMMH) which is supposed to forecast and prevent threats of mental and social epidemics. SMMH is a multi-disciplined complex monitoring aimed to reveal cause-and-effect link within the "environment-society-individual" system. It clusters core databases within a framework of integrated synergetic methodology, providing objective sight and dynamics of socially-important mental and behavioral trends. In the absence of this instrument, any programs of development and modernization will be very vulnerable.

The methodological base of mental medicine is Synergetics which is a cross-disciplinary scientific area studying development and self-organization of dissipative, energy-dispersive structures.

The synergetic approach in medicine contains vectors of *biopsychosociosp iritual model*: somato-, psycho-, socio- and animogenesis. Somatogenesis means the development of the systems and functions of the body; psychogenesis means the development of mental functions; sociogenesis means development of social roles and relations; animogenesis means the moral and spiritual development of a person.

Mental medicine basing on synergetic methodology combines mental health medicine and medicine of mental illnesses (clinical psychiatry). It is essential that mental medicine *in the framework of systemic synthesis integrate psychiatry and anti-psychiatry.*

Robert Webb-Johnstone expressed very succinctly the *anachronistical paradigm of bellicose anti-psychiatry* that has formed during the last 50 years. If we take his citation as a basis, we can modify it into a more generalized system version: "Neurotics build cloud-castles, schizophrenics live in them, psychopaths destroy them, and alcoholics guzzle away the ruins. Everybody enjoy the process and only the psychiatrists collect the rent." Such a disparaging appraisal is in direct proportion to the degree of stigmatization of our profession, although psychiatrists themselves are also concerned about these problems. It is not by coincidence that Carl Jung (1939) wrote: "To make a correct diagnosis and stop to look at a fence of a gloomy prognosis is not a substantial contribution to the art of medicine." Hopefully, it is Synergetics – cross-disciplinary, widely covering the methodological and phenomenological fields – that will be able to result in new etiopathogenetic breakthroughs in the studies of mental diseases.

The discussions of the problems of psychiatric diagnostics have recently intensified after the publication of DSM-5 (Diagnostic and Statistical Manual of Mental Disorders, 5th ed.) and wide debating about RDoC (a project of scientific classification based on neurosciences achievements – Research Domain Criteria). These classifications attempt to integrate an alternative approaches to diagnostics: categorical, dimensional, neurobiological, etc. The synergetic biopsychosociospiritual approach that we have suggested makes it possible to achieve the most integrative diagnostic platform and personalized model of treatment.

The first publication based on cross-disciplined synergetic methodology was implemented in "International Handbook on Alcohol and Culture» (Greenwood Press: Westport, Connecticut-London 1995). Then there was a release of a handbook "Addictologic preventology" (Genius-media 2005). And a year after there was the second, updated and revised edition (M. Medpress-inform 2006). The "Mental Medicine of post-crisis world," written jointly by an associate professor I. B. Yakushev, was released in 2011 (LAMBERT Academic Publishing). The handbook "Mental Medicine: Methodology and Practice," written jointly by a professor I. A. Novikova, was released in 2012 (LAMBERT Academic Publishing). The second edition was published by "Geotar-Media" publishing group in 2014. The present edition has been significantly updated and revised. The fourth dimension of animogenesis has been introduced in the synergetic methodology, for which reason all the chapters and parts of the book have been rewritten and widened. The second section of the handbook was prepared jointly by a general practitioner and a researcher of Northern State Medical University – Evgenia Sovershaeva.

All the chapters of the handbook are the articles published in the period between 2013 and 2015 in the journals of the “Genius-media” publishing house (CEO – D. A. Irishkin, science editor – professor I. L. Andreev,) and in the academic journal “Human ecology.”

I express deep gratitude to the reviewers and my long time friends – professors I. L. Andreev, V. V. Makarov and M. M. Burkin for the reviewing of the material presented in the handbook.

Invaluable assistance in preparing the book for publication was provided by research assistants of NSMU – Maria Zakharova, who has performed literary translation into English, and Evgenia Sovershaeva, a general practitioner, who has fulfilled the medical and scientific editing of the translation. I express the deepest gratitude to my esteemed colleagues for many years of selfless work.

I hope that in the upcoming tough years for the destiny of Russia it is Mental Medicine and Epidemiology that will enable to attract new resources for the mental health protection and mental illnesses treatment, for the effective guaranteeing of the Mental Ecology of national security of the country.

List of Abbreviations

AH	arterial hypertension
ANS	autonomic nervous system
BFB	biofeedback
BMI	body mass index
BP	blood pressure
BS	burnout syndrome
BA	bronchial asthma
CABG	coronary artery bypass graft surgery
CC	cerebral competence
CHD	coronary heart disease
CNS	central nervous system
DM1	diabetes mellitus type 1
DM2	diabetes mellitus type 2
DSM-5	Diagnostic and Statistical Manual of Mental Disorders, Fifth Edition
EEG	electroencephalography
ESR	erythrocyte sedimentation rate
GD	gallstone disease
GIT	gastrointestinal tract
HbAlc	glycated hemoglobin
HE	hypertensive encephalopathy
HNA	higher nervous activity
ICD	International Classification of Diseases
IGT	impaired glucose tolerance
ID	intellectual disability
MHS	mental health service
NCA	neurocirculatory asthenia
NSAIDs	non-steroid anti-inflammatory drugs
PU	peptic ulcer
QOL	quality of life
RF	risk factors
SFD	somatoform disorders
SMMH	system monitoring of mental health
WHO	World Health Organization

"Don't take life too seriously.
You'll never get out of it alive".

Elbert Hubbard
US writer, publisher and editor

About the Author and his mental immunity

Pavel Sidorov

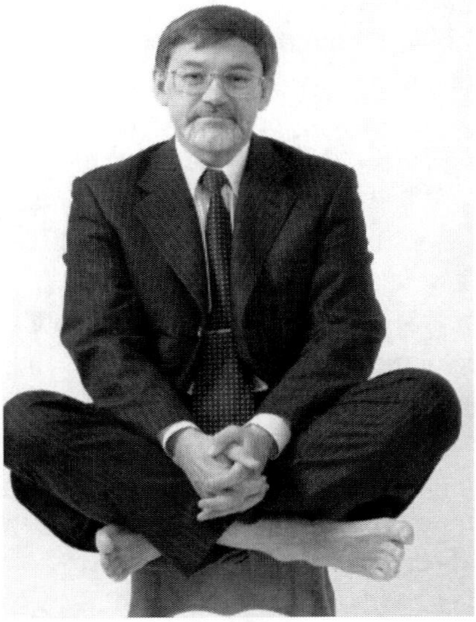

Education

Arkhangelsk State Medical Institute, Medical Faculty (1976).

The All-Russian State Distance-Learning Institute of Finance and Economics, Management (2000).

Degrees and titles

Doctor of Medical Sciences, Professor, Academician of the Russian Academy of Sciences.

Candidate's dissertation on "Clinical-Social Aspects of Alcoholization and Alcoholism in Teens and Adolescents (1979)".

Doctoral dissertation on "Pathogenesis of Alcoholism in Teens and Early Prevention Methods in the Northern European Environment" (1986).

Academic Career

In 1980, began to work as an assistant in the psychiatry department, of which he was made a professor in 1988, and in 1994, was the head of the department (until 2012).

In 1991, was made prorector of scientific work and in 1993, became rector of ASMI.

In 1994, changed the institution into an academy and in 2000, changed it to Northern State Medical University.

At NSMU opened twelve institutes, two research institutes for maritime medicine and arctic medicine, 18 specialties, nine areas of study for bachelor's degrees, and three international master's degree programs. This paved the way for the NSMU's multidisciplinary science, educational and practical innovation complex for integrated medicine based on a synergetic biology, psychology, sociology and spiritual technological platform. In 1992, the institution's economic development driver was Medipark (the medical analog of a technology park), uniting dozens of venture capital companies of varying forms of ownership and working under a public-private sector partnership (which was only legitimized in August 2009).

In 1991, opened the first doctoral dissertation council in Russia for new specialists of emergency safety, and it was the only one of its kind in the country for six years. Under the Russian Academy of Medical Sciences, in 1992 he organized the establishment of Human Ecology, a monthly practical science journal, and Narcology in 2002. He was the first Russian scientist admitted into the RAMS under the new specialty of human ecology; in 1995, became a Corresponding Member and in 2000 he became an Academician.

He developed and implemented in a number of pilot programs a systematic methodology for system monitoring, ranging from the ecological to the educational and from public health to public awareness. In 2007, after years of medical and ecological research into issues of safety at the Plesetsk Cosmodrome, Pavel Sidorov and his colleagues published a monograph on "System Monitoring of Rocket and Space Activity" (MEDpress-inform), which warned Roscosmos leadership of the increasing probability of catastrophe in the field due to the cumulative buildup of the effects of ineffective post-Soviet models of production and management.

In 2009, opened at NSMU the Mental Medicine Institute and in 2011, the Social Faculty of Mental Medicine was opened in a new kind of partnership with both the public and private sectors and with the Russian Orthodox Church and business community. The field of "mental medicine", developed by P.I. Sidorov as a psychiatric paradigm for integrated medicine, allows for the mobilization of new interdisciplinary resources in the management of awareness and health. Today, it is one of the priorities in the third stage of presidential initiatives involving "Strategies for the Development of Nanoindustry", set to begin in 2016 and develop over the next ten to twenty years.

P.I. Sidorov has been an advisor for the defense of 38 doctoral and 45 candidate's dissertations. He is the founder of mental ecology and medicine, mental epidemiology and preventology, the conception of a systematic monitoring of mental health and synergetic platforms for mental health services.

Academician P.I. Sidorov is a recognized leader in human ecology and social psychiatry, clinical psychology and disaster medicine, social epidemiology and conflictology, and the prevention of extremism and terrorism. Since 2012, has been the head research fellow at NSMU.

Honorary Titles, Awards and Prizes

In 1992, the Russian Association of Narcologists named Pavel Sidorov *The Narcologist of the Year*. He has been given the following honors: Distinguished Scientist of the RF (1997); Government of the RF Award for Science and Technology (2006) for the work on ecological system monitoring as a national security priority; 6 State Medals of the RF; Golden Badge of Honor of the Social Consciousness National Foundation; Golden Psyche Psychological Competition Winner; Lomonosov Foundation Regional Prize (for creating as native of the Kholmogorsky Region the Descendents of Lomonosov Association). Was awarded the Patriarch of Moscow and Russia Alexei II Certificate of Honor; the Albert Schweitzer Gold Medal; and the Polish Academy of Medicine Award for Healthcare Service. In 2009 the World Federation of Circumpolar Medicine awarded him the Jack Hildes Medal for outstanding contribution to the development of new synergistic paradigms in arctic medicine as a hybrid system of health safety in extreme environments.

Academic Interests

History of mental ecology and medicine, mental epidemiology and preventology, social psychiatry and narcology, clinical psychiatry and disaster medicine.

Academician P.I. Sidorov has made a fundamental contribution to the understanding and development of preventative systems for mental and social epidemics; the creation of original synergistic bio-psycho-socio-spiritual methodologies for evaluating and forecasting ontogenetic development; justifications for including terrorism and extremism within the group of polymodal and polymorphic related disorders; the conception of mental terrorism (commercial manipulation of consciousness by means of threats, sanctions, etc.) as a nonlethal weapon of mass destruction; the creation of sanogenetic therapy – adaptation of the bio-psycho-socio-spiritual management of consciousness and health (a priority since 1988); the validation of animogenetic (spiritual-moral) diagnostic and propaedeutic therapy and rehabilitation; the development of a multidisciplinary ideology and synergistic methodology of mental health care and system monitoring as an social awareness interface.

Scientific Publications

Pavel Sidorov is the author of over 900 works, including 56 books and monographs, 30 textbooks and manuals, 430 journal articles (120 published in foreign journals), and 31 invention patents.

Several of his books have won awards and prizes:

a) Psychology, Clinics, and Early Prevention of Alcoholism (1984, coauthor B.S. Bratus) – the RSFSR gold medal winner of the Republican Competition of Scientific Works. The book was dedicated to his teacher, Professor I.D. Muratov, who helped open the first teen narcology office in the USSR in 1974;

b) System Monitoring of Educational Environments (2007, coauthor E.Y. Vasilev) – best scientific work according to the All-Russia Competition Foundation for the Development of Domestic Education.

c) Personnel Management (2008, coauthor V.I. Starodubov and I.A. Konopleva), Narcological Preventology (2008) – winners in several thematic categories of the 2008 University Book competition;

d) Perinatal Psychology and Psychiatry (2009, coauthor N.N. Volodin, et al.) – winner of the all-Russia (VDNKh) and international (Paris) book exhibitions for academic literature for innovative education (2015).

Academician P.I. Sidorov has published the next generation of federal textbooks on clinical psychology (five publications), disaster psychology and disaster medicine (four publications), perinatal psychiatry (two publications) and medico-social work (three publications), personnel management and organization (two publications), addictological preventology (four publications) and social psychiatry (two publications), human ecology two publications) and maritime medicine (four publications), business communication (four publications) and system monitoring of educational environments (two publications), physiological foundations of human health (three publications) and psychosomatic medicine (two publications), adaptive professiogenesis (two publications) and medical law (three publications), all of which are written using a synergistic methodology of integrated medicine.

Academician P.I. Sidorov is the editor of a number of Russian translations of works on psychiatry and psychotherapy, psychology and disaster medicine from English, German, Swedish, Finnish, Norwegian, and Polish.

Over the last 20 years, he has developed a synergistic bio-psycho-socio-spiritual methodology of mental medicine which effectively provides an adaptive management of consciousness and health. He has taken part in the publication of a number of handbooks employing this methodology:

1. Sidorov P.I. Russian Alcohol Culture. International Handbook on Alcohol and Culture. Greenwood Press: Westport, Connecticut•London, 1995. P. 237-253.
2. Sidorov P.I. Narkologicheskaya preventologiya (Narcological Preventology). Rukovodstvo. 2-e izd. M.: MEDpress-inform, 2006. 720 p. [in Russian]
3. Sidorov P. I., Novikova I. A. Mental'naya meditsina (Mental Medicine). Rukovodstvo. 2-e izd. M.: GEOTAR-Media, 2014. 728 p. [in Russian]
4. Sidorov P. I. From bullying to pandemy of terrorism: synergetic bio-psycho-socio-spiritual methodology of Mental health protection. Handbook on Bullying: Prevalence, Psychological impacts and intervention Strategies. NY: NOVA Science Publishers, 2014. P. 177-214.
5. Sidorov P.I. Mental Terrorism of Hybrid Wars and Defense Synergetics. Handbook on New Developments in Surveillance Systems and National Security. NY: NOVA Science Publishers, 2015. P. 92-136.
6. Sidorov P.I. From mental epidemics to terrorism pandemic: synergetic bio-psycho-socio-spiritual methodology of public conscience protection. Handbook on Terrorism. NY: NOVA Science Publishers, 2015. P. 115-158.

Section I. Conceptual and Methodological Basis of Mental Medicine and Epidemiology

Chapter 1

Mental Ecology

1.1. Fundamentals of Mentality

Mentality is the way of outlook which is formed during the process of upbringing, education and gaining life experience in a particular cultural atmosphere. Mentality (from mens, mentis in Latin which means "reason, mind, intellect") refers to the concepts (for example mind in English) which do not have an exact equivalent in Russian.

V. E. Semyonov (2009, 2013) unveils polymentality within *the different versions* of *Russian mentality:*

- *the Russian Orthodox mentality*, which has a thousand year history of the Ancient Rus and Russia;
- *the collectivist socialistic mentality* which was formed during the years of the USSR and originates from peasant community, workmen's association and the activities of populists and socialists in the XIXth – early XXth centuries;
- *the individually capitalistic pro-Western mentality* which was formed in Russia beginning with the reform of Peter the Great and, notably, after the abolition of serfdom in 1861. It has been reviving during the last 25 years of Russian contemporary history, often in a twisted and extreme or a grotesque form;
- *the criminally mafia-style mentality* which has always existed, generated by human vices and social diseases. In the last decade of the XXth century in Russia it has turned into a phenomenon of "great criminal revolution" as one of the social epidemics that was destroying the country;
- *the mosaically eclectic* pseudomentality as a result of "mass culture," mass media and the Internet – the conglomerate of shatters and fragments belonging to all the specified mentalities.

Such understanding of mentality is close to the viewpoint of N. M. Rakityansky (2009) who identified three stages of its formation:

- *the implicit phase*, when the term has not yet been encountered in scientific works and when researchers use such concepts as "ethnical conscience," "national character," "nation's soul," "mental constitution," "nation's spirit," etc.;

- *introducing the concept into scientific terminology*, into imaginative writing, journalism, and spoken language;
- *the object of managing* information-and-psychological means since the 1990s.

Despite social manipulativity of the mentality N. M. Rakityansky (2009) still adheres to an idea that: "Mentality arises out of faith. As a basic mental function, faith stands out as some center piece where the entire person's structure or, at a broader level, the whole structure of the Russian national mentality, the political culture of its nationhood and so on is laid. It forms main and key human perceptions which determine his life, views, intentions and deeds. Faith is the primary system of knowledge, basis, and content of the mental matrix. Furthermore, it forms and determines the political power of the whole country, economy, morals, spirituality, life and destiny of nations, countries and each." Such a supreme politicization in understanding of mentality has been reflected in M. M. Reshetnikov's (2013) identification of the three Russian mentality traditions:

- *"the historical Russian dignity"* tracing back to the times of taking the first attempts at creating "the Third Rome" (or "the New Byzantine");
- *"the historical Russian expansion"* associated with the cultivation of Russia' special "messianic" role concerning the surrounding nations and countries;
- *"commitment to the top public official"* regardless of his official name, his declared historical goals or moral ideas and values.

At the maximum generalization level A. I. Yuryev (2013) identifies the collision of two mentalities in Russia: *liberal* (deterministic, behavioral) and *clerically patriotic* (conscious, spiritual) which develop from two different psychological paradigms of human ecology. It is the collision of such two paradigms which creates a unique design of mental ecology in modern Russia during the period of global crisis and system stagnation.

N. M. Rakityansky (2009) compared mentality with a special prism existing between us and the world. The contemporary associative array yet appears to be more informational. For instance, mentality may be compared with a web camera of our conscience which sets the possibilities to view the problems and nuances of the surrounding world. Collected billions of images and meanings in averaged format are accumulated on the hard disc of our conscience in both realized and unconscious forms. They are collectively focused in an individual mentality which has a complex architecture and a unique design of files and patterns. They are collectively focused in an individual mentality which has a complex architecture and a unique design of files and matrices. All the social educational institutes of the society also try to work with them using the "mental Photoshop" of mass media to the extent of understanding and motivated enthusiasm. For someone the perception of the world is important and for others the TV-involvement is sufficient.

But still, despite the huge variety of mindsets and mentalities, to avoid losing the so-called "informational wars" consistently one should constructively build his mentality which includes the reliance on new methodological resources of mental ecology and medicine, system monitoring and mental health service. It is important to understand the fundamental point in the process of such moral and spiritual construction – no illusively compensatory "cartoons and the Funnies" are involved in the creation of national Mental immunity. Only the creatively constructive activities backed by real results (for example, the Olympics) allow building the new Russian mentality.

1.2. Mental Health

In the last decades, problems of mental health have become particularly significant. And this is explained by the growing number of mentally ill patients, primarily, as a result of non-psychotic forms and also due to an increase in economic expenses connected with diagnostics, treatment, social and occupational rehabilitation among this category of patients.

According to WHO, the worldwide decline in working capacity and the possibilities of social functioning are related to mental and behavioral diseases in 12% of situations. In countries with high personal income level, this relation occurs in 23% of all cases. In many Council of Europe member countries, the expenses related to mental health amount to between 1/3 and 1/2 of the total healthcare costs (Kazakovtsev 2014).

The mental health represents one of the main values of an individual and the society. Human physical and social well-being that influence intellectual potential of the nation, are also included into the mental health concept. The development of production capacities and labor resources as well as the country's safety and defensive potential are also influenced by human physical and social well-being.

The term *"mental health"* was introduced by the WHO in 1979. WHO experts defined it as a psychic condition which encourages the most comprehensive physical, intellectual and emotional development of a person. "Mental health" was translated into Russian as "psychic health."

The psychic condition is the condition of a human mental sphere which is characterized by general peace of mind ensuring adequate behavior regulation and determined by the requirements of biological and social nature.

Mental health is a conventional concept which identifies only one of the human health components, and it can be classified as individual and public health. *Individual mental health* is such a state of individual psychic which is characterized by integrity and coordination of all mental organism functions, which provide the feel of personal psychic comforts, the ability to act purposefully and sensibly along with the perfect fulfillment of social functions. These functions should be adequate for typical human values and ethnocultural features of the group, to which the individual belongs. The term *public mental health* implies the level of the population's psychic health, i.e. the prevalence of psychic diseases, alcoholism and drug dependence, mental retardation, various forms of destructive behavior and the ratio between mentally healthy and ill people (Dmitriyeva, Polozhiy 2008).

The increasing multidisciplinarity and the public significance of neurosciences forced to expand substantially the nature of term "mental health" in XXI century without its restriction to the medicine-specific limits of "psychic health."

The WHO report "The condition of health protection in the world. Mental health: new understanding and new hope" (2001) contains a resolution for the support of scientific studies, which assist to understand the nature of mental health diseases and to elaborate efficient methods of their prevention.

Mental health refers to the human psychic well-being which allows him to realize his potential, helps to resist stress, work productively and contribute to the society's development (WHO 2001). It is crucially important to note that this term contains not only the classical biopsychosocial triad (Engel 1977) but also the moral component of "well-being" and "self-realization," "stress resistance" and "productive work" which are impossible without the ethics in business communication. The national civil component looks even more pathetical. It is represented by the appeal "to contribute to the society's development."

According to WHO, there is no "official" definition of the term "mental health" which is determined by cultural differences, subjective appraisals, and professional competing theories. At the same time, mental health is an essential condition of society's and country's development.

Mental health is the central component of individual and entire society's quality of life. This fact is substantially related to a sixtyfold growth of the number of mentally ill patients with non-psychotic diseases over the last century.

1.3. Mission of Mental Ecology

Mental ecology is a section of human ecology that studies relationships in the "environment – society – individual" system, factors and resources of mental health.

By meaning mental health, we imply the self-organizing synergetic system. It involves the relationship with nature which at first becomes the man's *environment* and then his *habitat* influencing his public health made up of somatic and moral, social and psychic trends. The created configuration in turn influences the surrounding world which, depending on the individual activities, becomes *the environment of survival, the environment evolution* or *the environment of prosperity* (Figure 1.1). Due to the integrity and interdisciplinarity of its interests, mental medicine lies at the center of this structure.

The aspect of *somatic* health is traditional and already explored in such a model of mental medicine composed of four equivalent biopsychosociospiritual components. It is related to the understanding and application of internist disciplines. For a long time, medicine was evolving having a materialistic concept of creation as its priority. This system has shaped the world medicine in its present form giving priority to this trend (it explains practical results and theoretic orientation of medical disciplines accentuated mainly on the *somatic* pathology which corresponds precisely to nozocentric principles). However, it is not the stylistics pathology of nozocentrism that matters, but *health,* which is what prevention deals with.

The social component has anti-nozocentric nature since it is supported by real condition and functional capabilities of a patient rather than the diagnosis. In the model of mental medicine, the potential growth of this component's actuality is defined by the latest trend. This pattern consists of resocialization and readaptation of a patient that means the shortening of hospitalization durations, the extension of therapeutic regimens and a gradual transfer to part-time inpatient facilities and other forms of out-of-hospital aid which is already observed in psychiatry today.

Moral health is characterized by morally-axiological and meaningful assessments of the quality of life, by the level of ethical competence and moral adaptation of the personality.

Psychic health remains a considerably underexplored field which is mainly investigated today by psychiatrists, narcologists, psychologists and philosophers. Psychology and Psychosomatics have developed as disciplines relatively recently. Due to that fact, first of all, there is an obvious methodological deficit experienced by this component of mental medicine; secondly, the practical appropriateness of further elaboration of particularly this field is realized; thirdly, a trend is clearly defined which suggests the necessity of further advancement in this direction.

The difference between *mental health* and the traditional psychic one lies in the content and the multidisciplinary biopsychosociospiritual integrity available for studying and practical implementation only within the scope of synergetic methodology.

The concept of "somatic medicine" exists nowadays whereas the lexeme of "mental medicine" has not yet even become a usual term. The disparity of somatic and mental health aspects is evident and indisputable. However, the traditional nozocentrism of modern psychiatry holds its development and capabilities which, in essence, does not meet the contemporary realias. Under such concept the preventive component is almost left out of psychiatry. With the entire up to date status of the "somatic" focus area and its clear orientation towards conventional determinism that is now experiencing system crisis it remains to be effective which undoubtedly does not mean the inefficiency of "mental" focus area. Besides, the "somatic" focus area has encountered problems (also because of its nozocentric concept) that have not been resolved at this stage despite the approaches different from methodological and theoretical aspects. Does not this condition mean that solving such problems may belong to other methodological spheres where mainly these trends are more effectively used in integral coordination?

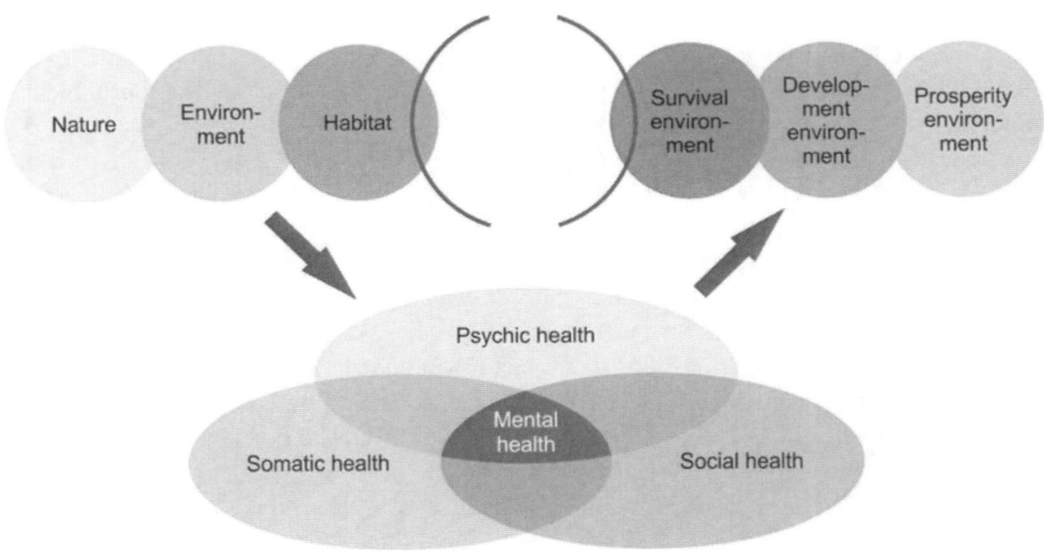

Figure 1.1. Mission of mental ecology in an interactive provision of civilizational trends.

The specifics of mental ecology mission involve interactive provision of civilization trends (Figure 1.1). Mental health integrates the potential of mental and moral, psychic, somatic and social health being a constructively creative resource of public perception and public health of the nation. The mental ecology mission considerably matches with the basic definition of psychotherapy as an interactive process of psychological arrangement of the past, the present and the future of an individual, a family, a group and the whole society for the sake of achieving a set goal (Makarov 2013). Another laconic definition of *psychotherapy as the science of adaptive control of individual and public conscience mentality* can be given within the scope of synergetic methodology.

Polymodal mentality represents the matrix or the target within individual and public perception on which mental and moral upbringing, education as well as a psychological and psychotherapeutic influence are focused.

In order to, figuratively speaking, measure a person's strength and moral potential, we (Sidorov, Novikova 2009) developed and patented the "Index of personal mental ecology," enabling to assess psycho-, socio-, somato-, animogenesis and ethical modalities of personal or group mentality in screening mode.

1.4. The Technique of Mental Ecology of Personality

The actuality of studying mental ecology is determined by the constant growth of mental pathology and the fact that most patients are the people of working age. We discovered no methods of evaluating personal mental ecology in the available literature.

As one alternative methodological toolset of system mental health monitoring, we suggested a proprietary methodology of assessing personal mental ecology (Sidorov, Novikova 2008).

During the elaboration of the methodology in 2008 three components of mental health were considered – psychogenesis, sociogenesis and somatogenesis – since the disorders occur within all the three elements almost from the very outbreak of the disease. The fourth block – animogenesis – was added to the methodology in 2013.

The checklist of personal mental ecology assessment included 252 questions divided into 3 blocks. Block I is related to psychogenesis assessment and contains 156 questions concerning the psychic component of quality of life; factors affecting mental health and symptoms of the 21 most popular mental diseases (neurotic, psychosomatic and addiction related) according to ICD – 10. Block II is related to sociogenesis assessment and includes 48 statements. By using this block it is possible to explore the social component of quality of life and the specifics of negative impact of social factors on human health. Block III is related to somatogenesis assessment and includes 48 statements and allows assessing the somatic component of quality of life as well as the factors that influence bodily health (biological, inherited, etc.).

We surveyed 90 mentally healthy undergraduates (with an average age of 21.1 ± 0.34 years), 30 somatically ill patients suffering from nonpsychotic diseases (with average age of 43.2 ± 2.26 years) and 26 patients with alcoholic dependence (with average age of 44.7 ± 2.51 years). The results of personal mental ecology assessment for different population groups are presented in Table 1.1.

Table 1.1. Indices of personal mental ecology assessment for different population groups (expressed in points)

Groups / Indices	Students without any mental pathology	Somatically ill patients with neurotic disorders	Alcohol-dependent patients
Psychogenesis	85.47 ± 1.12	53.95 ± 2.05	38.06 ± 2.46
Sociogenesis	77.05 ± 1.27	48.67 ± 2.31	44.11 ± 3.05
Somatogenesis	75.31 ± 1.02	35.61 ± 2.49	47.46 ± 2.98
Personal mental ecology	79.27 ± 0.91	46.08 ± 1.97	43.21 ± 2.82

Hence, it was established that when the value of own mental ecology index was between 68.2 and 100 points, the figure was evaluated as a good mental health of a surveyed person whereas index was between 0 and 68.1, it was evaluated as the presence of mental disorders. In future, the methodology will be supplemented with quantitative measurement of animogenesis.

High reliability and validity of the method were achieved in the process of its elaboration. The survey of 50 general education teachers demonstrated that the reliability level of predicting the presence of mental disorders or sanity constituted 96.0%.

Using the method of personal mental ecology assessment fulfills the following monitoring tasks: analyzing mental health factors; revealing psychic pathology and assessing the level of mental health; analyzing the nosological structure of psychic pathology; analyzing the structure of premorbid psychic pathology forms; evaluating quality of life and its impact on mental health.

1.5. Evaluation of Mentality as a Factor of Public Health

For the purpose of system mental health monitoring, we developed a method of screening assessment for health factors (Sidorov, Novikova 2010).

Health is one of the most necessary conditions for effective professional activity of a man. It represents the core and relatively casual dynamic basis of productivity for every aspect of work and overall human well-being.

The process of population's health formation over the last decades reflects general trends of the country's socioeconomic development. The most serious problems of population's health include the high rate of total mortality (especially among the working age men), low rate of fertility and negative population growth. Russia presently holds 134th and 100th world positions in terms of life expectancy index for men and women, respectively. *Such problems cannot be solved without developing a national strategy of health care and improvement.*

Human activities which are detrimental to personal health often contribute to unhealthy lifestyle and include such risk factors as smoking, alcohol consumption, psychoemotional stress, irrational nutrition and hypodynamia.

The condition of health among the country's population is evaluated according to demographic, socioeconomic and medical aspects as well as special surveys.

Population health is one of the integral indices of transformations which occur in the society. It is determined by the complex of sociopsychological and genetic characteristics of physical health as well as the psychophysiological standard of living. Healthy lifestyle formation, welfare growth and the development of health "industry" encourage the advancement of national health.

The concept of health must determine the abilities to perform main human functions considering the fact that the man is a living system based on physical and mental, natural and social, inherited and acquired principles.

Social health is perceived as a system of values, mindsets and motives of behavior in the social environment. Physical health is the current condition of functional capabilities of body organs and systems. Mental health is the state of human psychic sphere characterized by the general peace of mind, ensuring adequate behavior regulation and determined by the requirements of biological and social nature. Social and psychological health aspects determine the harmonic process of human inner world development, his relations with the surroundings and adaptation within the society.

Different approaches to assessing the contribution of various factors to health levels are presented in literature (Table 1.2).

Table 1.2. Health factors (%)

Factors / Authors	Lifestyle	Environment	Genetic factors	Healthcare
Lisitsyn 1987	49-53	17-20	18-20	8-10
Alexeev 1991	50-52	10-20	18-25	10-20
WHO 1992	50	20	20	10
Petlenko 1996	40-50	25	20	11
Khudoley, Mizgirev 1996	-	50-70	-	-
Savateeva 1998	-	25-50	-	-
Gichev 2000	-	40-60	-	-
Rubtsov 2005	50-55	20-25	15-20	10-15
Koreneva 2005	49-53	17-20	18-22	8-10

Despite some differences in the contribution of factors to overall human health most authors share the same opinion that such factors include lifestyle, environment, genetic factors and healthcare. Y. P. Lisitsyn (1987; 2012) views elements of such factor groups as shown below (Table 1.3).

At the same time, each of the four-factor groups includes a mental component. *For lifestyle* this includes smoking, alcohol, and drug abuse, taking medicines and toxicants, strained psychoemotional relations in the family and at work, growing absence of compensations and marginality, psychological illiteracy and hysterodemonic renaissance. *For the environment,* this is stressful situations and globalization of aggression, the compression of information environment and continuous flow mass culture. *For genetics,* this is a predisposition to psychoneurological and narcological diseases and *for healthcare* – inefficiency of psychoprophylaxis and psychohygiene.

In the overall hierarchy of the country's problems and its security system, one of the leading positions is held by the nation's mental health. It is a socially significant phenomenon which level and condition are used to judge the society's degree of evolution and well-being. Studying mental health is an objective requirement since it represents the most important element of public health which in many respects determines the economic and social well-being of the nation.

Table 1.3. Classification of risk factors

Risk factor groups	Estimated group contribution (relative share) to total morbidity, %	Some elements of this group
Lifestyle	49-53	Smoking, tobacco consumption Unbalanced nutrition Alcohol consumption Unhealthy working conditions Stressful situations Adynamia, hypodynamia Poor economic and household conditions Drug-taking, drug abuse Family instability. Loneliness Low educational and cultural levels Extremely high level of urbanization
Environment, natural and climatic conditions	17-20	Air, water and soil pollution caused by carcinogens and other substances Rapid changes in atmospheric effects Increased heliocosmic, magnetic and other radiations
Genetics, human biology	18-22	Predisposition to inherited diseases Predisposition to degenerative diseases
Healthcare	8-10	Inefficiency of preventive actions Poor quality of medical care Delay of medical care

The prevalence of mental disorders of a nonpsychotic level by far exceeds the official statistics data and makes up 27.3% of the adult population (1.4% as based on official data) (Churkin, Kasimova 2000).

Modern trends in examining the prevalence of mental health pathology are characterized by a shift in emphasis towards more universal ways that are based on presenting mental health as a combination of psychic, social and psychological well-being as well as the state of equilibrium between the individual and the environment. For example, N. K. Demcheva (2006) suggests considering the quality of life and social functioning as the criterion of population's mental health.

A trend towards a broader and multiple-aspect interpretation of mental health resulted in its definition as "person's psychic well-being which allows him to realize his potential, resist stress, work productively and contribute to society's evolution" given by the WHO. This definition establishes not only the absence of mental disease but also the high quality of social functioning, normative professiogenesis and interactive provision of civilization trends.

Furthermore, the concept of "mentality" has multi-aspect interpretation: "social thinking" as given by K. A. Abulkhanova-Slavskaya (1991), "criteria foundation of individual and public perception" as provided by B. S. Gershunsky (1996), "the system of behavioral norms" as given by I. G. Dubov (1997), “national character” as stated by N. O. Lossky (1991), “social representations” as given by S. Moscovichi (1996), “value-based orientations and social mindsets” as mentioned by D. V. Oborina (1994), “motives and preferences” as given by V. A. Sonin (1996) and so on.

Considering all the above mentioned it seems appropriate to add the fifth group – mentality –to the established four-factor groups which predetermine health.

We elaborated the “Health ecology assessment” method of screening that includes five blocks: lifestyle, environment, genetics, healthcare and mentality (Sidorov, Novikova 2014).

This method includes 50 questions with 10 questions in each of the five blocks. The index of lifestyle is evaluated according to questions concerning the presence of bad habits, regular nutrition, resting time rules and the presence of stressful lifestyle. The index of the environment includes the evaluation of climatic, ecological, informational, social and professional factors. The index of genetics is assessed according to the presence of inherited predisposition to psychic and somatic diseases. The contribution of healthcare to human health includes questions concerning quality and availability of medical care. The index of mentality is evaluated according to questions related to human mental and psychological condition.

Using this method of screening evaluation we surveyed 62 mentally and somatically healthy students (with the average age of 20.62 ± 0.78 years). As a result, we obtained the following data on the structure of health components (Figure 1.2).

The analysis of health components shows that a reasonably large share (18-21%) among the factors is given to mentality making the significance of factors related to lifestyle – which is the possible behavioral realization of mentality – half as great on the average.

The results obtained, using this method, enable to perform an analysis of factors influencing population’s health. It is possible to determine population groups with a high risk level of disorder development and to undertake preventive measures. The new method allows taking actions which prevent vocational disablement of population due to diseases and evaluating the prediction of mental and somatic disease dynamics within population.

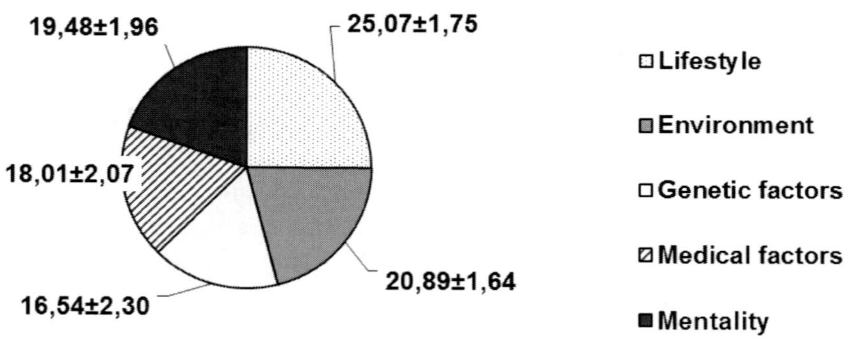

Figure 1.2. Health components according to the “Health ecology assessment” method (%).

Thus, by using the screening “Health ecology assessment” method that we developed, it is possible to establish the contribution of each factor to the health of an individual or a group. And therefore, to determine the factors which may be the cause of diseases, to optimize and to individualize the management of preventive care.

Chapter 2

Synthesis of Mental Medicine

2.1. Social Psychiatry

Recognizing the effect of social factors on the generation of mental diseases resulted in administrative, organizational innovations in the system of conventional classical psychiatry. In the middle of the XXth century, the authorities assumed taking care about human mental health continuing to implement society monitoring using the institutes of ψ-function. "The idea that a mentally ill patient represents an exception became a thing of the past. It is acknowledged today that most people suffer from a mental disease" (Porter 2008). By the middle of the XXth century, the number of mentally ill patients in USA hospitals reached 500.000 (about 150.000 in Great Britain).

The concept of *social psychiatry* was formed with the entire society being its subject of investigation and influence. In 1946, the USA President H. Truman signed the Law about the nation's mental health, which sanctioned the extension of functions performed by the Mental Hygiene Department under the jurisdiction of the Public Health Protection Service, which was reorganized into the National Institute of Mental Health in 1949. In 1956, the publication of the *International social psychiatry magazine* began. The first day hospital was organized for mentally ill patients in London. Further, on the intensity of psychiatric field governmentalization was enhanced. Organizational changes were taking place in the USA: in 1950, the Psychiatric fund, the National mental health fund and the National mental hygiene committee were united into a well-financed *National mental health association* conglomerate. In the *Message to the Congress regarding mental disease and retardation* made in 1963, J. Kennedy proposed a national mental health program which he named "one of the key directions of the American medicine" (Sas 2008).

The emergence and institutionalization of *social psychiatry* in the mid-XXth century defined the relevance of the new approach to the issues of mental diseases. Such approach which met contemporary challenges and the corresponding realities of the socioeconomic situation could eliminate the monopoly of biological determinism and the nozocentrism of classical psychiatry by demonstrating new potentialities and perspectives of psychiatric science which was focused not only on the biological but also on the social factor participating in the formation of mental diseases. However, the structure of the "social psychiatry" term describes the adjective "social" as particularly applicable to the key meaningful word "psychiatry." "Psychiatry," in turn, indicates the strictly auxiliary and servile nature of this definition, subject to the ideology of nozocentrism and biological factor supremacy in the contraction and clinical development of a mental disease. Social psychiatry continued to focus on the diagnosis and showed activity only with the affirmation of the disease, without trying to prevent it. Therefore, the appearance of social psychiatry did not change the fundamental status of classical psychiatry, becoming – in the absence of paradigm psychiatric science distinctness – a palliative which resulted in the same dead end.

Today qualitatively new dispersion and inversion of clinical and social psychiatry are taking place amid the global deethization of public conscience leading to the development of mental ecology and medicine based on the multidisciplinary synergetic methodology.

2.2. Anti-Psychiatry

Philosophical discrepancies of the mid-20th century led in the1960s to the appearance of a movement called anti-psychiatry within classical psychiatry that chose existentialism and socially critical philosophy as its basis. World Psychiatric Association President Mario May (2008) said the following about anti-psychiatry: “Anti-psychiatry is a reality in some countries. Our profession is unique in such a way that it can create its antibodies.”

The confirmation of cosmological string, superstring, dark matter and dark energy theories developed for multidimensional realities, which is expected tomorrow at the hadron collider in Bern may create chances for the new interpretation of conventional psychopathology. “There are approaches in psychiatry which attempt to present the concept of a mental disease as a tool used by general practitioners to put pressure on the so-called patients” (Lem 2006). Regarding its matter and time, this movement concurred with the ideology of descholarization aimed at the reformation of the school. Descholarization balanced the difference between the teacher and the student which was interpreted in this antisystem as the result of a repressive society. A similar story was taking place during the first years of the Soviet regime in the USSR.

The period of decline of empires in the post-war era generated anti-system tendencies in many spheres of human life. The traditional system of classical psychiatry was subjected to revision attempts from its opponents. Supporters of anti-psychiatry were aiming to “discover the truth hidden amongst the drivel,” and in the process almost doubting the status of classical psychiatry as medical science, protesting against its claims to qualify people as mentally ill.

Anti-psychiatrists: Ronald Laing, David Cooper, Thomas Szasz, and others thought that the decision not to treat patients was right and that their individual and social needs, including those expressed in psychotic motives, had to be satisfied. “Instead of psychiatric hospitals, these processing plants, we need places where people who went further than psychiatrists in their wanderings and consider themselves mentally healthy, would have a possibility to go even further in private time and space and return from there” (Laing 1969). Or, as clinical practice demonstrates, never come back.

American sociologist Erving Goffman highlighted the negative sides of psychiatric total institutions. In Italy Franco Basaglia, the initiator of de-institutionalisation of psychiatric hospitals became the leader of the anti-psychiatry movement. In the Netherlands Jan Foudraine led the student movement targeted against professional authority in psychiatric hospitals. Classical psychiatry was accused of having discrimination procedures within its regulations. A movement for removing a hospital structure out of psychiatric intervention appeared. That medical structure for almost two hundred years had been seen as treating psychiatric patients in a space isolated from society. In 1965, David Cooper, Ronald Laing and others created the Philadelphia association, aimed at "changing the perception of mental health and illness of the soul" (Baillon 1971).

Anti-psychiatry expressed fundamental criticism of the following:

a) illegal use of medical categories and methods regarding social and psychiatric phenomena;
b) conventional nature of nosologic categories in classical psychiatry, their highly provisional nature, dubious medical status;
c) not enough theoretical and clinical reasoning for distribution of these classes into rubrics in classifications;
d) toxicity and side effects of psychotropic medicine;
e) lack of a clearly and legally defined standard of the psychiatric norm;
f) use of non-voluntary treatment;
g) ignoring other approaches to the problem of psychiatric disorders;
h) compromising connections of classic psychiatry with pharmaceutical companies;
i) cruel treatment and tight control regarding the mentally ill.

Anti-psychiatry brought to the fore the following problems:

a) existential factors for psychiatric disorders;
b) pathological status of psychiatric disorders
c) place of the mentally ill in society;
d) institutionalisation and deinstitutionalisation of the mentally ill;
e) treatment regimens for psychiatric disorders;
f) personality suppression and functioning of the institutions of authority;
g) peculiarities of inter-personal interaction;
h) unconscious mechanisms of society functioning;
i) human rights protection for people with mental illnesses.

No one of the pioneers of anti-psychiatry developed a complete theoretical system. Laing and Cooper worked with phenomenological and existential concepts based on the theory of pathology of communication inside the family. Basaglia was concerned with politics, ideology, and revolutionary social reforms. Szasz's views were formed under the influence of Ludwig Binswanger and Freudianism. However, the anti-psychiatry movement influenced classical psychiatry, the nature of work of its institutions, and the quality of help for the mentally ill.

Thanks to the anti-psychiatry movement, starting from the 1960s, new methods and forms of working with the mentally ill became more widespread than earlier. Therapeutic communities (soterias) appeared and became popular again, but they were a modification of a method used by classical psychiatry in the 19th century. This approach supposed hosting patients in peasant families for their full social rehabilitation and labour therapy like in the Belgian town Geel and some other European locations. Stricter laws were passed that limited the use of non-human methods of treatment and the regulation of non-voluntary hospitalisation. A more liberal view of the mentally ill appeared, social and psychological methods became more frequent in their treatment and rehabilitation. Perceptions of ethical norms in classical psychiatry were being formed. The monopoly of the biological approach to psychiatry was broken; psycho-social approaches appeared and became more favorable.

Anti-psychiatry became the *antithesis* to the thesis of classical psychiatry, criticising its important concepts, achievements and theories, doubting its practical implementation and practicability. Anti-psychiatry attacked the foundation of nosology and epistemology of traditional psychiatry. A new opponent criticised the lack of satisfactory criteria for diagnostics and the objectivity of psychiatric methods. Anti-psychiatry doubted the very medical model of a mental illness accepted by the classical psychiatry and considered the nosological classification arbitrary. Anti-psychiatry criticised methods of therapy ("pharmacotherapy is chains locked from the inside") and prophylactics that did not take into account social conditions. The new school put the psychosocial aspect of the problem instead of the biological one to the foreground, regarding psychotherapy as social manipulation and control. Anti-psychiatry protested against obligatory hospitalisation, considering it a measure of segregating the mentally ill bereft of their human rights. Yet any "institution creates deformed, and progressive artificial societies which are caring like a mother, and sometimes they produce vestigial paternalistic pseudo-families. How can one prevent a chosen unit – even when it represents a peculiar institution – from generating a deformed society of tolerance, a group of mutual aid that hides real problems" (Deleuze, Guattari 2008).

The philosophical ideology of anti-psychiatry was also eclectic and cumulative, combining the philosophical concepts of the sentimental humanism of Jean-Jacques Rousseau, existentialism of Jean-Paul Sartre, and anarchism of Peter Kropotkin. Student riots in Paris in 1968 do not look coincidental in this context: readers of Sartre were prisoners of romantically viewed anarchism and Trotskyism. These riots were the first elemental experience of mental design and strategies, technologies and mechanisms of future man-made "color revolutions" replicating the synergetic methodology of "manageable chaos."

The difference between the authorities' thoughts on the forms of realising the ψ-function and peculiarities of its social use were expressed through psychiatric hospitals and mentally ill in socialist and capitalist countries. Inside the socialist system, the ψ-function came down to isolating this category of people in conditions where it was easy to conduct monitoring of this cohort. It is the totalitarian option of ψ-function implementation. Capitalist socio-economic formation featured the free choice, declaring human rights a priority and regulating psychiatric activity with this point of view in mind.

During this period, the problem with psychiatric hospitals in the West was solved by using the so-called "communities" which required much less financial expenses compared to the traditional psychiatric inpatient facilities. In 1961, the Ministry of Health in Great Britain declared the need to close down every psychiatric hospital of the old type. The hostile attitude expressed by M. Thatcher and R. Reagan towards the social policy of supporting disadvantaged population together with the government's commitment to cut down ("optimize") expenditure formed social politics in the style of limiting liberalization and moderated isolationism of the mentally ill patients. Hospitalization was no longer considered to be a priority measure in the process of their therapy. The number of patients at inpatient psychiatric facilities was decreasing during that time: in Great Britain, it dropped from 150,000 in 1950 to 30,000 by the early 1980-s. "Psychotropic revolution, movement in support of patients' rights and the fuss around falling apart foster houses were combined into a unified policy of *decarceration* promoted since 1960-s" (Porter 2008).

There was an explosion of popularity and the network distribution of such methods of psycho-correction and psychotherapy as group sessions, family psychotherapy, training, role games, and behavior modification among others. All of this became the prologue to the modern Era of Psychotherapy. Psychotherapy, having achieved the revolutionary breakthrough to the medical prenosological field, radically changed the focus of the ψ-mission of the state and society from mental illnesses to mental health. This shift secured dynamic development of the whole complex of neurosciences and sped up the development of social psychiatry and narcology, leading to the birth of mental ecology and mental medicine in the last decade.

2.3. System Synthesis of Mental Medicine

If it was possible to talk about long-term paradigms in philosophy and science (particularly in classical psychiatry) before the 20th century, then now, various concepts of philosophical directions that exist simultaneously, form a contradictory ontology and a perception of the worldview as unstable.

It is crucially important to note that this certainly does not entail perceiving "the reflections of ghosts of scientific illusions." The world is indeed losing its steadiness and stability with galloping speed. Terrorist acts performed by lone suicide bombers as well as network hacker attacks quickly exasperate global public perception demanding fundamentally new approaches to the protection of civilization's mental resources. Psychiatric "fences and railings" have become a perfect anachronism in the open global world. Humanity as a whole and each of us are so helpless that realizing this fact itself drives socio-stressful disorders.

Acceptance that the former canons of world scientific study turned insolvent became a frequent topic of polemic statements. Urgent desire for defenceless integration of classification systems in classical psychiatry today is accompanied by "the obvious futility of the announced methodological approach. Its lack of theory, change from nosological to syndrome level of clinical evaluations, bulkiness, inability to reflect cultural variety even when using the descriptive method, and eclecticism because of lack of theoretical principle" (Morozov, Ovsyannikov 2009).

Materialistic science and philosophy fully humiliate the person and the truth. The verdict of history refuted almost all empirical theories of the 19th and 20th centuries as strained and pretentious exhibits of vain erudition. Despite the significant number of historical, statistical, pseudo-experimental, clinical and other data, not a single unified theory was created. At best, they only restored in a vulgar and more primitive form the generalisations of the previous generations (Sorokin 1992).

This problem was formulated by Carl Gustav Jung concerning classical psychiatry and psychotherapy (Jung 1992): "Modern medicine can no longer understand the psyche as part of the body and thus is more and more considering the so-called psychic factor." "Practical loss of empiricism of modern culture is revealed in our growing inability to control humanity and the course of social and cultural processes" (Sorokin 1992). However, it is psychiatry that is the slowest in leaving behind the empirical period of scientific development.

In the context of a globally permanent and paroxysmally progressive crisis that fundamentally relates to the mental paradigm, modern possibilities for perfecting classical psychiatry and anti-psychiatry have almost been exhausted. "We are, seemingly, at the dusk of an era" (Lem 2006). But this "…imaginary dying agony is nothing else but the sharp pain from the birth of a new form of culture, labour pains, accompanying new creative forces" (Sorokin 1992), "a reassuring sign of possible deeper changes of the spiritual disposition" (Jung 1994).

"The 21st century will become the time of returning to continuity, to a broad understanding of common problems. The key will be technologies of a particular system integration, system synthesis" (Malinetskiy, Potapov 2006). "The main thing in the study of the living phenomena is not the elements that do not matter by themselves and do not exist, but something else – synthesis, form, idea" (Karsavin 1994). "Gradually the understanding that there is one humankind with one psyche is born and developed … would also do away with the awkward hypothesis of psychophysical parallelism and would afford us an opportunity to construct a new world model closer to the idea of the unus mundus" (Jung 1994).

The crisis of classical sciences in the 20th century generated the use of various interpretative and methodological systems in scientific methodology, which led to the understanding that it is necessary to utilise the principle of complementarity. "Being can only be described in part, as the other part remains at any given time unrecognised and unlimited. Life processes cannot be explained based on just the causality principle" (Jung 1995).

The rules of spiral civilization evolution whose form creates associations with DNA structure (and allows mentioning *genome and the program of human civilization*) indicate termination of another history cycle connected with the methodology of determinism. Following this route, the mental ecology of human life and destiny supported by a nonlinearity of self-organizing systems discussed by synergetics may become a gnoseological method of understanding the style and the content of the following paradigm. That will help to implement and shape a qualitative synthesis of a new type – "synthesis under advanced analysis which can be named as synthesis-analysis" (Gerasimova 2002) or "system synthesis" (Astafyeva 2008) using the immateriality of theocentrism paradigm and the cognitive achievements of scientific determinism model.

Today it is already acceptable to distinguish physical technologies engaged with physical time and space and humanitarian technologies (Ostrovsky 1998) correlated with informational space, internal time and subjective meanings. The former set the Space of the new paradigm whereas the latter harmonizes the relations between an individual and the society controlling the chances of implementing this paradigm's versions. To achieve optimum interaction physical and humanitarian technologies must be balanced forming, this way, "a new comprehensive history-generating trend and balancing it with the ability to manage the implementation of this trend" (Pereslegin 2006). That is exactly why the synergetic interpretation of today's vital problems has the chance to become a "productive hypothesis" (Udumian 2001) "that has the most chances to create a theory and a solution of long identified problems" (Chernavsky 2004) enabling to form the optimum of trend parity in mental medicine.

Contradiction unites into a whole the battle and the unity of opposites, and unity mutually supposes, and battle mutually exclude opposite sides. The fight of the thesis of classical psychiatry and the antithesis of anti-psychiatry brought these concepts to unipolar renditions in which both failures and achievements of these areas were subject to relativism from the opposing side. However, the thesis of classical psychiatry that was replaced by the antithesis of anti-psychiatry created conditions both for formation through the complementarity principle of a constructive synthesis of these contradicting concepts in mental medicine, promising a qualitatively new level of understanding and interpretation of mental health problems and mental illnesses (Table 2.1).

Table 2.1. System synthesis of mental medicine

Criteria	Clinical psychiatry (thesis)	Anti-psychiatry (antithesis)	Mental medicine (synthesis)
Philosophy	Positivism, neopositivism, scientism	Existentialism	Synergetics
Concept	Nosocentricity	Existential freedom of personality	Health-centricity
Priorities	Clinical	Social	Holistic
Trend	Biological	Socio-psychological	Bio-psycho-socio-spiritual and moral
Strategy	Treatment of mental illnesses	Individual mentality	Preventive correction, treatment, rehabilitation
Aims	Return of mental health	Implementing individual rights and freedoms	Improving quality of life and mental health levels
Tasks	Removing the symptoms	Maintaining the subject's right to his or her uniqueness	Preserving functions and mental potential
Objects	Sick person	Psychiatry as the ψ-functional institution of authority	Healthy person – client-patient
Focus	Mental disorder	Peculiarities of interpersonal interaction	Normal – changed – unbalanced mentality
Technologies	Treatment, rehabilitation	Communication	Preservation – optimisation - recovery
Process	Hospitalisation	Liberalisation	Adaptation – socialisation-humanisation – re-adaptation
Dynamics	Linear	Counter-linear	Multidimensional
Relationship	Paternalism	Protectionism	Partnership
Ethics	Stigmatisation	Presumption of mental uniqueness	De-stigmatisation
Forms of implementation	Hospital, clinic, care home	Therapeutic communities	Systematic monitoring of mental health

Internal contradictions of the thesis and antithesis are removed by the synthesis of old ideas, capable of using the new philosophical ideology of synergetics. A "system synthesis," "synthesis with the advanced analysis," which shows a meaningful combination of first methodological priorities and achievements, becomes a base for forming a new scientific discipline – mental medicine.

Synergetics that uses a complex approach, and has the complementarity principle among its most important systematic concepts, can creatively unite the achievements of classical psychiatry and anti-psychiatry, evading their shortcomings that first of all appear in their methodological relativism that denies the ideological priorities of the opposing side. The appearance of a new holistic philosophy inevitably generates new synthetic methodology, capable of retrieving the practical psychiatric science from the dead end of today's contradictory and irreconcilable concepts: theory will inspire practice. Elements of new useful trends are noticeable in the achievements of psychotherapy, narcology, and social psychiatry, with their more varied forms and methods of work, that fall outside the repertoire of traditional classic psychiatry. Mental medicine, whose polymodal structure is aimed at the wholesome, holistic approach to mental illnesses that considers not only nosological categories but also potential risks of their formation, can be the new base for implementation of the new synergetic philosophy in the mental health field.

Considering that mental illnesses consume up to 50% of the budget in developed countries' healthcare systems, the central task is the answer to the eternal question – what is more effective socially and economically, more clinically viable and humane. To preserve the subpopulations with mental disorders in their changed reality or to bring them to a true reality which they do not accept? Mental medicine provides the answer; it allows the strengthening of mental health in multiple scenarios and the treatment of mental illness. Mental medicine makes it possible to justify and implement a righteous care path and fate for any patient or client with specific resources of the polymodal mentality in an adequate for him or her multicultural or virtual hospital reality.

The dialectics of history in general and scientific research in particular are made up of the stages of "throwing away the stones" and their "gathering," meaning, respectively, processes of analysis and synthesis. However, in essence, they are just procedural thesis and antithesis, and this dyad demands its logical conclusion, which must be the third stage – construction of the new Cathedral of Science from the gathered stones. This stage can be called the system synthesis of mental medicine.

Chapter 3

From Nosocentric Psychiatry to Health-Oriented Mental Medicine

3.1. Mental Origins of the Global Crisis

The development and growth of socioeconomic capitalism formation system were arising from its possibility to derive extra profit and the increase in surplus value particularly caused by the deficit of goods in separate regions of the planet. Such deficit was at first historically created and then purposefully sustained. The surplus goods had to be transferred to the area where their deficit prevailed. The possibility of export goods actualized the importance of monopoly for a given type of production. Potentialities of excess profits became a critical argument for holding the development of own similar production in such regions. Retaining and growth of the product shortage were assisted by forming in such a way *anti-production* system which would not allow the development of countries which designated role was to be the sources of raw materials and the consumers of commodities. The selling race resulted in huge trends of socioeconomic capitalism development, which broadened the range of affected areas, financial productivity and profitability.

These changes led to the formation of imperialism. The following trend was developed: on the one hand, there was a growth of production and on the other hand, there was *the imposing of anti-production.* This situation was economically advantageous for the first category of countries and their compradors. Both processes were dependent on each other. They interacted within a single bimodal system. Goods were flowing in one direction. The flow of raw material and workforce resources representing the equivalent of merchandise payment means was coming from the opposite direction. The anti-production flow enabled to develop production processes involving cheap labor where "oil was obtained in return for food." The selling race on the one hand, and the means of the struggle for resources, on the other hand, have led to wars. Third world countries were the hostages of the system with differently directed production/anti-production flows.

The system where *the import of Resources and the export of Goods* represent differently directed flows that intersect its boundaries in different directions is working less and less effectively in the monopolar world. Today the number of territories where one can get cheap resources selling goods at a high price is becoming smaller and smaller. As a result, the deterritorialization of socioeconomic capitalism formation occurs losing the possibility to achieve extensive further development. "Capitalism, being always willing to expand its inner limits, continues to be under the threat of the outer limit which chance of splitting it rises internally with the expansion of the inner limits" (Deleuse, Guattari 2008).

The phenomenon of total overproduction emerges within the socioeconomic capitalism formation. This interrelation generates the problem of cheapening for those resources that are less and less needed. For the socioeconomic capitalism formation at this stage, unemployment turned out to be a significant issue about the economics. If labor shortage in the XIXth century resulted in the organization of psychiatric hospitals in the way they are today then now, when the capitalistic socioeconomic formation no longer requires the same labor quantities, the problem of excess proletariat generated the fundamentally opposite social dynamics of classical psychiatry. Processes of the 19th-century inverse dichotomy began, they were directed at the poor and the insane: now these social striations could be united which allowed to save funds and to conceal the economic component of such process by using medical rhetoric.

The social mission of classical psychiatry was radically changed. Nonetheless, the social nature of the ψ-function itself remained as an auxiliary means of production profitability regulation and optimization. The problems of socioethnic nature caused by the intensive import of cheap workforce during the last decades continue becoming sharper today which results in the growth of social tension and the prolongation of the global crisis.

The philosophical pluralism of the XXth century established the presence and deepening of system existential crisis which implied that critical problems requiring different solutions were actualized in the "nature – society – human (a subject of mental ecology)" system. At the moment, this "crisis is at the same time affecting almost the entire Western culture and society including all their key institutes. This is the crisis of art and science, philosophy and religion, law and morals, lifestyle and manners. This is the crisis of social, political and economic organization forms including the forms of marriage and family (children in same-sex partnerships). It is the crisis of the whole life, mind and behavior inherent to the Western society" (Sorokin 1992). Ethical and legal norms are devaluing, almost losing their prestige and lowering to the status of institutes used by authorities to manipulate the exploited majority. Moral imperatives almost do not affect human behavior. Their role is tragically weakening. All this leads to anomy, moral chaos and anarchy. This is exactly why the synergetically integrated four-dimensional model of ontogenesis which includes animogenesis and sociogenesis, psychogenesis and somatogenesis is becoming a popular methodology of mental ecology and mental medicine.

3.2. Crisis of Psychiatry and an Alternative to Mental Medicine

Any science evolves by grasping new ideas and forming the concepts that sometimes force to reconsider the ideas which seemed to be inviolable. At the same time, it becomes necessary to structure the acquired knowledge. International classification of diseases (ICD) is the system that the medical community is traditionally guided by. Therefore, its practical convenience, logical continuity concerning traditions and conceptual internal unity are so necessary.

The urgency of the problem of scientific and methodological system crisis in Psychiatry that found itself on the verge of exhausting traditional concepts often becomes a subject of discussion for experts. They propose changing paradigms in psychiatry (Nuller 2008; Krasnov 2014) as it appears to be a particular example of a more common difficulty faced by many modern sciences that have reached the end of another cycle of civilisation.The interdisciplinary nature of psychiatry determines the interest of various disciplines in this problem: natural sciences, humanities, technical sciences. It permits to apply a synergetic method in the present study.

It is remarkable that the countries, which use the diagnostic DSM system with its weaknesses decided not to change their traditions in the context of intensively varying psychiatric help including its ethical and legal aspect by adapting them to another ICD which, for this reason, cannot be considered "international."

Here it is appropriate to quote Igor Guberman who figuratively expressed the unproductiveness of discussions within the outworn methodology:

Amid rumors, stories, myths,
Simply lies and simply doubts
We fight harder than the Scyths
For diverseness of frauds.

In our opinion, the only solution is to find a new synergetic methodology which is likely to overcome, among other things, the "stigmatization damnation" of clinical psychiatry. For example, A. I. Skorik et al. (2014) distinguish the following motives of patients' evasion of collaboration with psychiatrists:

1) The fear of being registered with a psychoneurological dispensary.
2) The fear of losing their social status.
3) The fear of losing interpersonal relations at work and home.
4) Lack of information about psychoprophylactic care.
5) The fear of dependence on psychoprophylactic care.
6) The fear of dependence on the psychotropic medicine.
7) Weak attitude towards the obtaining of medical care.

To achieve the adaptive correction of public perception, it is suggested to reorganize psychiatric care on the basis of voluntariness, awareness-building and realizing the huge gap between the confabulated expectations of patients and psychiatric realias. However, the situation with stigmatization can only be overcome with the help of a radical rejection of psychiatric care branding in the opposite favor of organizing a mental health service based on the synergetic methodology.

Therefore, the features of deep *system psychiatric crisis* are as follows:

- Using up previous concepts and deficit of new ideas;
- Growing eclecticity and mechanicalness of approaches;
- Absence of a consistent stylistic and ideological concept of ICD-11;
- Globalization of approaches and classification criteria;

- Accumulating redundancy of information;
- Bifurcation into psychiatry of facts and psychiatry of values;
- Artificiality of new definitions and limited nature of classical terms;
- Conceptual non-implementation of growing multidisciplinarity and integrity.

Synergetics permits us to examine mental health and mental illnesses within a single methodology. The same group of professional psychotherapists, psychiatrists, clinical psychologists and social workers is using the same technologies and is working on both strengthening mental health of clients (who have difficulties in adapting in the absence of a diagnosis) and treating mental disorders of the patients. Such mental medicine is built on a synergetic interdisciplinary methodology which unites nosocentric clinical psychiatry and health-centric preventive mental health care.

Mental medicine is a science that studies etiopathogenesis and diagnostics along with the clinical picture and treatment of mental disorders, biopsychosociospiritual resources of personality and societal development, strategies and mechanisms of adaptation and professiogenesis based on a single synergetic methodology. This wording includes the classical definition of psychiatry in all the modes specified in the mental health definition by WHO (2001) and being the priorities of mental preventology.

Mental preventology is a section of general preventive medicine, a science that studies methods of achieving and maintaining the optimum level of mental health, psycho-hygiene and psycho-prophylactics on a systematic and interdisciplinary synergetic basis.

The main tasks are combining the classical psychiatry sphere of use with the field of interest of mental medicine. The latter apart from mental illnesses studies biopsychosociospiritual resources of personality development, mechanisms of socialisation and adaptive professiogenesis, and the search for a new health-centric concept that widens the possibilities for de-stigmatisation and the work of experts in the prenosological field.

Table 3.1. Mental medicine as a unified theory of improving mental health and treatment of mental illnesses

Criteria	Mental medicine	
	Clinical Psychiatry	Mental preventology
Concept	Nosocentricity	Health-centricity
Strategy	Illness Treatment	Prevention of pathology
Aim	Return of mental health	Raising quality of life
Task	Removing symptoms	Preserving functions
Object	Ill person	Healthy person
Focus	Psychiatric disorder	Normal function
Technologies	Treatment, rehabilitation	Preservation, optimisation
Priorities	Clinical	Holistic
Relationships	Paternalism	Partnership
Process	Hospitalisation	Socialisation
Dynamics	Linear	Multidimensional
Ethics	Stigmatisation	De-stigmatisation

In the light of the thoughts mentioned above, it seems relevant to compare and combine classical clinical psychiatry and mental preventology against the most important criteria for their content - direction and nature of functioning (Table 3.1) within unified mental medicine.

This table permits us to compare the direction of mental preventology and clinical psychiatry, outlining their mutual compatibility when solving tasks in strengthening the mental health of the nation. Integration in mental medicine of the traditional psychiatric nosocentricity with the growing health-centric trend of improving mental health became possible via synergetic methodology and interdisciplinary teamwork. This information casts doubt on the concept of viewing the psychiatric disorder as the main and only aim and task of psychiatry. In today's context, diagnostics, treatment, and prevention of psychopathology have become a tactical fragment of the common strategy and direction of mental medicine towards preserving and optimising a person's mental health and increasing his or her quality of life. Mental medicine becomes a unified science about mental health and mental illnesses.

Thus, more intensive development and research of branches of medicine, both already existing and those that have not been fully formed yet, are typical and relevant tasks of the modern science. Not only from a scientific determinism point of view, but also in opinion of other methodological approaches. Synergetics is one of them being the base for organisationally functional interdisciplinarity, capable of forming a new paradigm of mental medicine. Projecting it on the traditional field of classical psychiatry widens the area of use for specialist knowledge, directing it to situations that do not have a clinical interpretation yet. It demands to perfect mental health's efficient monitoring technologies that can complement and transform traditional clinical examination. Formalising the prophylactic monitoring activity of specialists (with the appearance of specialities like "preventive medicine," "control and strengthening health") is also of great importance. It seems necessary to form strategies for work in the prenosological field, screening mental health factors and resources. Multiplying potentials of trajectories of correctional prophylactic and treatment rehabilitation routes become a demand. Evaluating the quality of life and social functioning, in the end, secures better results in improving the mental health of the population.

Chapter 4

Synergetic Methodology of Mental Medicine

Synergetics is a multidisciplinary science about the development and self-organization of complex dynamic systems (including psychopathology development), the main functional principles of which are: non-linearity, non-stability, openness, dynamical hierarchy, observability. The methodology of synergetics is based on the integrative approach to the study of structures which are thermodynamically open, non-equilibrious, exchanging energy, information, a substance with the environment of dissipative structures.

4.1. Multiaspectuality of Scientific Cognition

The world's uniformity and diversity are the sources of two problems related to its awareness: *continuity and infinity*. Each of them has two aspects – one quantitative and one qualitative.

In the quantitative aspect, the first problem appears as continuity of the objective world's components. In the qualitative aspect, this condition is expressed in the continuity of its features. The second problem from the quantitative side appears as the spatiotemporal endlessness of the world and from the qualitative side it appears as the endlessness of its features and demonstrations. The latter condition assumes an infinite number of options that include an object (subject) in different systems, implying an infinite number of roles belonging to the same subject of observation. These problems conflict with the restricted abilities of human cognitive functions. Scientific analysis and synthesis methodology allow handling the situation. Analysis figuratively splits the indivisible, infinite world into subsystems each of which becomes the scope of a particular science study. Synthesis integrates knowledge into a cohesive cognitive complex.

Synthesis of simple evolving structures into a complex system occurs using identification of the overall rate of their evolution. A certain degree of lapping over the simple structures which make up a complex unified structure must occur to generate the latter. If the overlapping zone is small then the components will evolve indifferently from each other; if it is large, then the constituent trends will join into a single rapidly developing structure.

Table 4.1. The criteria of functional lateral asymmetry of human cogitation mechanisms

Lateral asymmetry / Criterion	Sinistrocerebral thinking	Interhemispheric (ambidextrous) thinking	Dextrocerebral thinking
Principle of information handling	Locality, tactics	"Input" strategy, "output" tactics	Globality, strategy
Direction	From details to the whole (Details specify the content of the whole)	Understanding the whole, elaborating details (Synchronism of multidirectional process)	From the whole to details (The whole specifies the nature of details)
Vector of actions	Consistent, single-line	Consistent, multidirectional	Inconsistent, multidirectional
Stylistics	Rationality of logics	Parity of the optimum	Irrationality of intuition
Semiotics	Theorem, law, figure	Task, regularity, dynamics	Axiom, paradox, word
Semantics	Polysemantics generating chaos and system disorganization	Dialogue generating synergetic constructivity of an open system	Monologue generating autization of a closed system
Circumstances of idea's genesis	Establishment of the fact	Creativity during dilemma selection	Productive hypothesis
Philosophical concept	Calculating the immanent	Realizing the transcendental	Approaching the transcendental
Methodology	Analyzing components, breaking up the object, induction of the implicit	Optimum of concept parity	Synthesis, deepening into the features of the whole object, deduction of the explicit
Level of information handling	Current paradigm	New paradigm	Change of paradigm
Way of object realization	One-dimensional determinism	Complementarity of methods	Holographic indeterminism
Possibilities	Objective search for right options	Creativity during options assessment and choice	Subjective "recognition," intuitive feeling of "hitting the mark"
External outline of actions	Constructive activity	Active selectivity	Meditative focus of external passivity
Level of activity realization	High	Very high	Admittedly low
Resolved tasks	Goal	Goal in the cause of meaning	Meaning
Results	Collecting empirical data, computation	Selecting the optimum of directories	Realizing "meanings," "brightening"
Level of actuality	The state of being essential, pragmatism	Effectivity, "tomorrow's" strategy	Eternity, impracticality
Role of time	Passive: development in real chronotope	Active: considering and using realias for a change of chronotope	Neutral: achronity
Freedom for…	Realizing an external action (logics of determinism)	Decision-making (constructivity of synergetics)	Internal thinking process (mysticism of indeterminism)
Acceptable limits	Internal	Appropriate	External
Perfect (logically arising from priorities) model of social organization	Anarchy of the Babylonian tower (ochlocracy)	Democracy	Totalitarianism, tyranny

The main differences between inductive, deductive and complementary scientific methods emphasize the multidirectionality of their priorities, tasks and vectors (provided the commonality of addressable strategies for which these methods are suitable from different perspectives) which are correlated with the functional lateral asymmetry of the human brain. In this context the sinistrocerebral arrangement will to a greater extent correspond with the first method, the dextrocerebral arrangement will correspond with the second method and the interhemispheric function of "system synthesis" which combines both mental trends will correspond with the third method (Table 4.1).

Functional asymmetry of human mentality reveals complementarity of sinistrocerebral and dextrocerebral types of thinking which synthesis is achieved due to interhemispheric links and interactions. Analytical sinistrocerebral thinking structures the scope of science, determining the inductivity of its methodology. Synthetic dextrocerebral thinking blurs demarcations between scientific schools, forming metadisciplinary trends (for example, philosophical metaphysics) which corresponds more with a deductive methodology. System synthesis which combines these functions provides constructive interaction between the first two types of thinking and implements interdisciplinary approach which allows constructively and productively uniting conventional methodologies that supplement each other and used to be almost incompatible with one another previously.

Therefore, disciplinary, metadisciplinary, and interdisciplinary scientific approaches turn out to be mutually complementary. The first one resolves a particular task of goals that emerged within the historical context of subject's development by using the methods of settled instrumentarium of the existing paradigm. The second one uses polymorphism of languages, search for analogies, poetical metaphoristics, circular causality (sometimes interpreting it mystically), demanding to modernize the concept of paradigm and attempting to resolve the complex task of symbols. The third one implements a holistically network method of structuring the reality, performing the interdisciplinary function which allows combining the first two methods of understanding the reality and assuming the solution of the goals in the cause of meaning task. Being an interdisciplinary science synergetics allows implementing the complementarity of traditional inductive analysis and deductive synthesis in psychiatry performing the qualitatively new gnoseological methodology of mental medicine.

4.2. Synergetic Biopsychosociospiritual Methodology

Synergetics views the human body as a complex open system with non-linear processes. Its behavior cannot be called determinate. The change of the system does not follow linear laws because of internal fluctuations that alter the trajectory of development.

Instead of numerous factors which determine the system's status, synergetics examines the few order parameters – in other words, the key variables that to a large extent determine the behavior of the system. By influencing just several variables we can direct system development at one or another attractor and in the future the cone of its attraction will level external and internal fluctuations of other variables.

When accumulating a large number of fluctuations, an exaltation of the system towards internal or external influences grows to such an extent that those variables which changes have not caused any significant influence on the system, start to affect change. Such points that the system passes (bifurcation points) make it possible to use the mechanism of a local increase in small fluctuations, which will enable change to the behavior and the trajectory of the system's development in the right direction (Figure 4.1). The term developmental "trajectory" of a condition or illness is often used in modern foreign and Russian literature. However, its use by A. B. Smulevich (2013) regarding "problems of personality disorder trajectory in the field of minor psychiatry" met reprimands from reviewers because it was deemed a "beautiful" term. From our point of view, the term "trajectory" is entirely justified and is borrowed from the synergetic methodology for describing development in multidimensional (at least three-dimensional) space, when traditional "flat dynamics" becomes incapable of describing the multi-modal relationships and scenarios with multiple options for development of modern evidence-based medicine.

The synergetic concept of ontogenesis that we developed presupposes interplay of equal factors:

- somatic health that forms as a result of biogenesis;
- psychic health that appears during psychogenesis;
- social health that develops in the sociogenesis process.
- spiritual and moral health that forms during animogenesis.

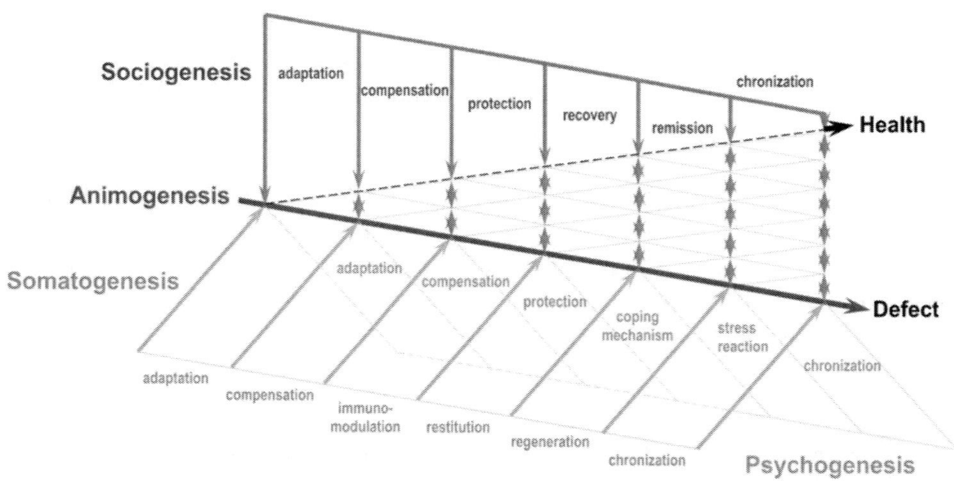

Figure 4.1. Fractal trajectory of states (diseases, epidemics) progress and protection mechanisms.

Anima, animus (from Latin anima – soul, animus – spirit) are concepts that in the Ancient Greek culture framed the phenomenon of spirit and acted as stages of evolution of spirituality understanding: if anima (soul) is inseparable from its material carrier, then animus (spirit) has an autonomous status.

Animogenesis refers to ontogenetic mental and moral evolution of a person. By integrating the ideas about soul and spirit, the term itself reflects polymodal mental health which is the core of the biopsychosociospiritual model of ontogenesis (Sidorov 2005). The four-dimensionality of the proposed model originates from the Albert Einstein's theory of relativity created for four-dimensional space.

The sum of individual parameters for a particular population provides an idea about the levels of its somatic, psychic, social as well as mental and moral functioning whereas the combination of obtained results allows performing system monitoring of public health level and public perception of the explored contingent.

Biopsychosociospiritual health of an individual (and public health) are impossible to imagine in isolation – independent of the effect of external factors, which in turn transform as a result of various influences on them from individuals, affecting the environment. These relationships lead to the formation of a complex, nonlinear, unstable, open, self-organising system of a dissipative type that conducts energy exchange and is defined in its development by the influence of multi-directional forces.

The synergetic approach can be visualized (Figure 4.2) through the main plains (vectors) of the bio-psycho-social model of ontogenesis: somato-, psycho-, and sociogenesis. Somatogenesis presupposes the development of systems and functions of the organism; psychogenesis is the development of psychic functions; sociogenesis is the development of social roles and relationships. The central part of the intersection and integration of the three vectors forms the fourth and the primary aspect – the spiritual and moral aspect of animogenesis, the core of which is a polymodal mentality. The model promotes an interdisciplinary and integrated approach to complex and complicated cause and effect relationships. The synergetic model is multidimensional and nonlinear, unstable and open. The developmental trajectories of the condition or the illness are set and corrected at bifurcation points, achieving spiral-like qualities and multiple possibilities. Nonlinear discretion and fractality replace linear and nososentric dynamics.

The main planes of ontogenesis penetrate each other, forming transit zones and a central zone that contains conscience, an integral part of mental health, the highest level of self-regulation and reflection of reality that accumulates spiritual and moral potential (picture 4.3). In the dynamics of ontogenesis, the amplitude and rhythm of the main aspects diminish and by the time they fade, the person's soul and conscience become the last relevant factors.

According to the synergetic concept, the development of any disorder has non-linear dynamics, the trajectory of which includes the following fractals: predisposition (family dysontogenesis); latent (diathesis); initial (functional disorders); clinical picture; chronicity (forms and types of the disease progress); outcome. In clinical medicine, a fractal is both progress and condition, uniting temporal and qualitative characteristics of the system and organism.

Multidisciplinary synergetics represents an optimum methodology for developing interdisciplinary mental ecology and mental medicine.

Synergetic methodology permits the systematic and successive integration of the whole variety of factors and resources of mental ecology to promote an optimal level of national health.

It is particularly the four-dimensional model of a *"synergetic person"* that enables to obtain maximum cumulative effect from the mobilization of biopsychosociospiritual resources of mental medicine as a psychiatric paradigm of integrative medicine.

Synergetics is a constructive basis which does not contradict with present diagnostics criteria as well as mental disorder therapy and which can be superposed by any clinical information that expands the degree of understanding the essence of mental diseases. Such information is optimized with the improvement of psychopharmacology, examination procedures, and psychological diagnostics. Distinguishing prenosological fractals and categories in mental medicine reduces diagnostic and prognostic uncertainty.

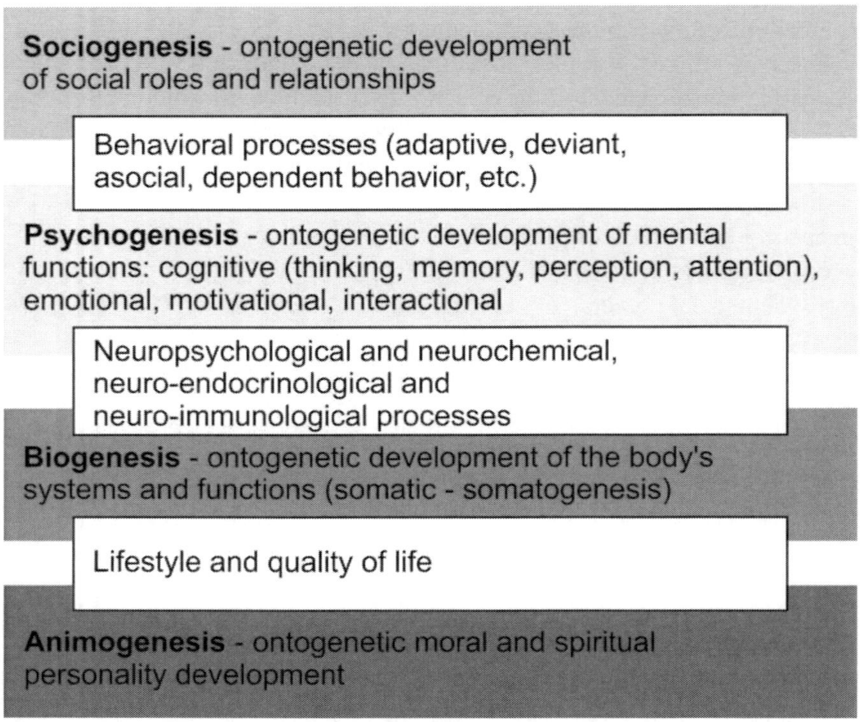

Figure 4.2. Biopsychosociospiritual model of ontogenesis.

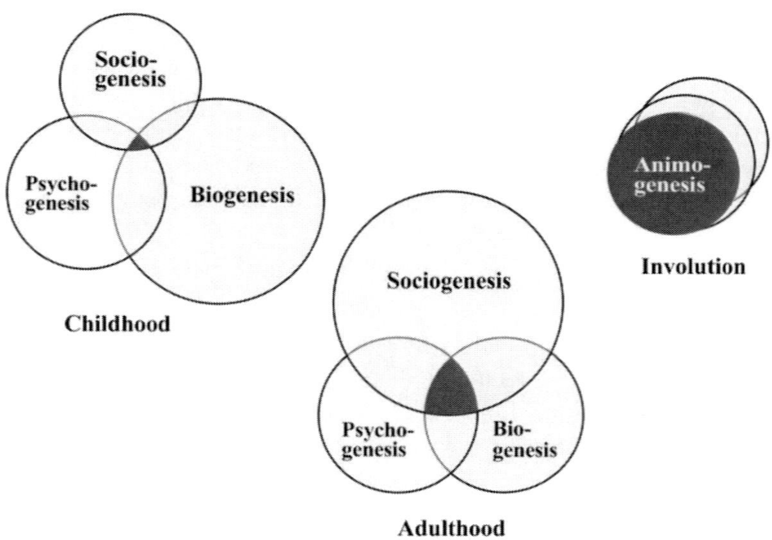

Figure 4.3. Dynamics of biopsychosociospiritual assimilation.

The synergetic methodology of mental medicine is far from a multipurpose “synergetic Esperanto” which can be equally applied to animo- and psycho-, socio- and biogenesis. Each of these four dimensions has its scientific methodology:

- *sociogenesis* is developed by sociology and social philosophy, management, and political science;
- *psychogenesis* – psychology and psychiatry, psychotherapy and addictology, neuropsychology and psychophysiology;
- *biogenesis* – biology and medicine;
- *animogenesis* – polymodal ethics from bioethics to orthodox ethics.

The synergetic methodology of mental medicine is a tool or, figuratively speaking, a “system administrator” of harmonizing and synchronizing the efforts of multiple specialties and approaches to the solution of specific tasks in strengthening mental health and curing mental diseases. It allows significant expanding of technological resources and clinical opportunities for the *morally personalized and genetically oriented medicine implemented in group forms of activities*.

4.3. Synergetic Functional Diagnosis

Clinical evolution of the classical biopsychosocial model (Engel 1982) into the practice of functional diagnostics emphasizes characteristics of biopsychosocial adaptation. The formation of screening quality of life assessment batteries and the construction of personalized assistance programs in national psychiatry are mostly conclusively implemented at the Department of biopsychosocial rehabilitation of the Saint-Petersburg Scientific Research Psychoneurological Institute n.a. V. M. Bekhterev (Kotsubinskiy et al. 2014).

The four-dimensional tetranuclear synergetic medico-psychosociospiritual model proposed by us (Figure 4.4.) requires justification of *moral diagnostics* and the characteristics of ethical competency and moral adaptation. The extension of the quality of life measuring tools to its moral and axiological and sense bearing appraisals also seems necessary. The expansion of practical care technologies from moral education and business communication ethic trainings to spiritual and moral correction and rehabilitation are required. In fact, this concerns clinical filling of the traditional bioethics apparatus with a development of a vast multidimensional field of ethical diagnostics and propaedeutics, treatment, and rehabilitation (Sidorov 2014). Handling this primary task is possible only by relying on a synergetic methodology of mental medicine. Integration of healthy style and moral meaning of living are becoming the most significant paradigm characteristic of mental medicine.

Present-day ideas about *psychological diagnostics* are mainly brought to the assessment of person’s psychological resources or “personal adaptation potential” (Posokhov 2008). The leading characteristic of such a potential is the structure of “Ego” that provides the coordination of diverse psychic functions, their management and identity preservation throughout the whole life (Ovchinnikov et al. 2010). The following must be investigated to analyze psychological resources of clients and patients. These are the specifics of personal structure, presence and nature of intrapsychic conflicts, details of personal adaptation and compensatory formations (forms of psychological defense, coping mechanisms, internal picture of the disease, etc.). These specifics have through-composed nature reflected in the phenomenology of clinical and social, moral and psychological diagnoses.

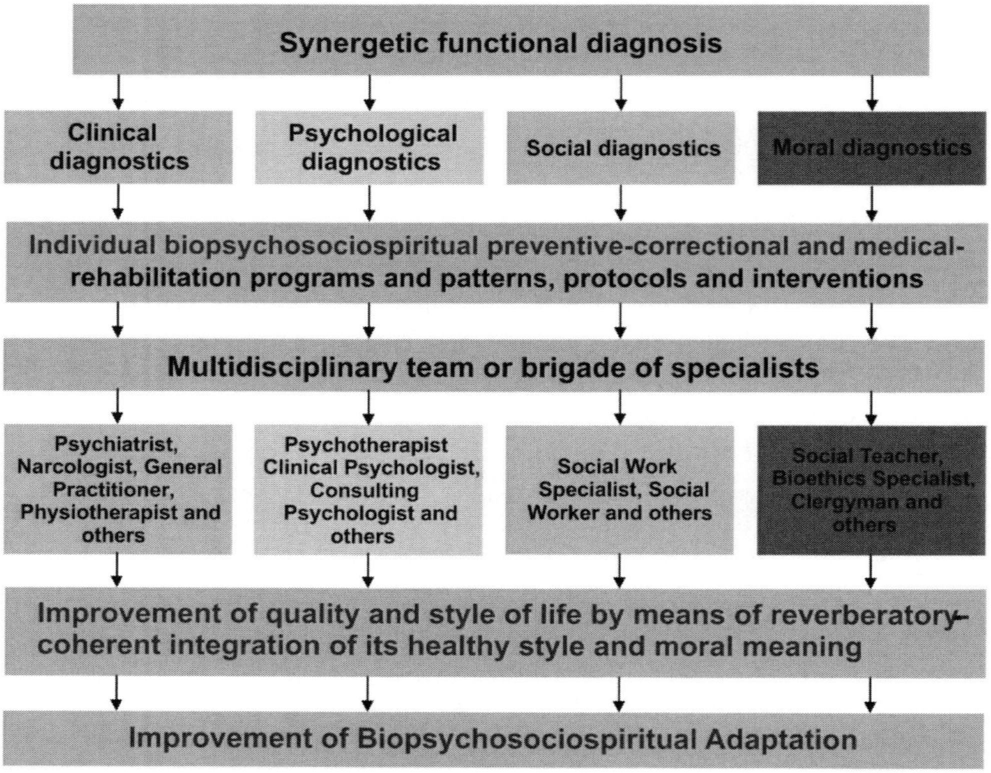

Figure 4.4. Synergetic and epidemiological functional diagnostics in mental medicine.

Social diagnostics reveal personal social resources and specifics of social identity, social competency and external social resources of an individual. The concept of social competency includes the existing human potential abilities to interact effectively with social environment (Schröder et al. 1978). Reduction or failure of social competency results in the exclusion of the mentally ill from the field of productive work and their loss of social links. When establishing social diagnosis, it is necessary to consider the dynamics of patients' social competency during the premorbid period and at this moment as well as the presence and the specifics of interpersonal conflicts in the family, at work, in partner relations and other fields of activities. Social diagnosis must also reflect external social resources which concern the characteristics of social potential of the family and peer surroundings.

The issues of traditional *clinical diagnostics* do not require any special discussion.

The formulation of clinical, psychological, social and moral diagnoses results in the development of *multipronged synergetic functional diagnosis* which is becoming an essential diagnostic tool in mental medicine. The "sinergeticity" of functional diagnosis involves the fact that it allows to validate and construct an individualized trajectory and a block-module multidisciplinary route of preventively-correcting and medically-rehabilitating support by using four-dimensional space for any conditions (diseases) and epidemic situations.

Chapter 5

Mental Epidemiology

Traditional epidemiology is the study of patterns of an infectious epidemic process.

Epidemiology of noncommunicable diseases considers patterns of occurrence and distribution, preventive measures, morbidity and mortality of noncommunicable diseases. Currently, in Russia, the percentage of infectious diseases is only 7%, while of noncommunicable – 93%.

Widespread use of epidemiological studies in the clinic led to the formation of *clinical epidemiology* – the basis of modern evidence-based medicine.

Forty years ago, English biologist Richard Dawkins (1976) proposed the idea of memes – ideas expressed verbally or in writing, circulating in the public conscience and forming an individual conscience. A quarter of a century ago, this idea on the associative model of computerization was developed by Dawkins in the *mental viruses* underlying mind contamination and information epidemiology, manifesting in a variety of "total madness" episodes. Subsequently, this resulted in the creation of new scientific disciplines – mental ecology and mental medicine, as well as in the appearance of a new series of journals (for example, "Human Ecology" in 1994, "Questions of mental medicine and ecology" in 1995, etc.).

Current sizes of the Global web as an interface of planetary and individual conscience has called for a rethinking of traditional social perception of social and mental epidemics, cyber virology and mental security. The relevant challenge was to find new resources and tools for adaptive protection of public conscience in the permanent information and hybrid wars. This task required the development of a multidisciplinary synergetic biopsychosociospiritual methodology of ontogenetic development and mental epidemic process.

5.1. From Psychic Epidemics to Mental Epidemics

In classical epidemiology behavioral epidemics are distinguished, and they are related to the power of suggestion or behavioral patterns (as opposed to penetration of microorganisms or physical impact). Clinical illustrations include dancing manias in medieval times, cases of mass fainting or seizure ("hysterical epidemics"), the panic of the crowd, the tides of fashion and enthusiasm. The nature of transmitted behavior was traced not only in personal contact between two people but also in group coercion (smoking, consuming alcohol or drugs). Behavioral epidemics were sometimes difficult to distinguish from organic diseases outbreaks, such as poisoning the environment with toxic substances. In psychiatry, such behavior has been called psychic epidemics.

Psychic epidemics (PE) as group contagious disorders started being explored in Russia in the second half of the XIX century. Formerly patients, being possessed by PE fell either under the patronage of church organizations as "victims of the devil," or under laws. From now on the given problem turned out to be in the focus of attention of philosophers and historians, as well as lawyers and ethnographers, public figures and doctors.

The majority of national psychiatrists in the second half of the XIX century regarded the phenomenon of psychic epidemics as predominantly psychosocial phenomenon. At the same time, psychiatrists did not deny that formation and manifestation of psychic epidemics can be influenced by national culture and ethnic traditions, adding fascinating details to the symptoms, but not changing development algorithms and clinical essence of this phenomenon. The fact that victims of psychic epidemics carry the pathology of specifically psychiatric nature was beyond doubt and ambiguity among psychiatrists. V. M. Bekhterev in 1908 spoke of the "collective or mass delusions and hallucinations," demon-obsession epidemics, hand-wringing (or hysterics), bad-spelling, psychotic manifestations of religious content, disseminating of panic reactions (Sidorov 2015).

Psychiatrist A. A. Tokarski (1893) divided the causes of psychic epidemics in *"predisposing and producing."* In the first group, he included "poverty of mental content, limited interests, the absence of criticism, ignorance"; in the second group – dominant in society ideas, external events, the tendency to imitate, psychic contagiosity, neuroinduction. This classification significantly coincides with the modern interpretation of personal and social identity of the subject, specifying universal trend of potential ways of occurrence of psychic epidemics.

Russian psychiatrists identified a set of "predisposing" and "producing by directly instilling ideas" prerequisites of psychic epidemics. The first group included: fanatical faith based on extraneous suggestion and influence of the inductor; the presence of a charismatic personality, which possesses the ability to inspire ideas (such inductor could be a mentally ill person); poor education, primitive culture, social ill-being. P. I. Jacobi wrote that psychic epidemic .".. develops only in nervous and exhausted, weakened physically, morally and mentally population" (cit. Schigolev 2001). Among the factors that influence the occurrence of psychic epidemics, some exogenous factors are actual as well: drugs and alcohol, poverty and hunger, fatigue and gathering of scores of people of same collective spirit, poor nourishment and repose, excessive physical stress and household inconveniences, sickness and frequent deliveries. State of mind of the subject and the level of personal reaction, the intensity of effects of doctrine dogmas on his psyche and current superstitions also play a significant role.

Most authors considered pumping of psycho-emotional tension (PET) among participants of the rite or process to be one of the leading causes of psychic epidemics. PET entailed narrowing of mind, leading to the inability of accounting for one's actions. The increase of PET potentiates suggestibility and autosuggestibility, melodramatization and demoralization, tendency to imitate and panic moods, becoming a factor affecting the life of the individual and the community in general. Influenced by suggestions a person loses individuality and initiative, becoming a part of the crowd and falling into a panic. “In the delirious crowd, each individual affects the others and is subjected to the similar effect” (cit. Schigolev 2001).

Psychiatrists have classified such factors as wars and revolutions, political upheavals and socio-economic reforms, potentiating uncertainty of social and political relationships and situations and enhancing neuro-psychic excitability, leading to a decrease in the stability of the central nervous system as “producing” causes of psychic epidemics.

Thus, polyetiological factor, which is the main criterion in shaping the ways of the emergence and spread of mass psychic viruses, was determined as the basis of occurrence of psychic epidemics. Socio-economic changes and crises affected the intensity of the emergence and spread of contagious phenomena of psychic character.

Polyetiological and polymorphic nature of PE in the XXI century required involving multidisciplinary synergetic methodology to estimate and predict the fractal dynamics of the epidemic process in four-dimensional space of psychogenesis and sociogenesis, somatogenesis and animogenesis that form the trajectory of the mental epidemic (ME) as the subject of mental medicine.

ME is the emergence of the cases (outbreaks) of mental disorders in the collective or on the territory at a rate significantly higher than normally expected. Mental epidemics pass into the category of destructive when they begin to threaten public conscience of the country as a whole. They can become pandemics, covering not only the country but also the continent.

MEs are contagious polymodal and polymorphic mental disorders and states. Inside an epidemic outbreak, it is possible to find groups not only with three prenosological fractals: predisposition, latent, initial but also with three nosological: developed clinical picture, chronization, and outcome. In the debut of ME prenosological and early forms of mental illness prevail; in destructive ME, threatening public conscience of the country as a whole – detailed clinical forms prevail, in pandemic ME – chronic, and outcome states prevail. Quantitative and qualitative measurement of the depth and intensity of the mental epidemic process can be obtained by using an index of mental ecology of the individual, socio- and psychometrics, scales of quality of life and human development.

Singular epidemicity of the modern world has transformed sporadic purely psychic epidemics into mental. Accumulating all the variety of registers and resources of public conscience, modulated by the global web, mental epidemics generalize stigmatization of mental contagiousness in new resonance-wave cascade architecture of the human brain mirror neurons. Reflecting the dynamics and rhythmics of noosphere shocks, these neurons change the old linear epidemicity of classical infectious processes into the multi-dimensional and multi-level synergetic dynamics.

And indeed, today's TV world news digests are increasingly approaching the psycho-manipulative design of the weather forecasts – apparently with the same, but in fact with noosphere typhoons and differential pressure zones, cyclones and anticyclones interconnected and interdependent on a global scale.

There is no doubt that in the case of a task assignment the whole earth will face quickly and quietly outwardly natural but essentially man-made another change “of noosphere poles!” Creators of such “noosphere weather” do not forget about the mental tolerance and social time polarity of the set of subpopulations for which the illusion of the old world picture is maintained by the sacramental light verse refrain stating that “there is always rain in Rainville.” And such a village exists anywhere in the world ... Although “globally rainy” World, long ago having become demoralized and dehumanized, promises to wash away the last islands of reason and morality in the future cloacal warming. This is certainly a metaphor, but only by dramatizing threats it is possible to achieve their actual perception.

5.2. Etiopathogenesis of Mental Epidemics

A long-term study of mental epidemics in the European North of Russia allowed us to identify the main characteristics of their etiology and pathogenesis (Sidorov 1976, 1990, 2015).

Sociogenesis of ME is marked by frequency of violations of the structure and functions of the family. Violations in personality socialization and social decompensation are usual problems. The coincidence of debut with conflict or stressful situation, disharmony and dysfunctionality of families are also among violations. Defects of upbringing and low level of education, sensory deprivation and social exclusion contribute to the development of the sociogenesis. Low mobility and professional incompetence, social-class homogeneity (poverty and marginality) influence sociogenesis. Inchoateness of socio-economic and political life, oppressive dullness of routine existence, and periodically bursting in flash MEs that give psycho-emotional discharge are all risk factors.

The modern socio-economic situation is characterized by the global crisis affecting virtually all aspects of human existence. Such social phenomenon as *anomie* of moral and psychological status of social and individual conscience develops, when the former system of values dissolves; contradictions between the proclaimed objectives and the inability to realize them in traditional for most people way deepen; isolation of the individual from society and depressive disappointment in life can be observed.

Anomie is manifested in three directions, indicating the potency of mental component growth:

interpersonal – strengthening of mutual mistrust and hostility, rivalry and aggression, reactions of exclusion and alienation, social stratification into subcultures – *filiations;*

cultural – collapse of the old cultural values and priorities, changing of established rules of interpretation of events, occurrence of conflict value systems, the state of identification emptiness in the absence of alternatives;

social – disintegration and polarization of society, crisis of confidence in public institutions.

All fields marked:

1) ascertain the potency of anomie influence on the formation and development of psychic epidemic disorders;
2) indicate etiopathogenic situation predisposing increasingly intensive appearance, epidemic development, and distribution of various mental disorders;
3) identify the obvious fact that the prevalence, severity and extent of psychopathological consequences of anomie transform the situation with the epidemic spread of mental disorders into a significant threat to public conscience and national security.

The situation of anomie contributes to the formation and spread of *permissive quality*, deblockation, and cancelation of prohibitions accepted in the society which are structuring ethical elements of society. In such circumstances, an individual may lose a foothold, losing the value system and ethical guidelines, appearing without the support of the formerly canonical principles, which structured pre-crisis society. The identity of the individual that relied on an outer frame of social norms dissolves in a chaotic welter of anomie, deforming mentality and rising sensitivity to mental epidemics.

Modern literature distinguishes two types of identities: *personal* and *social*. The first refers to self-determination of the individual regarding his physical, intellectual and moral traits. The second is "self-determination in terms of classifying oneself in a particular social group" (Burkovskaya 2005) – the knowledge of who you are and what your place in society is. Existentialist philosopher S. Kierkegaard wrote: "Man is a social animal; only in the herd is he happy. It is all one to him whether it is the most profound nonsense or the greatest villainy – he feels completely at ease with it – so long as it is the view of the herd, and he is able to join the herd" (Sas 2008). In essence, this is the formula of existential protection: either death under the hooves of the social herd or depersonalizing immersion in a mass psychogenic illness of the herd majority. M. Eliade said that .".. the man of the traditional culture sees himself existing only when it is no longer he, being content with imitation and repetition of gestures of the other. He is aware of his reality, adequacy for himself only when he refuses this adequacy." "Social psychology can not do without imitation" (Jung 1994), "mystic participation" (L. Levy-Bruhl).

A. G. Sanina (2014) highlights several angles of identity significant for mental epidemiology.

1) *The logical view of identity* determines its interpretation in various sciences.
2) *The philosophical view of identity* as a set of communication (including contagious) practices instead of the previous its understanding as a fixed datum.
3) *The psychological aspect of identity* as the basis of biopsychosociospiritual nature and adaptive human behavior (Erikson 1996; Sidorov 2015).
4) *Anthropological view of identity* as a cultural embodiment of traditions and customs.
5) *The sociological view of identity* as a meaningful product of communicative and epidemic development.
6) *System perspective on multidisciplinary identity* marks its important normative quality of self-reference, which is not affected by involvements in social networks and social positions. As one of the signs of spiritual immunity to mental epidemics, an individual identity can be considered. It is only through correlation with private individuality that the existence of multiple contexts of the multicultural environment is provided.

If the structure of society is destroyed or subjected to intense reforms and most social categories lost former value, there is a reassessment by the subject of a group belonging, and of a place in this group; traditional (old) social identification becomes difficult or impossible. Destruction of habitual relationship leads to the fact that the subject appears out of the stable and habitually familiar social system. Uncertainty creates discomfort and psychoemotional tension that are maintained among a significant part of the population by a radical change in all spheres of deformed by crisis society.

The role of unconscious and instinctual psychic phenomena and behavioral reactions grows increasingly reducing the potential of the analytical brain hemisphere. At the same time the feeling of loss of structuring ethical guidelines is enhanced, as well as the frustration of hopes and ideals, the desire of the miracle and its search in everyday life. Panic disorientation – such definition to the sense of a man living in the era of historical crises gives Spanish philosopher Ortega y Gasset (1997). "A man is disoriented with respect to himself, knocked out of the route, outside his limits, thrown into new circumstances extending for him an Unknown Land."

To feel like a part of the whole, like an element of the social system once again, the individual begins to search for a new social group, but the group life can dissolve his personality: "Identification with a social role is a generous source of neuroses. A person can not get rid of himself in favor of an artificial personality. Attempting this causes unconscious reactions, affects, phobias, obsessive representations and so on" (Jung 1994). Personal and social identification of the subject forms a kind of bimodal scheme, in which both components are in a dynamic relationship, determined by direct communication and feedback of components within the system. Sustainable prevalence of one of the trends can lead to disharmony in the dyad functioning, creating systemic problems and generating processes either of dissolution of authentic personality in society, or – of social nihilism. In the case of the first variant, the subject personal identity coalesces with the social. The man understands and appreciates himself only from the standpoint of belonging to a group, which under conditions of anomie can be almost any community – up to destructive or criminal organizations, as well as para-religious totalitarian sects currently experiencing a hystero-demonic renaissance.

In traditional perception anomie is the result and a symptom of system (paradigmatic) values deactualization, as well as of synchronous methodology, losing its monopoly of the uncontested comprehension of the existence meanings.

At the same time, many researchers note that the nature of anomie is becoming more complicated. So, R. Merton (1992) represents anomie as a consequence of dysfunctionality of social institutions. According to T. Parsons (2002), anomie manifests invulnerabilities to the self-sufficiency of society, which depend on the state of its internal integration and harmony of control. According to Erich Fromm (1998), anomie began to show itself in the approval of "sick societies" realities, becoming a criterion of civilizational mental health predetermining production of human destructiveness. Zh. T. Toshchenko (2013) treats anomie as the absence of norms and violation of social relations, manifested in centaurisms as a combination of incongruous. Thus, a paradoxical man creates a paradoxical and potentially epidemic explosive society.

Paradoxes, centaurisms, and antinomies came into the modern world not for a while, but forever. *Anomie, the quintessence of which is the absence of norms, itself became a permanently changing norm of everyday life.* S. A. Kravchenko (2014) proposed the concept of "normal anomie" as branching combination of vulnerabilities for society in the form of side effects of innovative and pragmatic, rational Human activity, as well as systemic crises. The main contours of this concept reflect the following:

1) Realities of normal anomie are caused by an objective process of formation of a complex society and by contradictory nature of its social and cultural dynamics.

2) Pluralism of social time with significant moral component dispersion becomes the norm (Prigozhin 2006).
3) Adiaphorisation is developing as an escape from the scope of the moral evaluation, resulting in established "moral blindness" (Bauman, Donskis 2013).
4) Simulation and simulacra become a factor not only of the dispersion of values and norms but also the basis of "total simulation era" as the latest global vulnerability.
5) Formation of normal processes of anomie influences virtualization (Debor 2000) and gamization (Kravchenko 2014) of society based on imitational and simulative democratic (nationalist, etc.) shows.
6) One of the essential characteristics of normal anomie has become a paradoxical combination of knowledge and ignorance, science and pseudo-science, the permanence of scientific revolution and short actuality of scientific paradigm.
7) Increasing paradoxicality of risks and threats, globalized and delocalized, innumerable and unpredictable, uncompensated and irreversible (Beck 2012). The meaning of risk definitions staging is becoming a force shaping nature of deviant conscience and paradoxical behavior.
8) Dispersion of traditional family relations is included in the field of stansard anomie.
9) For the analysis of normal anomie multidisciplinary methodology is required.
10) The normal anomie can not be "cured" by traditional rational-pragmatic means. Adequate humanistic strategies are necessary for approving new regulations of cosmopolitan ethics.

The latest international practice clearly shows that in answer to any lawlessness even a greater lawlessness can be found. We can say that "anomicity of anomie" creates a temporary illusion or a mental trap of stability and security, but this is only an initial fractal of tomorrow's destructive mental epidemic.

All this makes the synergetic biopsychosociospiritual methodology of mental medicine actual for analysis and correction of new crisis reality. Figuratively speaking, the growing "social madness" demonstrates helplessness of the traditional stigmatized clinical psychiatry and demands new resources and tools for adaptive protection of public conscience.

Translated from Greek, "stigma" is a brand that in the original meaning had purely pejorative sense. Gradually it began to expand and change, widely used in a Christian environment and biomedical research as a symptom of any hidden distinctive qualities of a person or an object, a phenomenon or a text (Goffman 1963).

Singular extension of an information field in modern society leads to the problem of its personal assimilation. A man is drowning in a boundless sea of information, much of which is simply not necessary or relevant. One of the mechanisms of social protection of people from excessive and unnecessary information is stigmatization with its verbal and conceptual, subject-iconic character (Elsukov 2014). So, Internet mental virology is embodied in new generations of public conscience stigmas, launching mental epidemics of hatred and hostility, extremism and fanaticism (for example, Ukranian "Ukrops" and "Colorados," etc.). As a result, this mental epidemic process leads to deformation of individual and social identity, becoming the non-lethal weapon of mass destruction. Stigmatization and autostigmatization appear to be mechanisms of development of modern mental epidemiology, which has no latency in the global and open world.

Epidemic stigmas or mental viruses of public conscience provide themselves with high contagiousness due to the special role and the actual value of such a mark, derogatory and concise label, originality and creativity, facilitating mass infection and expansion of mental epidemic.

The Internet can be considered as a prototype of conceptual realization and technological design of the noosphere theory of V. I. Vernadsky. Mental virology and epidemiology demanded complete antiepidemic protection, which today is carried out mainly by special services. And there is nothing special about it because the Internet itself emerged as a military innovation product 50 years ago. The requirement for personal privacy as a fundamental value of democratic world turned out not a fiction today, but a regulatory anomie. The meaning of a civil feat of Edward Snowden, a documentary about whom received "Oscar" in 2015, lies in demanding a radical strengthening of civil legal position in cyber defense of the public and individual conscience as an integral expression of mental health. This appeal is heard, and modern monitoring systems of mental health are based on the synergetic biopsychosociospiritual civil methodologies that take into account national security priorities.

Psychogenesis of ME is marked by the low intellectual level, hysterical and asthenic, conformist and epileptoid character traits in premorbid. Severe hereditary and psychotic forms of alcoholism with personality disorders and encephalopathies are present. An early acquaintance of children with the diseased and frequent witnessing of epidemic outbreaks take place. Patients' unconscious perception of ME as a defensive strategy of denial and avoidance can be clearly seen. Poor mental resilience and resistance to stress in endemic subpopulations are widespread. You can meet deep personal conflicts and complexes that are non-verbalized and insoluble in familiar microenvironment. High incidence of personality disorders, PTSD (posttraumatic stress disorder) and SSR (severe stress reaction) occur as well as somatoform and psychosomatic, dependent and anti-social disorders.

A characteristic feature of ME psychogenesis is *conformal subculture and mentality* manifested in the absence of criticism and ability of independent thinking, in banality and stereotypeness, in the tendency to "be like everyone else" and tremulous loyalty to any authorities. A. E. Lichko (1977) considered conformity to be an accentuation of character and dependence on referent environment. P. B. Gannushkin (1964) linked conformity with weak intellect and in the classification of abnormal personalities put them to the "constitutionally-foolish." D. Riesman (1993) referred a conformal personality to conservative type of character, committed to conservative traditions and customs. B. V. Voronkov (2014) notes that namely conformism as "environment-forming" factor gets the leading role in the spread of psychogenic epidemics though the mission of epidemic outbreak catalyst often performs hysteroid, paranoid and epileptoid personalities. It is also necessary to distinguish between conformity as the premorbid feature of the person and conformity as a way of adaptation (or pseudoadaptation for which a person will have to pay at least by psychosomatics) to a system of official values. The prevalence of teenagers' conformal personalities is 10 to 30% (Lichko 1977).

An essential role in ME psychogenesis plays media (mass media communications). M. A. Pushkina (2014) identifies a series of mechanisms of mass conscience destruction under the influence of media.

1) *Overload of human sensory systems* due to the technical capabilities of the media sphere: speed, volume, brightness, dynamism, etc. Sensory modulations increase the

sensitivity threshold of the viewer to any external stimuli, increase the speed of attention switching and reduce its concentration.

2) *Logical devaluation of reality,* consisting in inchoateness and primitivity of the proposed causal relationships between events and images.
3) *The emotional emphasis* with the exploitation of negative emotions – "a corpse animates the frame" (Nazaretyan 2011).
4) *Destruction of human models of behavior* accepted in society – everything is allowed, and everything is possible.
5) *Imposing of surrogate communication,* substituting ethics of real interpersonal interaction for immersion in TV-shows and media dependency.

All this affects the individual and social identity of the audience, facilitating the manipulation with public opinion.

Estimating possibilities of social psychotherapy in opposition to mental epidemics, I. S. Burikova (2014) notes the non-inclusion of television in this process. The author identifies four kinds of feedback applicable to the measurement of the interface of individual and public conscience:

1) *Increasing feedback* – spinup of the emotional degree of a problem, changes reinforce the initial.
2) *Increasing anticipation* – prevention of social epidemics.
3) *Balancing feedback* (information about upcoming changes falls back into the system and suppresses the change) – interest in social epidemics is lost.
4) *Balancing anticipation* – foresight or prediction of changes leads the system to the predictable state.

Today, TV rarely goes beyond the first type of increasing direct feedback – the spinup of a problem and less often – its prevention, and almost never – the third and the fourth kinds of feedback that can control the system of social epidemics. For the realization of the TV-mission and function of social psychotherapy, it is necessary to transfer the work to the plane of balancing feedback. Such fundamental issues affecting the political design of broadcasting and requiring significant financial resources can only be solved in the framework of "mobilization order" when very concretely and very literally, "Motherland will call!"

Animogenesis of ME is marked by limitations of interests and spiritual needs. The level of demands becomes low, and their differentiation weakens. The suffering is not perceived as humiliation anymore. Willingness to live and survive appears on a biological level and in the moral despair. There are troubles of the moral climate of the family, social and working environment, spiritual and moral ambivalence and deficiency of habitat and areas of residence. Formation and development of moral sentiments and moral image are violated. The moral position is early lost or immature. Conformism and indifference are present. Syndromes of demoralization and destructive professiogenesis are highly frequent. Behavior can be antisocial and illegal. Alcoholic customs and early formation of alcohol affirmations are prevalent. The level of culture and spiritual needs is low. Syncretism and sectarianism are widespread. There present high manipulative characteristics and absence of criticism to the hystero-demonic expansion of shamanism and sorcery. Society is dehumanized and demoralized.

Biogenesis of ME is affected by the genetic accumulation of somatic and mental pathology in endemic foci. Debut and epidemic outbreak coincide with reduced and altered reactivity in the spring and autumn periods, as well as with abortion and childbirth, pregnancy and menopause in participants of the epidemic core. The frequency of somatic and endocrine diseases increases. Neuroprocesses are violated, and somatoform dysfunctions appear as well as somatized disorders and psychosomatic illnesses. There appear treatment resistance and a high risk of recurrence.

In etiopathogenesis, pathoplastics, and pathokinetics of ME, mental medicine allows qualitative and quantitative measuring of the characteristics of psycho- and socio-, animo- and somatogenesis evaluating epidemic focus and predicting trajectories of its development.

5.3. Mechanisms of Development of Mental Epidemics

Many researchers noted the universality and unity of the epidemic mental base of alcoholism and drug addiction, extremism, and radicalism, sociopathies and psychosomatoses, somatoform and induced neuro-mental disorders, combining hurtlingly growing marginal subpopulations of "excluded" from the statutory social systems.

It is possible to allocate the following development mechanisms of mental epidemics.

The mechanism of anonymity is predetermined by the absence of the actual perception by the public conscience of mental epidemiology catalyzed by regulatory anomie and permissivity. The singular reality creates a kaleidoscopic phenomenological picture of demoralized and dehumanized "insane society." The traditional "patriarchal lattice" of ethical customs and traditions is replaced by virtualization and gamization, simulations and simulacra, centaurisms and antinomies. All this leads to the loss of traditional concepts and tools for assessing health and disease. In this situation, only synergetic methodology of mental medicine allows evaluating the quality of mental health and the degree of mental disorders, developmental trajectories and extent of mental epidemics.

The mechanism of generalization is manifested in violation of newer, more responsible and formally more punishable norms. So, banal alcohol abuse is predominantly immoral phenomenon violating the ethics in business communication. Later alcoholism becomes a psychiatric diagnosis, limiting certain rights of the patient and creating risks of administrative violations. Heavy alcoholic abuses or alcoholic psychoses with unlawful behavior provide a lot of reasons to get acquainted with the Criminal Code.

The mechanism of expanded reproduction is manifested in the high latency of mental illnesses. Thus, at best, only 1 out of 10 alcoholic patients and 1 out of 30 drug addicts are on file with a dependency clinic. The others with feasible enthusiasm continue to destroy themselves and their families, involving in the epidemic process more and more new generations of consumers, especially young people. The same situation is with psychosomatic and somatoform disorders when only 1 of 3-5 cases is detected. Correct statistics or even a hint of it on the real prevalence of mobbing and bullying, internet and gambling addiction, extremism and fanaticism, as well as many other problems, does not exist.

The mechanism of autonomy of mental epidemics is predetermined by the absence of a system monitoring of mental health and so far by insurmountable interdepartmental barriers in the organization of preventive-correctional and treatment-rehabilitation activities.

The mechanism of polymorphic deformation of mind is represented by various types and variants of timely and changed, narrowed and deformed states of mind arising from the use of dozens of previously described methods and techniques of manipulative influence, triggering and supporting mental epidemic process (Sidorov 2014, 2015).

The mechanism of identity destruction. Most of the "difficult" children and adolescents do not have normal family upbringing: no control over their learning, not enough encouragement for the development of intelligence and the formation of moral values. Therefore, they soon lose interest in learning, which inevitably leads to a lack of socially important affirmations, hobbies, and spiritual needs, and to a narrow circle and instability of interests, to avoiding critical situations and solutions. Such an orientation of the person is formed, which is based on the inability of complex activity, with the simplification and reorganization of the hierarchy of behavioral motives in the sense of readiness for manipulations and deviations, conformism and antisocial induction. Such a deformed person simply lacks inner resources for self-organization and self-development, as well as neurotic dissonance imposed by random antisocial roles. Thus, self-perception of the role will always be conformal, even if it is the mission of the hired killer.

The mechanism of induction is implemented largely due to the reaction of grouping and imitation. At the initial stage of addictive behavior formation it is permissible to talk about the psychogenic development of related disorders symptoms, forms of consumption and type of intoxication. Grotesque and induced symptoms of a "disease before clinic" imitate and potentiate initial biological manifestations of the disease. Mental epidemics of induced neuropsychiatric disorders are also developed by mechanisms of collective self- and mutual induction.

The mechanism of polymodal resonance is presented by biochemical, electromagnetic and ultrasonic "language of bacteria" exchanging information both with one another (quorum sensing) and with the host macroorganism (cross-talk). Microflora, even out of infectious process remains complete and relatively autonomous underlying system of human endoecology (Andreev 2015). In this context "communication" of microbes is carried out at the level of everyday vocabulary of human conversations, using not only several biochemical "languages" but also with the help of ultrasonic and electromagnetic signals. This fact is confirmed by the phenomenon of "whispering bacteria" when dying culture sends a signal that stimulates other cultures even separated from the first by a quartz glass (Nikolaev 2000). In mental medicine, the loss of resonance with the world and with oneself is read in a broad multidisciplinary endoecological context. Not by chance has I. I. Mechnikov singled out in variations and levels of human conscience states specific situational dysbacteriosis thinking, having shown the value of normal intestinal microflora (gastric brain) for psychoimmunology. Modern studies find in the etiopathogenesis of the fifth part of psychosomatic heart attacks and strokes pathogenic microorganisms (Dirton et al. 2007). That is why the current focus of microbiology is "social behavior" of bacteria in biofilms and colonies, cooperations in conglomerates, creating epidemic effects outside usual infectious processes.

Mindsight mechanism is the ability to perceive and realize feelings and thoughts of the self, as well as thoughts and feelings of the others through specifically focused and directed attention. The word "mindsight" is coined by Daniel Siegel (2014) and combines three components: 1) insight – literally breakthrough blasting both individual and public conscience; 2) empathy – the ability to feel and perceive both an individual and a mass; 3) integration – launching network chain reactions of mental epidemics. This mechanism is to a large extent represented even in the classical methodology of autogenous training. It is also the basis of developed by us thirty years ago technology of sanogenetic therapy – adaptive biopsychosociospiritual mind and health management of the patient or client (Sidorov 1988, 2015).

Highlighted mechanisms are the most universal and multi-disciplinary; in different ratios and proportions, they are presented in all the four planes of ME development: psychogenesis and sociogenesis, animogenesis and somatogenesis.

5.4. Systematics of Mental Epidemics

The following operational classification of mental epidemics can be considered:

1. *Mental epidemics of dependent disorders:*
   a) chemical: alcoholism, drug addiction, etc.;
   b) non-chemical: gambling, etc.;
   c) electronic: Internet and computer addiction, etc.;
   d) altered forms of eating behavior: dietary manias, anorexia, bulimia, manipulative nutraceuticals (dietary supplements), etc.;
   e) modified forms of interpersonal and group behavior: sectarianism and fanaticism, mobbing, etc.;
   f) altered forms of sexual behavior: group exhibitionism in public, hypercompensation sex parades, etc.;
   g) vicarious: a syndrome of demoralization, destructive professiogenesis (workaholism), etc.;
2. *Mental epidemics of induced disorders:*
   a) early hystero-demonical: Arctic hysteria or menerik, lishinka [a spell in Komi lands – *Translator's note*] and hernia, hand-wringing and sheva [mythological incarnation of the evil eye among the peoples of Komi – *TN*], etc.;
   b) hystero-demonical renaissance: shamanism and magic, witchcraft, etc.;
   c) induced neuro-psychic disorders: social phobias, anxiety-depressive, panic disorders, etc.;

3. *Mental epidemics of psychosomatic disorders*: arterial hypertension, coronary heart disease, bronchial asthma, diabetes, cancer, rheumatoid arthritis, skin diseases, overweight and others.

4. *Mental epidemics of somatoform disorders:* somatized, hypochondriac, conversion, and others.

5. *Mental epidemics of endoecological disorders:* schizophrenic and schizoaffective, depressive, and others.

Despite the fact that the search of viruses and prions that cause schizophrenia, has not so far been successful, many factors point to such a possibility, especially in the prenatal period.

Thus, many immune changes were detected, including IgA, IgG, and IgM. Furthermore, significantly more schizophrenic patients than expected, are born in the late winter and early spring, although close seasonal rhythmics is also noted in depressions and other mental disorders. It is also important to take into account data of the "Psychiatric genomic consortium" (2013). It suggests a genetic connection of the underlying mental illnesses, particularly schizophrenia and affective disorders, with some psychosomatic and neurological diseases such as rheumatoid arthritis, systemic lupus erythematosus, psoriasis, Crohn's disease, type 1 diabetes, multiple sclerosis.It is logical to assume commonness of etiopathogenic mechanisms of development of these disorders.

In the continuing situation of multiple etiopathogenic uncertainties, it seems appropriate to attribute mental epidemics of schizophrenia and depression to a group of endoecological mental disorders. Previously adopted term "endogenous" becomes too narrow.

The definition of schizophrenia as a polymorphic resonance-coherent mental disorder (Sidorov 2014) highlights its epidemicity. Biological evidence of at least the appropriateness of this approach is the study of NMDA-receptors involved in many important brain processes. They modulate the production of dopamine by neurons of the ventral tegmental area, modulate low-frequency oscillations of the brain by inhibitory thalamic interneurons, and processes of neuroplasticity and memory by the neurons of the hippocampus and the prefrontal cortex (Zhang et al. 2009; Hillman et al. 2011; Goff 2013). Synergetic terminology does not just mechanistically substitute axiomatic clinical categories such as autism as a resonance disorder or a defense mechanism and schisis as a coherent disorder. This terminology reveals fundamentally new extensive and methodological resources that allow combining different trends in their not arithmetic, but systemic interaction, creating *mental medicine as a psychiatric paradigm of the global trend of integrative medicine.*

We have previously cited Epidemical interpretation of induced and dependent, psychosomatic and somatoform disorders in the framework of fairly traditional social epidemics (Sidorov 2014). However, it is the synergetic biopsychosociospiritual methodology of mental medicine that provides the most comprehensive approach to the four-dimensional fractal dynamics of the clinical-epidemic process. Such multidisciplinarity becomes a requirement in the situation of simplified and ultra-fast access to the individual conscience (identity) of users of virtual social networks. The singularity of crisis reality transforms such seemingly banal communications into a new form of mental contagiousness and epidemicity. In this context, almost any mental disorder today can be seen as mental infection (instant, fast, slow, superslow, etc.) and mental epidemic. An urgent task is to study the characteristics and criteria of mental epidemicity threshold, as well as forms and types of singular progression and synergetic integrative assessment of the pest spot.

MEs are a threat to public conscience as an integral expression of mental health of the nation. When the magnitude of MEs becomes a danger to the public health of the region, they become *social epidemics*, developing into a *destructive social epidemic* in the case of a threat to public health of the country as a whole; further spread can be defined as a *social pandemic*, covering countries and continents.

A major role in attracting public attention to social epidemics played a bestseller of Malcolm Gladwell (The Tipping Point 2000), dedicated to a journalistic study of mechanisms of contraction and development, origins, and causes of personal typology and progress of social epidemics. The journalistic approach allows the author to refer rumors and fashion, syphilis and crime to homogeneous social epidemics. The scientific approach requires an evidence-based methodology for assessing and forecasting.

Attribution of the prevalence of psychosomatoses (diabetes, coronary heart disease, etc.) to social epidemics has become sufficiently habitual, although the quantitative determination of such epidemicity threshold has not yet been formulated. Attribution of alcoholism and drug addiction to destructive social epidemics is also quite clear. However, the epidemic spread of crime and terrorism must be more correctly described as *asocial epidemics* – destroying foundations of society.

It is possible to point out three main levels of synergetic epidemical process:

1) *Mental epidemics* measured by the amount of threats and damage to public conscience;
2) *Social epidemics* measured by the level of threats and damage to public health;
3) *Asocial epidemics* measured by the level of threats and damage to national security.

Thus, mental epidemic of bullying and crowding may develop into a social epidemic of radicalism and fanaticism, and then into the asocial epidemic of extremism and terrorism. Multidimensionality and multifactorness of such epidemic process require precisely multidisciplinary synergetic approach. Isolation of mental epidemics level seems important for focusing the attention on the possibilities of the earliest possible preventive-correctional interventions.

For example, terrorism is one of the most multimodal and multilevel varieties of asocial epidemics. At the primary level of mental epidemics, it is represented by mental terrorism of a mobbing nature that threatens public conscience of the collective or the village. The mental epidemic of mobbing becomes destructive when it begins to threaten public conscience of the whole country, acquiring this or that nationalist or religious ideology. Then mental epidemic evolves into social – threatening public health of the region and into a destructive social epidemic when the threat extends to the entire country. Phenomenologically this is described by syndromes of bullying and crowding. Subsequently, epidemic develops into asocial represented in all forms of terrorism. Depending on the extent and magnitude of threats to the national security of the country as a whole, it can become destructive. The final form is a pandemic of terrorism spanning countries and continents.

Today, the most famous pandemic of such a kind is "Islamic State" (IS). It is an international Islamic terrorist organization operating mainly in Syria and Iraq since 2013 as Islamic unrecognized quasi-state with the Sharia form of government. The merging preceded IS formation in 2006 of 11 radical Islamic groupings, headed by the local unit of "al Qaeda." By 2015, tens of thousands of volunteers from nearly 100 countries are fighting in the ranks of IS.

Tetranuclear and four-dimensional biopsychosociospiritual diagnostics in mental medicine allow giving qualitative characteristics of the epidemic process, evaluating and predicting the trajectory of its development, promptly mobilizing sanogenetic and therapeutic resources.

Mental epidemics that are the subject of mental medicine require the introduction of new preventive-correctional and treatment-rehabilitation resources of *system monitoring of mental health (SMMH) and mental health service (MHS),* the effectiveness of the pilot models of which has already been demonstrated (Sidorov 2014). The fundamental health-oriented position of MHS is that it is engaged both in the strengthening of mental health and in the treatment of mental illnesses, which prevents it from repeating "stigmatized curse" of nosocentric psychiatry. Pest spot of the mental epidemic, characterized by enormous polymorphism and polymodality of clinical and psychological, social and moral phenomenology can be effectively localized and sanitated only by multidisciplinary MHS.

Currently, there is an extremely popular and widespread in the scientific discourse interdisciplinary concept – an interface that is used to explain and design systems and mechanisms of selective non-destructive relationships in objects of animate and inanimate nature. Interface in the broad sense is defined by standards border between interacting independent objects. Interface, as an instrument of intersystem interaction, defines its parameters, procedures and specifications. SMMH can be described as an interface of individual and public conscience.

The main properties of the human mind, defining it as an interface between the subject and the world of physical reality, include:

1) *Selectivity of mind* to all forms of stimulation: physical and social, spiritual and psychological.
2) *Plasticity of mind,* providing creation, manifestation and limitation of degrees of freedom in the framework of an integrity of human personality and body.
3) *The universality of mind* that preserves functional properties changing content in different bodily forms.
4) *The individuality of mind* is determined by mechanisms of perceptual systems that create a subjective reality.
5) *Mirror transparency of mind* in which the subject does not distinguish constructs that arise in the mind under the influence of the world physical stimuli on the perceptual systems from the constructs created by the brain (Sergeev 2014).

Interface properties of mind and human perceptual systems must be considered when designing and implementing SMMH, and mental epidemics threats require a new quality of software and hardware systems MHS. The transition of humanity to new forms of a technological pattern associated with an intensive development of NBICS – convergence (nano - bio - info - cogno - socio) and artificial intelligence methods, leads to the total integration of the biopsychosociospiritual system of a person with society and a technogenic environment. Followed by the emergence of new forms of interface relations in integrative and, particularly, in mental medicine.

In summary, it can be noted that the infectious hypothesis of mental disorders has accompanied the entire history of psychiatry. From a very specific hystero-demonical spell and search for prion agents of schizophrenia to attempts of endoecological linkage of psychopathology with the "dark energy and dark matter," waiting for experimental confirmation on the Large Hadron Collider. Today, one can quantitatively and qualitatively measure the drift of identity and the mental drift (similar to the antigenic drift) against a cyber-virologic attack on the individual and group level. It is also possible to assess the mental shift of individual and social identity, to describe resources of mental resilience and mental attenuation (similar to the attenuation of the microorganism in the vaccine) of psycho-manipulative and social stress factors. Mental medicine can not only provide a synergetic functional diagnosis of the patient, but it can also give a multidisciplinary characterization of resources of *Mental immunity* of the client, as well as to purposefully form a resistance to the vast register of mental epidemics. This possibility just requires to build up and arrange systematically not so much a calendar of didactic mental "vaccination campaigns" as the style of the regular mental preventological "vitaminization" – i.e. resource-constructive and creative-pragmatist strengthening of public conscience and public health.

Whereas only one demographic trap is described in classical epidemiology, then in mental epidemiology there are hundreds of stressogenic mental traps requiring formation of adaptive strategies of mediation and ethics of business communication on a psychohygienic level of upbringing and education in mental preventology. At the same time the effectiveness of psychoprophylactic "vitaminization and vaccination" can be measured in renewable resources of mental resilience.

Using the terminology of clinical epidemiology, even mental epidemics can be described as hyperendemic, holoendemic and endemic diseases. Mental immunization and genetic engineering correction of forecasted mental illnesses tomorrow will be as usual procedure, as the modern vaccination against infectious diseases. Already today we can quantitatively and qualitatively measure the *mental virulence* of virtual simulacra infecting reality and *scan possibility of mental risk* of public conscience. In this respect, mental epidemiology on a new synergetic methodological level develops traditions of the *political epidemiology* engaged in research of political factors, processes, and conditions that affect public health (Porta, Alvarez-Darbet 1998).

Albert Einstein in a letter to Sigmund Freud (Caputh near Potsdam, 30.06.1932) sadly notes that "thirst of hatred and anger is located in a man himself." Then he asks: "Is it possible to control mental evolution of the human race in such a way as to make it sustainable against psychoses of violence and destruction?" In a response letter, S. Freud (Vienna, September 1932) confirms "reality of instinct of hatred and destruction, inherent in the very person who is manipulated by the instigators of war." Recognizing the lack of efficient technologies for prevention of aggression and self-destruction, he notes that only "everything that in one form or another is made for the development of culture – works against the war."

Over the lats 100 years mental engineering of public and individual conscience has done tremendous technological evolution, which today is set by a singular dynamics of mental virology of horrific epidemics of violence and terrorism. This necessitated the search for new resources of multidisciplinary protection embodied in the synergetic biopsychosociospiritual methodology of mental ecology and mental medicine, mental preventology and mental resilience, the development of mental health services and mental health system monitoring as an interface of the public conscience.

Chapter 6

Ethical Propaedeutics of Mental Epidemiology

After graduation from Medical Faculty of the University of Basel under the guidance of Professor Eugen Bleuler, Carl Gustav Jung (1991) wrote in his memoirs about his first years of work: "I isolated myself in the clinic like in a monastery to understand and learn better the world of mentally sick people. I wanted to find out how the human spirit reacts to its internal disorders." Henceforth he developed specific requirement to the professionalism of a psychotherapist as follows: "life embracing its soul" but only with the purpose to see and hear, feel and perceive better sufferings that souls of patients and clients experience.

According to the memoirs of V. J. Zavialov (2013), Prof. V. E. Rozhnov – the first chief psychotherapist of the USSR – called the profession of psychotherapist "priest for atheists" (literally – "priest of an atheistic century"). Prof. V. V. Makarov (2014) - successor of Prof. V. E. Rozhnov at the Department of Psychotherapy and founder of Professional Psychotherapeutic League - continues the same line more structurally, supporting the introduction of "spiritual dimension" to modern psychotherapy and involving into the League specialists in "religious practices." Thus, spiritual dimension is not a metaphor of the fourth dimension to biopsychosocial classics, but a necessary condition of "four-part model of psychotherapy."

The synergetic biopsychosociospiritual methodology of mental medicine and epidemiology that we have developed is not just four-nuclear, but also four-dimensional. There, a spiritual and moral dimension can be estimated psycho-sociometrically from the point of depth and richness of moral and axiological potential of the personality that is the chief human resource during a singular era of global demoralization.

Animogenesis as ontogenetic spiritual and moral development of the personality is a matrix for the majority of mechanisms of mental epidemic representation. For this reason, an actual task is the conceptual and methodological justification of resources and tools of ethical normalization and classification, syndromology and diagnostics in mental epidemiology.

6.1. Ethical Normal Cyclicity of Mental Epidemicity

"Norm" in Latin designates rule and sample. In the sociological encyclopedia, V. L. Abushchenko (2003) marks out the following meanings of the concept of a norm. First of all, a norm is an average value characterizing any mass-scale set of casual events or phenomena. Secondly, a norm is a concept designating borders within which the phenomena and systems, behavior and communication keep the qualities and functions setting their internal harmony. V. D. Plakhov (2011) allocates "norms-rules" or "norms-frameworks" as special structures intended to ensure functionally safety and activity of the system.

A. L. Katkov (2014) suggests considering the concept of moral standard in the following contexts:

1) through marking out the borders within which the phenomena and systems keep the qualities and functions;
2) through standards, rules, instructions, images and rules as specially created characteristics of any activity or condition of the system (Abushchenko 2003);
3) through the system of notions and mechanisms governing the relations and interaction inside the community (for example, scientific community) (Mirskii 2009);
4) through moral ideas and concepts of ethics in business communication (Sevastianova 1999).

For bioethical regulation, it is important to understand the heterogeneity of application of the notion of norm resulting from the polyvalence of the kinds of activities and discourses intertwining in it. So, there are "norms-rules" and "norms-instructions" that regulate the activity "from within" for the achievement of a result, these are so-called "technical norms." Standards regulating medical activity refer to them. Besides, there are rules acting "from outside" in relation to a kind of activity or discourse, synchronizing internal orderliness with other "orders." It is served by rules of logic, mathematics, grammar, etc. In this case, *the synergetics acts as the most polymodal instrument of system regulation.*

The structure of norm includes the following elements. *Content* – action or value which is the object of standard regulation. *Imperative* – the obligation force expressed in the form of permission or interdiction. *Disposition* – circumstances when the action must or mustn't be carried out. *Scale* – size of the group of individuals over which the norm is extended (Sidorova 2014).

"Measured" and "regulatory" character of the norm is accurately fixed in it. V. L. Abushchenko (2003) points at the dual fixing of the norm: in a sign form by way of statements (laws, rules, instructions, etc.) and in a social form as non-verbalized schemes of activity, behavior, and communication. The individualized form of the functioning of the norm is reduced to certain notions of "normality" of mental activity and thinking reproduced in this particular culture. The individualized level of fixing of norms is important for studying of normogenesis in bioethics. It is not incidental that moral and axiological measurements of the personality are essentially important in psychological consultation and psychotherapy when "the psychotherapist becomes the main working tool" (Kagan 2015).

Describing life stages of the norm as an element of the social system, V. D. Plakhov (2011) introduces the concept of a normocycle and includes in it the emergence, distribution, and revision of norms. L. V. Abushchenko (2003) allocates in the normocycle stages of rule-making, selection and falling of norms into a habit. Permanent normogenesis in bioethics represents the process of redefinition of the contents and function of a norm, before achievement of the legitimate level of moral conscience which accepts the established value as normal.

Dispersion and inversion of the described ethical normalization, projection of stages of a normocycle to fractal dynamics of an animogenesis of mental epidemics allow coming more closely to the allocation of critical ethical conditions and moral epidemic thresholds revealed by screening batteries and corrected by mental preventology.

Mental epidemicity of public conscience can be presented by the image of the River of Time which coasts have to be strengthened with standards as firm as a granitic rock. The speed of the current is to be regulated by the system of dams of the patriotic hydropower cascade. The quality of the movement of complex ideas and projects, of induced and natural needs is controlled by the systematicity and sequence of the dredging works preventing the emergence of epidemic rifts and terrible whirlpools or shallows and hursts, symbolizing stagnation as extra-mental desire to stop the Time… It goes at the level of mental traps of public conscience realized in numerous television shows (like “Your Face Sounds Familiar,” etc.). It seems as if this works quite well at the emotional level, but new generations demand new collective meanings and distinctive national idea. To replace a trend of Post-Soviet return (Transnistria, Abkhazia, South Ossetia, the Crimea), the rigid sanctions imperative of internal self-development and transformation comes. Social psychometrics of the millions of questions arrived at the Hotline with the President of the Russian Federation V. V. Putin (14.04.2016) convincingly confirms it.

6.2. Moral Risk Measurement of a Mental Epidemicity

The spiritual and moral typology of the personality is one of the priorities of ethic and psychological researches. L. M. Popov and A. O. Maksumova (2010) put two criteria in the fundamentals of the typology elaborated by them: *spirituality-inspirituality and transformation-contemplation,* allocating the following types on their basis: Apollo; Religious; Humanist; Fruitful (“Creator”); Aristocrat; Hero (Fair Fighter); Beloved; Guilty; Timeserver (Patient, Conformist); Doubting; Tiresome; Lost; Authoritative; Difficult; Commercial; Consumer; Avaricious; Greedy; Trickster; Angry; Destroyer (Destructive); Intriguer; Provoker; Cruel. The meaning of these types is in most cases can be obviously seen from their names.

A. B. Kupreichenko and A. E. Vorobiova (2010) allocate such types of *moral self-determination of the personality*, as 1) Theorist; 2) Detached; 3) Conformist; 4) Relativistic and Egocentric; 5) Advocate of Moral; 6) Committed to Ethical Standards; 7) Social and Standard. The authors make attempts of systematization from the point of view of psychology and their main object of study – morality. On the basis of the category of “moral self-determination” (of the personality, various social groups, etc.), in the structure of this phenomenon, they allocate a “moral core” and a plastic “cover” created by four segments which are formed by self-determination of the subject. The determination can relate to 1) morality and ethics; 2) objects and phenomena of the world around; 3) other people, groups, and society in general; 4) the subject itself. These segments reflect the resource structure of the spiritual immunity; its decrease or infraction facilitates the start of polymodal trigger mechanisms of mental epidemics.

The early revelation and forecasting of the moral typology of mental epidemicity risk are possible in case of developing of the synergetic screening batteries within the *systematic monitoring of mental health* that we have trained on the models of educational institutions. Such approach allows to see four-dimensional trajectories of the development of options and types of ethical syndromology in the prenosological fractals and to increase the efficiency of individual (group, subpopulational, etc.) preventive and correctional biopsychosociospiritual programs.

6.3. Ethical Syndromology of Mental Epidemics

Moral diagnosis must include the characteristics of ethical competency and moral adaptation, inner and outer mental and moral resources of an individual/group/society. The disintegration of lifestyle and life meaning becomes the most important characteristic of approaching the threshold of mental epidemicity.

As part of the ethically pedagogical and socially psychological methodology used by M. I. Volovikova (2010), it is suggested to distinguish *three fields of mental and moral evolution:* personal, public and government relations. Dispersion and inversion of normative characteristics applicable only in personal and family relations were usually used for diagnostic purposes.

The ethics of public and government relations was a priori excluded from the field of diagnostic interpretation of conventional clinical practice since it could have quite a diverse political arrangement. At the same time, the development of mental epidemics into social and asocial one (for example, the “Islamic State” and others) inevitably requires the attraction of religious-and-ethnic as well as the civil-and-political appraisals and characteristics displayed in ethical syndromology (syndrome of religious extremism, syndrome of terrorist demoralization, etc.). Undoubtedly, only the animogenetic vector alone is insufficient for functional diagnostics in mental medicine and epidemiology – a synergetic biopsychosociospiritual approach is required which, figuratively speaking, has a fourfold degree of protecting the rights of a patient/client. Ethical syndromology is also confirmed by trans and cross-cultural matches of diagnostic approaches.

For example, the phenomenology of the syndrome of existential despair (Sidorov 2014) or existential vacuum, according to V. Frankl (1990), corresponds to the anomic version of an identity crisis. The identity crisis was distinguished by B. S. Polozhiy (1996) and is characterized by the loss of living tonus and former interests, lower activity and a sense of purpose. Particular autization, predominance, and anxiodepressive mood are typical of this crisis as well as a lack of faith in one’s strengths, the feeling of self-insignificance and inability to resist the collisions of destiny.

Jerome D. Frank (1996) defined the demoralization as a sense of incompetence, experienced in a distressing situation, describing it as an “ethical shadow” of anxious depression:

- low self-esteem;
- a feeling of hopelessness and helplessness;
- a feeling of fear, anxiety, despair;
- psychophysiological symptoms, perceived as signs of physical health failure.

Just as mobbing (office wars) has changed from a disrupted moral socialization to a psychiatric syndrome, so demoralization condition is becoming a demoralization syndrome.

Demoralization syndrome is a disorder of formation and development of moral feelings and portrait, position and behavior.

This definition holds an ontogenetic approach. Disorders in the formation of underlying moral feelings are predetermined by a mentally-moral deficit in the family. Later, with disorders of moral socialization, a disharmony of a moral portrait appears and is then expressed in the loss of moral position, accumulated in motivationally-adjusting personality complex, which creates a possibility for amoral and illegal activity.

Within animogenesis, which is a core of the four-dimensional bio-psycho-socio- spiritual development, it is possible to highlight the following blocks of demoralization syndrome:

1) disorder of formation and development of morally-spiritual feelings:

- delay and disharmony in formation of the main moral sentiments:
  - conscience, duty, faith, and responsibility;
  - disorder of spiritual development;
  - distortion of self-esteem and misunderstanding of the meaning of life;
  - unpreparedness for sound individually-responsible behavior;
  - latent moral self-conscience of the personality and conscience;
  - undeveloped feelings of patriotism and civil solidarity;
  - moral irresponsibility for the family and society, country and future generations;

2) disorder of formation and development of morally-spiritual identity:

- delay and disharmony in the formation of the cores of a moral character:
  - patience and tolerance, mercy and humanism, honor and dignity, freedom and independence;
  - the deficit of creative potential in spiritual and objective-productive activity;
  - unpreparedness for social and professional mobility because of low moral motivation;
  - inability to continuous education "throughout the whole life";
  - wearing out and imperfection of self-culture and self-improvement mechanisms;
  - low tolerance and manipulability of national conscience, supported by nationalistic provocations, exploding interethnic peace and accord;

3) disorder of formation and development of a morally-spiritual position:

- delay and disharmony in the formation of the basis of a moral position and the ability to differentiate between good and evil, overcoming life difficulties and trials, expressing friendship and love;
- inability to accept basic national values, national customs, and traditions;
- lowering of the ability to express and argue one's personal point of view;
- non-critical evaluation of personal motives and settings, intents and thoughts;
- loss of view of life's perspectives, catastrophically-pessimistic view of the world and capitulation before difficulties;
- the inability to understand personal value of other people, a value of human life, mental health and spiritual safety of a person;
- the failure for conscious personal, professional and civil self-definition;
- devaluation of faith in people and country because of a deficit of personal responsibility;
- unpreparedness to jointly oppose external and internal challenges;
- incomprehension of the absolute value of family and its moral norms: love and mutual help, respect for parents, care for the young and continuation of the bloodline;
- disorder of spiritual, cultural and social succession of generations;

4) disorder in formation and developing of behavior ethics and communication:

- delays and distortions in the formation of morals as recognized by the individual
  - the necessity of a certain behavior, based on socially accepted notions of good and evil, proper and intolerable;
  - depletion of internal guideline of a person to act according to their conscience because of lowered moral motivation for freedom and will;
  - the inability to form personal moral obligations and perform honest self-control, give moral self-evaluation to personal actions and those of other people, demand from oneself fulfillment of moral norms and follow business communications ethics;
  - deformation and loss of personal and social identity;
  - dependency and irresponsibility of actions and activities;
  - heightened suggestibility and dependence, conformism and departure from a personal moral choice;
  - low ambition and industriousness, productivity and perseverance in achieving results;
  - devaluation of legal awareness and law abidance.

The secondary *child abuse syndrome (CAS)* becomes one of the dramatic primary *parent demoralization syndrome (PDS)* versions. It triggered hypogenesis and various disorders of neuropsychic, sociopsychological and mental-and-moral development.

The "battered child" syndrome was for the first time described in Paris by a professor of medicine A. Tardieu in 1868. His statement was based on the analysis of 32 dissected children who died from beating and burns. At the annual meeting of the American pediatrics academy in 1961 Henry Camp, the head of pediatrics department at the Colorado state medical university conducted a comprehensive analysis of battered child syndrome. He presented pediatric, psychiatric, radiologic and legal aspects of the problem in detail and for the first time provided statistical information on the spreading of child abuse in USA. Today not only physical and sexual but also psychic and emotional violence, as well as the multiple kinds of neglect or nonchalant attitude, expressed towards a child's needs are referred to child abuse. The term "battered child syndrome" is not used in modern literature since it implies only physical violence: the X revision of International classification of diseases (ICD) officially approved the term "child abuse syndrome."

Child abuse syndrome represents any form of mistreating a child under the age of 18 which is committed by parents, guardians, tutors or other people who are responsible for the child's well-being, a person that lives in the same flat or one of the parent's partner. Thus, not every case of violence or child battering refers to a CAS. For example, if children were beaten by random bypassers, children of the same age, parents' acquaintances and people who are not responsible for the child's well-being then the CAS is not registered. It is evident that the most vulnerable group of children is represented by infants living the first year of their life since their welfare entirely depends on parents, tutors, and babysitters.

In the CAS age structure, according to counsellings the share of infants less than one year of age does not exceed 1%, whereas 1/3 of the children who died from CAS were infants less than one year of age.

The main causes of CAS among children are as follows:

1) unemployment and low financial security of the parents;
2) alcoholism and drug addiction of one or both parents;
3) loneliness and split up marriage;
4) ressentiment of parents and disappointment in life;
5) physical or psychic overstrain among parents or guardians;
6) moral "immaturity" of parents;
7) selfishness of parents and pursuance of entertainment;
8) missing affection towards the child;
9) unwanted marriage (a motive or forcing to enter into marriage);
10) extramarital child;
11) a child with physical defects.

CAS classification (ICD X) includes the following:

T 74.0. Physical neglect.
T 74.1. Physical violence.
T 74.2. Sexual violence.
T 74.3. Psychological violence.
T 74.8. Other syndromes of abuse (mixed forms).

All of the listed types of violence are registered among children beginning with the first year of their life.

Physical neglect refers to the lack of providing necessary living conditions for a child: food, clothes, supervision and medical care.

Physical neglect may result in alimentary hypotrophy, diaper rush, vulvitis, pyodermia and other somatic diseases.

Physical violence refers to intentional infliction of bodily harm to a child. During the physical violence diagnosis, it is vitally important to conduct correctly the interview when parents or guardians request help for the first time.

The "shaken baby" syndrome represents one of the forms of physical abuse relating to infants living the first months of their life which is caused by shaking a child by his fixed shoulders (shaken baby syndrome). The baby's head is disproportionally big as related to its body and the neck muscles are weak. When the baby is shaken with force by holding its shoulders, his head is moved in a backward direction which results in the severe brain damage. It is known that every year up to 2.000 and 100 children die in the USA and Great Britain respectively in the result of shaking. This was reported at the I Congress dedicated to the "shaken baby" issue held in Edinburgh (2003) and at the 2004 seminar in Tartu (Estonia). Most children die in the result of the "shaken baby" syndrome accidentally, following parents' unawareness about the harm of shaking done to the infant baby. Most often intense shaking is a form of child abuse. The most frequent signs of the "shaken baby" syndrome include drowsiness; convulsions; muscle tone reduction; irregular breathing; hyperexcitability; vomiting; retinal hemorrhage; syndrome of hydrocephalus and sudden death syndrome.

The exact number of cases of incapacity and neuropsychic development disorders contained in the catamnesis of children who survived after "shaking" is unknown.

The scope of *sexual violence* expressed towards children is enormous. However, the term itself appears to be strange in the case of criminal responsibility for sexual children abuse although the growing public demoralization and dehumanization is initially demonstrated in the sexual upbringing of children. For example, in England today, 11-year-old schoolchildren must understand the meaning of "giving a freewill consent to have sex" whereas the latency of dissent is beyond any statistical records, which is clearly illustrated by the longstanding scandal with pedophilic Catholic priests.

Psychological violence is when the parents are unable to provide the environment where a child can fully develop when psychoemotional needs are neglected even when the child's physical needs are met. In such cases, the child is treated as the subject of care causing psychoemotional deprivation which results in emotional abandonment and disrupts neuropsychic development of the child.

A group of American researchers (Kross et al. 2011) demonstrated that pain and emotional stress caused by loneliness or unanswered love activate the same zones of the secondary somatosensory cortex and the insular lobe of the brain. The commonality of mechanisms that transform moral stress of a person into mental disorders and physical diseases emphasizes the efficiency of the synergetic biopsychosociospiritual methodology of mental medicine.

The obvious dramatic nature of diagnosis objectification of the *parents demoralization syndrome* is that it is manifested behaviorally in tortures concerning their children, usually distorting or destroying their inner world and human destiny. BCS – is the earliest "moral vaccination" of the future epidemic mental representation of aggressiveness and destructiveness in relation to society, allowing the child abuse. Wherever in the world, the army of homeless and neglected children, contributing orphanages and boarding schools, are the sociometry of mental epidemic of demoralization and dehumanization of society, providing a cyclical change in the new generations of PDS ↔ CAS.

Highlighting of *evil and immoral behavior* (Mendelevich 2014) as a special clinical form of all the types of deviant behavior is phenomenologically still the same demoralization syndrome, accompanying not only all the kinds of deviations but also psychogenious and endogenious, psycho-somatic and social-stress disorders. V. D. Mendelevich (2014) even supposes that shaping of psychopathological syndromes of paranoid specter is based not on the biological grounds, but on the individually-psychological and moral peculiarities of a person. He distinguishes four levels of values: totally human and personal, organism and household related, each of which is complemented by a definite form of a paranoid syndrome.

In the development of the demoralization syndrome 6 fractals of animogenesis can be distinguished. 1) *predisposition* - the spiritual and moral deficiency of the family. 2) *latent* - the strain of moral sentiments. 3) *initial* - disharmony of moral character. 4) *a full-scale clinical picture* - with a loss of a moral position (mental epidemic). 5) *chronization* – having different forms and types of immoral behavior, defined by the individual set of comorbid and associated disorders of somatic-, psycho- and social genesis (destructive mental epidemic). 6) *outcome* – noted by the risk of wrongful conduct (pandemic).

The multidisciplinary team implements an individual medical psychosociospiritual preventive correctional program (the first three prenosological fractals - the sphere of mental preventology) and the treatment and rehabilitation assistance (4-6 nosological fractals of clinical psychiatry). This program has in the spiritual and moral block the following fractal targets. 1) Identification and correction of "morale" of the family and the workforce. 2) Correction and harmonization of basic moral sentiments. 3) Correction of moral character. 4) Reconstruction of a moral position. 5) Reconstruction of moral behavior. 6) Spiritual and moral rehabilitation. For the tasks performing, the resources of the mental health service are mobilized and, in particular, the current mandate of the ethics committees activities, available in all health facilities.

The spiritual and moral prevention and correction, treatment and rehabilitation are the scopes of *logotherapy of* V. Frankl (1990). There are specific and non-specific application fields of logotherapy methods. The *specific application area is* the noogenic neuroses, generated by the loss of meaning in life. In these cases, a method of Socratic dialogue allows pushing the patient or the client for opening for them the adequate sense. A significant role is played here by the personality of the psychotherapist, although the imposition of his meanings is unacceptable. *The non-specific application field* of logotherapy - is the psychotherapy of all sorts of diseases, using the methods and techniques of existential analysis. For example, the using the technique of paradoxical intention and dereflexia for the treatment of phobias and obsessive-compulsive disorders, dependent and sexual disorders. The mechanism of action of these methods is based on two fundamental ontological characteristics of the person: the capacity for self-removal and self-transcendence. The first is expressed in a constant output of man beyond himself. The second - is the ability of man to rise above himself and the situation, to look at him from outside.

It is crucial to emphasize that the proposed characteristics of the demoralization syndrome fully complies the violation of modalities, provided in the definition of the WHO (2001) of mental health. Achieving prosperity and successful self-fulfillment, the stress resistance and productivity is not possible without the ethics in business communication and moral maturity of the person. The moral deformation is the earliest manifestation of the approaching to the mental epidemic threshold.

6.4. The Paradigm of Rights and Obligations as Moral Basis of Mental Epidemic Threshold

The Political Correctness (PC) became the central and fundamental reference point of morals, ethics and justice on Earth in the 20th century.

The pure essence of this new growth is that PC believes everybody to be equal to everybody in their rights: a woman – a man, a child – an old man, the Black – the White and so forth. Now sexual minorities have equal rights. General equal rights and total universal parity (ideally) have to make inexpressibly fine the lives of those oppressed by harmful patriarchy, primitive ethnic traditions, and vulgar world culture.

PC widely interferes in human affairs. From racial inequalities (the Black is not the Black now, but "Afro-American") and specific physiological features (thick is not thick, but "sound") – up to literature: politically incorrect words are deleted from the books of the American libraries. "Teenager" – as age-accenting features of an individual, "demons" – because of expressed religious and negative aspect, "insulted and humiliated " because of expressed pejorative and scornful shade. "Idiot" - for clear motives, and even the word "yacht" - because not everyone can buy a yacht and it overbrims a cup of sufferings of the "unfortunate," and that is not necessary to be reminded to such "sufferers." The desire to give new names to the things and phenomena finds a manipulativity and arrogance of the PC-activists assimilating themselves to the forefather of the mankind.

PC – is not a new invention. Several centuries ago the affected coquettish people with the "bulged little finger" invented euphemisms for designation of those things and phenomena which they considered too frank or obscene. So, the pregnant woman began to be called "a lady in a familiar way" (concerning this even A. S. Pushkin was indignant). However, as a rule, the destiny of these innovations was short or parodic: one of the known, although short Russian words during some time were designated by the Slavic name of its first letter. Finally, this option also became the word from the tabooed lexicon. After all, call as you might a small person "vertically anxious," his growth won't change. And the Russian saying says: "The Lord didn't make equal even trees," what can be said about people in this situation …

But PC-manipulators think too self-confidently that those groups of people that were traditionally considered in the past oppressed and suppressed, humiliated and offended need their defense and protectionism. They do not think of that such protectionism is more likely humiliating for the Blacks and the women, mentally sick and elderly people, especially, if carried out in such silly form. It is a poor Black who hesitates over the skin color of the ancestors; it is a stupid old man who is ashamed of his years; it is a shame to think that mentally unhealthy person is somehow worse than a healthy human. After all, if you do not think so, if you do not notice it or are indifferent to this circumstance, all these "affected PC-curtseys" are absolutely worthless! Moreover, politically correct neologisms unambiguously emphasize: I noticed that you are a hunch, but, being a politically correct person, I tactfully call your figure "non-standard." All these PC-inventions show in the brightest way an inferiority complex proper to the PC supporters who in the childhood were, probably, teased by their age-mates as "butterballs" or "four-eyes."

The persistence of the activists of the new ideology and their impenetrable dullness overcome all reasonable arguments of the opponents. Probably, somebody thinks correct to call terrorists and murderers – "guerrillas" or "insurgents." Probably, someone benefits from that all the people look up to the gold standard of average mind, average professionalism, and average abilities. The smart person is politically incorrect in relation to the blockhead, therefore, is doomed at least to moral deformation or deprivation.

Unfortunately, mental disorders, their specific clinic and social aspect of mental diseases also became the field of applications of PC. The sensitivity of many cultures and peoples regarding the patients with psychiatric pathologies is deemed to be a shy downtroddenness by the PC supporters. The fighters of the PC-front consider sacrality of a mental disease, its mystery and special position of such patients in many cultures (dervishes and foolish, visionaries and sorcerers…) a consequence of marginality, backwardness, and totalitarianism. Entering into a not-their ancient game with difficult rules a simplified equalization, they suggest to play chessmen at the giveaway, perhaps, sincerely considering these rules only reasonable and immutable.

The emergence of some movies about psychiatric clinics and their patients turned out to be a consequence of these good intentions.

Perhaps, the first movie dedicated to this subject was M. Forman's film "One Flew Over the Cuckoo's Nest," 1975. The Czechoslovak emigrant film director cinematized the book of the same name by K. Kesey, who was the great admirer of LSD and wrote some chapters of the book in a condition of drug intoxication. Kesey got his knowledge in psychiatry from a short hospital nurse's practice in a psychiatric office. The social delinquent behavior of the author of the book who even was arrested for storage and use of marihuana coincided with the "rebellious" spirit of the rough 60th epoch. (The book was written in 1962). Obviously, this is the source of the anarchical love of freedom that comes from the book of the 27-year-old author – a nihilist who represented the medical personnel to be sadists, therapy – sophisticated torture, patients –victims. The revolts against the orders existing in the society and the state were much popular among the western intellectuals of the 60s and student's youth who respected Sartre and Che Guevara. The character of D. Nicholson, for the sake of own entertainment, drew on to open revolt among the patients of the psychiatric office and slighted the senior nurse. This turned him into a hero, the revolutionary, the martyr and banner of anti-psychiatry. Forman's movie became a parable about existentialism, rights for self-identification and freedom of the person. In the course of philosophical and high humanistic sense searches during the movie, it was somehow forgotten that the main character was placed in the hospital for forensic psychiatric examination after a rape. The film received five "Oscars."

In 1988 the movie "Rain man" was shot in the USA; there D. Hoffman performed the autism patient. The film also claimed at being a comprehensive, thoughtful parable. Hoffman's character helped the morally unstable brother to humanistically "see the light." The process of personal "reforging" took about two hours of the screen time: unostentatiously, quickly and well. The citizens go home happily; they have seen the tale about the idyllic relationship of the sick and healthy. The movie about the conflict between the good and the fine received four "Oscars."

The movie “Forrest Gump” shot by Robert Zemeckis in 1994, based on the book of U. Grum, showed us the oligophrenic person – a very good (without irony) person whose story of life was imposed on the history of the USA of the last decades. It turned out that this is the average modern American who, despite the known intellectual inferiority, managed to become a symbol of the time, a mirror of the contemporary history, a sign of the development of progress and even nearly a standard of personal success. It is still unclear why the Americans offended themselves so much: they brightly showed a non-obligation of the full intellectual value and even that it is a complication for the achievement of significant success and wellbeing. Indeed, the low IQ of the protagonist of the movie did not discourage most of the characters of this film surrounding Forest Gump: they just did not notice his IQ. The imbecile became the hero of his and our time.

By the apt expression of N. E. Kravchenko (2015), it is the American version of the Russian fairy tale about Ivan the Fool. The artless ninny Forrest Gump, contrary to his imbecility and a set of ridiculous acts, becomes the excellent athlete and champion, a war hero and a rich man; he marries the beloved one and becomes a father of a clever son. Ivan the Fool and a holy fool, in essence, appear a synonym of blissful who demonstrates with his entire destiny that nothing depends on human mind and will, that all this is secondary and is not the most important in life. The main thing is to believe in God, in Good luck and the Case, to participate in Lotteries and Shows, relaying a classical mental trap about lucky little fools in a marginal consumer society. The movie took 6 “Oscars” and, besides, received seven nominations. Not incidentally, the U.S. Secretary of State John Kerry, addressing the students in Berlin, ironically and with pathos declared that each American has the right to be silly if he wants (27.02.2013. vz.ru).

In 1997, in Australia the movie “Shine” was shot – it is about a schizophrenic pianist – the real person. On a picture plot, the musician overcame the illness, having managed to adapt socially. However, tours of a prototype of the hero across the USA showed an essential exaggeration of musical talent of the pianist and underestimation of the extent of illness overcoming by him. However, political remedial curtseys in the movie were observed, the touching treacle spread on the screen, the audience learned again about mental diseases a lot of new and exciting.

The movie “A Beautiful Mind” was shot in 2001. It is based on a real history of the American mathematician John Nash. Despite being sick with schizophrenia for already about half a century, he managed “to adapt” to the illness and continued to study mathematics – up to the Nobel Prize award in 1994 for the application of the theory of games in the economy. A touching story about the victory of mind over pathology, about spousal support and fidelity, all-conquering love and rewarded hope received four “Golden Globes” and four “Oscars.” Being released for five weeks, the movie collected 77 million dollars. However, real events of the life of Nash did not find a place in the politically correct concept of the movie… Divorce with a loving spouse in 1963 who returned to the ex-husband, already Nobel laureate, just in 36 years. Homosexual relations of Nash, mental disease of one of his sons, the original content of hallucinations of the mathematician. Nash “received the encoded messages from aliens and was the Lord of the World” (in the movie the CIA agent slights him the Soviet threat). All this was superfluous, complicating and dramatic for an “Easter plot” with a pink bow of the kind end.

Ron Howard, the director of this movie, showed an interest in mental disorders as to a cinema plot, after acquaintance to professor of law of Yale University Loder, who, being the patient with schizophrenia, “saw” at the same time four various hallucinations. Loder managed to coexist with an illness for some time, continuing to hold a university course. However, the clinical record of professor ended in 1997 with the tragedy: after the death of his father who controlled take-in of psychotropic drugs, Loder ceased to get the supporting treatment and killed his pregnant wife.

Soon after the release of “Beautiful Mind,” the movie “I Am Sam” came to the screens where Sean Penn played again the oligophrenic person who could not independently make coffee and connect at least some words. His character appears in a position of a single father. His daughter is, naturally, clever and beautiful. (Is it possible to extrapolate Ch. Dickens into the XXI century?). The social officials anxious about the destiny of the girl want to place her in a normal family, but, despite the obstacles, the girl comes back to the real father. Everyone is sobbing. The end of the story.

The conceptual error of PC-manipulators, probably, is that they believe it is necessary to say that mentally sick people are “same as all other.” Thus, they place emphasis on the epithet, but not on the essence of the word “people” that is more important. The habit of playing sense of words led psycho-technologists to the loss of initial sense of a problem; but who can tell – whether it was not their purpose?

Politically correct equalization can imperceptibly result in the fact that the average arithmetic statistics from the virtual will turn into the real. It is already possible to meet on the street people without floor and age. Michael Jackson – not the man and not the woman, not the Black and not the White, not the child and not an adult, maybe not the complete fool, but not very clever – was the most striking example. It is obvious that PC-averaging of intelligence will lead to that the population of the planet becomes more foolish, because, after all, the clever are too little. Otherwise such PC-projects would not be discussed seriously.

The singular modern world becomes more and more paradoxical: comfortable and unfortunate, safe and dangerous. The pandemic of terrorism overflowed it with tragedies and shocks inconceivable earlier. So, America did not recover from the trauma of 11.11. For this reason, the world of harmonious death to which Patrick Swayze's characters in “Ghost” (1990) and Robin Williams went in “What Dreams May Come” (1998), was replaced by spiteful and aggressive reality. Such a reality is demonstrated in the series “The Walking Dead” (2010) – its subject recurrence has almost narcotic effect for already six triumphal seasons and 67 series (Belopolskaia 2015). Essentially, it is an example of engineering of public conscience and controlled mental epidemicity. The same tool became the series “Game of Thrones” (2011), where fantasy is not only a metaphor for terrestrial existence but also the shock therapy, feasible for conscience reconciling with a new reality of global terror and hopeless despair.

It is inadmissible to simplify a serious problem, turning the tragedy into the farce as Othello cannot become “Afro-Venetian.” Political correctness practically sees a standard in the average person whereas God, who not incidentally created a man “in His image,” can only be a standard. Moreover, only This image should be meant, seeking to improve the existing world because only such direction gives a prospect to movements not down and not sideways, but up.

J. M. Lotman (2002) said that the *culture is a system of a taboo.* Natural restrictions create civilizations and states, and permissiveness destroys them. So, the puppet that got rid of all threads constraining it powerlessly falls on a floor.

The tendency of modern life to speak about human rights as about a criterion of its advantage, in a separation from its duties, led to unexpected results. Such situation simulated if not permissiveness, then a broad interpretation of various rights and freedoms; while the taboo of duties, in general, was left in the basket of this discussion (probably, owing to the evidence about which, However, everyone forgot quite quickly). As a result, generations of people not remembering of their duties, but well knowing the rights appeared: after all, so many times they were told about them! *The moral design of the public relations lost its vernacular character, and, having become one-sided, warped.* It would be naive to think that all events are accidental. Too many financial expenses are involved in receiving the result which we have today.

Unfortunately, modern society, with its priority of material consumption extends the principles not only to goods but also to morals. To be more exact, the morals itself became in this society a good which is not well demanded. Application of regularities of the market system to ethical standards and rules was carried out imperceptibly, and nobody thought that today human rights are considered only, as something giving preferences and facilitating life in the broadest sense.

"Press the button, you will receive the result, and your dream will be fulfilled!" - a pop group sings. This is the ideal of the society of material consumption. (In the novel "Crime and Punishment" F. M. Dostoyevsky also reflected on the button, having pressed which it is possible "to fulfill dreams," but – at the cost of a life of a castaway Chinese tangerine). Is it permitted to dream of restrictions, taboo, and impossibility not to press this button – owing to any moral obligations? – It is unlikely – therefore, the culture follows from the modern society like from the overturned cup.

The separation of any human rights from his duties creates an infantile and marginal mass culture, of the society aimed only at consumption. In such culture the desire to carry out the rights becoming more and more primitive and aggressive, prevail over duties. The childish desire of Ivans-the-Fools to take what they need at any cost, in no way contacts with an understanding of the importance to give back what is necessary. Moral level of the society in this regard steadily decreases. It is much easier to operate such society, but its demoralization and dehumanization reduce a threshold of mental epidemics.

The infantile aspiration to acquire the rights (or candy – in this context it is the same – the mechanism is identical) speaks about purposefully created immaturity of moral bases of the society or moral stances of the subject. It is easy to reconstruct unripe structures in the direction necessary to "the knowing person," they fall in his hands. The convincing certificates to that are the pandemics of mental and social epidemics (from drug addiction and extremism to terrorism and "color revolutions" blazing with the civilization fires worldwide, from Ukraine to Yemen). Thus, they are as human-made as forest fires, habitual for Russia, and grassland fire, annually claiming hundreds of lives and destroying huge territories. If in Russia of Peter the Great, self-immolations of Old Believers were religiously motivated, nowadays modern mental epidemics of self-immolation can be explained as extra-mental suicidality of a syndrome of existential hopelessness…

The same problems of freedom and responsibility dialectics make a basis of the doctrine of V. Frankl (1990) about the free will of a person capable of finding and fulfilling the meaning of life even if the freedom is significantly limited under objective circumstances. The key moment of this doctrine is the question of a free goal-setting: freedom to make decisions and take responsibility for the destiny, hearing own conscience and remembering moral values. Essentially important is the balance of freedom and responsibility as freedom deprived of responsibility degenerates in an arbitrariness of mental epidemics. The responsibility of a man for his personal and professional, social and moral identity, for the correct finding and realization of the meaning of life, is embodied in his polymodal mentality and mental health the resources of which can be measured and predicted within a synergetic biopsychosociospiritual methodology of mental epidemiology.

Not incidentally, in many public lectures in the American universities, Victor Frankl urged to add the Statue of Liberty on the Easters coast with the Statue of Responsibility on the Western coast.

6.5. Happiness as a Fundamental Ethical Priority

Happiness is a state of a person which corresponds to the best internal qualities of life, its completeness, and intelligence, implementation of the human mission.

The succeeded tendency of the last time is *"ecopolicy of happiness"* as the instrument of creation of well-being for the society in general and each person separately (Popova et al. 2010). She declares the need of acceptance by the state the aspiration of a person to the happiness as the "gold standard" which is the cornerstone of all political decisions (Leyard 2012).

Economists also developed quantitative indices of *"the happiness level":* Index of Happy Life, Index of Happy Planet adopted by many international organizations – the UNO, the World Bank, the European Commission, Statistical Bureau of the European Union, the Organization for Economic Cooperation and Development, etc.

The attempts to allocate *the main components* of happiness are made in the psychology of happiness: positive emotions, involvement into the "stream" and meaning of life (Seligman 2013). Expanding this list, M. Argayl (2003) supplements it with the existence of the vital purpose, optimism and high self-assessment.

Depending on the *expressiveness of happiness and satisfaction with life* A. C. McKennel (1978) allocates four types of the personality:

1) "*reaching*" –both happy and satisfied person;
2) "*reconciled*" - satisfied with life, but unhappy;
3) "*directed*" - happy, but not satisfied;
4) "*unsuccessful*" - unhappy and unsatisfied.

Similar classification is offered by V. A. Hashchenko (2007); based on a ratio of subjective economic well-being and satisfaction with life, the author allocates four economical and psychological types of persons:

1) well-off, but dissatisfied;
2) the dissatisfied in need;
3) in need, but happy;
4) well-off and happy.

Satisfaction with life most often is considered as integrated satisfaction:

1) level of personal and family security;
2) financial position;
3) relations in family;
4) achievement of goals;
5) work and possibility of creative self-realization;
6) leisure-time activities;
7) weather, climate and ecology;
8) social status;
9) relations with friends;
10) level of social stability and confidence in the future;
11) health (Zhuravlev, Yurevich 2014).

The concept of happiness is often identified with *well-being* with the following major factors:

1) physical and mental health
2) knowledge and understanding of the world;
3) good work;
4) material welfare;
5) freedom and self-determination;
6) satisfactory interpersonal relations (Giovanini et al. 2009).

These parameters are supplemented with *psychological components of well-being:*

1) internal harmony (acceptance of oneself);
2) positive relations with other people;
3) independence;
4) control over circumstances;
5) existence of purpose in life;
6) personal growth (Ryff 1989).

There are other allocated elements of subjective well-being such as a good family, vital achievements, absence of depression and anxiety (Seligman 2013). Practically all indicators of satisfaction with life and its well-being, happiness and quality of life practically coincide; though demand the differentiated assessment in each ethnic, cultural case. For example, in Austria and Nigeria, there are close indicators of subjective well-being in a condition of essential distinction of the quality of life.

By convention, two main types of happiness are distinguished: *hedonistic and eudaimonistic*, connected with the orientation of the personality at the meaning of life, when the meaning of life is more important than life (Dzhidaryan 2013). Integrating both approaches, A. L. Zhuravlev, A. V. Yurevich (2014) offer the matrix of "*standard" structure of happiness* consisting of the following main components:

1) *positive affective balance* – quantitative prevalence of positive emotions over negative;
2) *certain perception of both*: pleasures as essential and natural, troubles as temporary and surmountable;
3) *positive cognitive balance* – quantitative prevalence of positively marked thoughts over negative;
4) *positive image of the world* in general;
5) *existence of the meaning of life* allowing to receive pleasures from life and at the same time perceive it as achievement of significant purposes;
6) *full-fledged semantic hierarchy* assuming a harmonious combination of personal and transpersonal meanings;
7) *general satisfaction* with all basic elements of life situation – health and work, relations with friends and family members, the situation in the country, etc.

Dependence of happiness on the existence of meaning of life is shown not only at the level of the certain person, but also at the level of the society demanding collective meanings and national idea, vision of prospects of development of the country and its new historical mission in the post-crisis world. These priorities are a basis of primary prevention of mental epidemics.

The romanticizing and poeticizing of psychotherapy the main working tool of which is still just a psychotherapist is represented very vulnerable in the society of total and cynical consumption. Only for ethical reasons, we will not call the surnames of dozens professional psychotherapists who successfully created the new cults and exotic business schools which became forms of mental terrorism – a mercantile manipulation of individual and public conscience. For this reason spiritual and moral characteristics of professional competence become the universal requirement for preparation of all *professional groups of Social service*: doctors and psychologists, teachers and social workers, priests and politicians.

Thus, dispersion and inversion of ethical normalization create the boundary and immoral, destructive and asocial behavioral phenomenology becoming an animogenetic pattern of a mental epidemics threshold. Imbalance of the rights and duties is possible to refer to the same epidemic threshold. The considered methodical approaches to systematization and classification of moral typology allow allocating target groups according to the risk of mental epidemicity.

Justification of applicability of all spheres of spiritual and moral development and the relations (personal and group, public and state) in mental epidemiology is represented essentially important during a singular modern era of global demoralization. It is shown in a specific feature of mental epidemics that differ in polymorphism and polymodality of ethical syndromology.

Allocation of fractal dynamics of trajectories of personality demoralization and scales of dehumanization of society allows differentiating epidemic targets and centers, to prove forms and methods of logo-therapeutic and psychologic-psychotherapeutic, biomedical and ethic - social correction. The unconditional priority of primary mental preventology is the happiness and well-being of people, healthy image and moral meaning of life.

The ethical propaedeutics of mental medicine and epidemiology is focused on allocation of diagnostic criteria within synergetic biopsychosociospiritual methodology of diagnostic process. Differentiation of norm and pathology in a vector of animogenesis is supplemented and corresponded to phenomenology in the planes of psychogenesis, somatogenesis, and sociogenesis, forming the integrated functional diagnosis. Synergetic multidisciplinary approach to substantiality of mental and behavioral phenomenology significantly raises possibilities of the objectification of diagnostics.

Section II. Mental Epidemics of Psychosomatic Disorders

Chapter 7

Synergetic Biopsychosociospiritual Concept of Mental Epidemics of Psychosomatic Disorders

The disorders are called psychosomatic when the leading role in their development and progression is played by psychotraumatic factors. Traditionally these disorders include: coronary heart disease, arterial hypertension, gastroduodenal ulcer, bronchial asthma, ulcerative colitis, rheumatoid arthritis, neurodermatitis and others. To a large extent, the psychosomatic component and a psychotraumatic factor may be found in the clinical picture of any disease. The galloping growth of psychosomatic mental epidemics in the present singular and stressful world requires a new multidisciplinary approach to the public conscience and health protection.

That is why the relevant task is to provide conceptual and methodological substantiation of synergetic biopsychosociospiritual concept of mental epidemics of psychosomatic disorders and to establish the systemic block-modular protection programs.

7.1. Etiopathogenesis of Psychosomatic Disorders

During the development of psychosomatic medicine, different theoretic concepts were dominating. The evolvement of Psychosomatics started from the creation of a rigid monolinear model gradually developing into the current multiple factor models.

The history of psychosomatic medicine knows more than 300 different concepts. There are several worth mentioning, namely:

- *psychoanalytic concepts,* based on S. Freud's theory (the conversion model where various bodily disorders are explained as symbolic expression of suppressed intrapsychic conflicts);
- *character-oriented,* aiming at explaining the nature of psychosomatic diseases through characterological and personal features;

- *psychophysiological,* based on systematic psychophysiological assessments for the explanation of the disease specificities;
- *personality-oriented,* based on personal development and, primarily, on protection mechanisms, maturity, personal regression, personal interaction with inner factors;
- *homeostatic,* originating from the modern homeostatic approach in psychology that unites theoretic concepts of self-psychology, developmental psychology theories, object relations psychology and physiology. Among these we could note prematurity pathology and objective relations theories, stating that functioning of the human psyche could be understood from the point of view of interpersonal relations – their development, as well as possible disruptions;
- *neurohumoral theories,* stating that psychosomatic pathology is the result of a general nonspecific adaptation syndrome and explaining diseases through the internal body environment disorders;
- *physiological* – cortico-visceral theory and others (Broitigam 1999; Alexander 2009; Kurpatov 2013).

Apart from these theories, we can also pinpoint *complex theories*, underlining the complicated nature of psychosomatic diseases and taking into account both psychological and somatic factors. Among them, *the clinical hypotheses of psychosomatic disorders formation mechanisms* by A. B. Smulevich (2011) and D. N. Isaev (2005) is worth mentioning. Thus, the evolution of psychosomatic medicine went its way from monolinear models to systemic, that take into account multiple interrelations between physiological and psychosocial factors. The majority of scientists nowadays adhere to the systemic models of psychosomatic disease development. It should be stressed that none of the previously established theories explain reliably and plausibly all the segments of the disease etiology and pathogenesis.

Recent studies become more and more convincing that psychosomatic epidemics are mostly just the inner picture or a virtual reflection of the stressful outside reality. Moreover, the ever speeded up and alleviated interactive and polymodal access to the individual and collective mind of the subpopulation in the global net requires new instruments for the protection of mentality and identity.

So, the American researchers P. Zoccola et al. (2013) have revealed that even the talks and thoughts about the negative and stressful events may exacerbate inflammatory response in the human organism, increasing significantly the level of C-reactive protein, which is the marker inflammation.

In the singular contemporary world, the Internet becomes the leading stress factor. The Swedish researchers S. Thomee et al. (2013) have been monitoring the health of 4 000 men and women at the age of 20 to 40 years for one year. They found out that those who surf the Internet for prolonged periods of time were significantly more prone to stress, depression, sleep disorders and pain syndromes. The same goes for a mobile phone that facilitates personal freedom deprivation and erases the borderline between work and rest, public and private life. In the end, all this provokes "the office syndrome" – the complex of symptoms that includes obesity, back and neck pain, headache, gastrointestinal and heart diseases.

The actively promoted view of multi- factor and multi- level nature of mental and psychosomatic disorders is surrounded with discussions on the degree of the influence of various factors on the onset of the disease and its progression, as well as on their registration during the organization of early prevention, treatment, and rehabilitation. For instance, N.

Ghaemi (2009) was critical of the suggestion of G. L. Engel (1977) on "the need to take into account all the three levels of the bio-psycho-social model while dealing with any medical task," and which "make almost the same contribution, irrespective of time and situation." However, rejecting this formulation of the three-core model, N. Ghaemi also disagrees with the orthodox views of biological reductionism, suggesting searching for the compromise between these two extreme points. One might agree with the opinion of G. Bolton (2013), who emphasizes that the cause-effect relations of etiopathogenesis and, subsequently, intervention may act on all three levels of the model, but this does not mean that all three are equal in their contribution to the disease progression.

The proposed by us extension of the model up to four-core model and filling it with the four-dimensional synergetic methodology sufficiently decreases the level of doubt in diagnostics and prognostication, enhances variability of approaches and evaluations, takes into account and accumulates the entire conceptual multidisciplinary diversity.

The synergetic biopsychosociospiritual methodology of mental medicine provides the widest and the most flexible approach to finding the mechanisms of psychosomatic diseases development and assessing the polymodal stress, which acts as the basis or performs the pathoplastic role in any nosology.

7.2. Synergetics of Psychosomatic Disorders

Synergetic model of psychosomatic diseases formation in general terms appears as follows (Table 7.1). Dynamics of psychosomatic diseases formation includes the fractals of predisposition – psychosomatogenic family, latent – psychovegetative diathesis, initial – functional disorder, full-scale clinical picture – psychosomatic disease, chronization – forms and types of psychosomatic disease course, outcome – somatoneurological complications.

The fractal of the *psychosomatogenic family* is the initial one in the psychosomatic disease development. Since childhood the process of a person's socialization takes place predominantly in the family and disruptions of family relations and roles' division may contribute to the development of this pathology.

E. G. Eidemiller (2007; 2015) and L. F. Kremneva (2007) spoke in favor of the psychosomatogenic family concept. They consider the disruptions of the main spheres of family life, in which a child grows up and develops, as the source of personal mental traumatization that leads to psychosomatic diseases.

The mechanisms of psychosomatogenic family development include 1) "binding" – a family with rigid communication stereotypes; children in such families become infantile, and their emotional development is lagging behind. The communication formula in these families is the following:

- "do as I say";
- "rejection (denial)" – a child rejects himself and his personality; he develops autism and tends to be autonomous;
- "delegation" – parents lose realistic perception of their children's achievements; they see their kids an extensions of themselves and hope that the kids will fulfill their broken plans (Kurpatov, Titova 2007).

Table 7.1. Conceptual model of epidemical development of psychosomatic disorders

Vector of ontogenesis	Prenosological fractals			Nosological fractals		
	Predisposition: psychosomatogenic family	Latent: psychovegetative diathesis	Initial: functional disorder	Full-scale clinical picture of the disease/ mental epidemic	Chronization: forms and types of the disease course/ destructive mental epidemic	Outcome: somatoneurological complications/ pandemic
Somatogenesis	Hereditary burden	Tendency to abnormal physiological reactions	Functional disorders	The disease	Forms and types of the disease course	Medical complications
Psychogenesis	Psychophysiological disposition	Premorbid personality traits	Psychosomatic reactions	Somatoform disorders	Psychosomatic disorders	Somatopsychic disorders
Sociogenesis	Disharmony of family relations	Disharmony of personality socialization	Violation of significant social relations	Transient social dysfunction	Social decompensation	Social disadaptation (invalidity)
Animogenesis	Spiritual and moral deficiency or ambivalence in the family	Disharmony of formation of the moral feelings	Deformation of the moral image	Loss of spiritual and moral position	Probability of immoral acts	Possibility of illegal behavior

Mental preventology — Clinical medicine (psychiatry etc.)

Mental medicine

There are five characteristics of psychosomatogenic families:

1) hyper-engagement of parents into their children's life problems, which impairs the development of independence and, therefore, the protection mechanisms grow weak and enable the development of inner conflict;
2) hypersensitivity of each family member to the distresses of the other;
3) rigid family relations with low ability to change the rules of interaction under the influence of changing environment;
4) tendency to avoid expressing disapproval and discuss the conflicts openly, that increases the risk of internal conflicts;
5) a child and his/her disease often act as a stabilizing factor in the hidden marital conflict (Isaev 2005; Eidemiller 2015).

Healthy expression of positive and negative emotions is not typical in psychosomatogenic families, where a child adopts the stereotypes of suppressing the negative emotions, what leads to their somatization. The suppression of negative emotions might be connected to the fact that an open reaction to pain is not acceptable in the family – the stereotype of enduring and referring to the disease as a state, which the sick person is the only one to be blamed for.

Psychosomatogenic family can have some pathogenic characteristics such as parents' (first of all, mother's) inability, unpreparedness and lack of education for early recognition of a child's bodily states and their attribution (the mother is unobservant and inattentive, or simply doesn't have enough time). The family, as an integral organism, is unable to resolve the conflicts verbally or with the help of any other constructive way and includes a child into their conflict. Usually, the child's bodily symptom appears at the time of conflict in the family, signifying an unfortunate attempt to resolve it.

Somatization of affects and emotions represents the family adaptation to difficulties and problems, a stereotype and a factor of failure avoidance and withdrawal from responsibility. The child starts to actively use his symptom for profit in various life situations in response to any kind of trouble.

Psychosomatogenic families have poor emotional health and prefer to deny the existent psychological problems. Parents may discourage or prohibit the demonstration of some psychologically determined emotions, considering them unacceptable. In this manner a child learns that the only way to get parental attention, love and support is to behave as if he is ill. The role of a sick person becomes even more attractive if a child is exempted of housework, without being blamed for it. An ill child may also bring a secondary benefit to his parents too, changing the relationships between them and steering away from the conflict that they don't want to acknowledge, in which case the situation in the family stabilizes.

The leading role in the early stages of the disease development belongs to the mother, who forms her child's body language. Traditionally, the psychosomatogenic mother is being described as authoritative and hyper-engaged, suppressing and dominating, anxious and latently hostile, demanding and obtrusive. The father in such family usually has a weak personality and is not able to confront the dominating and authoritative mother. He stands outside of this mother-child dyad. Any attempt of a child to separate from his mother or, in other words, to detach, is rejected by the mother. For the formation of psychosomatic pathology the most significant characteristic features of such mothers would be: high level of personal anxiety, presence of inner conflicts, i.e. disharmonious personality structure (neurotic mother); tendency of suppressing and controlling negative emotions, sense of guilt dominating the mother's mental sphere, ambiguous emotional attitude towards the family members; strong emotional response to troublesome situations resulting in disorganized activity (low stress resistance), as well as inability to resolve conflicts constructively, what leads to chronization and, therefore, to somatisation of mother's affect; disorganized personal activity during the child's illness due to heightened anxiety and fears, inability to make a radical decision; negative personal bodily experience of the mother, like the phenomenon of rejecting her own body or its parts relating to the early experience in the grandparents' family; disrupted mother-child relations on the early stage of development (Broitigam 1999; Alexander 2009).

There are two types of the mother's attitude towards her child: 1) hidden subconscious rejection, in which the child uses body language to get mother's attention (the mother stimulates her child to use this language more actively); 2) symbiosis – the mother tries to preserve body contact and suppresses the development of the next stages of interaction (Isaev 2015).

Thus, the psychosomatogenic family type is the first fractal of psychosomatic disease development.

The next fractal is *psychovegetative diathesis*. Psychovegetative diathesis is a violation of psychological adaptation of an organism or a borderline state that can transform into the functional psychosomatic state, and later on, under the influence of exogenous (stress) and endogenous (genetically-induced abnormalities and so on) factors transform into a psychosomatic disease. It represents one of the types of specific diathesis or predisposition in the general group of undifferentiated mental diatheses (Gindikin 2000).

"Mental diathesis" is a set of features describing the predisposition to mental pathology. Diathesis (from the Greek diathesis – disposition) is a constitutional predisposition of an organism to various diseases as the result of inherited metabolic peculiarities, physiological reactions and so on. Diathesis is a specific state of an organism, where metabolism and functions of an organism exist in a longstanding shaky balance because of hereditary, inborn or acquired features that provoke inadequate responses to an ordinary influence, the development of pathological reactions to the external harmful factors and define a more severe progression of the diseases possessed (Davidovskyi 1962). The exogenous factors of environment do lose their significance in a disease pathogenesis and transform into an "inner cause" of pathological states and processes, acting under a stereotype of all-biological principles.

S. Yu. Tsirkin (2009) considers mental diathesis as a general constitutional predisposition to mental diseases that has its own markers (attributes) of this predisposition (clinical and biological). Clinical markers include a wide range of functional mental disorders, like personality abnormalities, high vulnerability to developing reactive states and the presence of endogenous staging in their dynamics without forming a defect. According to the author, the specific markers of predisposition to a certain mental disease are not characteristic of the mental diathesis.

The psychosomatic dysontogenesis could be referred to psychovegetative diathesis. There are three variants of psychosomatic dysontogenesis:

The first variant – *lagging or delayed socialization of body functions* (in the psychosomatic development of a child). There is a late formation of body tidiness skills, prolonged use of body language as the main means of communication (until school age). Prolonged use of body language occurs when a child is covertly rejected, lives in a long-lasting symbiosis or is isolated from his closest relatives – residential care facility, day-and-night clinic. Normally, body vision develops in the process of ontogenesis: the development of the concepts about the body, its organs and functions; the vision of the body as a unity, "my body," body as an instrument.

The second variant – *regress in psychosomatic development* – as a reaction of a child to certain developmental conditions. These could be: sudden loss of mother (psychotrauma), displacement of a child from the family into a residential care facility or day-and-night clinic. The loss of skills of tidiness and body functions regulation, inability to fall asleep without assistance, means that the child is moving backwards to the earlier stages of development. This could be compensated later on. In this case – in case of regression – the child starts attracting adults' attention using body functions, learning to manipulate an adult using body language, due to the need of emotional acceptance, while lacking resources for organizing body comfort. This bodily way of influencing may become permanent (difficulties with falling asleep, headaches, etc.).

The third variant – *distortion of psychosomatic development.* This concerns the body "ego" as a whole. The vision of the body undergoes the process of formation and this "ego" might be distorted, developing a negative self-attitude to particular body activities – neurotic or psychosomatic dissociation. One of the variants could be the dissociation between self-esteem and self-attitude (Antropov et al. 2005).

Upon further psyche traumatization the person with psychovegetative diathesis develops *functional psychosomatic disorders*, which are functional in nature and are manifested through organ neuroses and other somatoform disorders. Isolated somatic complaints accompany organ neuroses. They include: cardioneurosis and hyperventilation syndrome (psychogenic panting), achalasia and irritable bowel syndrome, psychogenic itching, functional disorders of the biliary tract, and others. The disorder is predominantly located within one organ\system. The time span between the stressful event and the symptom occurrence could be from a couple of days up to a couple of weeks. Somatoform disorders are functional disorders accompanied by gastrointestinal, cardio-respiratory, conversion and pseudo-neurological symptoms and pain syndrome. There are characteristic recurrent and multiple clinically relevant complaints. These complaints are referred to at least four points or functions. The time span between the stressful event and the symptoms occurrence could be from a couple of days up to 2-3 months. This is *the initial state* for developing psychosomatic disease.

The common feature of this group of disorders is the occurrence of somatic complaints in the face of psychosocial stress, while the morphological changes in the corresponding tissues are absent (often disorders are nonspecific and functional).

The following disorders may be referred to as somatoform states: somatized disorder, undifferentiated somatoform disorder, hypochondriac disorder, somatoform vegetative dysfunction, chronic somatoform pain disorder (Paleev, Krasnov 2009). The pathogenic mechanisms of somatoform disorders' formation relate to conversion or transformation of the actual neurotic conflict into the functional somatic symptoms in the absence of organic background. The differential diagnostic criteria for the various forms of psychosomatic disorders are presented in Table 7.2.

Table 7.2. Differential Diagnostic Criteria for Clinical Epidemic Forms of Psychosomatic diseases

Criteria	Psychosomatoses Forms			
	Psychosomatic reaction	Functional psychosomatic disorders (“organ neuroses”)	Somatoform disorders	Psychosomatic diseases
Main symptoms	Elevated pulse rate; elevated blood pressure; changes in the breathing rate and depth; sudden muscle weakness and others	Cardio- and angioneuroses, hyperventilation syndrome and psychogenic panting, achalasia (cardiospasm), irritable bowel syndrome, irritable colon syndrome, painful bladder syndrome and others	Gastrointestinal, cardio-respiratory, pain, conversion and pseudo-neurological symptoms, pain syndrome and others	Arterial hypertension, coronary heart disease, bronchial asthma, ulcer disease, diabetes mellitus, rheumatoid arthritis and others
Somatic complaints	Isolated symptoms	One or multiple referred to one system	Multiple recurrent and clinically important complaints	Exact correspondence of symptoms with nosological form of the disease
Disorder localization	Limited to one organ’s function	Limited to one organ\system	Complaints referred to at least four points or functions	Depends on nosological form of the disease
Type of function disorders	None	Functional, reversible	Functional, reversible	Organic, irreversible
The time span between the stressful event and the symptom occurrence	A couple of minutes, days	From a couple of days to a couple of weeks	From a couple of days to 2-3 months	A couple of months, years
Duration of the disorder	A couple of minutes, days	More than six months	More than six months	Chronic progression (for entire life)

According to V. V. Marilov (2010), the emotional feelings that have not been acted out have a clear tendency to somatize, i.e., the pathology transforms from psychological into a somatic dysfunction of the organ or system through the vegetative nervous system. The phenomenon of post-stress psychosomatic vulnerability with protracted somatisation of emotions leads to a significant decrease in the stress reaction threshold in the person with a psychosomatic disease. The immediate consequence of lowered stress threshold is the amplification of psychosomatic reactions’ range together with the formation of polysystemic psychosomatic cycles, which leads to the development of secondary psychosomatic disorders.

If the stressful factor is still actual, this can lead to *the clinical onset of psychosomatic disease*. This is the group of diseases that manifests under the influence of mental and somatic factors interacting with each other and represents the somatized mental disorders and mental disorders reflecting the reaction to a somatic disease, or the somatic pathologies that are developed under the influence of psychogenic factors.

The nosological form of a psychosomatic disease depends on the hereditary predisposition, personal somatic state at the time of stress factor appearance (acute respiratory disease, gastritis, duodenitis, neurocirculatory dystonia and others), as well as on the other specific predisposing factors.

The next fractal is *different forms and types of psychosomatic diseases course,* which reflect a multidirectional nature of the disease progression. The form of a psychosomatic disease and its progression peculiarities depend on the influence of psychosocial and somatic factors. The course of the disease could be stable with rare exacerbations, or labile that leads to quick complications development.

Somatoneurological complications of psychosomatic diseases comprise the last fractal. They include mental disorders of neurotic and psychotic types that come as a consequence of a somatic disease influence on the mental state. Somatoneurological complications are the outcome of a long-lasting labile disease course.

The synergetic concept takes into account all the three conditions that are necessary for "launching" the disease (Alexander 2009): the psychological configuration; the "X" factor – vulnerable organs, the existence of which depends on the hereditary predisposition; the launching mechanism – a speeding up situation.

With the help of the synergetic approach, one could explain the psychosomatic diseases etiopathogenesis, irrespective of the nosological form, as well as the manifestation of the disease both in adults and children.

Thus, the synergetic concept takes into consideration all the exogenous and endogenous factors in the development of psychosomatic diseases. A psychotherapeutic approach based on this theory provides the possibility of a positive influence on the psychosomatic diseases progression, because it is targeted at the etiopathogenetic mechanisms of their manifestation, and thus opens new ways and perspectives in helping patients with psychosomatic pathologies. The synergetic biopsychosociospiritual model of psychosomatic diseases requires the introduction of multidisciplinary medical teams for the preventive and corrective organization of healthcare.

7.3. Medico-Psychosociospiritual Care

On the basis of the synergetic methodology of mental medicine (Sidorov, Sovershaeva 2015) we have proposed the program that includes four blocks: medical and psychological, social and spiritual and moral (Table 7.3). Preventive-correctional measures are taken in the first three prenosological fractals, while the medical rehabilitative are taken in the following nosological three, making up a uniform multidisciplinary protocol which is implemented by the brigade that includes general practitioners and psychiatrists, psychotherapists and clinical psychologists, social work and bioethics specialists.

The medical block in the vector of somatogenesis includes care provided by general practitioners and primary care physicians. *The psychological block* of care in the vector of psychogenesis presupposes participation of specialists in mental health: psychotherapists, clinical psychologists, psychiatrists. *Social care* is provided in the vector of sociogenesis together with social services specialists (social work specialists or social workers).

Table 7.3. Program of medico-psychosociospiritual care in mental epidemics of psychosomatic disorders

Blocks	Prenosological fractals			Nosological fractals		
	Predisposition: psychosomatogenic family	Latent: psychovegetative diathesis	Initial: functional disorder	Full-scale clinical picture of psychosomatic disorder/mental epidemic	Chronization: forms and types of psychosomatic disorder course/destructive mental epidemic	Outcome: somatoneurological complications/ pandemic
Medical	Inclusion of persons with hereditary predisposition in the risk group and their early preventive screening	Identification of persons with weak and unstable types of nervous system	Diagnosis; pharmacological and nonpharmacological intervention	Clinical diagnosis, administration of drug therapy, prevention of complications	Control of the somatic state; adequate drug therapy	Treatment of physical and mental complications of psychosomatic disorder
Psychological	Identification of persons brought up in somatogenic families and their inclusion in the risk group	Correction of premorbid personality characteristics, escalation of stress resistance	Correction of psychosomatic reactions, psychotherapy	Correction of psychosomatic disorders, psychotherapy, psycho-pharmacotherapy	Correction of psychosomatic disorders, psychotherapy, psycho-pharmacotherapy	Psychological rehabilitation
Social	Identification and correction of disharmonies in family relationships	Correction of family relations and harmonization of personality socialization	Harmonisation of significant social relations	Adaptation to the disease, correction of interpersonal problems	Professional and family adaptation	Social rehabilitation
Spiritual and moral	Screening and correction of the moral climate in family	Correction of formation and development of the moral feelings	Correction of the moral image formation	Reconstruction of a moral position	Reconstruction of moral behavior	Spiritual and moral rehabilitation

The spiritual and moral block in the vector of animogenesis presupposes participation of bioethics experts and consultants, clinical psychologists and social work experts, general practitioners that are familiar with the moral climate in the patient's family. Various psychotherapeutic and training methods, as well as coaching, are carried out to prevent the demoralization syndrome and destructive professiogenesis syndrome. Mediation is provided in conflict situations,

The patients are encouraged to participate in various public organizations' events that consolidate adaptive strategies in business communication ethics. These goals can also be fulfilled through the patients' involvement in voluntary and social movements, participation in the ethical-cultural events organized by the trade unions and veterans' organizations.

The religious-rehabilitative programs under the leadership of spiritual mentors of official confessions might be helpful to religious patients.

Primary preventive actions should be carried out in the *predisposition fractal (psychosomatogenic family)* already, where the measures are taken to find hereditary, psycho-physiological predisposition, and to harmonize family relations.

In *the latent fractal* the actions are focused on identifying the people prone to developing psychosomatic disorders (those that have weak and unstable nervous system, high level of anxiety, psychasthenic, asthenoneurotic, hysteric personality traits), on correcting personal moral socialization, as well as premorbid personal features.

The initial fractal, in the case of functional disorders, presupposes drug and drug-free therapy.

An early and efficient medical and psychological, social and spiritual and moral care should be provided in the fractal of *a full-scale clinical picture* of psychosomatic disorders.

Timely recognition and adequate diagnosis of psychosomatic diseases play an essential role in successful treatment and favorable disease prognosis *in the fractal of chronization and outcome*. In this regard, it seems quite reasonable to integrate the system of psychotherapeutic care into the somatic treatment, to open psychosomatic departments in the general somatic hospitals and to organize multidisciplinary mental health service.

Generalizing the published data, V. A. Domaratskyi (2014) highlights the following main targets in building the help for psychosomatic patients.

1) Internal conflict.
2) Motivation (provisional profit).
3) External suggestion effect.
4) Self-suggestion.
5) Organic speech elements.
6) Body language.
7) Identification.
8) Self-punishment.
9) Punishment of someone else.
10) The painful experience of the past.
11) Alexithymia.

The medical, psychological and social blocks of anti-epidemic program do not require a special discussion, as they are well presented in the specific guidelines (Smulevich 2011; Sidorov, Novikova 2014; Sidorov 2015).

The spiritual and moral block of the program starts with the screening and correction of the moral climate in the psychosomatogenic family. Screening and correction are performed in the process of family psycho and socio therapies, which fulfill the goals of ethical-psychological harmonization of interpersonal relations and spiritual and moral development of the family.

The correction of formation and development of the main moral attitudes and the moral image is applied to every personal modality that can be a source of demoralization syndrome and destructive professiogenesis syndrome. That is why, as part of the early intervention and mediation strategy, ethical committees and mental healthcare workers perform the supervision of adaptive professiogenesis and hold the training on business communication ethics to prevent mobbing, bossing, breaching of ethics and dehumanization of professional perception.

In the case of already formed demoralization syndrome the moral views and behavior reconstruction require coaching, sanogenetic and art therapies, ethical training and ethical-behavioral psychotherapy, spiritual and religious practices.

Spiritual and moral rehabilitation adds to the social-psychological one and fulfills the goals of correction of devastating pessimistic attitudes, forming the resourceful, optimistic view of life that strengthens mental resilience.

If personalized, multidisciplinary protocols of brigade care to patients have become a clinical reality, then containment of mental epidemics requires new strategies of fight based on synergetic methodology. The principles of the new paradigm of *adaptive protection of public health and public conscience from mental epidemics* are:

- synergetic integrativity of programs and projects;
- multidisciplinarity and multi-level nature of resonance-coherent efforts;
- instrumental-technological polymodality;
- interactive and systematic approach to sanitizing and correcting, therapeutic and rehabilitation communications;
- program-target and prognostic orientation;
- consistency and continuity of synchronous events;
- positivism and creative constructiveness;
- civil and patriotic national response;
- humanitarian and humanistic universally human refrain;
- transparent gender-age organizational and methodical association of approaches;
- block-modular design of therapeutic routes;
- variability of mental resilience of preventological programs;
- unity of healthy way of life and moral meaning of life;
- spiritual and moral dominant in building community and voluntary movements etc.

Systemic and efferent confrontation to mental epidemics can be a model for constructing the protection of public health and public conscience of Russia in modern crisis reality.

Chapter 8

Arterial Hypertension

8.1. Prevalence of Arterial Hypertension

Arterial hypertension (AH) is the main risk factor for cardiovascular morbidity (CVD) and mortality. The prevalence of AH has reached a pandemic level throughout the world. In 2000 the number of people with AH amounted to 972 million and, according to the prognosis, this figure will increase up to 1, 56 billion by 2025 (Kobalava et al. 2009).

On the whole, the AH morbidity varies between 30-45% of an entire population. About 40% of adult population in Russia suffers from AH. The AH morbidity increases with aging, reaching the rate of more than 60% at 60 years, 80% after 80 years. At the same time, it should be noted that the AH morbidity is growing among children and teenagers in the recent years. In 2001, the number of registered cases of elevated blood pressure (BP) among children and teenagers has increased by 6, 8% and made up 335, 6 thousand people (Putilina 2009).

The epidemiological data suggests that AH remains a state that is hard to control and the efficiency figure is not more than 30% in developed countries. However, an adequate level of adherence in patients enables to achieve hypertension control (Yoon et al. 2014).

8.2. Etiopathogenesis of Arterial Hypertension

The primary cause of AH development is not identified. In recent times, a more broad view of the nature of the disease prevails, but many questions remain open.

Traditionally, the main risk factors for developing AH include hypodynamia, overweight, dyslipidemia, insulin resistance, smoking, age-related neuroendocrine changes, heavy alcohol intake, genetic background, negative and chronic psychoemotional stresses, excessive consumption of salty food and others. For the patients with essential AH stressful, psychogenic and neurotic factors play a role in hypertensive crises development and pathogenesis in more than 2/3 of the cases (Lyusov et al. 2008; Volkov, Poselyugina 2011).

In the course of our study on the AH risk factor occurrence rate, it has been discovered that psycho-emotional stress was observed in 90% of the cases, which makes it the most usual one (Sidorov, Novikova 2014). So indeed, the meta-analysis that has united the results of 2 043 prospective and cohort studies showed that patients, who demonstrated both a strong response to the stressor and had a high sensitivity to stress, were much more predisposed to AH (Gasperin et al. 2009).

The AH patients' personality profile includes such traits as an intrapersonal conflict between aggressive impulses and need to be dependent on the people that are significant to them; perfectionism that is expressed in a desire to achieve high social goals and standards of social life (Lyuban-Plocca et al. 2000; Denollet 2000).

The view expressed by M. G. Pshennikova (2001) suggests that one of the significant factors that determine the result of emotional stress, as a factor of AH etiology and pathogenesis, is a genetical predisposition to stress-induced dysregulation of vascular tone. G. F. Lang (1950) maintained that not all people suffer from AH, but only those who have "certain characteristics" that predispose to this disease, like "the constitutional features of the nervous system," which take an important place among them. The sympathetic part of the nervous system (blood pressure, the level of noradrenaline in blood, muscle sympathetic nerve activity) of the people, whose parents suffered from AH, is highly responsive to stress due to genetics. Consequently, the genetically-induced or acquired predisposition has an important role in the pathological effect of emotional stress on the vascular tone regulation system, and the basis of predisposition lies in the dysfunction of the stress-limiting systems.

The level of BP and AH is the result of interconnection between multiple genetic factors, which are hereditary, and the factors of the environment. The genome analysis has allowed for identifying the chromosome sections, the genes of which may determine the AH development, such as α-adducin and angiotensinogen. However, most of the large-scale studies on the candidate genes did not give convincing data that would prove their role.

The main pathogenic mechanism that leads to the AH development under the influence of trigger factors is the sympathetic nervous system and renin-angiotensin-aldosterone system (RAAS) activation, which, in its turn, leads to some functional and structural consequences. Functional include endothelium dysfunction, change of cellular membrane's functions, insulin resistance, renal disorder, increased volume of circulating blood, functional constriction of arterioles and veins, an increase of pre- and post-load. Also, structural include remodeling of the cardiovascular system and specific target organs – myocardial and vascular wall hypertrophy, decreased number of nephrons and renal filtration surface, exhausted microvascular circulation.

Two groups can be pointed out among the theories of AH pathogenesis:

1) AH as a BP regulation disease;
2) AH as a result of adaptation disorder.

The approach uniting these two theories is the one that views AH as the result of adaptation failure under the condition of BP regulation disorder. Thus, on the background of unfavorable factors of behavior (smoking, hypodynamia, obesity, alcohol abuse) under the conditions of excessive stress reactions (urbanization, migration, and others) the BP of a person often gets elevated without a phylogenetic cause (i.e., without an intensified physical activity). The main mechanism of such BP elevation is the constriction of arterial resistance vessels, as the result of RAAS activation. If the BP regulation mechanisms have an extensive strength reserve, then the AH has a justified situational character. However, if the genetically predetermined dysregulation of BP is present, and first of all the endothelial dysfunction, then the proliferation of smooth muscle vascular cells and collagen accumulation take place, which inevitably leads to vascular remodeling and, consequently, to AH stabilization (Kobalava 2009).

A specific form of AH, and namely the neurogenic AH, is pointed out in the works of S. Mann (2003, 2012). Taking into account that the activation of the sympathetic nervous system under the influence of stressful factors plays the leading role in its formation, the approaches to medical treatment are different from the traditional ones. The other authors also emphasize that the activation of the sympathetic part of the central nervous system under the influence of a mental stress plays an important role in the genesis of essential AH. Thus, the sympathetic tone and noradrenalin system disorders, as a result of a stress situation, are observed in 50% of patients (Esler, Kaye 2000).

Therefore, according to the contemporary view, the AH represents itself as a multifactorial polygenic disease, the basis of which lies in the cumulative and cascade interconnection of genetic and psychosomatic, social and ethic factors that require a systemic synergetic approach.

8.3. Synergetics of Arterial Hypertension

The synergetic model of AH is presented in Table 8.1.

The primary fractal in AH is *hypertogenic family*. Family relations, the level of emotional acceptance and support can play a determining role in the development of AH.

According to the studies held by N. Peseschkian (1991), the hypertonic parents are often characterized as fastidious, controlling and not indulging in attention and support. They expect a child to be compliant and obedient under a rough and strict upbringing process. The relations between parents themselves lack tenderness and love, care and attention, support and commitment. The feelings, as well as the conflicts, are put away and hidden. The hypertonic people are characterized by rigid attitudes, that they have been inculcated in childhood like "be attentive," "brace yourself," "readiness means everything," "let the others in first" or "we love you only if you are amiable."

B. A. Namakanov et al. (2006) have expressed their opinion about the existence of a preclinical stage of family AH, which is characterized by genetic, as well as a psychological predisposition. In some cases, there is a noted linkage of a child's early experience, the relationships with parents in the early stages of life in particular, with the development of AH in the future life. The children, whose parents suffered from AH, are more aggressive with regards to others, but, together with the desire to impose their will on somebody, they feel the lack of confidence. Each and every family formulates certain rules between parents and children upon which the conflicts are resolved. In the families with hypertonic fathers, the children have less effective opportunities for enduring and resolving the conflict, which is why the negative verbal communication is predominant in such families (Broitigam et al. 1999).

The next fractal is *hypertogenic diathesis.* Diathesis (from the Greek diathesis – disposition) is a constitutional predisposition of an organism to various diseases as a result of hereditary metabolism peculiarities, physiological reactions and so on.

Table 8.1. Fractal dynamics of AH mental epidemics development

Vector of ontogenesis	Prenosological fractals			Nosological fractals		
	Predisposition: hypertogenic Family	Latent: hypertogenic diathesis	Initial: prehypertension	Full-scale clinical picture of AH/mental epidemic	Chronization: forms and types of AH course/destructive mental epidemic	Outcome: somatoneurological complications/ pandemic
Somatogenesis	Hereditary burden	Tendency to abnormal physiological reactions	NCA of hypertensive type	Arterial hypertension	Forms and types of arterial hypertension course	Medical complications
Psychogenesis	Psychophysiological disposition	Premorbid personality traits	Psychosomatic reactions	Somatoform disorders	Psychosomatic disorders	Somatopsychic disorders
Sociogenesis	Disharmony of family relations	Disharmony of personality socialization	Violation of significant social relations	Transient social dysfunction	Social decompensation	Social disadaptation (invalidity)
Animogenesis	Spiritual and moral deficiency or ambivalence in the family	Disharmony of formation of the moral feelings	Deformation of the moral image	Destruction of spiritual and moral position	Probability of immoral acts	Possibility of illegal behavior

Under the influence of exogenous or endogenous risk factors a person with hypertogenic diathesis develops the *initial fractal – the neurocirculatory dystonia (NCD) of hypertonic type (pre-hypertension)*. This is the central nervous system disorder of the functional nature and under the continuous influence of the latent phase factors, it can transform into AH. Out of 96 AH patients, we studied (31 men and 65 women; the average age of 49, 43±1, 14 years) 65, 3% of them had the NCD of hypertonic type preceding the AH development.

The criteria for the NCD of hypertonic type diagnosis are the following:

- BP exceeding 120\80 mm of mercury, but less than 140\90 mm of mercury;
- signs of hyperkinetic state of blood flow;
- signs of vegetovascular dystonia (vegetovascular crises, dizziness, headaches, low-grade fever, thermoregulation disorders, myodynia, sense of internal tremor);
- psychoemotional disorders (anxiety, uneasiness, irritancy, sleep disorders);
- asthenic syndrome (weakness, lowered tolerance to physical activity);
- benign progress without the signs of a serious pathology in the cardiovascular and nervous systems, or mental disorders (Makolkin et al. 2011).

It is important to note that pre-hypertension increases the risk of CVD development by two times, irrespective of its transformation into AH, and also increases the risk of death, especially because of cerebrovascular accidents (Guo et al. 2013; Huang et al. 2014).

The ICD-10 views the NCD as a somatoform vegetative dysfunction of the cardiovascular system (F 45.3) in the framework of a psychogenic vegetative dystonia syndrome. The later includes the somatic (vegetative) functions disorders that vary by their etiology and manifestation, and are predetermined by a disorder of their neurogenic regulation (Vein et al. 2010).

The continuous presence of the risk factors specific to AH may lead to the development of *a primary AH clinical picture*. A person that doesn't take in antihypertensive drugs is diagnosed with hypertension if the systolic BP is 140 mm mercury or more, and diastolic BP is 90 mm mercury or more. The diagnosis is established on the basis of a repeated BP level evaluation after not less than two visits with an interval of 1-2 weeks. The number of measurements during one visit should not be less than two.

Apart from the hereditary predisposition, personal somatic state, and stress factors, other specific factors play a role in predisposing to AH manifestation. Some of them are hypodinamia (people engaged in intellectual work only, not engaged in sport and physical activity), obesity, dyslipidemia, hormonal changes (linked to menopause), smoking, alcohol abuse. Each of these factors may contribute to the development of a disease.

The various forms and types of AH course in the chronization fractal reflect a multidirectional nature of the disease progression. The forms of AH and its course characteristics depend on the influence of psychological, social and somatic factors. The course of the disease may be stable with rare exacerbations, or labile that leads to complications.

The majority of prospective studies of AH patients show the high risk of mental pathology development before the disease, as well as after its manifestation. It is noted that during the CVD exacerbation period there is a high risk of interplay between psychopathological and somatic disorders. The severe course of AH may become the cause of nosogenic depressions of anxious and anxious-hypochondriac types (Smulevich et al. 2005).

Somatoneurological complications in the AH outcome include the somatic complications, as well as mental disorders of neurotic and psychotic types that come as a consequence of a somatic disease influencing the mental state. The somatoneurological complications are the result of a long-term labile disease course.

Making a step further, we shall take a closer look at each vector of the synergetic model of AH. The first fractal (hypertogenic family) of *AH somatogenesis* implies the presence of a hereditary predisposition, which takes one of the leading roles in the etiopathogenesis of AH. In the latent fractal of AH somatogenesis, there is a noted predisposition to pathologic physiological reactions, which may appear, for instance, in the form of an elevated BP in the case of stress. The factors predisposing to HT development that we've mentioned earlier become crucial here.

We define *NCD of hypertonic type or pre-hypertension* as a functional disorder because it may not transform into an extensive disease. The next is *a full-scale clinical picture* of a primary disease. *The forms and types of AH course* depend on the influence of exogenous and endogenous factors; that is why there could be a more or less positive progression of the disease, or labile, with frequent exacerbations. *Somatic complications* are the last fractal of AH somatogenesis. Among them, it is important to mention the cerebrovascular accident, coronary heart disease, hypertonic cerebropathy, acute myocardial infarction and others.

The AH psychogenesis in the first fractal is presented by a psychophysiological predisposition that implies the specific inborn features that may add to the development of a disease. Particularly, we have discovered the following psychophysiological features: weak or medium-weak types of the nervous system, low-grade ergic and tempo indexes, heightened emotions, emotional lability (Sidorov, Novikova 2014). The intensity of the physiological response to a stressor depends on the psychophysiological features. Those mentioned above may cause a more intense or even a pathological response to a stressor. The second fractal of psychogenesis includes premorbid personality features, among which we should note emotional instability, anxiety, suspicion, heightened susceptibility, excitability, restraint, apprehension, hypochondriac traits. The AH patients tend to be self-aggressive, which is the factor that encourages mental tension due to a long term fixated negative emotional experience (Medvedev 2007).

Most of people suffering from AH can be characterized as hardworking, accurate and conscientious. However, often these serve as a cover for ambition, aggression, and drive for contest. As the result of that, such patients may have internal and, sometimes, even external conflicts, as well as chronically suppressed aggression, specific modesty attitude, superficial shyness, suppressed needs. The AH patients often have internal and external conflicts that they cannot distract from emotionally, and they do not quite understand that they are ill (Sadock et al. 2007).

There is a possibility of psychosomatic reactions in the initial period of the disease, which manifest themselves in the form of complaints about the isolated symptoms in the somatic state (high pulse rate, elevated BP, change of respiration speed and depth, sudden muscle weakness and others). The disorder can last from a couple of minutes up to a couple of days and does not disrupt an organ's functions. On further psychological traumatizing the psychosomatic reactions transform into the somatoform disorders, which are still functional, but last longer (for more than six months) and are accompanied by reoccurring multiple and clinically important complaints. In this fractal, there is also the possibility of nosogenous responses to the fact of new disease onset that manifest themselves in the form of anxious, phobic and depressive symptoms.

In one of the wide studies (33.105 people) the patients were split into three groups: 1) patients that were informed about their AH diagnosis; 2) patients that were informed about their disease and received antihypertensive therapy; 3) patients that were unaware of their disease. It turned out that the high level of distress was observed in the group of patients that knew about their disease, as well as in the group that was already receiving the antihypertensive therapy on a long term basis. On the contrary, patients that were unaware of their disease did not demonstrate a scaled-up distress. Thus, the study emphasizes that the mere fact of being diagnosed with a serious disease may influence the psychological health of the patient (Hamer et al. 2010).

Later on, there could be a transformation into psychosomatic disorders that are chronic and irreversible in nature. The AH patients show symptoms of anxiety varying by intensity, which contribute to BP elevation and exacerbate the course of the disease.

The neurasthenic, asthenodepressive and asthenohypochondriac symptoms may occur in case of severe AH progression. The AH patients have a high or a medium level of personal and situational anxiety. One of the factors that may add to the development and further presence of arterial hypertension is the high level of personal anxiety as a rigid feature (Bunova et al. 2007; Smulevich 2014). The neurotic disorders interfere with the process of AH treatment and may serve as cause for patients to reject the adequate hypertensive therapy, as well as to avoid the diet therapy participation.

The somatopsychic disorders, being the mental result of a long-term influence of the disease, appear in the last fractal and mean the outcome.

Sociogenesis of AH starts with the disharmony in family relationships. The disharmony may stem out of one or more types of family relation problems:

- psychological (openness, trust, care for each other, mutual moral and emotional support),
- psychophysiological (sexual relations),
- social (family role division, financial dependence, authority, management),
- cultural (national and religious traditions and customs).

All these types of relations influence how a child is brought up in the family. The future disharmonious socialization of a person may appear as a result of disharmonious family relations. The majority of social relations that are present in a given society are adopted by a child exactly in the family. The disrupted family relations will be the model for adoption and may cause a disharmonious personality formation. Later on, in the adulthood, it could lead to the disrupted significant social relations acting as a stressful factor.

Transient social dysfunctions due to necessity of changing lifestyle may appear in the fractal of a full-scale clinical picture of AH. The severe AH course can cause social decompensation in the form of disrupted family, professional and other social relations. The outcome of the disease brings social disadaptation due to work incapacity, lost social status, professional and personal perspectives.

Animogenesis of the future AH is built up during the prenatal period on the level of possible moral-ethical family deficiency or ambivalence, which, in many cases, adds to its disrupted structure and functions. The premorbid "moral ground," accumulated in the family's cultural and moral values, traditions and customs is of significant importance for the formation of inadaptive behavioral strategies and business communication ethics that could come out tomorrow and pretty much determine the trajectory of one's destiny. Speaking generally and figuratively, the hypertogenic family predisposition comes as an elevated and unstable "pressure" affecting all the vectors of ontogenesis, including spiritual and moral sphere.

Latent fractal of hypertogenic diathesis may appear in the form of disharmonious formation of moral attitudes: credence and responsibility, sense of conscience and duty, honor and dignity. The spiritual and moral bringing up and development of a person start in the family. The family life values, adopted by a child in his early years, have a permanent significance for a person of any age. The family relations are projected into micro- and milli-, meso- and macro-society, forming a matrix of the moral image and moral viewpoint, manifested in a person's social behavior. The starting disharmony of moral attitudes formation and retranslation may determine the personal moral socialization disorder.

This is manifested in the first fractal already in the deficiency or devaluation of the moral image, notable for lack of restraint and patience, humanism and mercy, modesty and tact.

Further on, *demoralization syndrome* develops, the clinical picture of which in each specific case and fractal is complemented with co-morbid and associated manifestations of bio-, psycho- and sociogenesis. In the moral sense, the AH patients are safer, than those with addictive disorders, destructive professiogenesis or mobbing. However, it is essential to see the whole spectrum of modalities in the personal spiritual and moral sphere that are yet undeveloped or could potentially be disrupted and lead to demoralization.

The fractal of a full-scale clinical picture of AH appears as a deformed or lost spiritual and moral viewpoint, meaning the lowering ability to tell good from evil, signs of addiction from love, the refusal to fight and overcome hardships that have led to AH development.

The fractals of AH chronization and outcome are characterized by further aggravation of all the described definitions of demoralization syndrome and appearing risk of antisocial acts.

8.4. Medico-Psychosociospiritual Care

On the basis of a synergetic theory of AH development, we (Sidorov, Sovershaeva 2015) have worked out the program of medico-psychosociospiritual help that includes four blocks: medical, psychological, social and spiritual and moral (Table 8.2).

Synergetic theory of AH development requires the implementation of multidisciplinary and brigade forms of organization for prevention and correction, treatment and rehabilitation. The preventive-correctional measures are taken in the first three prenosological fractals, while the medical-rehabilitative are in the following nosological three, making up a uniform multidisciplinary protocol of care for AH patients in the framework of synergetic methodology of mental medicine.

The synergetic concept of the disease formation allows substantiating the organization of primary preventive actions in the *predisposition fractal (hypertogenic family)* already, where the measures are taken for finding the hereditary, psycho-physiological predisposition, harmonizing the family relations and its spiritual and moral development.

In *the latent fractal,* the actions are focused on identifying pathological physiological reactions, on correcting a person's professional and moral socialization, as well as premorbid personal features. Diagnosis of abnormal physiological responses should be to determine the level of blood pressure in patients with disorders of socialization of personality and premorbid personality traits.

For prevention of AH, when the NCD of hypertonic type has already occurred, *the initial fractal* presupposes drug-induced and drug-free treatment that prevents the disease developing. In case of pre-hypertension, there is a need for primary prevention strategy: elimination of hypodinamia, healthy lifestyle, bad habits cessation, harmonization of the spiritual and moral development of a person.

In the fractal of *a full-scale clinical picture* of AH, there is a need for an early and efficient medical and psychological, social and spiritual and moral help.

According to L. I. Vasserman et al. (2011) the nature of how the patients feel about their AH disease pretty much depends on the stage of the pathological process. The first stage is dominated by neurosis-like disorders in the general state, mood, and mental activity: somatic and mental discomfort, asthenic traits, lowered work capacity, irritancy. The patients mostly have mixed feelings about their disease, where the "harmonious" and "ergopathic" types (the adaptive variant) are combined with "anxious," "neurasthenic" and "sensitive" types.

The presence of these types of feelings about the disease is connected to the premorbid personal features of AH patients. Among them, it is worth to mention sentimentality, vulnerability, concern about the possibility of becoming a burden for the near and dear ones later on and lose all the social positions that were achieved during a lifetime and so forth. Interestingly enough, the last is more characteristic of men at the age of 40-50 that got into the hospital because of AH for the first time. The "apathic," "ergocentric," "paranoiac" and also the "anosognosic" (the tendency of ignoring the disease) types of feelings are registered quite seldom with the AH patients.

Positive attitude of the patient towards the treatment of AH and his compliance are important for increasing the therapeutic effect in *the chronization fractal.* The participation of AH patients in the drug-free therapy is significantly influenced by the mental status, personal features, deontology, attitude towards medical recommendations and ethics of patient-consultant relationships. The positive view of therapy is encouraged by medical awareness of the disease, social and moral well-being, the patient's participation in discussing the tactics of treatment and creation of constructive life strategies.

During this period, it is vital to give an adequate treatment in order not to let the disease move to the next fractal. The aim of AH patients' treatment is the maximum reduction of the overall risk of CVD and mortality, and this means not only the BP normalization but also correction of all risk factors revealed.

Drug-free ways of affecting the BP, being part of AH treatment, may be not less effective in relation to its prevention and should be recommended for implementation among the population as a whole. It is necessary to try to eliminate all the risk factors that can be corrected. The proven drug-free ways of lowering the BP and the risk of CVD include normalization of weight, limitation of alcohol, increased physical activity. Also restriction of salt, an adequate amount of potassium, magnum and calcium consumption is necessary. Besides, smoking cessation, reduction of animal fat, adaptive professiogenesis and personal spiritual and moral harmony are the best drug-free ways of the AH management.

Table 8.2. Program of medico-psychosociospiritual care for patients with arterial hypertension

Blocks	Prenosological fractals			Nosological fractals		
	Predisposition: hypertogenic Family	Latent: hypertogenic diathesis	Initial: prehypertension	Full-scale clinical picture of AH/mental epidemic	Chronization: forms and types of AH course/destructive mental epidemi	Outcome: somatoneurological complications/ pandemic
Medical	Inclusion of persons with hereditary predisposition in the risk group and their early preventive screening	Identification of persons inclined to pathological physiological reactions	Diagnosis of NCA of hypertensive type during periodic health examination; pharmacological and nonpharmacological intervention	Clinical diagnosis, administration of medical treatment, prevention of complications	Control of the somatic state; adequate medical therapy, prevention of complications	Treatment of physical and mental complications
Psychological	Identification of persons with specific psycho-physiological characteristics and their inclusion in the risk group	Correction of premorbid personality characteristics, escalation of stress resistance	Correction of psychosomatic reactions, psychotherapy	Correction of somatoform disorders, psychotherapy, psycho-pharmacotherapy	Correction of psychosomatic disorders, psychotherapy, psycho-pharmacotherapy	Psychological rehabilitation
Social	Identification and correction of disharmonies in family relationships	Correction of family relations and harmonization of personality socialization	Harmonization of significant social relations	Adaptation to the disease, correction of interpersonal problems	Professional and family adaptation	Social rehabilitation
Spiritual and moral	Screening and correction of the moral climate in family	Correction of formation and development of the moral feelings	Correction of the moral image formation	Reconstruction of a moral position	Reconstruction of moral behavior	Spiritual and moral rehabilitation

In the AH *outcome fractal*, due to the developed somatoneurological complications, the patients get through the medical, social, psychological and spiritual and moral rehabilitation.

The program of medico-psychosociospiritual care for AH patients that is worked out on the basis of the synergetic theory of the disease development includes medical and psychological, social and spiritual and moral blocks and implies the participation of multidisciplinary brigades in the process of prevention and correction, treatment and rehabilitation.

The medical block of the program in the vector of somatogenesis involves general practitioners and primary care physicians, cardiologists and, in the case of complications, by narrow specialists (neurologists, ophthalmologists, nephrologists).

The principles of medical treatment of AH are thoroughly specified in the recommendations of the European Cardiology Society (2013) and the recommendations of the Russian Medical Society of AT and the Russian Society of Cardiologists (2010).

The main goal of treating the AH is the maximum reduction of CVD complications and mortality risks. To achieve this goal, it is necessary not only to bring BP to the target level but also to correct all the risk factors that can be modified.

Nowadays there is a wide range of drugs that affect not only the somatic symptoms of AH but also the mental ones. It is important to lower the level of anxiety, as well as to boost up stress resistance, anti-anxiety mechanisms, mitigate the signs of depression and asthenia. For the treatment of AH affective disorders, one can use anxiolytics, antidepressants, and nootropics. The prescription of certain antidepressants and atypical antipsychotic drugs for treating the AH, progressing with BP elevations of psychogenic nature, results in lowering the average "working" BP and minimizes the elevation rate.

The psychological block of the program in the psychogenesis vector presupposes the participation of specialists that deal with mental health: psychotherapists, clinical psychologists, psychiatrists.

In the AH therapy, an important role is given to psychotherapeutic methods. The most common methods are relaxation, personal and group psychotherapy, a psychotherapeutic influence that has a symptom-, person- and socio-oriented direction (Ababkov, Karvasarskyi 2012).

The task of the family and social psychotherapy in the context of AH is to make a patient realize his emotional problems and situations that support these unconstructive reactions in the family, and behavioral stereotypes that lead him away from his emotional problems. One of the psychotherapeutic techniques that can be recommended for being one of the most suitable for the purpose is the method of "constructive argument" by G. Bach – E. Kratochvil that helps in solving marital and interpersonal conflicts (Eidemiller 2015).

The method of psychotherapy is chosen on the basis of concrete personal features of the patient and a clinical-pathogenic variant of the disease. It is important to use adequate ways of conducting psychotherapy – adequate to the disease and patient's features. Autogenic training is good for neuromuscular relaxation, gestalt therapy – for personal problems reformulation, neuro-linguistic programming – for modifying mentally traumatizing situation, and others. The result of psychotherapy is the most successful in the early stages of HT, but, at the same time, it is individual. Thus, there is no need for restricting its implementation only to the early stages of the disease.

The social block of the program is implemented in the sociogenesis vector together with the specialists of social services.

Currently, the fact that social factors have a considerable influence on the disease manifestation, progress peculiarities, treatment resistance, outcome and complications development is well-known (Hansel, Von Kanel 2012).

The importance of positive social environment and social support since the early stages of life or childhood is emphasized by American scholars, who view it as a significant and independent factor that lowers the risk of CVD development in adulthood (Appleton et al. 2013).

The mechanisms underlying the connection between social support and CVD prognosis have not been studied sufficiently, However,, the possible explanations are: improved engagement of patients into treatment, change of lifestyle (for instance, cessation of smoking after a myocardial infarction), and also protection from stress (Rozanski et al. 2005).

The prospective cohort study conducted in Japan showed that the low level of social support is associated with the high risk of cerebrovascular accident for men, which is one of the most serious complications of AH (Ikeda et al. 2008).

The researchers note that for increasing the success of AH treatment the patient's positive attitude towards therapy is essential. Such factors as the number of drugs prescribed, the lack of trust in the patient-doctor relationships influence the patient's attitude towards treatment in a negative way. The patient's participation in the drug-free therapy of AH is affected by the mental status, personal features and the negative attitude towards medical recommendations.

The positive influence and compliance (adherence to medical recommendations) are provided by the family that supports the patient during a long-lasting treatment process. Moreover, the medical awareness of the disease, social well-being, patient's engagement in the discussion of the therapy tactics is also useful for improving the attitude.

Educational programs for AH patients, organized on the primary level of healthcare, were proven to be effective in educating the patients and improving their compliance.

The spiritual and moral block of the program is implemented in the animogenesis vector together with the family and referent people of the cultural environment in the framework of contemporary forms of adults' training and education, coaching and personal development trainings, engagement of experts and ethical committees' consultants in case of impending professional conflicts and need for mediation, spiritual advisors of official confessions, public organizations, relatives, social and voluntary movements, trade unions and veterans' organizations.

The connection between faith and the state of well-being or ill-being of the population is currently the subject of interest for the scientists.

The religious faith is crucial for many patients and comes as a positive coping resource. Irrespective of how deep the religious experience is, those beliefs represent an important part of patient's culture. Another adaptive factor of religion is its intransient nature and spiritual integrity (Carone, Barone 2001; Powell-Wiley et al. 2013).

Animogenesis is the core of our four-dimensional synergetic biopsychosociospiritual model of ontogenesis. Spirituality becomes the fourth dimension of perceived reality not by its significance and value, but by the chronology of assessment of its role in pathoplastics and pathokinesis of mental medicine, after the development of biological, psychological, social and clinical-diagnostic units. One can say that spirituality is the fourth dimension of the four-dimensional space, for which Albert Einstein suggested his theory of relativity.

Screening and correction of the “moral climate” in the family are performed in the course of family and social psychotherapy, aimed at achieving the goals of ethical-psychological harmonization of interpersonal relations and spiritual and moral development of the family.

The correction of formation and development of the main moral attitudes and moral image as a whole is applied to every modality of personal spiritual and moral development that was specified as disrupted in animogenesis, taking into account the individual features of a real patient and his micro-society.

The more complicated and wider tasks of reconstructing the moral viewpoint and behavior are dealt with in the framework of multidisciplinary protocol implementation, involving the resources of moral-social training and spiritual practices.

The spiritual and moral rehabilitation is performed in the form of supportive therapy that is aimed at forming the optimistic and resourceful life strategy, that allows finding and keeping Faith, Hope, and Love, irrespective and in defiance of the hardships and complexities of the somatic state.

Thus, the medico-psychosociospiritual care for AH patients is based on the synergetic methodology of mental medicine and allow substantiating the individual medical-rehabilitative routes and organizing the disease prevention on the prenosological level already.

Chapter 9

Coronary Heart Disease

9.1. Prevalence of Coronary Heart Disease

Coronary heart disease (CHD) is a burning mental epidemic of the contemporary world. At the maximum level of generalization, it can be considered as a stress-producing mental trap of singular reality.

Prevalence of coronary heart disease (CHD) is the highest in the economically developed countries, particularly in the US and the UK. This fact reflects the level of health culture and proper diagnostics materially.

In middle adulthood, women are more amenable to angina pectoris than men, probably due to the higher prevalence of a functional CHD (e.g., microvascular angina) among women, whereas the situation is reversed for older ages. With age, the prevalence proportion of angina pectoris increases for both sexes: from 5-7% in 45-64 years to 10-12% in 65-84 years for women, and from 4-7% to 12-14 % for men of the same age group. More than half of patients with angina pectoris suffer from symptoms which seriously limit their activities of daily living and often lead to untimely loss of function (Chazov 2014).

CHD is the leading cause of disability and death of the working population in all countries. In Russia the prevalence proportion of CHD is increasing, and we have a world lead in mortality caused by CHD – 58% of our fellow citizens die untimely and suddenly with exacerbation of cardiovascular diseases (Smulevich et al. 2015).

The increase of cardiovascular morbidity is particularly noticeable during the systemic crises that require the mobilization of all multidisciplinary adaptational social and personal resources. This is precisely why the **task** is to provide conceptual and methodological substantiation of synergetic biopsychosociospiritual CHD paradigm and new strategies to confront the cardiac pandemic as a mental trap of "crisis social ischemia."

9.2. Etiopathogenesis of Coronary Heart Disease

Understanding of etiopathogenesis of coronary heart disease improves as soon as new data of fundamental, clinical and epidemiological studies become available. Nowadays it is referred to a multifactorial etiology of CHD. There are external and internal factors that contribute to the CHD progression. Today more than 30 of them are characterized. The main risk factors include hypercholesterolemia, arterial hypertension (AH), smoking, diabetes mellitus (DM), sedentary lifestyle, neuropsychic strain, overweight, male gender, elderly age, genetic predisposition, personal and behavioral characteristics (type A), alcohol abuse, thrombus formation. Any combination of factors has especially negative value. Thus, with the 3-4 risk factors combination the probability of CHD is several times higher (Oganov 2006).

Due to the negative trend of increasing morbidity and mortality from coronary heart disease in Russia, it is necessary to study in depth psychological and behavioral factors (increased stress reactivity, hostility, type A behavior) that reveal the connection with CHD formation and progression. The role of these factors increases even more regarding the socioeconomic crisis.

Psychoemotional stresses are among the leading risk factors of CHD. Among these factors are adverse life situations and repeating stresses, mental strain, mental fatigue. Instability and unpredictability of the socio-economic status and level of social relationship, the quality of the interpersonal relationship, the unexpectedness of life events, contradictory awareness of the own health and the attitude toward it can also be attributed to stress factors.

Numerous studies prove the impact of stress factors on the CHD contraction. The majority of patients with CHD relate the disease onset to neuro-emotional strain, caused by acute or continuous irritants in the professional sphere. Family conflicts often accompany conflicts in the working sphere.

Myocardial infarction develops immediately after acute psychic trauma or prolonged psychoemotional stress in more than one-third of cases. In 80% of cases, men aged up to 50 years have the acute myocardial infarction after a two hours emotional strain often coming from working overpressure and great responsibility. In 20-30% of cases, the myocardial infarction progression was preceded by acute psychic trauma and in 80% of cases – by prolonged psychoemotional strain. The important role of psychoemotional strain in the development of unexpected death of patients with CHD has been proved (Smulevich 2011).

Often CHD develops within six months or sooner after various situations, such as loss of a loved one, loss of a job, moving to a new place. Sometimes patients recall not only one major event but a long period of sleep and calm deprivation due to the difficulties that caused their helplessness.

In 66% of cases before the disease formation, psychosocial situations preceding the onset of clinical CHD symptoms take place. Among them: 1) family difficulties: conflicts with family members, divorce, etc.; 2) fatigue as a result of intensive work, high professional responsibility; 3) intense professional life, conflicts with superiors, subordinates, and colleagues, change of position; 4) lack of professional and family changes during the month preceding the first manifestation of the disease. The greatest role in CHD plays the stress at work. Repeated powerful psychoemotional experiences along with anxious, phobic and thanatophobic syndrome are the important factor in the development and progression of CHD (Garganeeva et al. 2010).

The population showed a high level of personal anxiety and weakening of social ties, which possibly bears evidence of the tension presence in the psychoemotional sphere, which is a link in the etiopathogenesis of CHD. One of the other factors predisposing to CHD can be alexithymia, which is diagnosed in more than half of patients with CHD (Chazov 2014).

Type A behavior is a CHD predisposing factor. This type includes people with a high-strung nervous system, feverish desire to a rivalry, permanent psychoemotional strain. Type

A has an increased amount of low-density lipoprotein, serum cholesterol, triglycerides, 17-hydroxycorticosteroids which are CHD risk factors. Cardiovascular diseases occur more frequently among those representatives of type A, who during a relatively short time before the development of the disease felt strongly pronounced excitation, motor anxiety, excessive nervousness which then gave way to despondency and depression. There is stability in the dynamics of the type A behavior which changes hardly (Evsyukov 2010).

Multidisciplinary approach in cardiology requires a full-scale mobilization of synergetic methodology in a systemic crisis. Closures of enterprises and mounting unemployment, intense competition and intensification of labor, ruble devaluation and growing collapse of the banking system are the components of this crisis. Social security decrease and loss of vision of life perspectives, growing dramatics of the perception of sharp society differentiation as consistent with socioeconomic, religious and national affiliation – all this leads to the explosive change in the style and quality of life, causing the stressful social situation and triggering a psychosomatic cardiac pandemic.

The dominant etiopathogenetic feature of the cardiac pandemic is a stressful mental trap that consists in a progressive increase in the basic level of psychoemotional strain as a consequence of a singular civilizational trend, which outruns the adaptational organizational and functional resources of society and the individual sanogenetic resources. It is no mere chance that I. L. Andreev and L. N. Nazarova (2013) propose to rank the entire spectrum of cardiac pathology class to the systemic and complex "diseases of homeostasis" pathology that are determined by the lack, surplus or inadequacy of adaptive body systems.

9.3. Synergetics of Coronary Heart Disease

Dynamics of development of coronary heart disease (Table 9.1) includes following fractals: predisposition – cardiogenic family; latent – cardiogenic diathesis; initial – dystonia of the cardiac type (cardiac neurosis); a full-scale clinical picture – mental epidemic of CHD; chronization – destructive mental epidemic: forms and types of course of CHD; outcome – pandemic: somatoneurological complications of CHD.

The fractal of a *cardiogenic family* is a primary in the formation of IHD. Breach of family relationship and roles may contribute to the formation of the pathology.

Psychological factors related to the family, to the interpersonal relationship in the family, to the level of emotional acceptance and support can play an important role in the early formation of coronary heart disease. In the family of the patient with CHD, there is often a lack of mother love due to separation or death. Father is not an authority or an assistant. Conflict of dominance often characterizes the relationship between parents. Communicating with people outside the family is limited. Parents` hopes are focused on the children`s achievements. Potential patients with myocardial infarction experience a loss as a rough narcissistic resentment and social catastrophe since childhood (Sadock et al. 2007).

The following fractal is *cardiogenic diathesis* – violation of psychic adaptation to the environment or borderline state, which can be transformed into the disease under the influence of exogenous (stress) and endogenous (genetically determined abnormalities, etc.) factors. It represents one of the variations of specific diathesis or predisposition in the general group of undifferentiated mental diatheses.

Table 9.1. Fractal dynamics of CHD mental epidemics development

Vector of ontogenesis	Prenosological fractals			Nosological fractals		
	Predisposition: cardiogenic family	Latent: cardiogenic diathesis	Initial: NCD of cardial type	Full-scale clinical picture/ CHD mental epidemic	Chronization: forms and types of the course/destructive mental epidemic of CHD	Outcome: somatoneurological complications/ pandemic
Somatogenesis	Hereditary burden	Tendency to abnormal physiological reactions	Cardiac neurosis	Coronary heart disease	Forms and types of CHD course	Medical complications
Psychogenesis	Psychophysiological disposition	Premorbid personality traits	Psychosomatic reactions	Somatoform disorders	Psychosomatic disorders	Somatopsychic disorders
Sociogenesis	Disharmony of family relations	Disharmony of personality socialization	Violation of significant social relations	Transient social dysfunction	Social decompensation	Social disadaptation (invalidity)
Animogenesis	Spiritual and moral deficiency or ambivalence in the family	Disharmony of formation of the moral feelings	Deformation of the moral image	Destruction of spiritual and moral position	Probability of immoral acts	Possibility of illegal behavior

Cardiac type of NCD (cardioneurosis) develops in people with cardiogenic diathesis under the influence of external or internal risk factors – it is a disorder of the central nervous system, which is of functional nature and future impact of negative factors can lead to the transition from a latent phase to a large-scale disease. Among 99 examined patients suffering from CHD (57 women and 42 men; average age 52.72 ± 0.91 years) in 45.5% the formation of CHD was preceded by the cardiac type of NCD (cardioneurosis).

The criteria for cardioneurosis are (Vein et al. 2010):

- continuous and recurrent during ≥ three months symptoms: a sense of discomfort or pain in the chest; changes in the strength and rate of heartbeat (accelerated heartbeat, tachycardia, premature ventricular contraction);
- intensification of symptoms due to stressful situations or during periods of hormonal changes (puberty, menopause, pregnancy);
- signs of autonomic dysfunction (local sweating, mottled skin or coolness of extremities, persistent white dermographism); lability of heart rate with a tendency to tachycardia; labile blood pressure;
- lability and nonspecific changes of the termination of the ventricular complex; positive ECG-testing with potassium chloride, with β- adrenergic blocking agents, hyperventilation and also changes in orthostasis; a temporary reversion of the T wave during the exercise tolerance test.

Chronic psychogenic cardialgia can be relegated to cardioneurosis. About 80% of patients on outpatient reception hours are suffering exactly from psychogenic cardialgia. They are often found in the structure of affective and autonomic nervous system disorders, and for this reason, they are viewed within the psychovegetative disorders (Solovyova et al. 2007).

The criteria for the diagnosis of psychogenic cardialgia by DSM are 1) prevalence of prolonged pain; 2) absence of organ pathology; 3) temporary connection with psychotrauma; 4) avoidance of excessive activity; 5) use of pain as a factor in achieving social support.

The impact of specific for CHD risk factors may lead in the future to the development of the *clinical picture of the primary CHD*. Other specific and predisposing factors also play a role in the CHD formation in addition to genetic predisposition, the physical state of a person, stress factors. The leading ones among them are: smoking, arterial hypertension, hormonal changes (menopause), hypercholesterolemia, type A behavior, age. Each of these factors may contribute to the progression of the disease.

Different forms and types of CHD reflect multiple paths of the disease development. Characteristic properties of the course and form of CHD depend on the effects of psychological, spiritual and moral, social and physical factors. The course of the disease can be stable, with occasional exacerbations, or labile leading to the rapid development of complications.

Somatoneurological complications of CHD include somatic as well as psychic disorders of neurotic and psychotic levels which are results of the effect on the psyche of a somatic disease. Somatoneurological complications are the outcome of a long-term disease with a labile course.

Among the somatic complications and severe cases of CHD, one may mention myocardial infarction, arrhythmia, acute cardiac failure, cardiogenic shock, thromboembolic complications, pericarditis, aneurysm, ventricular fibrillation, sudden cardiac death (Belenkov, Oganov 2010).

We shall focus on each vector of a synergetic model of CHD.

Somatogenesis of CHD presupposes in the first fractal the presence of hereditary predisposition. Almost 1/3 of the patients had an inherited predisposition for CHD, more often among parents, elder sisters, and brothers. In the latent fractal of CHD somatogenesis, the presence of tendency for pathological, physiological reactions can be noted. This can be manifested in, for example, tachycardia and high blood pressure during stressful situations. Here the previously mentioned factors predisposing to the development of CHD are very important.

In the analysis of the incidence of CHD risk factors we (Sidorov, Novikova 2014) found that in 2/3 (70.4%) patients, the disease appeared on the background of already existing arterial hypertension. At the time, 2/3 female patients with CHD showed age-related hormonal changes. A little more than ½ (53.9%) of patients had the onset of the disease after 50 years. Type A behavior, characterized by the assertive behavior with the desire of rivalry, is present in almost half (43.8%) of patients. Phenomena of dyslipidemia, overweight, and physical inactivity were observed in every third patient (37.4%).

In 1/5 patients (19.1%) smoking was indicated as a risk factor; 2/3 of examined men (64.5%) smoked. In 1/10 of patients (11.3%) the presence of the 2nd type of diabetes mellitus or glucose intolerance were observed, that revealed metabolic disorders.

We defined a cardiac type of NCD (cardioneurosis) as a functional disorder, as it probably can not pass to the stage of a large-scale disease. Afterward, a full-scale clinical picture of the primary disease follows.

CHD proceeds in different clinical forms: stable angina, unstable (progressive) angina, painless (asymptomatic, "dumb") myocardial ischemia, vasospastic angina pectoris, "X" syndrome (microvascular angina), myocardial infarction, sudden death and chronic cardiac failure.

Forms and types of CHD course depend on the impact of external and internal factors and, therefore, the relatively favorable course of the disease or labile with frequent exacerbations is possible. The final fractal of CHD somatogenesis includes somatic complications, among which are the arrhythmias, cardiac failure, thromboembolic complications, etc.

Psychogenesis of CHD is presented in the first fractal by the psychophysiological disposition which assumes the presence of specific innate characteristics that may contribute to the progression of the disease. Particularly we have found the following psychophysiological characteristics: weak and moderately weak types of nervous system, low values of vitality, tempo, high emotionality, and emotional instability. The intensity of physiological response to the stressor depends on the psychophysiological characteristics. Enumerated psychophysiological peculiarities can cause more pronounced and pathological reaction to the stressor. The second fractal of psychogenesis comes with premorbid personality traits, among them are anxiety, suspiciousness, increased susceptibility, isolation, and hypochondriacal features.

During the initial period of the disease, the psychosomatic reactions are shown as complaints about individual symptoms of the physical state. Such symptoms may be tachycardia, increase in arterial blood pressure, change in the frequency and depth of breathing, sudden muscle weakness, shot-run altered defecation pattern, etc. Usually, these symptoms last from few minutes to few days, without dysfunctions of the organ. With further mental traumatization, there is a transformation of psychosomatic reactions into somatoform disorders, which are also functional, but are more longstanding (more than six months) and are accompanied by repeated, multiple and clinically significant complaints. In this fractal nosogenic reactions to the primary disease, manifesting in worried, asthenic, phobic, depressive symptoms are also possible. In future the transition to psychosomatic disorders which are already chronic and irreversible is possible. In the case of severe progression of CHD neurasthenic, asthenodepressive and asthenohypochondriac symptoms can probably be present.

CHD is a disease with serious prognosis, objectively life-threatening, so depending on personality characteristics the range of psychological reactions to the illness can be quite broad. More than 70% of patients suffering from angina pectoris do not have any significant signs of misadaption due to the disease and the attitude towards it is composed of the "ergopathic" and "harmonious" types; approximately in 5-10% of cases, anosognosic type appears (Ardashev, Loskutov 2011).

Clinical features of CHD course associated with hypernosognosis and hyponosognosis include both variants and characteristics of the patient state at the time of the examination. Thus, hypernosognosis is significantly higher in cases where: myocardial infarction became the first manifestation of CHD; the patient suffered from several myocardial infarctions (2 or more coronary catastrophes); disability in the middle age (up to 65 years). On the contrary, hyponosognosis is associated with the onset of CHD, with stable angina pectoris or with cardiac arrhythmia non-hazardous for life; with only one myocardial infarction in the anamnesis or with an absence of coronary catastrophes in the past, as well as disability in older age (65 years and older).

CHD can cause the depression that in turn worsens the prognosis of CHD because of the inherent in affective pathology compliance decrease. Regarding psychosomatic interrelation, depressions observed in patients with CHD are divided into those that have a close pathogenic connection with cardiovascular disease (type I depressions – nosogenic, somatoform). And, depressions, which are formed with the complicity of endogenous mechanisms or exhibiting affinity for personality disorders (type II depressions – manifest within cyclothymia, dysthymia, affective phases within the personality disorders) (Smulevich 2011).

Patients with CHD who have adaptive neuropsychic reactions have high rates of compliance. Reduction of compliance of CHD patients is observed along with the appearance of mental misadaptation, specific to people with painful forms of myocardial ischemia (Biriukova et al. 2008).

The upcoming coronary artery bypass graft surgery (CABG) for patients with CHD is more often a significant and indefinite event regarding future, a stressful situation. The decision to initiate the operation, means for the patient a waiting stage that emerges full blown emotional pain, cognitive processing reflecting on strategies for overcoming behavior stress. While waiting for an operation, in 81.1% of cases, destructive forms of response are observed. They are a denial of real threat (4.95%); dominance of the emotional component of attitude to the disease (46.5%); cognitive component of attitude to the disease (17.8%); behavioral component of attitude to the disease (11.88%) (Belokrylova et al. 2007).

In the very last fractal, speaking about the outcome of the disease, somatopsychic disorders are arising from the impact on the psyche of the long-term disease.

Sociogenesis of CHD starts with the disharmony of family relations. Disharmony may be linked to the impairment of one or several kinds of family relations. They may be psychological (openness, trust, caring for each other, mutual moral and emotional support), psychophysiological (sexual relationship), social (role structure, material dependence, authority, leadership), cultural (national and religious traditions and customs). All these types of relations affect the upbringing of the child in the family. Further personality socialization disharmony can occur due to the disharmony of family relations. It is in the family that the child learns most of the existing social relations. Broken family relations will be a model to follow and will lead to the formation of personality disharmony. In future, this can result in the disruption of significant social relations in adulthood, which will become a stress-producing factor.

In the phase of a full-scale clinical picture of CHD temporary social dysfunction linked with the necessity of lifestyle change may occur. In the case of severe course of CHD social decompensation is possible which manifests in violation of family, professional and other social relations. During the outcome of the disease, there is a social misadaption associated with the disability, loss of social status, professional and personal perspectives.

Animogenesis of CHD can start in a fractal of predisposition with spiritual and moral disharmony, deficiency or ambivalence of family relations creating chronic psychosocial strain.

Latent fractal of cardiogenic diathesis is presented by the disharmony of formation and development of basic moral feelings: faith and responsibility, conscience and duty, honor and dignity. This is manifested in the slowdown and breach of moral socialization and development of the personality in any age group.

In the initial fractal deficits and devaluation of the moral image, manifested in the lack of endurance and patience, humanity, and mercy, modesty and tact become distinguishable. Afterward, demoralization syndrome starts forming, with clinical picture in each case and fractal complemented by comorbid disorders in the bio-, psycho- and sociogenesis.

The fractal of a full-scale clinical picture of CHD can be manifested in deformation and loss of spiritual and moral position: by the reduction of ability to distinguish good and evil, to manifest affection and love, by the refusal of the struggle and continuation of the trials of life.

Fractals of chronization and outcome of CHD are characterized by the increase of all selected definitions of the demoralization syndrome within the patient's personality typology.

9.4. Medico-Psychosociospiritual Care

On the basis of the synergetic concept of CHD formation, we (Sidorov, Sovershaeva 2015) have developed (elaborated) a program of medico-psychosociospiritual care for patients, including four blocks: medical, psychological, social, spiritual and moral (Table 9.2).

The synergetic concept of disease formation admits justifying the organization of primary preventive measures even in a *predisposition fractal* (cardiogenic family), where measures are aimed at identifying genetic, psychophysiological predispositions and at the socio-psychological and spiritual and moral harmonization of family relationships.

Table 9.2. Program of medico-psychosociospiritual care for patients with coronary heart disease

Blocks	Prenosological fractals			Nosological fractals		
	Predisposition: cardiogenic family	Latent: cardiogenic diathesis	Initial: NCD of cardial type	Full-scale clinical picture/CHD mental epidemic	Chronization: forms and types of the course /destructive mental epidemic of CHD	Outcome: somato-neurological complications/ pandemic
Medical	Inclusion of persons with hereditary predisposition in the risk group and their early preventive screening	Identification of persons inclined to pathological physiological reactions	Diagnosis of NCD of cardial type during a periodic medical examination; pharmacological and nonpharmacological intervention	Clinical diagnosis, administration of medical treatment, prevention of complications	Control of the somatic state; proper medical therapy, prevention of complications	Treatment of physical and mental complications
Psychological	Identification of persons with specific psychophysiological characteristics and their inclusion in the risk group	Correction of premorbid personality characteristics, escalation of stress resistance	Correction of psychosomatic reactions, psychotherapy	Correction of somatoform disorders, psychotherapy, psycho-pharmacotherapy	Correction of psychosomatic disorders, psychotherapy, psycho-pharmacotherapy	Psychological rehabilitation
Social	Identification and correction of disharmonies in family relationships	Correction of family relations and harmonization of personality socialization	Harmonisation of significant social relations	Adaptation to the disease, correction of interpersonal problems	Professional and family adaptation	Social rehabilitation
Spiritual and moral	Screening and correction of the moral climate in family	Correction of formation and development of the moral feelings	Correction of the moral image formation	Reconstruction of a moral position	Reconstruction of moral behavior	Spiritual and moral rehabilitation

The latent fractal activities are aimed at identifying abnormal physiological reactions, correction of socialization of personality, premorbid peculiarities. The diagnosis of abnormal physiological reactions should determine the quantity of heartbeats and the level of blood pressure in individuals with disorders of the moral socialization of personality and premorbid personality traits.

In *the initial fractal* for the prevention of CHD, progression medicated and non-medicated impacts hampering the development of the disease are assumed under the NCD of cardiac type. The strategy of primary prevention (elimination of hypodynamia, healthy lifestyle, refusal of bad habits, and prevention of demoralization syndrome) is needed.

In *fractal of a full-scale clinical picture* of CHD early highly qualified medical and psychological, social, spiritual and moral care is required.

Today for the CHD diagnosis the following methods are used: clinical evaluation of angina attacks; ECG at rest; 24-hour ECG monitoring; cycle ergometer test (stress test under the ECG control); echocardiography (at rest); stress echocardiography; myocardial perfusion scintigraphy; coronary arteriography; exercise radionuclide arteriography.

The data of various studies give evidence of the fact that the development of CHD can be prevented by influencing the modifiable risk factors.

Treatment of stenocardia pursues two main objectives. The first is to improve prognosis and prevent the contraction of myocardial infarction and to increase longevity. The second is to reduce the frequency and to decrease the intensity of stenocardia attacks for the improvement of the quality of life. Priority is given to therapy that is aimed at reducing the risk of complications and death.

The main aspects of non-medical treatment of angina pectoris are patient informing and education; individual recommendations on permissible physical activity and nutrition; smoking cessation.

Medications that improve the prognosis for patients suffering from angina pectoris are recommended for all patients with the diagnosis of stenocardia in the absence of contraindications.

Compliance and positive patient`s attitude to treatment are important to improve the effectiveness of the CHD treatment. Significant impact on the CHD patients participation in non-medical therapy have mental status, personality traits, ethics of relationship of the patient with a multidisciplinary brigade of specialists. Medical awareness about the disease, social well-being, involvement of the patient in the discussion of treatment tactics and his spiritual and moral harmonization also improve the attitude towards therapy.

During this period adequate treatment to prevent the transition to the next fractal becomes very important.

During *the outcome of CHD* with the development of somatoneurological complications patients are given medical and social, psychological, spiritual and moral rehabilitation.

The medical block of the program does not require a detailed discussion in the article as it is represented in special cardiac manuals (Belenkov, Oganov 2010; Chazov 2014).

For the treatment of comorbid psychic disorders psychoactive drugs can be used. Obviously, the therapy of CHD patients with affective disorders is not effective enough and cannot be considered rational without using such medications. Inclusion in the scheme of complex treatment of patients with coronary heart disease and comorbid anxiety and depressive disorders the administration of afobazole, tenoten and pirazidol can be recommended. Afobazol and tenoten are usually used in the case of the prevalence of anxiety component in the structure of the affective disorders, and pirazidol is used in the case of a more pronounced depressive component. Intake of these drugs improves the quality of life of patients (Minakov, Kudashova 2009).

Abroad as well as in our country in recent years, anxious and depressive disorders of mild and moderate severity in cardiac patients are successfully treated by cardiologists and general practitioners.

Effective and timely treatment of psychopathological disorders in patients with CHD may be considered an integral part of the modern complex approach to treatment. In addition, all groups of psychotropic medication are used in clinical practice. However, peculiarities of the dynamics of psychosomatic cardiovascular disorders dictate the distinctness of therapeutic intervention: patients with psychopathological disorders should take psychoactive drug indirectly stabilizing physiological parameter (anxiolytics, antidepressants, antipsychotics, somnifacient, nootropic) along with somatotrophic therapy. Besides, when psychotropic drugs are administrated the following requirements should be considered: minimal evidence of undesirable neurotropic and somatotropic effects, limited signs of behavioral toxicity, low probability of undesirable interactions with cardiotropic and vasoactive drugs, ease of use (the appointment of a flat dose or a minimum need for its titration). Finally, the main difficulties in the prescription of psychotropic therapy in general medicine are patient's stigmatization and contradictory ideas about the possibility of prescription of psychotropic medication by non-psychiatrist (Medvedev 2010).

Such a wide range of problems and requirements to drug therapy determine the relevance of constant search for the optimal drugs for relief (and prevention) of psychic disorders in the department of cardiology (cardiac hospital). In this regard, promising is the use of new generation of nootropic drugs – neuroprotectants possessing a broad spectrum of psychopharmacotherapeutic activity including not only direct activating effect on cognitive functions (learning, memory, intellectual functioning, etc.) but also anxiolytic, antiasthenic, thymoleptic, stimulating and other effects. Nootropic drugs are already exhibited for treating somatogenic, asthenic depressions, asthenic and hypersomnic states as well as for relief and prevention of cardioneurotic and asthenoneurotic symptom complexes.

Absence or lack of effectiveness of drug therapy, progressive course of angina pectoris are indications for the coronarography and aggressive approach. The frequency of psychogenic disorders in the preoperative CABG period, according to various authors, is 40-60%. Postoperatively it is from 13 to 64%, and in about half of the cases, there is a persistence of psychogenic disorders within 6-12 months after surgery (Smulevich 2005, 2015).

The psychological block of the program. Nowadays patients with CHD widely use the modern psychotherapeutic techniques, which, according to studies, can significantly affect psychic and physical indices. In the case of CHD body relaxation techniques, transcendental meditation, rational psychotherapy, hypnotic techniques and autohypnosis are successfully used.

One of the possible ways to increase the effectiveness of rehabilitation programs for patients with acute myocardial infarction is a behavioral therapy that is used to correct psychological problems.

In the treatment of patients with myocardial infarction, such psychotherapies like autotraining, hypnosuggestive therapy, and art therapy are used. Their administration contributes to the transformation of type A behavior to type AB behavior, to the positive dynamics of the level of personal anxiety. In the case of acute myocardial infarction, rational therapy and vegetostabilizing auto training can be successfully carried out. In such a way patients have the compensation of adaptive possibilities, disappearance of hypochondriacal, hysterical and anxious symptoms, reversal of affect rigidity and depressive and psychasthenic symptoms, initiative and optimism appears, as well as confidence in the life prospects and joy of recovery.

Almost necessary the psychotherapeutic assistance became after cardiac surgery. Patients with CHD who underwent CABG surgery showed a pronounced increase in exercise capacity after the auto-training. After the transcendental meditation program, they have less ischemic responses to physical activity which are accompanied by a lower hemodynamic response to comparable as well as to maximal strain.

A structured program of medical and psychological support for patients with CHD who underwent CABG surgery, comprising the methodology of the treatment process, strengthening of the motivation for treatment, patient lifestyle change, organization of close cooperation between a doctor and a patient was worked up. The program is based on a combination of methods of a group and individual psychotherapy. Moreover, the program also includes the methods of autogenous training and physical training, which allows extending the range of medical and preventive impacts, intensifying therapeutic effect (Klimko 2009).

The course of group psychotherapy allows developing after CABG rather a high level of motivation to carry out medical recommendations and to realize self-control of one's state. Patients show active, conscious perception of physician's instructions, internal agreement with them, a higher level of analysis of the real situation; individual habits of psychological self-help depending on the particular condition appear, as well as tendency to take actions aimed at achieving goals and conviction in the successful outcome of treatment. Improving of the general state is observed in 94.4% of cases. According to the character research test, there is a decrease of inner tension, reduction of anxiety and painful fixation on the state of health. The program of medical and psychological support helps to change behavior and lifestyle of patients, resulting in improved life quality (Klimko 2009).

Psychotherapy CABG complex involves rational, symptom-oriented psychotherapy (sessions of Ericksonian hypnotherapy during the preoperative period to relieve anxiety, stress, agitation and fear for the future), elements of positive, cognitive-behavioral and Gestalt therapy and neurolinguistic programming – in the postoperative period.

Psychotherapeutic treatment is beneficial from the economic point of view as well. Thus, patients with myocardial infarction, who underwent rehabilitation with the inclusion of psychotherapeutic methods, had less and shorter hospitalizations in next five years, and it helped to reduce significantly the cost of the medical care.

The social block of the program helps to overcome the one-sidedness of social orientations and preferences of patients. During the sessions of social and family psychotherapy patient with the help of relatives or association of patients learns to enlarge the range of social roles by acquiring and deepening the images of "father" and "husband," "mother" and "wife». It is particularly important to overcome the emotional detachment of the patient from his family and to transfer the style of his professional relations into the family. In the early stages of family and social psychotherapy there is an attempt to find an "ally," that is the family member who is the most interested in solving the situation. Most often, the "ally" of psychotherapist and social worker in searching the alternative family relations is the partner of the patient, but they can be also children. Then the psycho- and sociotherapeutical work with "allies" is carried out to improve their social competence. Partner independently seeks out ways to improve the attractiveness of family life for the patient. Such program is long, it begins in the hospital and requires its continuation in the extramural conditions (Eidemiller 2015).

Individual changes of way and style of life with the correction of existing risk factors are carried out most consistently and effectively in the "Schools for patients and their relatives." Graded and multidisciplinary personalized cardiac rehabilitation programs can significantly reduce the frequency of hospitalizations and acute coronary events, as well as total cardiovascular disability and death.

Spiritual and moral block of the program is implemented on the general algorithm for all psychosomatic disorders (chapter 7.3).

In such a way, the synergetic methodology of mental medicine in case of CHD considers all the internal and external factors of the disease formation and allows organizing the earliest prevention already on the prenosological level.

Chapter 10

Peptic Ulcer

10.1. Prevalence of Peptic Ulcer

Peptic ulcer (PU) is a chronic recurrent disease developing in response to a break in the lining of the stomach or duodenum. It may evolve into the progressive disease as well as cause severe complications.

The prevalence proportion of peptic ulcer estimates 5-15% (on the average 7-10%) of the adult population in different countries. Duodenal ulcers are four times more common than gastric ulcers. Duodenal ulcer is more common in men than in women whereas the occurrence of gastric ulcer disease is similar in men and women (Ivashkin 2009).

Urban population suffers from the disease more frequently than rural people. Men aged 25 – 40 are more likely to get ill. Women are more likely to get ill after menopause. Almost 10% of the population aged up to 60 suffers from a gastric ulcer or duodenal ulcer. Peptic ulcer often includes exacerbations, severe complications, and results in a long period of incapacity (Vasilyev 2002).

The modern experimental and clinical researches proved the infectious theory of peptic ulcer. The decrease in the occurrence of Helicobacter pylori-associated peptic ulcer disease and stomach cancer has become the best confirmation of the infectious theory. Developing and implementation of so-called eradication therapy in different countries mainly located in Europe, the USA, and Australia contribute to the primary goal – total elimination of Helicobacter pylori infection in a gastroduodenal region. The downward trend in the incidence of PU is so reliable that mathematical modeling of the process makes it possible to predict the disappearance of Helicobacter-associated PU (Ivashkin 2013).

The relevant task is conceptual and methodological substantiation of the synergetic biopsychosociospiritual concept of PU and effectiveness of a systematic approach to treatment and preventive care.

10.2. Etiopathogenesis of Peptic Ulcer

Modern medicine considers peptic ulcer as a multifactorial, genetically and pathogenetically heterogeneous disease. Heredity is an important causative factor resulted in the developing of peptic ulcer. However, it is the predisposition to the disease that is inherited, not the disease itself (Simonenkov 2008).

Several genetic factors that may result in the disease development are established: inherited abnormally large parietal cell mass, their hypersensitivity to gastrin; insufficient mucus secretion, an insufficient release of IgA and prostaglandin; 0 (1) blood type, Rh positive, HLA antigens B5, B15 and B35 and others.

The following negative impacts may contribute to genetic predisposition: Helicobacter pylori contamination, nutritional disorder, the effect of local irritators, drug administration (nonsteroidal anti-inflammatory drugs), smoking, alcohol consumption, emotional stress.

The peptic ulcer has a multifactorial genesis. However,, infectious agent Helicobacter pylori is known as the major causative factor of gastric and duodenal ulcers. Epidemiological data from different countries demonstrated that almost 100% of duodenum ulcers and more than 80% of stomach ulcers are connected with H. pylori persistence. However, 5-10% of patients with duodenum ulcers and 15-20% of patients with stomach ulcers may experience health decline without Helicobacter pylori involvement. Primarily it refers to symptomatic gastroduodenal ulcers (Ivashkin 2013).

The main point in the pathogenesis of peptic ulcer is imbalance between the factors of aggression and the factors of stomach and duodenum mucous protection.

Factors of aggression include: intensification of hydrochloric acid and pepsin secretion; gastrointestinal motility dysfunction, duodenogastric reflux.

Factors of protection include: resistance of mucus membrane to aggressive factors; secretion of mucus in the stomach; efficient production of bicarbonates; rapid mucus membrane epithelial tissue regeneration; efficient blood supply to mucus membrane; sufficient amount of prostaglandin; an immune system defense mechanism.

The majority of factors of aggression and protection are genetically determined. Efficient functioning of the neuroendocrine system that comprises cerebral cortex, hypothalamus, peripheral and endocrine glands and gastrointestinal hormones, peptides contributes to the balance between the mentioned factors.

The imbalance between factors of aggression and protection may differ in every certain case.

In our study, we (Sidorov, Novikova 2014) have examined 60 patients (30 women and 30 men; the average age was 48, 23±1, 83) to determine the risk factors for peptic ulcer. Psycho – emotional stress was widespread (95, 6%). It was more likely to be an initiating etiological agent. Nearly 2/3 of patients were infected with Helicobacter pylori (66, 3%). Almost 2/3 of patients (63, 2%) suffered from peptic ulcer due to the already existed diseases of the digestive tract (GIT) (chronic gastritis, duodenitis, cholecystitis, and pancreatitis). Half of the patients noted nutritional and behavioral disturbances as well as imbalanced nutrition (53, 2%). About 2/5 of those examined (43, 4%) had O (I) blood type. 17% of the patients suffering from arthropathy took drugs like nonsteroidal anti-inflammatory one. In 1/6 of the patients (16, 4%) strong hereditary factors of peptic ulcer were noticed. One in ten people experienced the influence of local physical, chemical or thermal effects (12, 8%). Craniocerebral trauma (4, 3%), thyroid diseases accompanied by hyperthyroidism (8, 5%) causing dysfunction of a pituitary-hypothalamic zone and break in the endocrine system were rare among risk factors.

Five top risk factors (general informative value 70,7%) were discovered during the factor analysis. The 1st factor – the largest in size (20, 2%) including smoking and alcohol abuse was primarily common for men. The 2nd factor (14, 4%) included genetic predisposition to the peptic ulcer and 0(I) blood type. The 3d factor comprised stress and digestive tract diseases (13, 4%). The stress factor accompanied digestive tract dysfunction. The 4th factor included nutritional disorder and taking nonsteroidal anti-inflammatory drugs (11, 9%). The 5th factor (10, 7%) comprised craniocerebral trauma that was considered to accompany with hypothalamic dysfunction.

In the course of multiply regression analysis, we presented a regression equation that allows predicting the magnitude of the peptic ulcer risk taking into consideration the risk factors. To build a regression model the survey data of patients who do not have psychosomatic disorders is used. The regression equation:

A = 0,007 + 0,678●stress + 0,155●alcohol + 0,142●nutritional disorders + 0,222●Helicobacter pylori

The patient was given a score for each symptom and 0 for lack of them.

A coefficient in multiple regression (R) = 0,883. The equation explains 77, 9% (R^2 = 0, 779) of dependent variable variation. All the coefficients of the equation are significant at the level (p-level) ≤0, 023. Limitations: age from 17 to 57. In case of 0, 007-0, 406 the risk is estimated as low; 0, 407-0, 804 – as medium risk; 0, 805-1, 204 – as high risk.

10.3. Synergetics of Peptic Ulcer

Dynamics of the PU development includes fractals like (table 10.1): predisposition – ulcerogenic family, latent – ulcerogenic diathesis, initial – preulcerous state, full - scale clinical picture of PU, chronization – forms and types of PU course, outcome – somato-neurological complications of PU.

The fractal of the ulcerogenic family is the initial point of PU development. The break in the family relationships and family roles may contribute to the development of the pathology.

Family plays an important role in PU development. Break in family relationships in childhood results in disruption of interpersonal communication, hard period of adaptation, an increase of emotional tension and anxiety that in its turn greatly influence adult family relationships.

76, 6% of the PU patients have actual psychogenia, 27 – 30% experienced psychogenia in childhood time and among those living in big cities, there are 60%. PU patients experienced childhood psychological trauma because of constant conflicts in the family or parents' divorce, cruel methods of education like "detachment." PU patients witnessed and sometimes unwillingly participated in parents' quarrels and conflicts in their childhood. Parents put a restriction on child's freedom and hardly took care of them. Those children suffered bitter mortification from their friends; barely adapted in the army; were dissatisfied with chosen profession and as a result changed their work quite a lot herewith having no enjoyment of the work. There are a lot of inharmonious marriages among those having suffered from PU, these people often stay at home, and they are unsocial in all spheres of their life (Cimmerman, Schyotkin 2002).

Table 10.1. Fractal dynamics of the PU mental epidemic development

Vector of ontogenesis	Prenosological fractals			Nosological fractals		
	Predisposition: ulcerogenic family	Latent: ulcerogenic diathesis	Initial: preulcerous state	Full-scale clinical picture of PU/mental epidemic	Chronization: forms and types of PU course /destructive mental epidemic	Outcome: somatoneurological complications/ pandemic
Somatogenesis	Hereditary burden	Tendency to abnormal physiological reactions	Preulcerous state	Peptic ulcer	Forms and types of PU course	Medical complications
Psychogenesis	Psychophysiological disposition	Premorbid personality traits	Psychosomatic reactions	Somatoform disorders	Psychosomatic disorders	Somatopsychic disorders
Sociogenesis	Disharmony of family relations	Disharmony of personality socialization	Violation of significant social relations	Transient social dysfunction	Social decompensation	Social disadaptation (invalidity)
Animogenesis	Spiritual and moral deficiency or ambivalence in the family	Disharmony of formation of the moral feelings	Deformation of the moral image	Destruction of spiritual and moral position	Probability of immoral acts	Possibility of illegal behavior

With a break in emotional connections in childhood, a child develops an early peptic ulcer. It is characterized by severe acute course, frequent exacerbations, complications and severe pain.

Alexithymia is an important psychological feature of the PU families. The degree of severity of the disease is varying among the family members. Pathologized methods of upbringing, great hyper (indulgent) protection accompanied by disconfidence in upbringing methods and childish behavior contribute to family dysfunction. Such families show a high level of the general family anxiety and inefficient stress management.

The next is the *fractal of ulcerogenic diathesis* – a break in a psychological adaptation of the organism to the environment or a borderline state that may transform into a disease under the influence of exogenic (stress) and endogenic (genetically inherited defects and others) factors. It represents one of the variations of specific diathesis or predisposition in the general group of undifferentiated mental diatheses.

A person suffering from ulcerogenic diathesis may experience a pre-ulcer state under the influence of external or internal factors. Acute or chronic duodenitis or gastritis may be referred to it. In our study, 63, 2% of examined PU patients earlier suffered from acute or chronic inflammation of duodenum (Sidorov, Novikova 2014).

Influence of risk factors specific for PU later may result in the development of *primary PU clinical picture.* Specific and contributory causes like Helicobacter pylori, smoking, and alcohol, as well as genetic predisposition, a somatic state of a person and stress factor, contribute greatly to PU development. Each of the factors may result in the disease development.

Different forms and types of PU course reflect multivariate features of disease development. Features of the disease progression depend on psychological, social, spiritual and moral and somatic factors. The course of a disease may be stable with rare acute exacerbations or instable rapidly resulting in a variety of complications.

Somato-neurological PU complications include somatic complications, psychic disorders of neurotic and psychotic levels arising from somatic disease influence on the mind. Somatic and neurological complications are the results of long- term disease accompanied by acute exacerbations.

PU somatic complications include bleeding, pyloric obstruction, perforation, penetration, malignization of an ulcer.

We shall focus on each vector of PU synergetic model.

Somatogenesis of PU presupposes heredity burden in the first fractal. The results of our PU patients' survey prove this fact. Almost 16, 4% of patients showed a PU heredity burden. Latent fractal of PU somatogenesis shows the tendency to abnormal physiological reactions such as nausea, increased stomach motility under stress. Already mentioned risk factors contributing to PU development play an important role.

Preulcerous state as a functional illness may not be developed into the advanced stage of a disease. Acute or chronic duodenitis or gastritis may be referred to a preulcerous state. Next goes a full-scale clinical picture of a primary disease.

PU disease has different clinical forms. The light form has one exacerbation per 1-3 years and moderate abdominal pain, which stops in 4 - 7 days. The moderately severe form has two exacerbations per year and severe abdominal pain, which stops in 10 - 14 days. Severe form is characterized by frequent exacerbations (more than two times a year and severe abdominal pain, which stops in more than 10 - 14 days, complications are not rare.

Forms and types of PU course depend on external and internal factors. They may lead to relatively favourable course of the disease or instable with frequent exacerbations. The final fractal of PU somatogenesis includes already marked medical complications.

The first fractal of *the PU psychogenesis* includes psychophysiological disposition that presupposes inborn defects contributing to the development of the disease. Physiological response to stressor depends on psychophysiological characteristics. We have revealed the following psychophysiological characteristics of PU patients: weak and relatively weak types of nervous system, low values of ergicity and tempo, emotional instability. The mentioned psychophysiological characteristics may cause pathologic response to the stressor (Sidorov, Novikova 2014).

The second fractal of psychogenesis includes premorbid personality traits. Anxiety, suspiciousness, hypochondriacal traits, constriction of thinking, uncommunicativeness and pessimism may be referred to it.

Psychosomatic reactions are possible in the first stage of the disease. They are presented as individual symptoms of the somatic state (abdominal pain, nausea, etc.) with the duration of the disorder from a few minutes to a few days taking into consideration that they do not disturb the organ functions. With further mental trauma, there is a transformation of psychosomatic reactions into somatoform disorders which are also functional but last more than six months. They are accompanied by repeated, multiple and clinically significant complaints. Nosogenic reactions to the fact of a primary disease are also possible in this fractal. They become evident with asthenic, phobic and depressive symptoms. Further, we may see a transition to psychosomatic disorders which are already chronic and irreversible. In the case of severe PU, hypochondriacal, hysterical and depressive symptoms may occur (Smulevich 2011).

In the last fractal, the outcome of the disease is presented, and somatopsychic disorders are arising from the impact of the long-term PU on the psyche.

Sociogenesis of PU begins with the disharmony of family relations. Disharmony may be associated with a break in one or more kinds of family relationships: psychological (openness, trust, caring for each other, mutual moral and emotional support), psychophysiological (sexual relationship), social (roles, money dependence, authority, leadership), cultural (national and religious traditions and customs). All these types of relationships affect the child upbringing in the family. Due to the disharmony of family relations later disharmony in personal socialization may appear. It is in the family where the child learns most of the existing social relations. Broken family relationships will be a model for learning and will result in the personal disharmony. In future, this can cause a disruption of significant social relationships in the adult stage.

In the case of a full-scale clinical picture of PU social dysfunctions associated with the need to change lifestyle may occur. Severe cases of PA may result in a social decompensation which becomes evident in a violation of family, professional and other social relationships. The outcome of the disease is accompanied by social exclusion connected with disability, loss of social status, professional and personal perspectives.

Animogenesis of PU starts in a predisposition fractal with moral and spiritual disharmony, deficiency or ambivalence in the family relationships contributing to conscious or unconscious emotional stress.

Latent fractal of ulcerogenic diathesis demonstrates disharmony and break in formation and development of basic moral feelings: faith and responsibility, conscience and duty, honor and dignity. This causes slowdown and violation of moral socialization and personal development at any period.

Initial fractal shows diminishing or deformation of moral character that results in a lack of endurance and patience, humanity and mercy, modesty and tact. Further, the syndrome of demoralization develops. It is formed and supplemented by associated and comorbid disorders in the bio-, psycho- and sociogenesis in the certain case and fractal.

Fractal of a full-scale clinical picture of PU demonstrates destruction and loss of spiritual and moral values: decrease in ability to distinguish between good and evil, expressions of devotion and love, to struggle and overcome life trials, associated with the PU perception by a patient.

Fractals of chronization and outcome of PU are characterized by an increase of all presented definitions of demoralization syndrome.

10.4. Medico-Psychosociospiritual Care

We (Sidorov, Sovershaeva 2015) have proposed a program of medico-psychosociospiritual care for patients with PU based on the synergetic concept of PU development. The program includes four blocks: medical and psychological, social and spiritual and moral (Table 10.2).

The synergetic concept of the disease development enables to establish the organization of primary preventive measures already in a predisposition fractal (ulcerogenic family), where special measures are aimed at identifying the genetic, psychophysiological predisposition and harmonization of social, psychological, spiritual and moral aspects of family relationships.

Activities during the latent fractal are aimed at identifying pathologic physiological responses, at correction of personal socialization and premorbid features. Diagnosis of pathologic physiological responses should involve the examination of patients' gastrointestinal complaints as well as disturbances in the moral individual socialization and the premorbid personality traits.

The initial fractal presupposes pharmacological and non-pharmacological treatment as a preventive measure for PU in the case of the preulcerous state. The primary prevention strategy (healthy lifestyle, giving up bad habits and prevention of demoralization syndrome) is needed.

Early qualified medical, psychological, social, spiritual and moral care is required in the fractal of a full-scale clinical picture.

The main clinical symptom of acute PU is abdominal pain, which can radiate to the left side of the chest and left shoulder blade, thoracic or lumbar spine. Functional dyspepsia may also accompany the clinical picture of PU. Following symptoms are not rare: acid reflux, heartburn, nausea, vomiting, and constipation.

Acidic gastric content vomiting is a typical symptom.

Radiological and endoscopic methods are the main methods in diagnostics of PU. The search for Helicobacter pylori in gastric mucosa is of great importance in order to choose the further treatment strategy.

Different studies suggest that the development of PU may be prevented by influence on the modifiable risk factors.

Table 10.2. Program of medico-psychosociospiritual care for patients with peptic ulcer

Blocks	Prenosological fractals			Nosological fractals		
	Predisposition: ulcerogenic family	Latent: ulcerogenic diathesis	Initial: preulcerous state	Full-scale clinical picture of PU/ mental epidemic	Chronization: forms and types of PU course /destructive mental epidemic	Outcome: somato-neurological complications/ pandemic
Medical	Inclusion of persons with hereditary PU predisposition in the risk group and their early preventive screening	Identification of persons inclined to pathological physiological reactions	Diagnosis of acute and chronic gastritis and duodenitis during periodic health examination; pharmacological and nonpharmacological intervention	Clinical diagnosis, administration of medical treatment, prevention of complications	Control of the somatic state; adequate medical therapy; prevention of complications	Treatment of physical and mental complications
Psychological	Identification of persons with specific psycho-physiological characteristics and their inclusion in the risk group	Correction of premorbid personality characteristics, escalation of stress resistance	Correction of psychosomatic reactions, psychotherapy	Correction of disorders, psychotherapy, psycho-pharmacotherapy	Correction of psychosomatic disorders, psychotherapy, psycho-pharmacotherapy	Psychological rehabilitation
Social	Identification and correction of disharmonies in family relationships	Correction of family relations and harmonization of personality socialization	Harmonisation of significant social relations	Adaptation to the disease, correction of interpersonal problems	Professional and family adaptation	Social rehabilitation
Spiritual and moral	Screening and correction of the moral climate in family	Correction of formation and development of the moral feelings	Correction of the moral image formation	Reconstruction of a moral position	Reconstruction of moral behavior	Spiritual and moral rehabilitation

Principles of acute phase treatment mean to inform the patient about his or her disease, to fix the motivation to comply with diet, healthy lifestyle and to adhere to treatment recommendations, as well as patients' education to achieve a partnership in the treatment. It is known that the readiness and willingness of the patient to follow the doctor's prescriptions strictly are the key factors of treatment efficiency.

The basic principles of PU treatment are (Ivashkin 2013):

1) correction of aggressive and/or protective factors;
2) in case of PU disease associated with Helicobacter pylori – eradication is required;
3) treatment with drugs that eliminate dyspeptic and/or neurotic symptoms if necessary;
4) adjustment of medical treatment taking into consideration the concomitant diseases;
5) taking into account the individual characteristics of patients (age, weight, tolerance to various drugs, activity, etc.);
6) taking into account the financial capacity of a hospital and individual patients if treatment is done in outpatient setting.

In case of treating elderly and senile patients suffering from PU disease you should also consider the following additional principles:

1) treatment with medications that improve blood circulation, regeneration and protective mucosal barrier;
2) reduction in conventional drug dosage based on patient age;
3) preferably treatment with fast dissolving drugs for weak patients.

Appropriate treatment to prevent the transition to the next fractal is extremely important in this period.

Taking into consideration somatic and neurological complications in the outcome of PU the patient is provided with medical, social, psychological, spiritual and moral rehabilitation.

The medical block is represented in special manuals of gastroenterology (Ivashkin 2009, 2013) and does not require detailed discussion in the article.

Psychotropic drugs may be introduced to correct comorbid psychiatric disorders. The choice of medicines should be individual taking into account the severity of the PU, complications, comorbidities and tolerability.

The psychological block. Patients suffering from PU disease require psychotherapeutic treatment together with somatotropic therapy. For example, 36% of PU patients need active therapy aimed at correction of mental health and psychosocial factors (Spahn 2002).

There is data about effective use of various methods of psychotherapy for PU patients, such as rational psychotherapy, hypnotherapy, autogenic training and group psychotherapy.

Rational psychotherapy not only improves psycho-emotional state, but contributes to the reduction of vegetative reactions intensity as well as pain. Hypnosuggestive therapy especially at a young age - at the 1st and the 2nd stages of hypnosis, and at maturity – at the 3d stage is effective. Elderly patients have a low effectiveness of hypnotherapy. Patients with duodenal ulcer demonstrate more positive results.

A patient with "neurotic character" "disperses" aggressive emotions contributing to negative attitude from family members and others. This negative reaction increases the patient's desire to express aggression, which forms a "vicious circle." There is a technology of a "constructive dispute" to overcome this problem (Ababkov, Karvasarskyi 2012).

A group pathogenetic therapy is an effective way of psychotherapeutic correction of broken relationships and should be aimed at the development of primarily emotional components of PU patients' relationships.

The need for a group pathogenetic psychotherapy during the complex treatment of PU patients is predetermined by a significant role of psychological factors in the etiopathogenesis of the disease. Particularly this is a distortion of the emotional deprivation in the intrapersonal relationships meaningful to the patient, as well as a distortion of gender-role behavior patterns in the interpersonal interaction that requires effective correction.

The technique of group psychotherapy in the case of PU disease is aimed at restoring broken relationships affecting all the main components of these relationships: cognitive, emotional and behavioral in a psychotherapeutic group (Martens et al. 2010).

A specific feature of psychotherapeutic work with PU patients is the possibility of emotional provocation of the disease exacerbation. This provocation makes it impossible to use special techniques based on the emotional stress in the initial stages. Another feature of patients is their sustainable social status and corresponding to it behavioral patterns that limit the range of self – actualization. This feature provides a kind of "psychological defense" with a tendency to the opposition, critical attitude and mistrust. These features predetermine the psychotherapist's group management.

With the purpose of psychological correction of significant emotional relationships of the PU patients psychotherapeutic work should be aimed at achieving the following objectives:

1) developing emotional interaction – increasing of emotional sensitivity, empathy level, adequacy of the reflection and expression of their emotions and feelings;
2) identifying and analyzing individual psychological problems of each member of a therapeutic group taking into account his or her behavioral and emotional pattern;
3) expanding a range of behavioral patterns to overcome rigid and maladaptive stereotypes and to form an individual effective behavior and emotional response for every person

Specific psychological features of patients with PU should be taken into consideration while working with them. Common factors in psychotherapeutic interaction with PU patients are emotional contact and mutual support of group members; overcoming social exclusion associated with the fixation on the disease; cathartic release of emotions and a corrective emotional experience; providing each other with a feedback and confrontation with their psychological problems; formation of new social skills. 25-30 lessons once a week for 1, 5-2 hours in the out-patient department is the most appropriate method for psychotherapeutic work. The constant work allows patients to realize their psychological problems and apply acquired group communication skills in everyday life (Solovyova 2007).

Thus, different methods of psychotherapy may be implemented for treatment of patients with PU. The methods contribute to improving patients' psychological condition, motivation and mentality, as well as the reduction of severity of somatic symptoms. The methods emphasize the need for their use in combination with medication.

The social block. Supportive therapy is used for PU patients with a passive personality type. When this therapy treats the patient, he/she is to be free to express one's need for dependence without fear of negative evaluation by a physician. If he/she does not hide his/her aggressive impulses with guilty, then he/she will perceive a doctor as a positive figure of a parent and will feel free to speak about masked fears. Thus, there will be an opportunity to verbalize the socio-psychological conflict and discuss problems rationally. Family involving in the therapeutic process enhances the effectiveness of social therapy. Family confrontation is used for this purpose. A sick person often becomes «a carrier» of family conflicts in the integral family structure. Involving family in the therapeutic process is also valuable because the PU history often burdens patients. Relationships with a partner or children are a source of multiple conflicts. Family confrontation also helps to prevent social and psychological «inheritance» of ulcer disease. This is true because elimination of the difficulties in understanding and intrafamily conflict can prevent the typical for a PU patient early interaction disturbance for children in future generations.

Family and social therapy in the case of "tyrannical patient" is aimed at understanding the root of the fear and situations with an extreme range of fear and desire to get away from this experience with the help of tyrannical behavior. The classes should be conducted on the "here and now" principle using gestalt therapy technique. The patient and his family members use the "turncoats" technique. It means that they change their roles from "aggressive" and "tyrannical" to "scared" person. The analyzed social and psychological problem is formed in the parental home of the patient where either both or one of the parents found the desire for domination and suppression. Parents' behavior made children feel fear and introduce further socio-psychological defense reaction in the form of tyranny. Such a tyrannical behavior used to form in the patient's married couple. Family and social therapy should contribute to family members' empathy and an introduction of social interaction alternative standards (Eidemiller 2015). The most effective social therapy is implemented in so–called "Health Schools" (educational programs) for patients with PU.

The spiritual and moral block of the program is implemented on one and the same algorithm for all psychosomatic disorders (chapter 7.3).

Thus, care for patients with PU based on the synergetic methodology of mental medicine contributes to the implementation of the modern biopsychosocialspiritual approach involving multi-disciplinary teams of specialists, including gastroenterologist, psychotherapist, clinical psychologist and specialists in social work and bioethics.

Chapter 11

Bronchial Asthma

11.1. Prevalence of Bronchial Asthma

Bronchial asthma (BA) (from Greek asthma – panting) is a chronic recurrent disease mostly affecting bronchi, resulting in their hyperresponsiveness that is determined by specific (immunological) and\or nonspecific (non-immunological), inborn and\or acquired mechanisms. The main inseparable symptom is asthma attack and\or status asthmaticus arising from bronchial smooth muscles spasm, hypersecretion, dyscrinia and mucous membrane edema.

BA affects people of all ages and comes as a serious medical problem for healthcare throughout the world. Expansion of asthma grows in Russia, as well as in other countries. The recent epidemiological studies show that 4-10% of an entire world population suffers from BA of various severities. In the last 20-30 years, there is a noted severe progression of BA, often leading to death, and there is a clear disease proliferation tendency. Judging by epidemiological studies more than 9% of children and 5% of adult population in Russia demonstrates the symptoms of this disease. However, officially the disease is registered in 1 out of 4-5 patients (Chuchalin 2009).

Regardless, 300 million people do already suffer from asthma and, according to some suggestions, 100 million more will develop it by 2025. Prevalence of BA in Moscow is 6, 4% of men and 6% of women, in St. Petersburg it is 7, 3% of the adult population (Fedoseev 2006). The highest rates are in Moscow and St. Petersburg, and also in Altai region. In these regions, there are pulmonology centers that conduct a planned work on BA epidemiology. Therefore, one can say that the information generated there is objective enough. According to the epidemiological data obtained among the teenage population, the rate of BA is more than 9% (Chuchalin 2008).

Incidence rate, mortality and disability due to BA are observed together with an intensive introduction of new antiasthmatic drugs and rapid development of new treatment methods. Alongside with the common explanations, this fact might also be the consequence of bad ecology, low qualification of medical staff, ill-timed medical assistance, poor communication between medical staff and patients, patients showing insufficient adherence to medical recommendations and lacking the knowledge about their disease.

The increase of BA dictates the interest in early diagnostics and new treatment methods. The complexity of BA pathogenesis, the growing rate of disease forms that are unresponsive to treatment suggests finding a solution to this problem at the junction of interests of various science disciplines.

The financial expenses with regards to asthma are estimated to be higher than those on tuberculosis and HIV\AIDS combined. In the US, the annual financial burden due to asthma is estimated to be 4 billion USD of direct healthcare expenses and indirect ones (lost labor productivity). The volume of healthcare expenses in Great Britain and Australia due to asthma has amounted to 1, 8 billion and 46 billion USD accordingly (Masoli et al. 2004).

11.2. Etiopathogenesis of Bronchial Asthma

BA is a classic example of a multiple-factor disease in which various somatic and psychic, social and spiritual and moral factors interplay. These are all sorts of allergens, some drugs, infections, physical activity, meteorological, professional, endocrinal, psychogenic, social stressful and moral factors.

The current form of BA progression stands out for its severity, resistance to applied treatment, more frequent status asthmaticus, increased disability and mortality rates. To a large extent, this is determined by the fact that BA falls into the group of psychosomatic diseases, because of multiple factors that, intertwining with each other, create complex cause-effect connections.

Bronchial asthma is a chronic persistent inflammatory disease of respiratory passages irrespective of progression's severity. The signs of immune inflammation are found even in the case of mild disease progression, and also during a remission period. The inflammatory process in its turn leads to bronchi hyper-reactivity, obstruction and onset of respiratory symptoms. This thesis is of principle importance for the modern disease concept as it substantiates the need for a long-term, and sometimes even constant basic BA therapy, irrespective of whether the disease is acute or not.

According to many researchers' data, stress factors play an essential role in BA etiopathogenesis (Krasnorouteskaya 2009; Chuchalin 2014). BA is referred to the "classic" psychosomatic diseases (Alexander 2009). During the process of psychosomatic disorders development, it is impossible to point out any one-way vector of mental or somatic influence, as they can only be looked upon in their interconnection (Smulevich 2014). As reported by V. I. Kurpatov and V. V. Titova (2007), the multidisciplinary approach to psychosomatic disorders stems out of the bio-psycho-social model of examination, where the disrupted crucial personal relations lead to "classic" mentally-induced psychosomatic diseases.

To find out the risk factors that are specific to BA, we (Sidorov, Novikova 2014) have conducted a study of 52 patients (35 women and 17 men; the average age is 46.41±2.27 years). The most frequent etiological trigger factor was psychoemotional stress (94.4%). 77.8% of the patients had an infectious allergen, either viral (acute respiratory disease, influenza) or bacterial (pneumonia), before the disease manifestation. 61.1% of them had allergic diseases (allergic dermatitis, Quincke's edema type of reactions, vasomotor rhinitis) prior to the BA manifestation. Nearly half of the patients (44.4%) were hypersensible to atopic allergens (plant pollen, vegetable and animal protein, drugs). Every third patient, before BA developing, was exposed to meteorological and physical factors, some of which include: temperature and air humidity fluctuations, and also atmospheric air fluctuations. It is not a coincidence that the majority of BA patients develop a disease during autumn or spring when the weather is far more unstable. The hereditary predisposition to BA was diagnosed with 1\4 of the patients. Another quarter of patients, before the BA manifestation were exposed to mechanical or chemical factors (acid and alkalis fumes, inorganic dust). For most of the patients, the presence of such allergens was connected to their hazardous labor activity (colourer, welder, cleaner, fuel servicer, work at pulp-and-paper plants and waste treatment facilities). Every tenth patient developed BA after an intensive physical activity.

Conducting a multiple regression analysis we have established a regression equation that allows prognosticating the risk level of developing BA on the basis of risk factors present. The assessment data of patients without any psychosomatic disease was used for creating a regression model. The established regression equation appears as follows:

A = 0.136 + 0.544•stress + 0.189•atopic allergens + 0.253•infectious allergens + 0.275•physical and meteorological factors + 0.255•allergic diseases.

The presence of each attribute was marked by 1 point, absence – by 0 points. The coefficient of multiple regression (R) = 0.908. The equation explains 82.5% (R^2 = 0,825) of dependent variable alternations. All the coefficients are significant at $p \leq 0.009$ level. The model is valid for the age of 16-50. The risk is estimated as low in the value range of 0.136-0.369; 0.370-0.874 – as a medium; 0.875-1.380 – as high.

Tracking, estimation and prognostication of BA risk factors actualization for each patient in the framework of our synergetic biopsychosociospiritual model allows forming controlled and manageable parameters of living style and quality, and personifies the preventive-correctional strategies of mental resilience.

11.3. Synergetics of Bronchial Asthma

The BA dynamics includes the following fractals (Table 11.1): predisposition – asthmogenic family, latent – asthmogenic diathesis, initial – pre-asthma, a full-scale clinical picture – BA, chronization – forms and types of BA course, outcome – somatic BA complications.

The fractal of an *asthmogenic family* is the primary one in BA formation. Therefore, the disrupted family relations might contribute to the development of this pathology.

The psychological factors related to the family may play a certain role in BA manifestation. The main role in BA development is played by a mother, who suppresses her child's emotional expression – shouting, crying and the like – in the early years of life. The parents of BA patients are characterized as reserved in their emotional expression; these parents seek to control and suppress their child's initiative and block unapproved emotional expression (Eidemiller 2015).

Table 11.1. Fractal dynamics of BA mental epidemic development

Vector of ontogenesis	Prenosological fractals			Nosological fractals		
	Predisposition: asthmogenic family	Latent: Asthmogenic diathesis	Initial: preasthma	Full-scale clinical picture of BA/mental epidemic	Chronization: forms and types of BA course/destructive mental epidemic	Outcome: somatoneurological complications/ pandemic
Somatogenesis	Hereditary burden	Tendency to pathological, physiological reactions	Bronchitis, pneumonia, allergic diseases	Bronchial asthma	Forms and types of BA course	Somatic complications
Psychogenesis	Psychophysiological disposition	Premorbid personality traits	Psychosomatic reactions	Somatoform disorders	Psychosomatic disorders	Somatopsychic disorders
Sociogenesis	Disharmony of family relations	Disharmony of personality socialization	Violation of significant social relations	Transient social dysfunction	Social decompensation	Social disadaptation
Animogenesis	Spiritual and moral deficiency or ambivalence in the family	Disharmony of formation of the moral feelings	Deformation of the moral image	Destruction of spiritual and moral position	Probability of immoral acts	Possibility of illegal behavior

The psychodynamic conflict factor that leads to BA is a strong subconscious need for tenderness and protection on the part of a mother or somebody fulfilling her duties. The mother or this somebody should dominate, be caring and perfect, watch at patient's bedside and protect him. If the support is not provided, there comes the BA attack. Some BA children have recovered from the disease in case they had to part with an emotionally cold and indifferent mother (Alexander 2009).

BA teenagers have the following family communication peculiarities that determine a family dysfunction: divorces in generation lines, hyper-normative family members, unexpressed emotions. Having a brother or a sister only complicates family communication, resulting in one sibling marginalizing the other, or self-exclusion out of the conflict zone. "Dominating hyper protection" in the case of BA is a pathologizing type of family upbringing (Biletskaya, Melnikova 2010).

The next fractal is *asthmogenic diathesis*, which is a mental, environmental adaptation disorder or a borderline state that can transform into the disease under the influence of exogenous (stress) and endogenous (genetically-induced abnormalities and so forth) factors. It represents one of the variants of a specific diathesis or a predisposition in the general group of undifferentiated mental diatheses. The psychosomatic diathesis is a set of features describing the predisposition to a corresponding pathology.

Under the influence of exogenous or endogenous risk factors a person with asthmogenic diathesis develops *preasthma.* It can have the form of respiratory passages' mucous membrane vasomotor disorder, acute or chronic bronchitis, pneumonia with the elements of bronchial spasm, vasomotor rhinitis, allergic symptoms (urticaria, Quincke's edema). Under the continuing influence of negative factors, these disorders could, later on, transform into a full-scale clinical picture of BA. Preasthma is the last sign of impending BA.

Under the influence of the risk factors that are specific to BA, this may lead to the development of a *full-scale clinical picture* of primary BA. Apart from the hereditary predisposition, personal somatic state and stress factors, there are other specific and predisposing factors that play a role in BA development, the main of which would be: atopic allergens, infectious allergens, physical and meteorological factors, hormonal disruptions, exposure to chemicals, allergic diseases. Each of them might encourage the development of this disease.

Various forms and types of BA course reflect a multidirectional nature of the disease development. The forms and course characteristics of BA depend on the influence of psychosocial and somatic factors. The progression of the disease could be stable with rare exacerbations, or labile.

There are five degrees of BA course severity: mild and intermittent; mild and persistent; moderately severe and persistent; severe and persistent; severe persistent and steroid-dependent. The establishment of BA diagnosis is performed on the basis of the following data: complaints, clinical symptoms and disease anamnesis, results of physical assessment, the study of external respiratory function, sputum and\or bronchial mucous eosinophilia (obligatory attribute), blood eosinophilia (supplementary attribute), allergic status.

The *somatopsychic complications* of BA include pulmonary complications: pulmonary emphysema, respiratory failure, pulmonary collapse, pneumothorax and others; extrapulmonary: myocardial dystrophy, pulmonary heart, heart failure and others; and also mental disorders of neurotic and psychotic types, being the consequence of a somatic disease influencing the mental sphere. The somatic complications are the result of a long-lasting labile disease course.

The BA patients have neurotic disorders occurring over the mechanism of nosogenies (Smulevich 2011). Among them prevail: the hyperventilation syndrome, anxious phobic reactions, panic disorder, generalized anxiety disorder (Drobishev, Makuh 2007). The more intense the psychoemotional disorders are, the harder is the course of BA (Feldman et al. 2009).

The synergetic theory of the disease formation fits into the current view of a multiple-factor nature of BA.

We shall take a look at each vector of the synergetic BA model.

The somatogenesis of BA in the first fractal implies the presence of a genetic predisposition. The hereditary predisposition is found in 25.4%-46.3% of the patients. Notably, it is more intense in the atopic form. There is a suggestion about the recessive mode of BA inheritance with 50% penetrance (Fedoseev 2006).

In the latent fractal of BA somatogenesis, there is a notable liability to pathological, physiological reactions, which may, for instance, manifest themselves in the form of bronchial spasm due to a stressful situation. At this point, the factors predisposing to developing BA that we have discussed above are very important. We consider preasthma as a functional disorder because it may or may not transit to the stage of primary manifestation. Further on comes the full-scale clinical picture of the primary disease manifestation. The forms and types of BA course depend on the influence of the exogenous and endogenous factors, and that is why there could be a more or less positive progression of the disease, or labile, with frequent exacerbations. The somatic complications are the last fractal of BA somatogenesis, among which we should mention the pulmonary heart disease, myocardial dystrophy and so on.

The BA psychogenesis in the first fractal is presented by a psychophysiological disposition that implies the specific inborn features that may add to the development of a disease. Particularly, we have discovered the following psychophysiological features: weak or medium-weak types of the nervous system, heightened emotions and emotional lability (Sidorov, Novikova 2014).

Along with BA, there is a psychovegetative syndrome being formed, the core of which is the parasympathetic direction of vegetative tone and reactivity, insufficient vegetative supply. These shifts are combined with an excessive uprising nonspecific activation and anxious-hypochondriac changes in the personality structure. Thus, due to BA the formation of the dissociated psychovegetative syndrome takes place when the dysfunction of suprasegmental parts of the vegetative nervous system is characterized by the insufficiency of uprising nonspecific influences coming out of the limbic-reticular structures.

Psychophysiological characteristics determine the intensity of the physiological response to a stressor. The psychophysiological peculiarities noted above can cause a more intense and even pathological stress reaction.

The second fractal of psychogenesis involves the premorbid personal features, among which we should note the high levels of personal anxiety and alexithymia. In the initial period of the disease, there is a possibility of psychosomatic reactions, occurring in the form of complaints about the isolated symptoms in the somatic state. Such disturbances can last from a couple of minutes up to a couple of days and does not disrupt an organ’s functions. The data, suggesting that a neurotic disorder precedes BA in the form of organ neurosis proves this statement.

On further psychological traumatization the psychosomatic reactions transform into the somatoform disorders, which are still functional, but last longer (for more than six months) and are accompanied by multiple, reoccurring and clinically important complaints.

In this fractal, there is also the possibility of nosogenous responses to the firstly discovered disease that manifest themselves in the form of anxious, phobic and depressive symptoms. Later on, there could be a transformation into the psychosomatic disorders that are already chronic and irreversible in nature.

On the stage of forming the neuropsychic mechanism of pathogenesis the hysteria-like and neurasthenia-like reactions are common for the patients with BA. They show the tendency of lowering self-acceptance in their microsocial environment due to the actualized conflict of personal importance. Immediately after the attack, there could be low mood, petulance, irritancy, hyperexcitability, exhaustibility, mood instability, neurasthenic and phobic disorders. The BA patients typically have a high level of reactive and personal anxiety and depression (Ilyashevich 2007).

In the case of severe BA progression, there is a possibility of asthenodepressive, hypochondriac and anxiodepressive symptoms. We have established that BA patients are prone to low mood, body ego fixation and displacement of mentally-traumatizing factors, heightened anxiety, frequent phobias, restraint, low work capacity (Sidorov, Novikova 2014). The somatopsychic disorders, being the mental result of a long-term influence of the disease, appear in the last fractal and mean the outcome.

The chronic and recurrent disease course clearly influences the nature of attitude towards the disease. On the background of relatively high and stable adaptive components of personal reaction to the disease, there is an obvious constantly low mood, anxiety and anticipation of the new asthma attack. The high values on the scale of "anxious" type are combined with close values on the scales of "hypochondriac," "neurasthenic" and "sensitive" types (Vasserman et al. 2011).

The sociogenesis of BA starts with the disharmonious family relations. This disharmony may stem out of one or more types of family relation problems. They are the psychological (openness, trust, care for each other, mutual moral and emotional support), psychophysiological (sexual relations), social (family roles' division, financial dependence, authority, management), cultural (national and religious traditions and customs). All these types of relations influence how a child is brought up in the family. The future disharmonious socialization of a person may appear as the result of disharmonious family relations. The disrupted family relations will be the model for adoption, and that may cause a disharmonious personality formation. Later on, in the adulthood, it could lead to the disrupted crucial social relations acting as a stressful factor. Transient social dysfunctions connected with the necessity to change lifestyle may appear in the fractal of a full-scale clinical picture of BA. The severe BA progression could cause social decompensation in the form of disrupted family, professional and other social relations. The outcome of the disease brings social disadaptation due to work incapacity, loss of social status, professional and personal perspectives.

Inability to participate in social relations according to the patients' age and socio-economic status should be considered as the worst possible outcome of BA. Anxious anticipation of attacks and vital threat constantly frustrates patients, disadapts them socially and bars from building up family relations and plans for future life. Obsessive fears and concerns appear attached to the attacks. The disease "swallows" the person. The BA patients have a distinct tendency to overcome the disease. They constantly search for the new and more effective ways of treatment and consult with highly qualified specialists.

The BA animogenesis starts in the predisposition fractal with the spiritual and moral disharmony, deficiency or ambivalence of the family relations that create a conscious or unconscious psychoemotional tension.

The latent fractal of asthmogenic diathesis is represented by disharmonious and dischronous formation and development of the main moral attitudes: credence and responsibility, conscience and duty, honor and dignity. This appears in the form of impaired and disrupted moral socialization and personal development at any age.

In the initial preasthma fractal, there are obvious early deformations of the moral image, occurring in the form of restraint and patience insufficiency, as well as insufficiency of humanism and mercy, modesty and tact. Going forward, these develop into the demoralization syndrome, the clinical picture of which in each concrete case and fractal is formed and supplemented by the co-morbid and associated disorders in bio-, psycho- and sociogenesis.

The fractal of a full-scale clinical picture of BA represents a destructed spiritual and moral attitude, meaning the lowering ability to tell good from evil, to display friendship and love, lowering resistance and a possible refusal to fight and continuingly overcome hardships that are related to BA in the patient's perception.

The fractals of BA chronization and outcome are characterized by the further accumulation of all the aspects of the demoralization syndrome and the appearing risk of immoral and unlawful behavior.

11.4. Medico-Psychosociospiritual Care

On the basis of the synergetic methodology of BA development, we (Sidorov, Sovershaeva 2015) have worked out the program of care that includes four blocks: medical and psychological, social and spiritual and moral (Table 11.2).

The synergetic theory of the disease formation substantiates the organization of the primary preventive measures in the predisposition fractal (asthmogenic family) already that are aimed at identifying the hereditary, psychophysiological predisposition and at ethical-psychological harmonization of family relations.

In the latent fractal, preventive measures are aimed at identifying the pathological, physiological reactions, personal socialization and premorbid features correction. The diagnostics of pathological, physiological reactions has to be performed in the form of studying the allergic status and respiratory function of the persons that have moral socialization disorders and premorbid personal features.

In the initial fractal, when preasthma – the state preceding BA – has already occurred, there is a need for timely diagnostics and correction of lifestyle and cessation of bad habits, and for correction of the primary complex syndrome of professiongenesis and demoralization.

Table 11.2. Program of medico-psychosociospiritual care for patients with BA

Blocks	Prenosological fractals			Nosological fractals		
	Predisposition: asthmogenic family	Latent: asthmogenic diathesis	Initial: preasthma	Full-scale clinical picture of BA/mental epidemic	Chronization: forms and types of BA course/destructive mental epidemic	Outcome: somatoneurological complications/ pandemic
Medical	Inclusion of persons with hereditary predisposition in the risk group and their early preventive screening	Identification of persons prone to pathological physiological reactions	Diagnosis of allergic diseases, bronchitis and pneumonia with symptoms of bronchial obstruction during preventive examinations; pharmacological and nonpharmacological intervention	Clinical diagnosis, administration of medical treatment, prevention of complications, studying at "Asthma School"	Control of the somatic state; adequate medical therapy, prevention of complications	Treatment of somatic complications
Psychological	Identification of persons with specific psychophysiological peculiarities and their inclusion in the risk group	Correction of premorbid personality characteristics, escalation of stress resistance	Correction of psychosomatic reactions, psychotherapy	Correction of somatoform disorders, psychotherapy, psycho-pharmacotherapy	Correction of psychosomatic disorders, psychotherapy, psycho-pharmacotherapy	Psychological rehabilitation
Social	Identification and correction of disharmonies in family relationships	Correction of family relations and harmonization of personality socialization	Harmonisation of significant social relations	Adaptation to the disease, correction of interpersonal problems	Professional and family adaptation	Social rehabilitation
Spiritual and moral	Screening and correction of the moral climate in family	Correction of formation and development of the moral feelings	Correction of the moral image formation	Reconstruction of a moral position	Reconstruction of moral behavior	Spiritual and moral rehabilitation

On the instance of allergic diseases, for the purpose of BA prevention, it is suggested to use drug-induced and drug-free treatment. There is a noted possibility of using desensitizing therapy for BA prevention. The program of primary prevention is considered to be a strategic direction in fighting BA. Having said that, at this point, the implementation of this project is only of scientific nature. The peptide derived from Mycobacteria vaccae is used for the primary BA prevention. It possesses a high immune-modulating property, which allows preventing neonatal allergic reactions. This study needs acquiring the long-term data.

In the fractal of a full-scale clinical picture of BA, there is a need for early and efficient medical and psychological, social and spiritual and moral care.

First of all, the measures are taken to exclude the influence of any given allergen on the patient's organism. For instance, the avoidance of contacts with plants during their blossom period, the use of the so-called special elimination diets in the case of food allergy, stable employment in the case of professional allergy, and others). On the identification of patient's reaction to certain allergens, a specific hyposensitization could be performed to decrease the organism reaction to a given allergen.

During this period, it is very important to give an adequate treatment in order not to let the disease move to the next fractal. The therapy must be performed according to the recommendation presented in GINA, taking into account the severity of the disease when the patient is stable.

The treatment of BA is realized through the step-by-step approach, where the therapy's intensity increases in accordance with increasing severity of BA. The goal of this step-by-step approach is to achieve control over BA, but using the least possible number of drugs. The volume and dosage frequency increases if the BA progression gets worse, and decreases if the progression gets under control. The transition from one step to another is possible only on the basis of a successful control over BA during three months (Chuchalin 2009).

In the outcome stage of BA, due to the developed somatopsychic complications, the patients go through medical and social, psychological and spiritual and moral rehabilitation of patients.

The medical block of the program is presented in the pulmonary guidelines and does not require a special discussion in the framework of this article (Fedoseev 2006; Chuchalin 2009). Anxiolytics, antidepressants and nootropics gained widespread use for the purpose of correcting the co-morbid mental disorders in the psychoemotional sphere predominantly (hypochondria, depression, high level of anxiety, nosophobia and others) (Smulevich 2011).

The psychological block of the program. The introduction of psychotherapy into the system of medical-rehabilitative measures regarding BA facilitates the improvement of the patient's somatic state. Moreover, it contributes to the prevention of exacerbations, because the reconstruction of patients' disrupted relations and proper social functioning is an important segment of the chain of distress prevention that often plays a significant role in BA manifestation and course. There are various methods of psychotherapy that are being used for this purpose: hypnotherapy, autogenic training, rational psychotherapy, group psychotherapy.

The correction of disorders in the framework of family psychotherapy should be performed in two directions. The first considers the development and intensification of emotional communications in the family using nonverbal techniques. The second touches upon situational role play in the aspect of behavioral family psychotherapy on the following matters: "request," "demand," "gratitude" and others, which are discussed later on. Such psychotherapy, implemented in combination with the other treatment procedures, leads to better control of disease progression and a significant cut in the number of bronchial spasm attacks, as well as to the reduction of nervous-psychic mechanisms of pathogenesis in 92.1% of BA patients (Ababkov, Karvasarskyi 2012).

Together with somatotropic treatment BA patients should receive adequate psychotherapy, the choice of types and forms of which depends on the peculiarities of the disease course and a patient's personality.

The social block of the program. Informing the BA patients about their disease is of particular relevance. The regular group education at "Asthma School," partner-like doctor—patient relations, patients' adherence to the medical recommendations come as a new form of social help.

The spiritual and moral block of the program is implemented through the same algorithms for all psychosomatic disorders (chapter 7.3).

Thus, the synergetic methodology of BA mental medicine allows organizing the earliest possible disease prevention on the prenosological level already and, in the case of manifestation, early complex treatment with the help of a multidisciplinary brigade of specialists: pulmonologist, psychotherapist, clinical psychologist, social work and bioethics specialists.

Chapter 12

Diabetes Mellitus

12.1. Prevalence of Diabetes Mellitus

Diabetes (DM) is a burning medical-social epidemic of the contemporary world. At the maximum level of generalization, it can be considered as a hedonistic mental trap of "dolce vita" of the consumer society.

Diabetes mellitus is one of the most pressing health and social problems, which has acquired epidemic proportions among all non-communicable diseases in the world. Pandemic DM characteristics make it a civilizational challenge for all countries – both industrialized and developing.

During the last 30-40 years, there has been a significant increase in the incidence of diabetes, especially in industrialized countries where diabetes affects 6-10% of the population. The incidence of diabetes is doubling every 10-15 years, assuming the character of an infectious pandemic. According to the World Health Organization (WHO) currently in the world there are 285 million patients with diabetes, and by 2025, their number will be 380 million, and 435 million by 2030. On the 01.01.2010 Russia registered the figure of 3.121.318 patients with diabetes. It made 2156 patients for 100 thousand people, of whom 297.794 – patients with diabetes mellitus type 1 (DM1) and 2.823.524 – patients with diabetes mellitus type 2 (DM2) (Ametov 2009; Dedov, Shestakova 2011).

Diabetes is the most common endocrine disorder. In most countries, diabetes takes 3-4 place in the overall mortality structure (after cardiovascular diseases and malignant tumors), being a leading cause of blindness and visual impairment in the adult population. About half of cases are between the ages of 40-60 years, but However, quite often the disease touches young adults as well.

Since 1988, WHO has been collecting standardized information on the prevalence of diabetes and impaired glucose tolerance (IGT) among the population of the world. In populations of Caucasoid origin indicators of diabetes and IGT are in the range of 3-10% and 3-15%, respectively. The incidence of diabetes in Switzerland is 1, 19%, in France – 1.3%, in Belgium – 1.64%, in Sweden – 1.7%, and in Italy – 2.2%. In Finland DM1 occurs 50 times more frequently than in China and Korea. In European countries, 2-5% of the population suffers from DM2.

The above data does not accurately reflect the actual prevalence of diabetes because it does not take into account all the people with a mild form of DM2 that does not require medical treatment, as well as individuals with IGT and impaired fasting glucose (IFG) as the two options of prediabetes. The Third National Health and Nutrition Examination Survey (NHANES III), conducted in the US revealed a high prevalence of undiagnosed DM2 among the population – on average it is 2.7%, and among men and women aged 50-59 – 3.3 and 5.8% respectively.

The incidence of diabetes is increasing annually worldwide by 5-7%. The number of annually recorded new cases of DM1 per 100.000 population in different countries varies considerably. In Finland – 28.6; in Sweden – 22.6; in Norway – 17.6; in the United States – 14.7; in Scotland – 13.8; in Denmark – 13.7; in Canada – 9.0; in the UK – 7.7; in Israel – 4.3; in France – 3.7; in Japan – 0.8. Epidemiological studies on the prevalence of diabetes in Moscow say that the greatest number of patients is observed in the age group of 40-49 years, and the actual prevalence of DM2 in the most working-age population (30-50 years) is 3-4 times higher than the registrable. One person seeking medical advice accounts for 3-4 people with blood glucose 7-15 mmol/l, unaware of their diabetes (Dedov, Balabolkin 2006).

DM leads to early disability and increased mortality among the population, the main cause of which are late vascular complications. Among patients with diabetes death rate from heart diseases and cerebrovascular accidents is 2-3 times higher, blindness occurs ten times more often, nephropathy 12-15 times more often, gangrene with amputation of limbs – 20 times more often than among the population as a whole. Of the 120.000 amputations carried out each year in the United States more than 50% fall on patients with diabetes. Up to 80% of patients diagnosed with DM in childhood, die within 20-30 years after the onset of the disease. All-Russia Association of the Blind by 60-80% consists of patients with diabetes.

Despite the dramatic situation with the course of the disease, achievements in the field of DM and its late complications allow to be optimistic about the possibility of reducing the incidence of DM, prolonging and improving the quality of life of patients with late complications.

12.2. Etiopathogenesis of Diabetes Mellitus

DM is a polygenic multifactorial disease. Mechanisms of development of the pathological process in DM1 and DM2 are different: cell death conditions the leading cause of DM1 disease in islet apparatus resulting from autoimmune reactions that are induced by environmental factors; DM2 is a change in the function of β-cells and the development of insulin resistance.

DM develops as a result of an interaction of different genetic mechanisms and nonspecific environmental factors. In each person, the disease occurs under the influence of combined factors. A significant number of researchers are inclined to the viewpoint that socio-economic factors and disadvantaged living conditions significantly affect the incidence of DM in the population (Ametov 2009).

In the occurrence of DM1 following etiological factors may play a role: genetic predisposition, viral infections, autoimmune disorders, nutrition, emotional stresses, while of DM2: a genetic predisposition, obesity, overeating, emotional stresses.

Regardless of the initiating factors and the primary development mechanisms of DM1 (virus-induced, autoimmune, or slowly progressive) degradation and progressive reduction in the number of β-cells are observed at later stages in the islets of the pancreas, up to their complete disappearance and development of the absolute insulin deficiency.

Genetic predisposition plays a more significant role in DM2. Obesity and pregnancy (gestational DM) can serve as triggers. It is shown that in patients suffering from obesity, weight loss reduces the initial concentration of glucose and insulin in response to a food intake. Patients' turning to excessive eating again is accompanied by hyperglycemia and hyperinsulinemia on an empty stomach, as well as the deterioration of insulin secretion in response to a food intake.

The development of DM2 is conditioned by insulin resistance and dysfunction of b-cells. The ratio of these two components of DM2 pathogenesis varies both in selected populations and among patients of one particular population. However, it is unclear which of these two defects is primary in DM2. One thing is certain – the causes of insulin resistance in DM2 are heterogeneous.

Currently, clinical and experimental studies have shown that one of the reasons for the manifestation of insulin resistance to a greater extent is the glucose toxicity, which is a state of prolonged hyperglycemia. We describe the three main socio-psychological mechanisms that induce alimentary hyperglycemia, leading to the development of DM (Dedov, Shestakova 2011).

1. Intrapersonal conflicts and needs to satisfy oneself compensatory by an act of eating according to the formula: "food – love." Intense appetite and a tendency to obesity lead to stable hyperglycemia, which weakens the functional activity of the islets of Langerhans.
2. When there is a reductionistic identification of food with love, destruction or deformation of the implementation of this emotional affirmation leads to the experience of the state of hunger, which is enhanced regardless of the meal, forming a "hungry" metabolism.
3. Strengthening of stress in modern life style makes hyperglycemic load the easiest means of "escaping from problems" substituting meaningful fight with their causes. At the same time, the sources of psychoemotional tension cannot be removed, while hyperglycemia becomes a factor of addictive behavior, resulting in DM.

Highlighted illusory-compensatory mechanisms of induced hyperglycemia or mental trap of "the sweet life" launch DM mental epidemics.

It is known that attainment of happiness is possible only when you find the meaning of life and incarnate it livingly. Not by chance in the existential analysis of V. Frankl pleasure principle and hedonistic motivation are not related to the normative goal-setting of human aspirations. They are only the result and a side effect of achieving the goal, which structure the meaning of life: .". if there is a reason for happiness, it follows from that place automatically and spontaneously" (Frankl 1990). The hedonistic mental trap of "the sweet life" lies in the fact that making happiness the object of one's desires and aspirations, one inevitably loses sight of the underlying causes of moral values, that create this happiness and happiness escapes. New attempts to extend the illusory joy on the background of hyperglycemic loads lead to self-destructive consequences, launching incurable diabetes.

According to I. L. Andreev, L. N. Nazarova (2014), diabetes should be considered as a complex systemic syndrome, as "a disease of homeostasis" regarding synergetic cooperation of hormonal-humoral and neuropsychiatric regulation systems of human activity. That is why we attempt to build the synergetic biopsychosociospiritual concept of diabetes.

12.3. Synergetics of Diabetes Mellitus

Synergetic model of diabetes formation is shown in Table 12.1.

In DM somatogenesis, the fractal of a *diabetogenic family* is the initial the formation of the disease, as most of the socialization in humans occurs from birth in the family, and the violation of family relationships and distribution of roles may contribute to the formation of this pathology.

Psychological factors associated with the family, interpersonal relationships in the family, the level of emotional acceptance and support can play a role in the occurrence of diabetes. In connection with the traditional trend in the framework of psychodynamic direction, equating food with love, lack of love, leading to the experience of the state of hunger, creates "hunger" metabolism corresponding to the metabolism of DM patients. Violation of the role structure and emotional component of relations in families worsen the condition of patients.

The following is a fractal of *diabetogenic diathesis*. Diabetogenic diathesis is a violation of mental adaptation to the environment or a borderline state which can be transformed into the disease under the influence of exogenous (stress) and endogenous factors (genetically caused anomalies and so on). It represents one of the options of a specific diathesis or predisposition in the common group of undifferentiated mental diatheses.

A person having a diabetogenic diathesis, when exposed to external or internal risk factors, develops IGT (*prediabetes*) – a violation of carbohydrate metabolism, which is a functional and under the further impact of factors from the latent phase may go into a full-scale disease. IGT is diagnosed by an oral glucose tolerance test. The criteria for diagnosis are fasting glycemia (capillary blood) <6.1 mmol/L, glycemia 2 hours after a load of 75g. of glucose ≥7.8 and <11.1 mmol/l. Pre-diabetes also includes IFG, which is also diagnosed after oral glucose tolerance test. The criteria for diagnosis are fasting glycemia (capillary blood) ≥ 5.6, but <6.1 mmol/l, glycemia 2 hours after a load of 75g. of glucose <7.8 mmol/l (Dedov, Shestakova 2011).

The impact of risk factors that are specific to type 1 diabetes and type 2 diabetes may lead to the *development of the clinical picture* of primary diabetes. In the event of diabetes, except for genetic predisposition, the somatic state of a person and stress factors other predisposing factors are highlighted: in type 1 diabetes these are autoimmune disorders, viral infections, toxic effects; in type 2 diabetes – obesity, dyslipidemia, hormonal disorders, excess food. Each of these factors may contribute to the disease. Thus, almost 60% of diabetic patients began the disease soon after a severe psychic trauma, 30% mentioned a long psychic experience (Dedov, Balabolkin 2006).

The next fractal is *different forms and types of DM course*, reflecting multivariate features of the disease development. Features of DM progress and shape depend on the impact of ethical-social and psychosomatic factors. The course of the disease can be stable with occasional aggravations or labile, leading to the rapid development of complications.

Table 12.1. Fractal dynamics of DM mental epidemics development

Vector of ontogenesis	Prenosological fractals			Nosological fractals		
	Predisposition: diabetogenic family	Latent: diabetogenic diathesis	Initial: prediabetes	Full-scale clinical picture of DM/mental epidemic	Chronization: forms and types of DM course/destructive mental epidemic	Outcome: somatoneurological complications/ pandemic
Somatogenesis	Hereditary burden	Tendency to abnormal physiological reactions	IGT and IFG	Diabetes mellitus	Forms and types of diabetes course	Medical complications
Psychogenesis	Psychophysiological disposition	Premorbid personality traits	Psychosomatic reactions	Somatoform disorders	Psychosomatic disorders	Diabetic encephalopathy
Sociogenesis	Disharmony of family relations	Disharmony of personality socialization	Violation of significant social relations	Transient social dysfunction	Social decompensation	Social disadaptation (invalidity)
Animogenesis	Spiritual and moral deficiency or ambivalence in the family	Disharmony of formation of the moral feelings	Deformation of the moral image	Destruction of spiritual and moral position	Probability of immoral acts	Possibility of illegal behavior

The following fractal comprises *somatoneurological complications of diabetes*. These include macro and microvascular somatic complications as well as psychiatric disorders of neurotic and psychotic levels arising out of effect on the psyche that physical illness produces. Somatoneurological complications are the outcome of a long-labile course of the disease.

Changes in personality traits resulting from chronic psychological stress are caused by the awareness of one's severe illness, often – by forced change of profession and disability. These patients have a typical structure of "diabetic type of personality": reduced overall mood, emotional lability, frequent neurotic reactions, indifference, failure to make an independent decision, irritability, sharpening of traits inherent to patients before the disease, asthenic condition (Kaplan, Sadock 1994).

Synergetic concept fits into currently existing view of the autoimmune nature of type 1 diabetes. Thus, at the present moment, 6 stages in the development of type 1 diabetes are distinguished: 1) genetic predisposition due to the presence of gene haplotypes of HLA-system, of the I, II and III classes, as well as other genes associated with type 1 diabetes; 2) impact of various external environmental factors that trigger the beginning of autoimmune processes leading to the development of insulitis; 3) development of immunological disorders; 4) stage of expressed immunological disorders; 5) manifestation of the disease; 6) complete destruction of β-cells.

Let us dwell on the analysis of each of the vectors of a DM synergetic model.

Somatogenesis of diabetes involves hereditary predisposition in the first fractal. In particular, this is confirmed by the results of our (Sidorov, Novikova 2014) 84 polling patients with type 1 diabetes (mean age 30.72 ± 1.44 years), and 91 patients with type 2 DM (mean age 54.22 ± 0.69 years). Diabetes in close relatives was noted in 13.4% of patients with type 1 diabetes and in 27.3% patients with type 2 DM. In the second fractal of diabetes somatogenesis, a tendency to pathological, physiological reactions can be noted that may, for example, manifest in hyperglycemic reactions in stressful situations. In this fractal previously mentioned factors predisposing to the development of diabetes become very important. The third fractal is represented by two forms of prediabetes: IGT and IFG. This state is indicated by us as functional as it cannot go to the stage of a full-scale disease. This is followed by a detailed clinical picture of the primary disease. Forms and types of DM progress are the next fractal in the disease somatogenesis. Depending on the external and internal factors relatively favorable course of a disease is possible or labile, with frequent exacerbations. The final fractal of somatogenesis is medical complications of diabetes, among which it is important to note diabetic retinopathy, nephropathy, neuropathy, diabetic foot syndrome, and others.

Psychogenesis of DM, involving the development of mental disturbances during the formation of the disease, is represented by the same fractals. The first fractal – psychophysiological disposition, supposing the presence of specific innate characteristics that may contribute to the disease development. In particular, we have found the following psychophysiological features of patients: weak or medium-weak unbalanced type of nervous system, high emotionality and emotional instability. The severity of the physiological response to the stressor depends on psycho-physiological characteristics. Reported psychophysiological features can cause a more pronounced pathological reaction to a stressor. The second fractal of psychogenesis comprises premorbid personality traits, among which are high personal anxiety and high level of alexithymia (Koshanskaya 2010). In an initial period of the disease, psychosomatic reactions are possible; they are manifested by single symptoms of the somatic state (increased heart rate, increased blood pressure, changes in the frequency and depth of breathing, sudden muscle weakness, short violations of intestinal habits etc.). The duration of such a disorder can last from a few minutes to several days, not disrupting functions of the body.

With further mental traumatization the transformation of psychosomatic reactions to somatoform disorders takes place and these disorders are also functional, but are more continuing (more than six months) and are accompanied by repeated, multiple and clinically significant complaints. In this fractal nosogenic reactions to the fact of the disease, detected for the first time, are possible, and they are manifested in alarm, phobic and depressive symptoms. In 40% of patients with type 2 diabetes symptoms of depression are observed, and in 30% of patients – symptoms of asthenia. In patients with DM, there is a low stress tolerance, the predominance of destructive ways of coping with stress over the constructive, high personal anxiety, low self-esteem and low level of subjective control (Garganeeva et al. 2007; Starostina et al. 2014).

Further psychosomatic disorders develop, which are already chronic and irreversible. In severe DM asthenodepressive, hypochondriacal and anxious-depressive symptoms may occur (Vinokur, Koshanskaya 2008). In the latest fractal of the disease outcome diabetic encephalopathy occurs, which is a consequence of an impact on the psyche of a current long-term disease that leads to a decrease in elastic-tonic properties of a vascular wall, worsening cerebral circulation. However, organic brain damage in case of DM1 is nonspecific, and there is no interconnection between such damage and the level of glycated hemoglobine, as well as with acute and chronic vascular complications of DM (Starostina et al. 2014).

Sociogenesis of DM that is the development of social roles and relations in the course of the disease includes several fractals. The first fractal is disharmony of family relations. It may be associated with impairment of one or more kinds of family relationships. These are psychological (openness, trust, care for each other, mutual moral and emotional support); psychophysiological (sexual relations); social (distribution of roles, material dependence, authority, leadership), and cultural (national and religious traditions and customs). All these types of relationships affect upbringing of a child in the family. Due to disharmony in family relations disharmony of socialization can further appear. A child learns most of the existing social relations and social roles in the family. Deformed family relationships will be a model for learning and will lead to the formation of personality disharmony. Later this could lead to disruption of important social relationships in the adult state, which will become a stressogenic factor. Under the expanded clinical picture of DM transient, social dysfunctions may appear, associated with the need to change a lifestyle. During a severe course of DM, social decompensation is possible, which manifests itself in violation of family, professional and other social relations. In the outcome of the disease, social disadaptation appears associated with obtaining invalidity, loss of social status, professional and personal perspectives.

Animogenesis of DM begins in a predisposition fractal with moral and spiritual disharmony, deficiency or ambivalence in family relations that create reportable or unreportable psycho-emotional stress. Not by chance, the real or falsely perceived the excess calories often compensate the lack of love or attention as the quickest and most easily accessible attribute of a “sweet (i.e., happy) life.”

Latent fractal of diabetogenic diathesis is represented by disharmony and dischronosis of formation and development of basic moral feelings: faith and responsibility, sense of conscience and duty, honor and dignity. This manifests itself in slowdown and violation of moral socialization and personality development at any age period.

In an initial fractal, the early deformations of moral image become apparent, manifesting itself in the lack of endurance and patience, humanity and mercy, modesty and tact. Further the syndrome of demoralization develops which clinical picture in each specific case and fractal is formed and supplemented by comorbid and associated disorders in somato-, psycho- and sociogenesis.

Fractal of a full-scale clinical picture of DM is manifested in the destruction of spiritual and moral position. The ability to distinguish between good and evil decreases, as well as manifestations of friendly affection and love. There is the reduction in the resistance and a possible rejection of struggle and continuation of the trials of life, conjugated in patient's perception with severe complications of DM.

Fractals of chronization and outcome of DM are characterized by an increase of all manifestations of the syndrome of demoralization and the emergence of the risk of immoral and illegal behavior against the background of diabetic encephalopathy.

Figurative expression of spiritual and moral paradigm of diabetes, as well as of any other psychosomatic disorder can be the words of Clive Lewis: "God whispers to us in our pleasures, speaks in our conscience, but shouts in our pains: it is His megaphone to rouse a deaf world" (cit. Epple 2012). In this context, DM is a version of "moral autism", with the forced or voluntary withdrawal from the productive human moral self-assertion into illusory world of hyperglycemic intoxication by "sweet either life, or death." DM is civilization ailment of a modern "hybrid world" affected by "leprosy" of dehumanization and deethization of public conscience.

Thus, synergetic methodology of mental medicine takes into account all the external and internal factors of both types of DM and allows you to organize the earliest prevention of the disease still at preclinical level.

12.4. Medico-Psychosociospiritual Care

Multidisciplinary program of care for patients includes four blocks: medical, psychological, social and spiritual and moral (Table 12.2).

Synergetic model of diabetes formation requires implementation of multi-disciplinary brigade forms of organization of prevention and correction, treatment and rehabilitation. Preventive and corrective measures are implemented in the first three prenosological fractals, and treatment and rehabilitation – in the three nosological, forming a single multidisciplinary block-modular protocol of care for patients with DM within the synergetic methodology of mental medicine. The brigade includes an endocrinologist, a psychotherapist, a clinical psychologist and a specialist in social work and bioethics (Sidorov, Sovershaeva 2015).

The medical block in the vector of somatogenesis includes care by general practitioners, physicians, endocrinologists, and in case of complications – by narrow specialists (neurologists, ophthalmologists, cardiologists). *The psychological block* of care in the vector of psychogenesis assumes participation of specialists involved in mental health: psychotherapists, clinical psychologists and psychiatrists. *Social care* is provided in the vector of sociogenesis with the participation of specialists of social services. *The spiritual and moral block* in the vector of animogenesis is implemented with the participation of family and reference surrounding in micro social and working environment. Modern methods and forms of education and training of adults are used, coaching and training of personal growth, the participation of consultants of corporate mental health services and ethical committees in cases of threat of destructive professiogenesis (mobbing, bossing, labor disputes and so on). In the case of need for mediation, spiritual mentors of the official Russian confessions, participation of patients' relatives in programs of public organizations, in volunteer and social movements, trade unions and veterans' organizations.

The synergetic concept of formation of disease enables us to justify the organization of primary preventive measures even in a *fractal of predisposition (diabetogenic family),* aimed at identifying the genetic psycho-physiological predisposition and at ethical and psychological harmonization of family relationships.

In the latent fractal measures are aimed at identifying pathological, physiological responses, correction of socialization of personality and premorbid features. Diagnostics of pathological, physiological responses should lie in the determination of the level of glucose in individuals with disorders in the moral socialization of personality and premorbid personality traits.

In the initial fractal in case of IGT and IFG for the prevention of diabetes medication and non-drug interventions are offered, hindering the development of the disease. The package of early intervention includes correction of lifestyle and diet, avoiding harmful habits, conducting nutrition therapy, prevention of symptom complex of destructive professiogenesis and demoralization syndrome.

In the fractal of a full-scale clinical picture of diabetes early qualified medical and psychological care is required, as well as social, spiritual and moral support both in type 1 diabetes, and in type 2 diabetes. Specificity of life situation under DM1 is determined by a sudden onset of the disease at a young age and by its incurability; by the presence of a vital threat connected with the risk of acute hypo- and hyperglycemic states, as well as the by development of late complications; by the risk of disability due to the development of late complications; by the need for strict adherence to the control of the disease; by the risk of lowering a social status due to illness, lack of social protection. In the case of type 2 diabetes reactions to the fact of the disease are more reserved, because it often occurs in adulthood and old age, but it is a chronic incurable disease which requires constant monitoring and self-control, regular treatment that, of course, affect the patient's mind (Vasserman et al. 2011).

Adequate treatment for prevention of complications is very important in *the fractal of chronization.* Existing differences in the mechanisms of pathogenesis of diabetes define approaches to DM drug therapy – replacement therapy under type 1 diabetes and oral hypoglycemic – under type 2. It should be noted that in protected cases of type 2 diabetes and in the event of ineffectiveness of antidiabetic drugs insulin is also used. Other components of treatment, such as diet, physical activity, control and self-control of carbohydrate metabolism, use of antioxidants and drugs aimed at prevention of vascular complications are virtually identical in patients with type 1 diabetes and type 2 diabetes.

In the outcome of a long course of DM with the development of somatoneurological complications patients are provided with medical and social, spiritual and moral and psychological rehabilitation.

The medical block of the program is represented in special guides on endocrinology (Dedov, Shestakova 2011) and does not require a detailed discussion.

Table 12.2. Program of medico-psychosociospiritual care for patients with diabetes mellitus

Blocks	Prenosological fractals			Nosological fractals		
	Predisposition: diabetogenic family	Latent: diabetogenic diathesis	Initial: prediabetes	Full-scale clinical picture of DM/mental epidemic	Chronization: forms and types of DM course/destructive mental epidemic	Outcome: somato-neurological complications/ pandemic
Medical	Inclusion of persons with hereditary predisposition in the risk group and their early preventive screening	Identification of persons inclined to pathological physiological reactions	Diagnosis of impaired glucose tolerance during periodic health examination; pharmacological and nonpharmacological intervention	Clinical diagnosis, administration of medical treatment, prevention of complications	Control of the somatic state; adequate medical therapy	Treatment of physical and mental complications
Psychological	Identification of persons with specific psychophysiological characteristics and their inclusion in the risk group	Correction of premorbid personality characteristics, escalation of stress resistance	Correction of psychosomatic reactions, psychotherapy	Correction of somatoform disorders, psychotherapy, psycho-pharmacotherapy	Correction of psychosomatic disorders, psychotherapy, psycho-pharmacotherapy	Psychological rehabilitation
Social	Identification and correction of disharmonies in family relationships	Correction of family relations and harmonization of personality socialization	Harmonisation of significant social relations	Adaptation to the disease, correction of interpersonal problems	Professional and family adaptation	Social rehabilitation
Spiritual and moral	Screening and correction of the moral climate in family	Correction of formation and development of the moral feelings	Correction of the moral image formation	Reconstruction of a moral position	Reconstruction of moral behavior	Spiritual and moral rehabilitation

The psychological block of the program. The primary goals of psychotherapy for DM are: restructuring of the stereotype of food, development of necessary affirmation on forbidden foods, adaptation to new conditions of life, lifestyle changes, increased psychological roles, awareness of one's possibilities and ways of their implementation, change of attitude towards stressful situations, restoration of personal and social status, building of psychological competence, as well as reduction of blood glucose. Important priorities are: formation of right attitude of the patient towards himself and his disease, restructuring of the internal picture of disease and the development of affirmation on a healthy lifestyle. Correction of psychological disorders in diabetes, normalization of psycho-emotional state, elimination or mitigation of neurotic complications and correction of behavioral disorders are also essential.

In working with patients with diabetes, the following types of psychotherapy are used: suggestive, emotional stress, hypnotherapy, autogenous and emotionally-volitional variety of training, rational, person-centered, using the techniques of group discussion, cognitive-behavioral therapy, gestalt therapy, psychodrama, relaxation, creative therapy of self-expression, positive psychotherapy. Psychotherapy in diabetes should be comprehensive, systemic and can be either individual or in groups, as well as in the form of work with a family.

The peculiarity of psychotherapy for DM is the need to consider the role of emotional stresses, which worsen the disease.

The aim of positive psychotherapy when working with diabetic patients is a change in the patient's perspective and a more distanced and differential attitude towards the existing conflict. Psychosomatic disorders in positive psychotherapy are viewed as one-sided differentiation of basic human capabilities. From the positive side, DM is interpreted as the "ability to impart oneself with one's warmth"; i.e., to compensate the lack of warmth (attention) from others using hyperglycemia), and such an interpretation makes it possible to move from discussion of somatic symptoms only to the patient's life situation as a whole.

For patients with type 1 diabetes and type 2 diabetes specialized psycho-correctional programs are developed and applied, they are carried out in line with the person-centered approach, using group discussion techniques, cognitive-behavioral therapy, gestalt therapy, psychodrama and relaxation.

In the case of mild depressive syndromes, people suffering from DM and their family members at the beginning of the treatment are provided with advice, information, explanations and practical support. In more resistant cases specific methods of psychotherapy can be applied, such as therapy aimed at solving problems, cognitive-behavioral therapy or psychotherapy applied in violation of interpersonal relationships.

The inclusion of diabetic patients in the illness-centered group therapy is justified. Especially effective is family psychotherapy with children and patients with diabetes, because families can have serious difficulties in overcoming the disease and a variety of communication disorders, which sometimes become a cause of DM exacerbations.

During the psychotherapeutic treatment of patients with diabetes an improvement of the psycho-emotional state is marked, as well as reduced internal stress, decrease in anxiety, disappearance of depressive syndrome, reducing the need for help and support from the outside, improving of the socio-psychological competence and lowering of blood glucose.

Psychotherapy in patients with diabetes should be used as a catalyzer for the reorganization of personal styles closely connected to somatic response, as a means of intensification of medical therapy and as an effective way to improve the quality of life and to improve social and psychological functioning.

The social block of the program to a large extent is represented by training in the "School of diabetes." In the groups, there is a friendly atmosphere of "round table," where anyone can comment on the proposed topic: nature and manifestations of the disease, insulin therapy, physical activity in diabetes, vascular complications, pregnancy problems and diabetes. Successful implementation of the training program depends largely on the stage of the disease and intellectual capacity of a patient; on such characteristics of conducting activities as simplicity, credibility, visibility; on the financial capacity of a patient, determining the acquisition of assets of self-monitoring equipment; on a variety of motivational factors. During the training, it is important to align external and internal pictures of the disease, which allows a patient to have a more responsible attitude to the disease.

Education of patients in the "School of diabetes" convinces them of the need for self-monitoring of glucose, proper diet and insulin treatment, and forms a kind of "acceptor of an action result" (Atamanov 2007).

The shift of the locus of control on the internal side and improvement of therapeutical compliance contribute to diabetes compensation. It is important to teach patients to variate control and therapeutic regimens independently in accordance with the actual level of glycemia, physical activity, the presence of concomitant diseases and peculiarities of life. Adaptation of patients with diabetes to chronic course of the disease is possible with activation of one's personal resources to develop active life position, to correct value orientations, to change the system of relationships with others and to remove emotional intensity associated with the disease (Koshanskaya 2010).

The spiritual and moral block of the program is implemented on the same algorithms for all psychosomatic disorders.

Thus, the synergetic methodology of mental medicine in diabetes allows ensuring high efficiency at the expense of a multidisciplinary team (endocrinologist, psychotherapist, clinical psychologist and specialists in social work and bioethics), as well as of cumulative, resonant and coherent mechanisms. This includes the adaptive management of the patient's conscience and health, destabilization of stable pathological state, activation of the body reserves and resources of the individual, restoring and harmonizing the structural and functional systems of life. These processes are fulfilled in the course of multichannel and multimodal preventive and corrective, treatment and rehabilitation impact taking into account the effect of biogenetic, socio-psychological and spiritual moral factors. Such multidisciplinary programs form the basis of *personalized sanogenetic therapy*. Sanogenetic therapy is one of the tools of mental medicine. Essentially, mental medicine is the development of mental health in the health-oriented field and in the nosocentric field. It is the development of mental illnesses (psychiatry, psychosomatic medicine) of the modern concept of a personalized (individualized) medicine (Dedov 2012; Ushakov, Bogomolov 2014), that reveals the potential and adaptability of the human body, increasing the duration and improving the quality of active life.

Chapter 13

Oncological Diseases

13.1. Prevalence of Oncological Diseases

Oncological diseases (OD) keep its place in the top leading causes of death and disability. As a rule, they predominantly affect the most economically active part of the population, leading to substantial financial damage and loss of qualified workforce. OD are a group of polygenic diseases, and their incidence relies greatly on demographic and environmental factors. That is why the actual task is conceptual and methodological substantiation of the synergetic biopsychosociospiritual concept of OD and a multidisciplinary care program.

13.2. Stress and Cancer Pathology

The connection between the risk of OD development and stress has been demonstrated in various studies. It has been noted that the beginning of tumor growth is often preceded by a life full of stress, especially with a sense of loneliness and loss, which is typical for cervical cancer, leukemias and lymphomas. The beginning of bladder cancer is preceded by a period of slowly developing negative events. Numerous studies attempt to determine the connection between personality features and cancer susceptibility. It has been noted that patients with lung cancer are less able to release their emotions, they do not tend to quick expression of their emotions. Other researchers believe that patients with OD overuse their protective mechanisms of denial and regression. Psychosocial factors play an important role in mediating immunological mechanisms of predisposition to tumors and neoplastic development (Moiseenko, Chulkova 2007; Chissov, Davydov 2014).

A major meta-analysis based on 165 studies has shown that stress-mediated psychological factors are associated with a higher incidence of tumors in a healthy population. Severe life events, sensitivity to stress, negative emotional reactions, and low quality of life are associated with a higher incidence of OD, as well as with a lower survival rate. The study has also shown that psychological factors are associated with a higher incidence of lung cancer and with an unfavorable prognosis for breast, lung, head, neck, and hepatobiliary cancer, for leukemias and lymphomas (Chida et al. 2008).

There is a link between personality and the onset of cancer or resistance to the disease. The risk of cancer is associated with such personality characteristics as emotional instability, extroversion, suppression of feelings, depression and loss of hope. Anxiety and neuroticism protect against tumor diseases. Acute stress, which reduces the efficiency of the immune system, contributes to the development of cancer. Increased levels of corticosteroids, which are typical for depression, result in impaired cellular immunity and promote the development of tumors. On the contrary, corticosteroid hormones, associated with anxiety and neuroticism, contribute to the reinforcement of host defenses. Individual differences and genetic factors may have a significant impact on the manifestation of the corresponding indicators.

Depression contributes to the onset of OD. Psychological factors «pave the way» for the development of cancer. According to P. Revidi, breast cancer is often a "passive suicide" resulting from feelings of guilt and depression. Among the etiological factors of breast cancer one can name emotional restraint, as well as the suppression of sexual instincts. Insomnia, lack of self-confidence, psychic traumas can lead to the development of cancer within a period from 1 to 15 years. OD may be considered as the result of adaptation to stress and immunosuppression. Breast cancer is often preceded by a chronic depression and dysphoria. These patients are more often childfree and have inhibited sexual desire (Sidorov, Velikolug 2006).

In adults, OD manifest the loss of hope to achieve one's goals in life, as well as problems related to sexuality, marriage and motherhood.

The specificity of psychological phenomena and psychopathological disorders, associated with OD of different localization has been studied for many years. For example, it has been found that patients with lung cancer have a long latent painful period and the absence of certain neuro-psychic phenomena. Afterward, patients rapidly develop a sense of anxiety, fear and apathy. Patients with exophytic cervical cancer describe a feeling of suddenly getting older. Hepatobiliary cancer is accompanied by oneiric and hypnagogic phenomena while gastrointestinal tumors are more often associated with enduring hypochondriac attitudes (Pitceathly et al. 2013).

Psychogenic reactions are observed in women who suffered from neurosis and vegetal instability in the past. Along with anxiety-depressive syndrome and low mood, the main trauma is the feeling of losing one's attractiveness and fear of the breakdown of their family.

Severe psychological stress accompanies breast cancer. Such patients feel as if they have lost their femininity and, as a result, see themselves deficient and inferior. The patient experiences a threat to life and fears possible social exclusion. Each of these patients has to deal with the challenge of adapting to a new situation and forming an adequate attitude to health. OD lead to changes in attitude to life, which transform a patient's motivational sphere. The main sense-making motive on the diagnostic stage is survival; for the preoperative stage, this is saving health and survival; for the postoperative – social survival; for the late stages of treatment - social rehabilitation of the patient. A patient's awareness of OD is mediated by the attitude of social microenvironment towards the disease. Inappropriate relationships tend to result in the disruption of social connections and contacts, advantage by illness and isolation. An important role is played by sexual dysfunctions in case of genital tumors and after radical surgery of such tumors.

Psychic overload, which forms the basis of psychoimmunologic dysfunctions in the processing of emotional stress, in combination with personal characteristics, develop the psychosomatic factors in the etiology of cancer. It has been established that emotionally significant, stressful life events and an insufficient overcoming of the internal conflict have an impact on the immune system. Carcinogens and psychosocial factors have a synergistic relationship: they complement and reinforce each other.

13.3. Synergetics of Oncological Diseases

The synergetic model of OD formation is presented in Table 13.1.

The fractal of an *oncogenic family* is the initial in the OD formation. Disrupted family relationships and dysfunctional family roles may contribute to the formation of this pathology.

The term "*cancerous family*" was introduced in 1913. Napoleon's family was listed among "cancerous families." Many generations of ancestors and descendants of the French emperor died of gastrointestinal cancer. They became a classic example of a "cancerous family", which is included in all course books on oncogenetics (Akulenko, Ugarov 2011).

The following is the fractal of *oncogenic diathesis*, which involves dysfunctional mental adaptation to the environment or a borderline state, which can transform into OD under the influence of exogenous (stress) and/or endogenous (genetic anomalies) factors. It is one of specific diathesis, or predisposition, in a common group of undifferentiated mental diathesis.

When a person who has oncogenic diathesis is exposed to external or internal risk factors, precancerous states develop. For example, a precancerous disease of the gastrointestinal tract includes three components. The first is a *pre-cancerous disease* of the stomach (atrophic gastritis, hyperplastic gastritis, untreated gastric ulcers, stomach polyps, especially multiple, hypertrophic gastritis). The second is a precancerous intestinal disease (polyps of small and large intestine, especially multiple, ulcers and pseudopolyps in cases of ulcerative colitis, persistent inflammation of the colon — proctitis and anal fissures). The third component is a pre-cancerous pancreatic disease (pancreatic adenoma, cysts, chronic pancreatitis).

Later, the impact of specific OD risk factors may lead to the development of a clinical picture of a *primary* OD.

Risk factors of OD development include chronic stress, negative emotions, depression; smoking; eating disorders; contact with carcinogens (arsenic, asbestos, dioxins, heavy metals, polyvinyl chloride, etc.); radiation exposure.

Different *forms and types* of the OD course reflect the multivariate specifics of the disease development. Types and forms of OD depend on the impact of psychological, social, ethical and somatic factors. The disease can progress slowly or rapidly, in the latter case, leading to the outcome within a short time.

Somatoneurological complications of OD include somatic complications, as well as psychic disorders of neurotic and psychotic levels that result from the impact of physical illness on the psyche. Somatoneurological complications result from a long-term course of OD.

We are going to focus on each of the vectors of the synergetic model of OD.

Somatogenesis of cancer presupposes in the first fractal the presence of hereditary predisposition.

There are about 50 recognized hereditary forms of cancer. These forms may also be non-hereditary, but sporadic. Highly penetrant mutations that demonstrate Mendelian inheritance cause strong genetic predisposition to OD. In such cases, the disease tends to emerge at a younger age than the sporadic forms. There are various forms of hereditary cancers known: carcinomas of different localization, neuroblastomas, neurofibromatosis, multiple endocrine neoplasias (Chissov, Davydov 2014).

A tendency to develop pathological, physiological reactions in stressful situations can be noted in the latent fractal of OD somatogenesis.

We have classified premorbid disturbances as a functional disorder, as it may not lead to the next stage of a full-scale clinical picture of the OD.

The course of OD depends on the impact of external and internal factors, and, therefore, it can be relatively favorable or labile, with frequent exacerbations. The final fractal of OD somatogenesis is cancer stage IV.

Psychogenesis of OD in the first fractal is presented by psychophysiological disposition, which suggests the presence of specific inherent characteristics that may contribute to the development of the disease. Premorbid personality traits characterize the second fractal of psychogenesis. Among them are emotional lability, extraversion, excessive suppression of feelings, as well as depression and hopelessness.

Possible psychosomatic reactions may characterize the initial period of OD manifested as somatic symptoms, with the duration from a few minutes to a few days and without dysfunctions of the organ. Further mental traumatization results in the transformation of psychosomatic reactions into somatoform disorders, which are also functional, but continue for a longer period (more than six months) and are accompanied by repeated, multiple and clinically significant complaints. This fractal can also be characterized by nosogenic reactions to the fact of the diagnosis with OD, which are manifested by anxiety, as well as asthenic, phobic and depressive symptoms.

The prevalence of nosogenic reactions in cancer patients varies widely, from 20 to 100%. Nosogenic manifestations in cancer patients have a complex syndromic structure that reflects the "double" type of reaction with different proportions of anxiodepressive and dissociative disorders. Nosogenic reactions differ among various forms of cancer pathology. For example, the dominating type of nosogenic reactions in patients with gastric cancer is dissociative with mild symptoms of latent anxiety, while in cases of uterine and ovarian cancer nosogenic affective reactions are predominate (Wise et al. 2013).

In future, the state may progress into psychosomatic disorders, which are chronic and irreversible.

In the last fractal, which refers to the outcome of the disease, somatopsychic disorders emerge, which are caused by the impact of the long-lasting OD on the psyche.

In the last fractal of the disease outcome astenodepressive states (41.2% of all reasons for a visit to a doctor), abnormal family climate (31.1%), acute psychotic disorders and fear of death (5.1%) are presented (Smulevich et al. 2015).

Sociogenesis of OD begins with disharmony in family relationships. Disharmony may be associated with the impairment of one or more kinds of family relationships. These are psychological (openness, trust, caring for each other, mutual moral and emotional support), psychophysiological (sexual relationships), social (distribution of roles, material dependence, authority, leadership) and cultural (national and religious traditions and customs). All these types of relationships have an influence on the child's upbringing in the family. The disharmony in the family relations can further result in the disharmony of the person's socialization. Disrupted family relationships become a role model and lead to the disharmony of the child's personality development that in the future can lead to the disruption of significant social relationships in adulthood, which will become a stress-producing factor.

The stage of a full-scale clinical picture of OD may be characterized by temporary social dysfunctions associated with the need to change lifestyle. Social decompensation may develop in cases of a severe course of the disease, manifesting itself in the disturbed family, professional and other social relations. The outcome of the disease is characterized by social disadaptation associated with leaving one's job due to disability, loss of social status, professional and personal prospects.

Animogenesis of OD develops through the same algorithms for all psychosomatic diseases (chapter 8.3).

Thus, the synergetic methodology of mental medicine makes it possible to take systematically into account all the internal and external factors in the development of OD and organize timely preventive and corrective care already in the prenosological fractals.

13.4. Medico-Psychosociospiritual Care

On the basis of the synergetic methodology of mental medicine (Sidorov, Sovershaeva 2015) we have elaborated a multidisciplinary program of care for patients with OD, which consists of four blocks: medical, psychological, spiritual and moral and social (Table 13.2).

Synergetic model of OD development requires the participation of multidisciplinary medical teams for prevention and correction, treatment and rehabilitation. Preventive and corrective measures are implemented in the first three prenosological fractals, whereas treatment and rehabilitation are carried out in the three nosological ones, constituting a single protocol of multidisciplinary personalized care for OD patients. Such multidisciplinary team should include an oncologist, a psychotherapist, a clinical psychologist, a social worker and a specialist in bioethics.

This position is also supported by the authors of the international manual "Psycho-Oncology" (2013), who are all convinced that adequate management for cancer patients can only be provided by a multi-professional brigade, which includes not only oncologists but also psychiatrists, psychologists, psychotherapists and palliative care physicians. Close multidisciplinary integration is only possible within the framework of the methodology of psychosomatic medicine. Which is implemented through the advisory model (consultation-liaison) and is supported by international research, practical and educational projects that promote patients' compliance and adherence and reinforce the links between the patient and his/her family member acting as a caregiver. It is important to recognize the phenomena of demoralization ("feelings of hopelessness and objective incompetence") and depression, which are to be regarded not as "psychologically clear" states but as a reason to conduct timoanaleptic therapy.

The synergetic concept of the disease development enables to organize primary preventive care already in the predisposition fractal, where measures are aimed at identifying genetic and psycho-physiological predisposition, as well as at ethical and psychological harmonization of family relationships.

Table 13.1. Fractal dynamics of OD mental epidemics development

Vector of ontogenesis	Prenosological fractals			Nosological fractals		
	Predisposition: oncogenic family	Latent: oncogenic diathesis	Initial: precancer states	Full-scale clinical picture of OD/mental epidemic	Chronization: forms and types of OD course/destructive mental epidemic	Outcome: somatoneurological complications/ pandemic
Somatogenesis	Hereditary burden	Tendency to abnormal physiological reactions	Premorbid disorders	OD development	Forms and types of a disease course	Medical complications
Psychogenesis	Psychophysiological disposition	Premorbid personality traits	Psychosomatic reactions	Somatoform disorders	Psychosomatic disorders	Somatopsychic disorders
Sociogenesis	Disharmony of family relations	Disharmony of personality socialization	Violation of significant social relations	Transient social dysfunction	Social decompensation	Social disadaptation (invalidity)
Animogenesis	Family spiritual and moral deficiency	Disharmony of formation of the moral feelings	Deformation of the moral image	Destruction of spiritual and moral position	Probability of immoral acts	Possibility of illegal behavior

Table 13.2. Program of medico-psychosociospiritual care for patients with oncological diseases

Blocks	Prenosological fractals			Nosological fractals		
	Predisposition: oncogenic family	Latent: oncogenic diathesis	Initial: precancer states	Full-scale clinical picture of OD/mental epidemic	Chronization: forms and types of OD course/destructive mental epidemic	Outcome: somato-neurological complications/ pandemic
Medical	Inclusion of persons with hereditary predisposition in the risk group and their early preventive screening	Identification of persons inclined to pathological physiological reactions	Diagnostics of premorbid disorders during periodic health examination; pharmacological and nonpharmacological intervention	Diagnosis of OD, administration of therapy, surgical treatment, prevention of complications	Control of the somatic state; adequate medical therapy, prevention of complications	Somatoneurological rehabilitation and/or palliative care
Psychological	Identification of persons with specific psychophysiological characteristics and their inclusion in the risk group	Correction of personality characteristics, escalation of stress resistance	Correction of psychosomatic reactions, psychotherapy	Correction of somatoform disorders, psychotherapy, psycho-pharmacotherapy	Correction of psychosomatic disorders, psychotherapy, psycho-pharmacotherapy	Psychological rehabilitation and/or palliative care
Social	Identification and correction of disharmonies in family relationships	Correction of personality socialization	Harmonisation of significant social relations	Adaptation to the disease, correction of interpersonal problems	Professional and family adaptation	Social rehabilitation and/or palliative care
Spiritual and moral	Screening and correction of the moral climate in family	Correction of formation and development of the moral feelings	Correction of the moral image formation	Reconstruction of a moral position	Reconstruction of moral behavior	Spiritual and moral rehabilitation and/or palliative care

In the latent fractal, the activities are carried out to determine pathological, physiological responses and to correct the person's socialization and premorbid features. Diagnosis of pathological, physiological responses should include the study of the somatic status, existing abnormalities in the moral socialization of a person and premorbid personality characteristics.

Primary prevention of OD includes normalization of diet and lifestyle, fight against smoking, prevention of exposure to carcinogens, increasing the body resistance to harmful factors in apparently healthy people (Bespalov 2001).

In the initial fractal of the development of precancerous states, it is important to provide timely diagnosis and correction, including the prevention of destructive professiogenesis syndrome and demoralization syndrome. Regular periodic health examinations and screening are necessary for the purpose of early detection/prevention of OD.

In the fractal of a full-scale clinical picture of OD, it is necessary to provide qualified care, including medical, psychological, spiritual, moral and social components.

In the case of terminal phase (outcome) of OD, which is accompanied by the development of somatopsychic complications, patients receive palliative care.

The medical block of the program is presented in the practical manuals of oncology (Chissov, Davydov 2014; Wise et al. 2013) and does not require special discussion.

The correction of comorbid psychic disorders can be realized with the use of psychotropic drugs.

For patients with OD, good results in the treatment of various forms of depressive disorders are achieved by using various classes of antidepressants, including tricyclic antidepressants (TCAs), monoamine oxidase inhibitors (MAOIs), selective serotonin reuptake inhibitor (SSRI). The treatment of anxiety and depressive disorders in patients with malignant tumors can include the use of efevelon (venlafaxine) and escitalopram – antidepressants with a clear anxiolytic effect. These medications have favorable tolerability and a high level of safety. Therapy of nosogenic anxiety reactions in cancer patients undergoing treatment in the hospital can be carried out with the use of afobazole (Ivanov 2009; Smulevich 2011).

Diagnostics of mental and psychosomatic disorders, psychopharmacotherapy and teamwork, should be conducted from the perspective of comprehensive categorical and dimensional approach (Biondi, Pasquini 2013). For example, for the treatment of "depression/demoralization" dimension it is proposed to use antidepressants of a tricyclic group - serotonergic, dual-action (venlafaxine, duloxetine, mirtazapine, mianserin). Anxiolytics (mostly benzodiazepine-type) are recommended for correcting disorders of "anxiety/stress" dimension. For disorders of the "irritability/compulsiveness" range, fluoxetine or low doses of amitriptyline or clomipramine are used in combination with psychological intervention. For cutting off "delirium/confusion" disorders, it is recommended to use antipsychotics (low and medium doses of the standard medications like chlorpromazine, haloperidol, or modern ones: risperidone, olanzapine, quetiapine, aripiprazole). In the case of obsessive disorders and hypochondria, serotonergic antidepressants or low/medium doses of clomipramine are recommended.

Due to its depressogenic properties, chemotherapeutic treatment requires the use of antidepressants for preventive purposes. D. Kissane, M. Doolittle (2013) recommend paroxetine and sertraline to prevent depression, which usually develops after administration of interferons in the treatment of melanoma. Serotonin syndrome is regarded as a serious complication of the treatment with antidepressants (monoamine oxidase inhibitors) used in combination with opioids. Attention is paid to hematological side effects of tricyclic antidepressants and some serotonergic ones (fluoxetine, sertraline), which reinforce neutropenia associated with chemotherapy. Additional prescriptions for antidepressants and neuroleptics in oncology are the enhancement of analgesic efficiency (venlafaxine, duloxetine, tricyclic antidepressants). New medicines should deal with hot flushes that occur during hormone therapy in men and women (venlafaxine and mirtazapine). They should reduce nausea and vomiting, normalize appetite and body weight, which prevents cancer cachexia (haloperidol, olanzapine). They should lessen the severity of itching in the case of renal failure or cholestasis (paroxetine, mirtazapine). It is stressed that tamoxifen and irinotecan used in chemotherapy can be safely combined with venlafaxine and mirtazapine, whereas the use of selective serotonin reuptake inhibitors (fluoxetine, paroxetine, sertraline) as a part of combination therapy is undesirable.

The approaches to the use of psychotropic drugs for certain categories (demoralization, tension) are chosen on the basis of some fairly controversial criteria and psychological patterns that cannot be the target symptoms or targets for the prescription of psychotropic drugs. For example, tension may be observed in both delirium syndrome and in anxiety disorders that require different treatment approaches: in the former case, antipsychotic agents are preferable, in the latter – anxiolytics and antidepressants with anxiolytic properties (Myasnikova 2013). The proposed multidimensional medico-psychosociospiritual methodology of mental medicine can dramatically improve individualization and efficiency of any preventive/corrective or treatment and rehabilitation route.

The psychological block of the program. A new group of challenges that psycho-oncology has to deal with is psychotherapeutic support of genetic counseling and detection of predisposition to hereditary forms of cancer, preventative medical and surgical treatment to reduce the risk of the OD (for example, Angelina Jolie). A. Burton-Chase et al. (2013) emphasize that not only identification of cancer in a patient, but even the information that he or she has mutations in certain genes and, therefore, the risk of cancer (e.g., some types of melanoma, breast cancer and ovarian cancer, prostate cancer, colorectal cancer, etc.), can adversely affect the quality of life of the person. In this context, it becomes clear why some relatives of patients with hereditary forms of cancer are reluctant to undergo genetic tests. Correction of such dysfunctional behavior requires more intensive psychological-psychotherapeutic and psychoeducational activity that can reduce the level of anxiety and depression in such potential patients.

The use of behavioral and realistic approaches in psychotherapy is widely known in oncology. The effectiveness of group psychotherapeutic methods is proved in working with patients with cancer pathology to correct psycho-emotional disorders, to manage pain, anxiety, vomiting and other symptoms.

In general, in clinical practice, the predominant approach to medical care for cancer patients is eclectic, including the elements of supportive-expressive grief therapy and existential therapy, as well as psychodynamic, cognitive-behavioral and interpersonal therapy (Levin, Kissane 2007). Cognitive-behavioral therapy is very effective in the case of fear of a recurrence, coping with indecision and behavioral approaches to the treatment of phobias and traumatic symptoms, whereas behavioral therapy is more suitable for coping with changes, a transition to new roles, a new meaning of life and interpersonal relationships. Earlier models of care for OD patients include family therapy aimed at anger management, adaptive coping and resilience.

Various components of verbal, rational and suggestive psychotherapy have to be in harmony with the sense of empathy, a sympathetic attitude, emotional self-possession and ethics. Group therapy can contribute to the development of the realistic personal understanding of the disease, can assist in changing negative attitudes, and help to get rid of depressive mood, reduce personal anxiety and find new positive values and goals.

The work with patients can also include transpersonal approach aimed at the development of psychological and spiritual awareness of the inevitability of death as a reality. The model is based on the juxtaposition of death and on the presumption that the patient has some degree of transpersonal development. Such a development is usually related to the level of awareness and personal view of death, and the ratio between these two aspects can play a major role in psycho-social reality when the patient is experiencing his or her juxtaposition of death.

Various suggestive techniques are widely recommended. The use of hypnosis is very effective for the purpose of relieving pain in the terminal stages of the disease and improving emotional state in case of anxiety and depression, guilt and anger, the fear of death and pain (Sidorov, Velikolug 2006).

The combination of psychotherapy (cognitive therapy aimed at creating an adequate internal picture of the disease and relaxation techniques for relieving emotional stress) and reflexology (laserpuncture, auricular acupuncture, electropuncture) is also effective. Progressive muscle relaxation, work with the direction of mental images and relaxation training with biofeedback may be useful. There is data describing the benefits of music therapy. Music resonates with emotional and life experience and contributes to pain mitigation (Wise et al. 2013).

As a cost-effective strategy, C. Pitceathly et al. (2013) propose the four-level system of psychological and psychotherapeutic support in oncology that exists in the UK. In the first stage, psychological support and assistance are provided by the entire healthcare workers and social workers. The healthcare workers also identify the patients who need psychotherapy and psychiatric care. In the second stage, trained specialists provide psychosocial support with the use of certain methods (group or individual supportive therapy, etc.). In the third stage, if the preceding treatment did not have an effect, assistance is provided by highly qualified professionals — psychologists who have special certificates and had training in specific fields. And finally, the fourth stage is established for patients who need to be monitored and treated by psychotherapists and psychiatrists. The range of psychotherapeutic methods includes cognitive-behavioral, cognitive analytical therapy and hypnotherapy.

Positive psychotherapy is also useful for terminal cancer patients. The hospice patients were found to have positive changes in mental and emotional status, reduction of pain syndrome, improvement of family relationships. In the group of terminal cancer patients, the priority task becomes to provide individual and family psychotherapy, as it is these patients who are most likely to develop mental self-isolation, cutting themselves off from contacts with people around them. If the psychologist and the palliative care physician are aware of the «repertoire» of psychological defenses peculiar to a particular patient, it helps to predict the patient's personal response to the news of the approaching death effectively. It would also be helpful in providing necessary assistance based on the available social support for the patient, the patient's initial spiritual level, socio-cultural context and the remaining time (Stiefel, Krenz 2013).

Therefore, all types of psychotherapy are highly in demand in case of cancer: they can significantly improve patients' emotional state, reduce the symptoms of pain and other physical symptoms associated with the disease, normalize family relationships and improve the quality of life.

The social block of the program. It is very important that OD patients undergo active medical and social rehabilitation. It includes such issues as the selection and administration of painkillers and medications for other syndromes, administration of chemotherapy, hormonotherapy, radiotherapy, and palliative surgery. Several social issues must be taken into account. The patient should be taught to eat, perform the daily hygienic procedures, clean gastro- and tracheostome. Patient household activities and leisure time should also be organized during this period. All the activities related to palliative care and psychosocial rehabilitation have a definite effect, it is possible to extend the life of some of the patients and improve their quality of life.

Family support is an essential and fundamental factor in the rehabilitation of patients with cancer pathology. The role of family relationships increases in cases when cancer patients have psychological problems and mental disorders. Persons receiving chemotherapy require warmer relations in families compared to patients undergoing tumor surgery. The husband's support is essential in cases of mastectomy. It was observed that sexual and aesthetic factors can cause inadequate reactions from the husband and provoke psychogenic mental disorders (Mendelevich 2014).

A priority target for sociotherapy is the patient's family, the process of its adaptation to the disease as "a series of hopes and disappointments." The leading role here belongs to "family resistance" or "family resilience." The family is a dynamic system, affected by numerous factors that may either decrease or increase a family's inherent resistance to the serious disease. Among the various communication styles aimed at reducing tension in the family, L. Bilder (2013) underlines the universality of "active listening." It encourages the patient to be open and willing not to draw the curtain on the "vexed questions" for the fear of "upsetting the loved ones" or hurting them.

One of the possible strategies of psychosocial support for hospice patients and their families is a model based on positive psychotherapy. Psycho-social rehabilitation can be classified into such general areas as work with patients, work with the patients' families, work with employees. The concept of positive psychotherapy considers all the activities of a person as self-actualization in the following areas: "Body/Feelings," "Work/Achievement», "Family/Contacts", "Fantasia/Future." This concept is the basis for the development of a psychosocial rehabilitation program.

The main complaints that make patients seek social and psychological assistance are fear, anxiety and emotional lability, problems with partners and family relations that are changing because of the disease. During the work with patients, the four areas of activity are discussed in relation to specific issues.

Another area of rehabilitation and/or palliative care is working with patients' families. It is important not to lose contact with the family of a deceased patient because this is the time when relatives are very susceptible to depression. Assistance also involves medical consultancy for the families, including the promotion to help patients living nearby, which helps one to rediscover spiritual harmony.

The specifics of the working conditions have a significant impact on the healthcare workers. It is not uncommon that all the burden of emotional support is on their shoulders. Psychoprophylactic care to the employees also constitutes an important area of work.

The positive approach gives opportunities for the most comprehensive and systematic development of rehabilitation routes, which correspond to the patients' urgent psychological, medical and social requirements.

The spiritual and moral block of the program. The ethics of the physician-patient relationship in oncology means that the doctor who informs the patient about the diagnosis has to forecast the patient's reaction, as well as to estimate the needs and expectations of the patient and his/her family. The doctor also has to assist in the development of the best plan of action that provides patient with independence rather than excessive support; the doctor should also recommend some online resources related to the problems of the particular patient and those that help to mobilize adaptive behavioral strategies (Baile, Constantini 2013).

Screening and correction of the moral climate in an oncogenic family is performed in the course of psychological and social family therapy intended to deal with the task of ethical and psychological harmonization of interpersonal relations, spiritual and moral development of the family.

Correction of the formation and development of the basic moral senses and moral character is performed in respect of all the spiritual and moral modalities of personality which may give rise to demoralization syndrome and destructive professiogenesis syndrome, taking into account the patient's individual character traits and his/her micro-environment, co-morbid and associated disorders. As a part of the early intervention and mediation, support is provided in the area of adaptive professiogenesis, prevention of bossing and mobbing, loss of the ethic basis and dehumanization of professional thinking.

Reconstruction of moral position and behavior in cases when demoralization syndrome is already presented requires the use of such resources as social training, coaching and spiritual (religious) practices, therapies that involve creative expression.

The task of spiritual and moral palliative support is to overcome pessimistic-disastrous attitudes.

The effectiveness of dignity therapy is proved. This is a unique short-term form of psychotherapy for terminal patients. This method provides a quick reduction of psychological and moral distress and leads to significant increase of life quality and positive changes in intrafamily relations (Chochinov et al. 2013).

The most studied aspect of demoralization is the stage when the patient goes far beyond the gloom, to an area that is described as "surrender", where loss of meaning and purpose of life can reinforce the longing for death to come sooner along with helplessness and subjective incapacity that accompany this state, (Graudi et al. 2013). Demoralization with the sense of loss of the meaning of life in the period of palliative treatment, after heart transplantation in endocrine disorders, motor neuron diseases or cancer is found in 14-38% of cases (Clarke et al. 2013).

According to the recommendations, the correction of the demoralization syndrome should be performed with existential psychotherapeutic interventions: supportive-expressive, humanistic and meaning-centered (Constantini et al. 2013).

Thus, systematic approach to care for patients with OD within the synergetic methodology of mental medicine makes it possible to arrange this care taking into account individual ethical-psychological and medical-social characteristics of patients. Personalized block-modular protocols and routes make up a unified program for counteracting social oncoepidemics.

Chapter 14

Overweight and Obesity

Overweight and obesity are defined as abnormal condition and an excessive amount of body fat harmful for health. Body mass index (BMI) is the most popular tool to evaluate obesity. The index calculates the ratio of weight in kilograms to height in meters (kg/m^2). According to WHO (2014), BMI: ≥ 25 – overweight; ≥ 30 – obesity. Overweight presupposes 6-14% weight gain, obesity – 15%.

The relevant task is to propose conceptual and methodological basis of the synergetic biopsychosociospiritual concept of obesity and multidisciplinary program to struggle against the mental pandemic of the hedonistic and alimentary destruction of consumer society.

14.1. Prevalence of Overweight and Obesity

According to the WHO approximately 2, 3 billion of adults will have overweight and more than 700 million will suffer from obesity by 2015. In Europe, about 50% of the population has overweight, and 30% suffers from obesity. Overweight raises the risk of arterial hypertension (AH) and diabetes mellitus type 2 (DM2), atherosclerosis and coronary heart disease (CHD), gallstone disease, some types of cancer as well as mental illnesses. Most overweight middle-aged people are 71% more likely to develop dementia after 65 years compared with people with normal weight (Xu et al. 2011).

Obesity reduces life expectancy considerably: on the average from 3-5 years with a slight excessive fat content and up to 15 years with severe obesity. At the same time the number of people suffering from obesity progressively increases (every ten years by 10%). Such a rapid growth is associated with modern lifestyle, demographic, social, cultural and biological reasons (Dedov 2011).

In Russia overweight was diagnosed in 25-30%, obesity – in 15-20% of the population. In some age groups, these figures are significantly higher. For example, 75% of women aged 35-55 years are overweight and about 50% are obese (Butrova, Berkovskaya 2008).

WHO regards obesity as an epidemic. This problem has affected all the social groups regardless of social and professional status, age and sex, residence and nationality.

14.2. Etiopathogenesis of Overweight and Obesity

Obesity refers to polyetiological diseases. Poor diet and decreased physical activity being exogenous factors often contribute to the development of the disease. Nutritional factor (especially fat content in the diet) presents a fundamental importance for the development of all obesity types; others have only minor significance.

Obesity is a multifactorial process. Genetic, metabolic, individual and psychodynamic, spiritual and moral, social and economic, as well as cultural factors, contribute to the development of the disease. Genetic predisposition is recognized to play a great role in the development of obesity.

The pathogenesis of obesity is rather complicated. The main factors creating this pathology can be grouped into 1) genetically determined phenomenon (with a probability of 16% - 85% as regards to BMI); 2) overeating in childhood may form functional and morphological basis for the expression of a genetic phenomenon and the development of obesity as a pathophysiologic process; 3) endocrine dysfunction due to an increase in basal metabolism resulted in irregular eating habits; 4) reduced physical activity contributes to overweight and aggravates obesity (Sidorov et al. 2004).

Lack of protein in the diet that weakens specific dynamic action of food contributes to obesity. Generally, obesity with an equal caloric excess develops faster if breaks between meals are great, and the portions are plentiful. High concentration of insulin is preserved in the organism due to such kind of a diet. Nyctophilia contributes to obesity; it is a shift of feeding activity to late evening. Here we can observe a tendency to disruption of daily rhythms typical for hypothalamic dysfunction.

Specific breaks in a hormonal link between adipose tissue and hypothalamus represent a key mechanism of obesity. Those breaks result in a changing of patient eating behavior, his psychology and lifestyle. The hypothalamus is a central point to regulate homeostasis, specific centers that are in charge of the constant amount of adipose tissue both due to changing the direction of biochemical processes in the body and regulation of appetite.

I. P. Pavlov was the first to express the idea of a "food center" as an automatic regulator of food intake in 1911. He regarded that there was a functional organization of cells sensitive to the degree of stomach fullness and chemical signals providing a food intake control in the cerebral cortex and the lower parts of the central nervous system. Later hunger (appetite) and satiety centers were found respectively in the ventrolateral and ventromedial nucleus of the hypothalamus. The components determining emotional and behavioral correlates of eating are located in the cortical part of a limbic system as well as in amygdala.

The regulation of metabolism and body fat mass includes central and peripheral components. Thus, a central element is a set of hypothalamic hormones divided into lipogenic and lipolytic ones according to their effect. Equilibrium of their antagonistic effects is aimed at maintaining energy homeostasis in the body.

Lipogenic factors include neuropeptide Y, which stimulates feeding behavior, transhypophysial and parahypophysial modulation of some endocrine glands, production of insulin and fat accumulation in adipocytes. Reduction of neuropeptide Y production results in loss of appetite. In these conditions body's energy wasting is reduced to a minimum while lipogenic processes significantly outweigh lipolytic ones. Carbohydrate metabolism considerably contributes to body energy supply. A similar function is performed by orexin – hypothalamic substance that can fully compensate a lack of neuropeptide Y.

Fat mobilization from adipose tissue – lipolysis – is a process with complex multi-stage neuroendocrine regulation. Hormone-sensitive lipase is its key enzyme. It is a substrate to an activating phosphorylation involving c-AMP-sensitive protein kinases. Sympathoadrenal activity increases between meal times and also speeds up lipolysis. Thyroid hormones and adenohypophysis stimulate lipolysis in adipocytes. Hypothalamus hormones like corticotropin releasing factor, melatonin, urocortin and central neurotransmitter – serotonin make the same effect. Increased production of these substances leads to the suppression of hunger centers, activation of the sympathetic nervous system and resulting in increased lipolysis (Zaichik, Churilov 2007).

Adipocytes are essential peripheral regulator of metabolic homeostasis. Adipocytes are active cells secreting various hormones, growth factors and cytokines. Leptin is one of the major hormones of adipose tissue. Leptin production in adipocytes is stimulated by insulin and in a less degree by glucocorticoids and depends on the size of fat cells. Leptin causes satiation and production of inhibitory signals from hunger center, increases thermogenesis, activates noradrenergic lipolysis in adipose tissue.

There is a sort of "addiction" of central receptors of the lipid metabolism to the excessive concentration of peripheral mediators with a constant excess of food intake. Then the organism starts to require a greater amount of leptin and insulin because of increasing sensitivity in the centers of the hypothalamus. All these contribute to deactivation of lipolysis.

Obesity syndrome should be considered as a state of total metabolic resistance to lipolytic effects. Development of insulin and leptin resistance results in abnormal activation of lipogenesis because of reactive hyperinsulinemia.

Obesity promotes the formation of a vicious circle where intake of many nutrients is not balanced with opposite effects of lipogenesis processes. Moreover, nutrients are transformed into a metabolically inert fat mass, and the organism increases food intake in order to provide increasing obesity metabolic requirements. Obesity is often accompanied by the development of insulin resistance resulting in a fall of glucose utilization despite the abnormally high levels of glucose in the blood. Metabolic syndrome is formed in the body of the patient very soon. The syndrome may be one of the major causes of cardiovascular diseases and type 2 diabetes (Dedov, Shestakova 2011).

Obesity can be considered as an outcome of a consumer society hedonistic mental trap called "alimentary happiness." Food poisoning destroys individual and social identity, deforms mentality and marginalizes public conscience, increases the risk of early dementia. Obesity pandemic is one of the arguments that show the exhaustion of the old postindustrial paradigm of social development and the need to strengthen humanitarian and humanistic components of a singular civilizational trend. Spiritual and moral creativity should supplement clear requirements for physical activity. Indeed, the Man becomes obese if his Soul stops working. That is why synergetic biopsychosociospiritual paradigm of individual and social development seems to us the most systematic modern model in opposition to any mental pandemic including obesity.

14.3. Synergetics of Overweight and Obesity

Synergetic model of obesity is presented in Table 14.1.

The fractal of an *adipogenic family* is the initial one in obesity formation because socialization of a person occurs mainly in a family from the early birth. As a result violations of family, relationships may contribute to the formation of the pathology.

Obesity can be caused by those parents who often offer food to their child when he expresses a self-actualization need. Moreover, parents express their love depending on how a child eats. Such a vicious structure of family relationships leads to a lack of "ego strength" causing the break in frustrations. As a result, frustrations should be washed away by "snacking" or food intoxication.

People suffering from obesity are often close to their mothers. The dominance of the mother in a family where the father plays only a subordinate role as well as extreme mother's care may contribute to child's unreadiness for social contacts, and finally it results in fixing the passive and receptive position of the child.

The second fractal is *adipogenic diathesis.* Diathesis (from Greek: diathesis – location) is a constitutional predisposition of the organism to certain diseases due to the inborn characteristics of metabolism, physiological responses, etc.

Adipogenic diathesis is a break in mental body adaptation to the environment or a borderline state which can be transformed into the disease under the influence of exogenous (stress) and endogenous (genetic) factors. It is one of the specific diathesis types or a predisposition in a common group of undifferentiated mental diatheses. *Overweight* is developed in case of adipogenic diathesis under the influence of internal and external risk factors.

The reasons for eating disorders can be the following (Sidorov et al. 2004; Voznesenskaya 2009): genetics and body type (the specifics of cerebral regulation of feeding behavior and fat metabolism, peculiarities of neurotransmitter regulation accompanied by dysfunction of serotonergic systems in brain). Also it can be the traditions (national, family), specific features of upbringing (from early childhood food is perceived as encouragement, reward and relief), underdevelopment or less importance of other motivations. Living in a state of chronic stress and severity of affective states (obese people are more vulnerable, touchy and sensitive than those with normal weight) and personality traits (infantilism and marginalization, psychological immaturity and dependence) can as well contribute to eating disorders.

Oral fixation, oral regression and overvalued attitude to food are among psychodynamic factors. Bulimia may also refer to the factors. In addition, a self-neglect and poor feeding in early childhood sometimes contributes to obesity (Sadock et al. 2007).

Obese patients with their food needs are under greater influence from the outside world as compared to the internal physiological stimuli. Patients do not know when they are hungry. Instead, their appetite is caused by external factors and various forms of ill-being. Patients' desire to eat or sudden severe famine are not connected with the «real» nutritional needs. Patients are likely to regress when face conflicts and personal problems grabbing an opportunity to resolve them with the help of food like in early childhood. Food becomes an illusory-compensatory substitute for unmet emotional needs. Additional risk factors may result in the development of a *clinical picture of primary obesity.*

Table 14.1. Fractal dynamics of obesity mental epidemics development

Vector of ontogenesis	Prenosological fractals			Nosological fractals		
	Predisposition: adipogenic family	Latent: adipogenic diathesis	Initial: overweight	Full-scale clinical picture of obesity/mental epidemic	Chronization: forms and types of obesity course/destructive mental epidemic	Outcome: somatopsychic complications/ pandemic
Somatogenesis	Hereditary burden	Violation of neural processes	Overweight (pre-disease)	Overweight	Forms and types of a disease course	Somatic complications
Psychogenesis	Psychophysiological disposition	Premorbid personality traits	Psychosomatic reactions	Somatoform disorders	Psychosomatic disorders	Somatopsychic disorders
Sociogenesis	Disharmony of family relations	Disharmony of personality socialization	Violation of significant social relations	Transient social dysfunction	Social decompensation	Social disadaptation (disability)
Animogenesis	Spiritual and moral deficiency or ambivalence in the family	Disharmony of formation of the moral feelings	Deformation of the moral image	Destruction of spiritual and moral position	Probability of immoral acts	Possibility of illegal behavior

Different forms and types of obesity course reflect multiple paths of the particular disease development. Types and forms of obesity depend on the impact of psychosocial and physical factors.

Somatopsychic complications of obesity include diseases and syndromes like type 2 diabetes, arterial hypertension, coronary heart disease, anxiety and depressive disorders and others.

Obese patients are 4.5 times more likely to experience arterial hypertension. Sodium retention, an increase in activity of sympathoadrenal and renin-angiotensin-aldosterone system (RAAS), insulin resistance contributes to the risk of arterial hypertension in obese patients.

Coronary heart disease is 2-3 times more prevalent in overweight and obese patients. The incidence of coronary complications is increased by 10% with increasing BMI by 1 unit.

The risk of type 2 diabetes increases by 25% for each unit of BMI. Resistin production in adipose tissue is of great importance, as well as TNF-alpha, adiponectin and production of other substances affecting the sensitivity of peripheral tissues to insulin and cellular mechanisms of glucose utilization.

Obesity is a part of the metabolic syndrome. Criteria: an increase in waist circumference (specific for gender, country and ethnic group); plasma triglycerides ≥1.7 mmol/l (≥150 mg/dl) or receiving drug therapy for hypertriglyceridemia; HDL-C <1.29 mol/l (<40 mg/dl) for men and <1.04 mol/l (<50 mg/dl) for women or receiving drug therapy for reduced HDL-C; BP ≥ 130/85 mmHg or antihypertensive therapy; fasting glucose ≥ 5.6 mmol/l (≥ 100 mg/dl) or receiving drug therapy for hyperglycemia. Any three of these five criteria prove the diagnosis of metabolic syndrome.

Obese patients are 2-2.5 times more likely to experience cholelithiasis. It is associated with a disorder of cholesterol metabolism, change of the physicochemical bile properties and problems with biliary excretion.

Patients with III degree of obesity often suffer from Pickwick syndrome – sleep apnea due to hypoventilation, violation of the respiratory center sensitivity to hypoxia, hypercapnia and pulmonary hypertension (Dedov, Shestakova 2011).

Synergetic concept of the disease formation reflects a modern view of multifactorial nature of obesity. The last one is essentially diathesis of almost all psychosomatic disorders.

We shall focus on each of the vectors of obesity synergetic model.

Somatogenesis in the first fractal implies hereditary predisposition.

Pathological tendency to physiological reactions may be noted in the latent fractal of obesity somatogenesis. We define overweight as a functional disorder because this condition may not transfer to the full scale clinical picture of the disease. Then we have a detailed clinical picture of the 1st case of the disease. Forms and types of obesity course depend on external and internal factors. Medical complications are included in the final fractal of obesity somatogenesis.

Psychogenesis is presented in psychophysiological disposition in the first fractal. It presupposes specific inborn characteristics that may contribute to the development of the disease (a weak, unbalanced type of nervous system, high emotional level and emotional instability).

The severity of physiological response to stressor depends on psycho-physiological characteristics. Mentioned psychophysiological characteristics may cause pathological stress reactions.

Studies show the priority of psychological factors in the genesis of obesity and psychosomatic nature of the disease (Markov 2006; Smulevich 2011). Thus, psychological factors are of great importance for hyperphagic obesity associated with overeating. The study conducted among 10 000 women with clinical signs of alimentary-constitutional obesity (aged 18 - 55), anamnestic analysis of eating behavior has revealed a variety of psychological factors that contribute to hyperphagic responses. 84% of patients responded to the emotional stress by overeating caused by conflicts in the family and at work, displeasure in everyday life. 72% of patients noted increased appetite at the sight of delicious food. 32% of patients noted overeating after drinking alcohol. 20% of patients noted increased appetite after severe physical and mental activity (Rogov, Medvedev 2004).

The second fractal of psychogenesis is known for premorbid personality traits. High personal anxiety and high levels of alexithymia are among them. Psychosomatic reactions are possible in the initial period of the disease. The reactions are presented by individual somatic symptoms, with the disorder duration from a few minutes to a few days and without organ dysfunctions. Functional disturbances in the processes of motivation accompany overweight and obesity. In particular disturbances of the hypothalamic feeding center contribute to characteristic feeding behavior. For the majority of obese patients alternating episodes of increase and decrease in body weight always clearly depend on the extent of mental stress. Overeating during the stress becomes not a sign of hunger, but a means of distraction. Episodes of bulimia during the aggravation of conflict can be considered as a kind of an inadequate form of psychological defense. It becomes real because of the dominant character of a food motivation, stereotypic relief of emotional stress by means of eating and a certain set of personality traits: passivity and suggestibility, dependence and rigidity, tendency to anxiety phenomena and mental infantilism (Voznesenskaya 2009).

There is a transformation of psychosomatic reactions in somatoform disorders with further mental trauma. Disorders are also functional but long-term (more than 6 months) and are accompanied by repeated, multiple and clinically significant complaints.

Nosogenic reactions to the fact of primary disease are also possible in this fractal. The reactions are presented by anxious, phobic and depressive symptoms. In future, a transition to psychosomatic disorders is possible, which already have chronic and irreversible character.

Sociogenesis and *animogenesis* develop through common algorithms for all psychosomatic disorders (chapter 8.3).

Fractal block-modular components of the biopsychosociospiritual dynamic model allow diagnosing and predicting multivariate trajectories of disease development. The synergetic methodology of mental medicine always takes into account all the internal and external factors of obesity pathoplastics and pathokinetics and proposes complex individual preventive, correctional, treatment and rehabilitation measures in the framework of a multidisciplinary program.

14.4. Medico-Psychosociospiritual Care

On the basis of the synergetic methodology of mental medicine, we (Sidorov, Sovershaeva 2015) have developed a multidisciplinary program of care. The program includes four blocks: medical and psychological, social and spiritual and moral (Table 14.2).

Table 14.2. Program of medico-psychosociospiritual care for patients with obesity

Blocks	Prenosological fractals			Nosological fractals		
	Predisposition: adipogenic family	Latent: adipogenic diathesis	Initial: overweight	Full-scale clinical picture of obesity/mental epidemic	Chronization: forms and types of obesity course/ destructive mental epidemic	Outcome: somatopsychic complications/ pandemic
Medical	Inclusion of persons with hereditary predisposition in the risk group and their early preventive screening	Identification of persons prone to overweight	Diagnosis of overweight; pharmacological and nonpharmacological intervention	Clinical diagnosis of overweight, administration of medical treatment, prevention of complications	Control of the somatic state; proper medical treatment, prevention of complications	Treatment of physical and mental obesity complications
Psychological	Identification of with specific psychophysiological characteristics and their inclusion in the risk group	Correction of family relations and personality socialization	Correction of psychosomatic reactions, psychotherapy	Correction of somatoform disorders, psychotherapy, psycho-pharmacotherapy	Correction of psychosomatic disorders, psychotherapy, psycho-pharmacotherapy	Psychological rehabilitation
Social	Identification and correction of disharmonies in family relationships	Correction of family relations and harmonization of personality socialization	Harmonisation of significant social relations	Adaptation to the disease, correction of interpersonal problems	Professional and family adaptation	Social rehabilitation
Spiritual and moral	Screening and correction of the moral climate in family	Correction of formation and development of the moral feelings	Correction of the moral image formation	Reconstruction of a moral position	Reconstruction of moral behavior	Spiritual and moral rehabilitation

Primary preventive activities should be carried out already in a *fractal of predisposition (adipogenic family)* where they are directed at identifying genetic, psychophysiological predisposition, at ethical and psychological harmonization of family relationships.

The latent fractal activities are aimed at identifying individuals who are prone to overweight, at correction of individual moral socialization, premorbid features.

Initial fractal offers pharmacological and nonpharmacological intervention to stop development of the disease in case of overweight.

Fractal of a full-scale clinical picture of obesity requires timely, qualified medical, psychological, spiritual, moral and social care, which is then established as an individual treatment and rehabilitation program.

The medical block of the program is represented in specialized manuals (Sidorov et al. 2004) and does not require a special discussion in this article, aimed at developing the synergetic design of prevention and care programs. Synergistic cascading and cumulative mechanisms demonstrate multiple increases in sanogenetic efficiency, significantly higher than the arithmetic sum of interdisciplinary efforts due to the resonance and coherent adjustment of preventive, corrective, therapeutic and rehabilitation work of the medical brigade.

The psychological block of the program. The inclusion of psychotherapeutic methods in the rehabilitation process for obese patients stems from the concept of psychosomatic nature of the disease.

Psychotherapy in the case of overweight should be aimed at changing dietary behavior patterns, person's adaptation to reduce overweight, changing self-identity, correction of social factors contributing to hyperphagic reactions.

The tasks of psycho-correctional work in case of obesity depend on the age and personality, psychosocial and motivational factors. Psychotherapy should be focused on the role of psychosocial factors in obesity development, adequate mechanisms of mental adaptation, on teaching the patients to be more constructive in their behavior. Much attention should be paid to a motivational sphere of personality during the psychotherapy. Here the patient perceives rational diet not as a limitation but as the only possible and natural diet.

Acquired and recognized skills, changed motives during the psychotherapy, and strong emotions can cause a reduction or suppression of the functional activity of the food center, as well as of other instincts.

Some researchers suggest their original methods of dealing with obesity patients. There is a group technique, which consists of three late-night therapy sessions (total 24 hours), which involves rational, trance and transpersonal psychotherapy, elements of autosuggestion, programming and hypnoanalysis as well as psycho-techniques to reduce appetite. The purpose of the technique is to form new, stable attitude to a body and health, develop dominant on weight loss and further maintenance of the body weight at the level appropriate for psycho-physiological mechanisms (Rogov, Medvedev 2004).

Methods of group behavioral psychotherapy, stress psychotherapy, psychosomatic programming and other methods are used to treat obesity (Sidorov, Novikova 2014)

The patient's awareness of the connection between his personal characteristics and obesity contributes to the success of the therapy as well as to the effectiveness of body weight correction and the long-term results of therapy.

The social block of the program. Treatment and rehabilitation measures for obesity patients are deficient without affecting the psychosocial component of the disease. At the stage of social rehabilitation, the main objectives include improving social adaptation and correction of disturbed social relations. Changed appearance of an obese patient has an adverse impact on his ability to fulfill social functions, especially in the field of communication. Due to the treatment, patients' health and metabolism have improved. Body weight reduces and the appearance changes. However, behavioral patterns stay the same. Methods of group and family social therapy, training and coaching are the most appropriate at this stage. New behavioral and social stereotypes are effectively formed in a variety of schools of health and fitness clubs.

The spiritual and moral block of the program is implemented through common algorithm flop all the psychosomatic disorders (chapter 7.3).

Thus, within the synergetic methodology of mental medicine, medico-psychosociospiritual care for adipogenic patients provides systematic and multidisciplinary, early and effective individual routes of treatment and rehabilitation and organizes prevention campaign of obesity pandemic.

Chapter 15

Rheumatoid Arthritis

15.1. Prevalence of Rheumatoid Arthritis

Rheumatoid arthritis (RA) is a chronic, progressive autoimmune disease that is characterized by synovial inflammation, autoantibody production, cartilage and bone destruction, and systemic features, including cardiovascular, pulmonary, skeletal and also psychological disorders (Nasonov, Nasonova 2010).

The average prevalence of RA in populations of developed countries is 0,5 – 1,0%, and the primary incidence reaches 0,02%. Women get sick more often than men by 2 – 5 times. The disease can occur at any age, but most often it is detected at the age of 40 – 50 years (Folomeeva et al. 2010; Uhlig, Kvien 2005).

RA is associated with systemic complications, progressive disability, early death and socioeconomic costs. On the one hand, the disease is characterized by a high level of painful sensations, functional disorders, and on the other – with serious disorders in the psycho-emotional sphere (Lain et al. 2011).

Various forms and types of the course of RA reflect multivariance of the disease origin. Peculiarities of the RA course depend on the somatic and social, psychological, spiritual and moral factors.

Despite significant advances over the past decade in the study of pathogenesis and approaches to medication, many questions remain open, and the development of the synergetic concept of RA helps to mobilize multidisciplinary resources.

15.2. Etiopathogenesis of Rheumatoid Arthritis

According to modern views, the pathogenesis of RA is comprised of defects of T- and B-cell immune responses that lead to overproduction of some proinflammatory cytokines and a wide range of organ-specific autoantibodies inducing inflammation and destruction of the joints and other tissues of the body (Nasonov et al. 2012).

So far, the etiology of RA remains unknown. The trigger role of a wide range of exogenous (e.g., stress, smoking), infectious (Epstein-Barr virus, parvovirus B19, retroviruses, etc.) and endogenous (citrullinated proteins and peptides) factors, as well as genetic factors in disease development, was studied (Scott et al. 2010).

F. Alexander and F. Dunbar were the first who stated the psychosomatic nature of RA in the 20-ies of the XX century, which was the starting point for numerous studies of psychological aspects of the incidence and development of the disease.

It is known that in response to stressful stimuli the body simultaneously activates its three major systems, that is: nervous, immune and endocrine, which in turn leads to the development of somatic diseases as well as mental disorders (Lisitsyna et al. 2013).

Stress and breakdown of immune homeostasis together with a chronic inflammatory process – is a possible way of RA development as a psychosomatic pathology. In cases where mental stress is not presented in the onset of RA, the subsequent chronic, disabling disease course still poses some complex social and psychological problems for a patient, influencing through the regulatory mechanisms of immunity and inflammation on the course of the pathological process itself (Dube et al. 2009).

The role of stress factors in the development and progression of RA is proved by statistically significant clinical advantage in patients treated with anti-stress psychotherapeutic intervention in comparison with patients not receiving such intervention (Sharpe 2013).

According to the data of several studies, the incidence of anxiety-depressive spectrum disorders (ADSD) in RA patients is 13 – 43% (Kekov et al. 2011; Margaretten 2011). Based on the results of Russian studies 93, 6% of patients with the RA have ADSD (Lisitsyna et al. 2013). Among ADSD depression and dysthymia occur, as well as adjustment disorders and generalized anxiety disorders. Half of the patients with ADSD were diagnosed with cognitive impairments (CI) (Lisitsyna et al. 2011).

The psychological state allows some patients to adapt safely to the new living conditions while others develop psychiatric states requiring medication and psychotherapy. At the same time, it is a mistake to consider all mental and primarily depressive disorders only as a consequence of the severe chronic course of the RA.

ADSD and CI in RA patients are associated with increased levels of proinflammatory cytokines such as tumor necrosis factor α (TNFα), interleukin 1β (IL1β) and interleukin 6 (IL6), which confirms the role of chronic inflammation in the pathogenesis of ADSD and CI in RA. The high level of TNFα and IL1β is typical for RA patients with clinically significant fatigue and severe pain

It is necessary to take into account the psychoanalytic importance of young female patient's hate to their body, acquired unconsciously due to mechanisms of induction from mothers. This mechanism manifests itself in violation of identification and mental representation in early forms of the RA (Linda 2014). Mechanisms of induction of self-destructive auto-bullying may be the core of the etiopathogenesis of RA (Sidorov 2014). Interesting to note that in schizophrenia, when the patient hates own personality, RA does not almost occur (Fuller 1996).

Thus, psycho-traumatic stressful situations play an important role in the etiology and pathogenesis of RA, which only occurs under a combination of factors: genetic predisposition and immunological conflict; susceptibility to affective aggression and stressful situation with depression, sense of guilt leading to self-aggression (Korshunov et al. 2011). The disease can be considered as a disease of disadaptation with a primary disruption of central mechanisms of regulation of homeostasis under the influence of exogenous and endogenous factors.

15.3. Synergetics of Rheumatoid Arthritis

Synergetic model of RA is presented in Table 15.1.

Fractal of an *arthritic family* is the first in the formation of RA. The development of this stage may be induced by disturbed family relations, early psychological traumas and deprivation. Thus, some studies demonstrated a significant increase in the risk of developing of autoimmune diseases in adults after two or more traumatic events in childhood (Spitzer et al. 2013).

The results of the Russian works demonstrated the presence of early childhood mental traumas, mainly deprivation, in 81% of patients with juvenile rheumatoid arthritis (JRA) and 77, 6% of patients with RA, while in the general population this figure was only 20% (Drozhdina et al. 2012).

Deformations of family relationships in childhood lead to impairment of interpersonal communication skills and difficulties in adaptation, increased emotional stress and anxiety that inevitably affect the family relationships in adult life.

Some studies show the influence of early childhood mental traumas on the formation of predisposition to the stress response with the development of depressive disorders. For example, psychological stress has an impact on the disease course in 80% of cases. However, about 90% of patients associate the onset or exacerbation of the disease with acute and 10% - with a chronic psychogenic situation. Development of the disease is often preceded by the loss of loved ones, and in the childhood such patients have serious psychological problems. The frequency of life stress for the year before the disease in a group of women with RA was significantly higher than among the general medical population of patients (Straub, Kalden 2009; Stojanovich 2010).

The next is a fractal of *arthritic diathesis* - disturbances of mental adaptation to the environment or borderline state, which can be transformed into disease under the influence of exogenous (stress) and endogenous (genetically determined abnormalities, etc.) factors.

Under the influence of external risk factors *prearthritic state* develops – a functional disorder, which may or may not go to the stage of a full-scale disease. Stress, hypothermia, and some infectious agents can trigger the development of a clinical picture of the disease at this stage.

In future, the impact of significant risk factors of RA may lead to *the clinical onset* of the disease. Psychoemotional tension is observed in patients in a pre-disease state in 30-87% of cases, and during exacerbation (Sidorov et al. 2002). Under distress the composition of the connective tissue changes, the immune system is suppressed, as well as hormonal functions of the body; while the stabilization of the mental state leads to positive changes in the immunological status, influencing the course of the disease, in the *chronization fractal.*

Somatoneurological complications of RA include medical complications, as well as mental disorders of neurotic and psychotic levels, resulting from the impact on the mentality of physical illness. Somatoneurological complications are the long-term disease outcome.

Patients with RA in the acute phase showed signs of socio-psychological disadaptation, including asthenic and depressive syndromes. In the remission phase, active forms of adaptation dominate (Nemirovskyi et al. 2010).

Table 15.1. Fractal dynamics of rheumatoid arthritis development

Vector of ontogenesis	Prenosological fractals			Nosological fractals		
	Predisposition: arthritic family	Latent: arthritic diathesis	Initial: prearthritic state	A full-scale clinical picture of the RA/mental epidemic	Chronization: forms and types of the RA course /destructive mental epidemic	Outcome: somatoneurological complications/pandemic
Somatogenesis	Hereditary burden	Tendency to abnormal physiological reactions	Prearthritic state	Rheumatoid arthritis	Forms and types of rheumatoid arthritis course	Medical complications
Psychogenesis	Psychophysiological disposition	Premorbid personality traits	Psychosomatic reactions	Somatoform disorders	Psychosomatic disorders	Somatopsychic violations
Sociogenesis	Disharmony of family relations	Disharmony of personality socialization	Significant problems with socialization	Transient social disability	Social decompensation	Social disadaptation (invalidity)
Animogenesis	Family spiritual and moral deficiency or ambivalence	Disharmony of formation of the moral feelings	Deformation of the moral image	Destruction of spiritual and moral position	The probability of immoral acts	The possibility of illegal behavior

We shall review each vector of the RA synergetic model.

Somatogenesis of RA in the first fractal involves genetic predisposition to altered immunological reactivity. There is a close correlation between the development of rheumatoid arthritis and antigens of histocompatibility complex HLA DR_1 DR_4, DRW_4, DW_4, DW_{14}. The association with the human leukocyte antigen (HLA)-DRB1 locus has been confirmed in patients who are positive for rheumatoid factor or anti-citrullinated protein antibody. The presence of these antigens encoding immune response of the organism can modify the cellular and humoral immune response to various infectious agents and contribute to the development of RA. Family-genetic predisposition to RA is proved by an increased rate of disease among relatives, especially monozygotic twins (Scott et al. 2010).

In the latent fractal of RA somatogenesis, pathological, physiological reactions may occur that may manifest itself, for example, in the presence of short-term joint pain in stressful situations.

The prearthritic state is a functional disorder, as it may not go to the stage of a full-scale disease.

This stage is followed by a full-scale clinical onset of RA.

There may be three types of the disease course: a slowly progressive, rapidly progressive and without noticeable progression.

The final fractal of the RA somatogenesis is medical complications. RA begins with joint damage, but eventually systemic extra-articular manifestations of RA occur.

Psychogenesis of RA in the first fractal is presented by psychophysiological disposition, assuming the presence of specific innate characteristics that may contribute to the development of the disease. Among them are: the weak and moderately weak types of the nervous system, low values of ergic and tempo, high emotionality and instability. Psychophysiological characteristics are the base for severity of physiological response to a stressor. Marked psychophysiological peculiarities can cause a more pronounced and pathological reaction to the stressor.

Some researchers have suggested that psychological stress is significant only for patients with RA, who have psychodynamic conflict. In these cases, the disease begins suddenly and progresses rapidly (Lichtenberg et al. 1984; Pow 1987).

It is established that a valuable role in the pathogenesis of RA belongs to extreme vital events (loss of a loved one, intrafamily problems, financial difficulties), which are marked a year before the manifestation of RA in 30-75% of cases. The most frequent adverse psychological effects are connected with relationships in the family and personal life, more rarely - with business relations (Smulevich 2011).

The high frequency of psychological stress, before the disease, is detected (47.7%). Into account were taken only obvious intractable and unsolvable conflicts, frustrating patients. Researchers do not insist on the fact that mental distress was the causative factor in all these cases, but simply a condition for the realization of other unknown cause of RA. In 1/3 of cases, when the onset of the disease was preceded by mental stress, the onset was acute. In RA, the most common adverse mental effects were associated with the relationships in the family and personal life, more rarely - with business relations (Korshunov, Rechkina 2005).

Most traumatic situations in patients with RA are in the field of personal and family life. Various psychological traumas, interpersonal conflicts, accompanied by psycho-emotional stress, were observed in patients with premorbid or in the further course of the disease in 71.1% (Kurygina, Uryvaeva 2006).

The second fractal of psychogenesis is characterized by premorbid personality traits, among them are the anxiety and suspiciousness, hypochondria and pessimism.

Personality characteristics in conjunction with the external circumstances may form the internal conflict, which places a heavy burden on the adaptive system of the body and hits genetically vulnerable structures, causing disruption of homeostasis, including immune. Thus, stress and breakdown of the immune system together with a chronic inflammatory process mainly at the level of the musculoskeletal system is one of the trajectories of the RA development as a psychosomatic pathology.

In an initial period of the disease, psychosomatic reactions are possible, and they are shown by single symptoms of the physical state (joint pain, fever, et al.), with the duration of the disorder from a few minutes to a few days and without organ dysfunctions.

With further mental traumatization a transformation of psychosomatic reactions takes place. They are transformed in somatoform disorders that are also functional, but last over a longer period (more than six months) and are accompanied by repeated, multiple and clinically significant complaints. This fractal is also known for possible nosogenic reactions to the fact of onset of the disease manifested in alarming and asthenic, phobic, and depressive symptoms.

There is evidence that the adaptive abilities of patients with RA are limited due to the reduced intensity of most of the major types of psychological protection in comparison with healthy people. At the same time, the more active rheumatoid process is, the more increasingly possibilities of using psychological defense become narrower (Savelyeva 1995).

Symptoms of borderline neuropsychiatric disorders (fatigue, tiredness, apathy, irritability, sleep disturbances, tremors, etc.) occur in most patients, but they are not considered leading clinical phenomena, as opposed to a joint syndrome. In the future, transformation to psychosomatic disorders is possible, which already are chronic and irreversible.

In RA, there are borderline mental disorders that may be manifested in neurotic syndrome, individual neurotic symptoms, and personality changes. 45.9% of RA patients revealed a combination of various mental disorders. The most frequently observed are affective disorders, sleep disorders, included in the structure of asthenic syndrome, and psychovegetative disorders. Affective disorders are most obvious in comparison with other mental disorders (Korshunov et al. 2010).

In the case of severe course of RA hypochondriac, depressive and hysterical symptoms may appear.

In the last fractal of a disease outcome, somatopsychic disorders occur, resulting from the impact on the mentality of a long-term disease. RA patients have a significant change in the physical and psychological status and are subject to the psychosocial deprivation and decompensation.

Sociogenesis of RA begins with disharmony of family relations. It may be associated with problems in or more types of family relationships: psychological (openness, trust, caring for each other, mutual moral and emotional support), psychophysiological (sex), social (roles, material dependence, authority, leadership) cultural (national and religious traditions and customs). All these types of relationships affect the education of the child in the family. Due to family relationship problems, further socialization disharmony may appear as being in the family a child learns most of the existing social relations. Disturbed family relationships will be a model for learning and in mental representation will lead to the formation of disharmony in a person, deformation of important social roles and relationships, becoming a chronic stressor.

The greater the duration of RA is, the clearer the influence of psychological factors is in the development of disease and its exacerbations. Half of patients with RA detect various psychosocial problems. Although in the frequency of occurrence the first place took the problems within the scope of career, their significance was low. The problems of loneliness, family and sexuality are very relevant for patients. We found no relationship between the severity of the problems and social status of the patient (employed, disabled, retired, student). Patients with higher education compared to patients with secondary and secondary professional education, have a tendency to decrease the significance of psychological problems; the same situation is with patients whose disease experience is more than 10 years, compared to those whose illness is not so long-termed yet (Sidorov, Sovershaeva 2014).

In the stage of a full-scale clinical picture of RA transient, social dysfunctions can occur, and they are associated with the necessity of changing a lifestyle. In the case of severe disease progression, social decompensation may be presented and can manifest itself as problems in the family, professional and other social relations.

The RA outcomes depend on the biomedical and physiological, behavioral, and social factors. Willpower, stressful situations, socioeconomic status and role in the family act as independent factors that predict the somatic state of the patient.

In the outcome of the disease social exclusion occurs, it is associated with an acquisition of a disability status, loss of social status, professional and personal perspectives.

Animogenesis of RA begins in predisposition fractal from moral and spiritual disharmony, deficiency or ambiguity of family relationships that create conscious or unconscious psychoemotional tension.

Latent fractal of the arthritic diathesis is presented by disharmony and dischronosis of formation and development of basic moral feelings: faith and responsibility, conscience and duty, honor and dignity. This is manifested in impaired moral socialization and personality development in any age period.

In the initial fractal, early deformation of moral image becomes apparent and is manifested in the failure of endurance and patience, humanity and mercy, modesty and tact. This creates prerequisites for the possible development of the syndrome of demoralization and destructive professiogenesis, the clinical picture of which in each specific case and fractal is formed and supplemented by comorbid and associated disorders in somato-, psycho-, and sociogenesis.

Fractal of the full-scale clinical picture of RA manifests in the destruction of spiritual and moral position: a decrease ability to distinguish between good and evil, between manifestations of friendly affection and love, possible abandonment of struggle with illness, fear and despair because of continuing trials of life.

Chronization and outcome of RA fractals are characterized by an increase in all manifestations of the demoralization syndrome and the emergence of the risk of immoral and illegal behavior.

Thus, the synergetic methodology of mental medicine enables to take into account all the internal and external factors of the RA pathoplastics and pathokinetics systematically and to build up comprehensively individual preventive and remedial, treatment and rehabilitation algorithms in the framework of a multidisciplinary program.

15.4. Medico-Psychosociospiritual Care

Based on the synergetic methodology we (Sidorov, Sovershaeva 2014) have developed a multi-disciplinary program of care for RA patients (Table 15.2), which includes four sections: medical and psychological, spiritual and moral and social. Preventive measures are implemented in the first three prenosological fractals, and treatment and rehabilitation - in the three nosological fractals, constituting a single multidisciplinary protocol of care for RA patients according to the synergetic methodology of mental medicine. This protocol is realized by a team composed of a rheumatologist, psychotherapist, clinical psychologist, social work and bioethics specialists.

Primary prevention activities should be carried out already in the *predisposition fractal* (arthritic family), for identifying of hereditary, psychophysiological predisposition and ethical and psychological harmonization of family relationships.

In the *latent fractal* measures aim to identify abnormal physiological responses, correction of moral socialization and premorbid personality traits.

In the *initial fractal* when a prearthritic state appears, pharmacological and nonpharmacological interventions are assumed for the prevention of RA, hampering the development of the disease.

In the fractal of a *full-scale clinical picture* of RA, early qualified medical and psychological, spiritual, moral and social care is required, which later develops in an individual treatment and rehabilitation program implemented in *chronization and outcome fractals.*

The medical block of the program within the framework of somatogenesis contains medical care provided by rheumatologists, general practitioners, physicians, and if complications arise - by narrow specialists (cardiologists, neurologists, etc.).

Pharmacological treatment of RA is considered in detail in specialized guidelines (Nasonov et al. 2014; Smolen et al. 2013) and does not require special discussion in this article.

The inclusion of new antidepressants in the complex treatment of patients with RA and comorbid depressive disorders improves the functional state of the musculoskeletal system, which is manifested in a significant reduction of pain, morning stiffness and a greater improvement in functional indexes than in the comparison groups without antidepressants (Lisenko, Tkachenko, 2007).

The psychological block of care under the psychogenesis framework assumes participation of psychotherapists, clinical psychologists and psychiatrists.

Recently, the attention of researchers is increasingly attracted by the use and effectiveness of psychotherapy in RA. In RA psychotherapy techniques of self-regulation are applied (biofeedback through temperature or electrical activity of muscles, combined with relaxation exercises) and various behavioral approaches, the ultimate goal of which is to train patients the ability to cope with pain. The use of hypnosis in RA reduces the manifestations of pain syndrome and promotes the disappearance of neurotic symptoms (Kremleva 2007; Ababkov, Karvasarsky 2012).

It is proposed to use predominantly cognitive psychotherapy, which allows "destroying" existing stereotypes of assessment of what is happening (Kurygina, Uryvaeva 2006).

Table 15.2. Program of medico-psychosociospiritual care for patients with rheumatoid arthritis

Blocks	Prenosological fractals			Nosological fractals		
	Predisposition: arthritic family	Latent: arthritic diathesis	Initial: prearthritic state	A full-scale clinical picture of the RA / mental epidemic	Chronization: forms and types of the RA course/destructive mental epidemic	Outcome: somatoneurological complications
Medical	Inclusion of persons with hereditary predisposition in the risk group and their early preventive screening	Identification of persons inclined to pathological physiological reactions	Diagnostics of prearthritic states during periodic health examination; pharmacological and nonpharmacological intervention	Clinical diagnosis, prescription of drug treatment, prevention of complications	Control of the somatic state; adequate drug therapy, prevention of complications	Treatment of physical and neurological complications
Psychological	Identification of persons with specific psycho-physiological characteristics and their inclusion in the risk group	Correction of premorbid personality characteristics, escalation of stress resistance	Correction of psychosomatic reactions, psychotherapy	Correction of somatoform disorders, psychotherapy, psycho-pharmacotherapy	Correction of psychosomatic disorders, psychotherapy, psycho-pharmacotherapy	Psychological rehabilitation
Social	Identification and correction of disharmonies in family relationships	Correction of family relationships and harmonization of personality socialization	Harmonisation of significant social relations	Adaptation to the disease, correction of interpersonal problems	Professional and family adaptation	Social rehabilitation
Spiritual and moral	Screening and correction of the moral climate in family	Correction of formation and development of the moral feelings	Correction of the moral image formation	Reconstruction of a moral position	Reconstruction of moral behavior	Spiritual and moral rehabilitation

Group psychotherapy helps patients with RA to normalize disturbed interpersonal relationships through an emotional enactment of conflicts in the group. Family psychotherapy is aimed at optimizing family relationships, which is very important for patients with RA since disability arisen due to illness often significantly modifies the position of the person in the family.

Despite the scarcity of publications devoted to the application of psychotherapy in RA, we can say that it contributes to positive changes in the psychological and psychosomatic status of the patients.

Under pharmacologically controlled rational psychotherapy in young female patients it has become possible to achieve catharsis and sustained remission over the understanding of the transfer of hatred for their bodies from their mothers. Correction of auto bullying induction mechanisms through family psychotherapy can produce significant sanogenetic effects (Sidorov 2014).

Social care is provided under the vector of sociogenesis with the participation of specialists of social services (social work specialists, social workers).

Educational programs are designed to raise awareness of patients about the disease, its course, methods of treatment, prognosis, also to strengthen their motivation to receive prescribed medication and to adhere to treatment compliance. Such programs should teach motor skills, form a correct behavioral pattern, teach the basics of physical therapy, methods of psychological adaptation to the disease and self-regulation. All this is essential to prevent functional impairment of joints and progression of deformations, to preserve the ability of self-servicing and performing household activities and professional work; to correct psycho-emotional disorders, maintaining the patient as an active social identity and to improve the quality of life (Orlova et al. 2012).

Individual rehabilitation programs for patients with RA improve the functionality and the locomotor activity (compression force of hand, power, symmetry of movement, load distribution) and quality of life. Furthermore, they can maintain high compliance of disease modifying anti-rheumatic drugs use, reducing the need for symptomatic medications, and increasing physical activity. Taking into account the reduction of training effect after six months, such programs are recommended to realize at least once every six months (Shafieva et al. 2008; Masiero et al. 2007).

In patients with RA, group and family sociotherapy are successfully applied to the rehabilitation, as well as art therapy, music therapy and therapy of creative self-expression (Sidorov et al. 2002).

The spiritual and moral block under the vector of animogenesis is implemented with the participation of the family and the referent surrounding in the micro social and professional environment, using modern methods and forms of education and training of adults and children, coaching and personal growth training, together with mental health experts and consultants from ethics committees, especially in cases of a destructive professiogenesis threat (mobbing, bossing, bullying, crowding, labor conflicts, etc.). Also there is a need for mediation and spiritual leaders of the official confessions; it is necessary for RA patients and their relatives to participate in programs of community organizations, in volunteer and social movements, in trade unions' and veterans' organizations.

In recent years, interconnection between religionism and the state of health or illness of the population has become the subject of intense scientific interest. Religious belief is important for many patients with severe chronic illnesses, appearing for them as a positive coping resource. Spiritual beliefs are an important part of the culture of patients, regardless of their degree of awareness. Another adaptive religious factor is the everlasting belief in the spiritual integrity (Carone, Borone 2001; Bekke-Hausen et al. 2012; Peres et al. 2012; Powell-Wiley et al. 2013).

Screening and correction of the moral climate of an arthritic family are carried out in the course of family psycho- and sociotherapy that solve ethical and psychological problems of harmonization of interpersonal relations, spiritual and moral development of the family.

Correction of formation of basic moral feelings and the moral image is conducted through all the spiritual and moral personality modalities. These modalities usually develop the syndrome of demoralization and destructive professiogenesis. This is carried out taking into account individual characterological peculiarities of a patient and his microenvironment, as well as comorbid and associated disorders. Within the framework of strategies for early intervention and mediation, maintenance of adaptive professiogenesis and ethics in business communication are provided, as well as prevention of ethics loss and dehumanization of professional conscience.

Reconstruction of a moral position and behavior within the generated demoralization syndrome requires the use of resources from business communication ethics training, coaching and spiritual (religious) practices, therapies of creative self-expression. Spiritual and moral rehabilitation is carried out to maintain optimistic durable attitudes.

Spiritual and moral rehabilitation is carried out in the framework of maintenance therapy that realizes the task of leveling pessimistic and catastrophic affirmations and maintaining optimistic durable attitudes.

Thus, the proposed synergetic biopsychosociospiritual concept of RA allows mobilizing new resources and launch effective resonantly coherent mechanisms of therapeutic and preventive care.

Section III. Mental Epidemics of Somatoform Disorders

Chapter 16

Somatoform Disorders

Since the time of identifying neuroses by W. Cullen in 1776, the somatoform disorders have been described as psychic disorders that proceed with autonomic stigmas. Later on, a group of neuroses with the different terminological descriptions were being identified: vegetative, viscera-vegetative, systemic neuroses, cardio psychoneuroses, and vegetative-vascular dystonia In the ICD-10, these disorders are put into the class of "somatoform disorders" (SFD) that are diagnosed on the basis of constant somatic symptoms, while the objective pathology is absent, as well as severity and continuity of complaints that are inadequate to the nature of a diagnosed somatic disorder. The patients are demanding more assessments, in spite of the negative findings, their distrust and disregard of the doctors' opinion about the absence of a physical basis for the symptoms.

In the American DSM-5, issued in 2013, the SFD category was substituted by "somatic symptom disorder." Other synonyms of these disorders are "medically unexplained symptoms" and "functional somatic symptoms" (Greed 2010). The multifaceted and polymodal nature of SFD was acknowledged many times (Voigt et al. 2010; Schröder 2011), and this does not allow to build an acceptable block-modular patterns of etiopathogenesis, to determine the mechanisms of pathokinesis and pathoplastics and the instruments for evaluating and predicting the trajectory of clinical and epidemic development. That is why the task is to conceptually and methodologically substantiate the synergetic biopsychosociospiritual model of mental epidemics of SFD, to determine the development and design mechanisms of multidisciplinary programs of medical and preventive help.

16.1. Prevalence of Somatoform Disorders

Prevalence of SFD among population varies between 0,8% and 6% (Wittchen, Jacobi 2005; Escobar et al. 2010). The risk of developing the disorder during a lifetime amounts to 20% (Jacobi 2004; Hiller 2006). According to the international studies the frequency of SFD among the patients of primary medical care is 15-40% (Steinbrecher 2011), which corresponds to Russian researchers' data (Smulevich 2011).

Different groups of healthy and ill people are diagnosed with the *SFD*. The somatized symptoms are detected among 10-80% of physically healthy people, which makes them somewhat concerned and anxious about their health. The patients with the subjective complaints about their health that do not correspond to the objective findings make up 40% of disability cases. However, only a quarter of such patients seeks medical attention (Van der Boom et al. 2010), which makes the mental epidemic uncontrollable.

According to the National Ambulatory Medical Care Survey in the United States, out of 90 thousand visitors to the general practitioners, 72% of the patients with the psychiatric diagnosis had one or two somatic symptoms that were their main complaint. Out of 4 thousand patients examined in the general medical network, 30% had somatic disorders, as part of a mental pathology in the form of the anxiety-depressive disorder. On the whole, 30% of the people seeking medical attention are diagnosed with mental disorders and somatic symptoms are observed in half of the cases (Dimsdale et al. 2011).

Various diagnostic and treatment procedures cause sufficient economic expenditures. The cost of endless clinical and paraclinical assessments, of ineffective therapy, is so high, that the ill-timed diagnostics of somatized disorders is considered to be a socio-economic problem for any society. The amount of time being spent on every such patient is much bigger, compared to the true somatic patients. The significant financial expenditures are caused by the fact that often doctors, treating the SFD patients, do not have a sufficient competence in this exact sphere (Pribytkov et al. 2014; Sidorov, Sovershaeva 2015).

All the mentioned above requires the epidemic approach to the evaluation of the SFD prevalence, validating the criteria and characteristics of the epidemic threshold, and the new forms of organizing the multidisciplinary mental care.

16.2. Etiopathogenesis of Somatoform Disorders

In developing of SFD, the main etiological value belongs to the three groups of factors (Smulevich 2014; Sidorov, Sovershaeva 2015; Voigt et al. 2010):

- *hereditary-constitutional:* constitutional and typological features of the central nervous system (CNS) and the characteristics of personality accentuations;
- *psycho-emotional* or psychogenic: acute or chronic factors of external influence mediated by the mental sphere, and having both cognitive and emotional value and thus playing a role in psychogeny;
- *organic factors:* various premorbid organic (traumatic, infectious, toxic, hypoxic) discredity of integrative cerebral systems of a suprasegmentary level, first of all, of the limbic-reticular complex.

With the help of magnetic resonance imaging the Japanese researchers (Komaki et al. 2013) estimated the neural response to the painful electrical stimuli and also the response to the warning signs, inducing a high or a low level of anxiety. The acquired data indicates that anxiety takes part in disturbing neural links, including the hippocampus. According to the authors, the correlation between the anxiety disorders and the processes of modulating a sense of pain is the basis of the SFD manifestation.

This hypothesis is also proven by the psychopathological model of the SFD, according to which the disorders that imitate a physical pathology represent paired psychopathological formations corresponding to the two levels of mental activity organization being damaged: auto- and somatopsychic (Smulevich 2014).

16.3. Synergetics of Somatoform Disorders

The synergetic model of the SFD formation is presented in Table 16.1. The SFD dynamics includes the following fractals: predisposition – somatoform family, latent – somatoform diatheses, initial – primary SFD, full-scale clinical picture – SFD, chronization – forms and types of SFD progression, outcome – somatopsychic complications.

The somatoform family fractal is a primary level in developing the SFD. Troubled family relations may contribute to the development of this pathology.

In the contemporary concept of the SFD etiopathogenesis, the crucial role is given to a person's troubled significant relations. The unfavorable family climate lasting since the early childhood may decompensate even a healthy person. The SFD is a peculiar clinical-psychological phenomenon that is being developed throughout one-three generations – grandparents, parents and children. The family turns out to be the direct source of psychological well-being or ill-being of its members. There is an interconnection between dissatisfaction, tension in the family or a conflict on the one hand, and various neuropsychic disorders in children on the other. As the psychogenic diseases of a developing personality, the SFD in its affective-accentuated form is a reflection of various problems in personal relations, first of all, of understanding and communication between people, finding a personal identity and optimal ways of self-expression, self-affirmation, acknowledgment and love (Karvasarskyi et al. 2012).

If a child is being brought up in the family that can be characterized as "somatoform," with conflicts and emotional tensions between its members, he is deprived of a possibility to acquire adequate communication skills. His ability to correct his emotional reactions on the basis of experience is blocked, which limits the range of his emotional and cognitive potential actualization.

The somatoform family is characterized by a disharmonious spiritual and moral education as the result of neurotic parents.

The next is the fractal of *somatoform diathesis.* Diathesis (from the Greek diathesis – disposition) is a constitutional predisposition of an organism to various diseases as the result of inherited metabolism characteristics, physiological reactions and so on.

The somatoform diathesis manifests itself in disharmonious formation and development of the main moral attitudes, which can later on predetermine the moral socialization and personal development disorders for those having a low adaptation potential.

Under the influence of stressful factors a person that has diathesis develops *the primary somatoform reactions (initial fractal),* which manifest themselves by psychosomatic complaints about isolated symptoms in a somatic state (high pulse rate, elevated blood pressure, change of respiration speed and depth, sudden muscle weakness and others). The disorder can last from a couple of minutes up to a couple of days and does not disrupt an organ's functions. These reactions are not rigid and are short-term in nature. In this fractal, a dysfunctional personality comes into being, which may manifest itself through nonspecific asthenic and anxiety symptoms.

In animogenesis, the primary somatoform reactions appear as a multifaceted and personality-related deformation of the moral image. This image lays the foundation for the future development of demoralization syndrome and destructive professiogenesis syndrome, the clinical picture of which in each and every case is formed and added to the co-morbid and associated disorders in somato-, psycho- and sociogenesis.

The transformation of psychosomatic reactions into the SFD occurs during further psychological traumatizing *(fractal of a full-scale clinical picture).* These disorders are not already functional, they last longer (for more than six months) and are accompanied by reoccurring multiple and clinically relevant complaints. In this fractal, there is a possibility of personal decompensation in the form of anxiety, phobia and depression symptoms. Animogenesis of SFD is manifested in the destruction of the spiritual and moral position of the person that is shown in the development of the syndrome of demoralization (Sidorov, Sovershaeva 2015).

In the *chronization fractal,* it is necessary to view the forms and types of somatoform disorder progression. Most frequently it manifests itself as a somatized disorder, undifferentiated SFD, somatoform pain disorder. There is a possibility of rigid personal disorders, social and spiritual and moral decompensation, including the risk of immoral behavior.

Later on, there could be a transition to *somatopsychic complications* of the SFD, which are chronic and irreversible in nature, and lead to reduced work capacity in patients. In animogenesis, there is a growing evidence of demoralization syndrome.

Thus, the synergetic methodology of mental medicine allows taking into account all the internal and external factors of the SFD pathoplastics and pathokinetics, to create integral block-modular conditions of individual preventive-correctional and medical, rehabilitative routes in the framework of the multidisciplinary program.

16.4. Medico-Psychosociospiritual Care

On the basis of the synergetic methodology of mental medicine we (Sidorov, Sovershaeva 2015) have worked out a program that includes the following four blocks: medical and psychological, social and spiritual and moral (Table 16.2).

Primary preventive actions must be done in the *predisposition fractal* already, and they should be focused on finding hereditary psycho-physiological predisposition and ethical-psychological harmonization of family relations.

In the *latent fractal,* the actions are focused on finding people that are prone to developing the SFD (those having weak and unstable nervous system, high level of anxiety, psychasthenic, asthenoneurotic, or hysteric accentuations of personality traits), on correction of a person's moral socialization and premorbid features.

The *initial fractal* presupposes pharmacological and nonpharmacological treatment that prevents the SFD development.

In the *fractal of a full-scale clinical picture of the SFD,* there is a need for an early efficient medical and psychological, social and spiritual and moral help.

Table 16.1. Fractal dynamics of SFD mental epidemics development

Vector of ontogenesis	Prenosological fractals			Nosological fractals		
	Predisposition: somatoform family	Latent: somatoform diathesis	Initial: primary somatoform reactions	Full-scale clinical picture of SFD/mental epidemic	Chronization: forms and types of SFD course/destructive mental epidemic	Outcome: somatoneurological complications/ pandemic
Somatogenesis	Hereditary burden	Violation of neural processes	Psychosomatic reactions	Somatoform disorder	Forms and types of SFD course	Somatopsychic complications
Psychogenesis	Somatoform family	Premorbid personality traits	Dysfunctional personality	Personality decompensation	Persistent personality disorders	Complications of personality disorders
Sociogenesis	Disharmony of family relations	Disharmony of personality socialization	Violation of significant social relations	Transient social dysfunction	Social decompensation	Social disadaptation
Animogenesis	Spiritual and moral deficiency or ambivalence in the family	Disharmony of formation of the moral feelings	Deformation of the moral image	Destruction of spiritual and moral position	Probability of immoral acts	Possibility of illegal behavior

Table 16.2. Program of medico-psychosociospiritual care for patients with somatoform disorders

Blocks	Prenosological fractals			Nosological fractals		
	Predisposition: somatoform family	Latent: somatoform diathesis	Initial: primary somatoform reactions	Full-scale clinical picture of SFD/mental epidemic	Chronization: forms and types of SFD course/ destructive mental epidemic	Outcome: somato-neurological complications/ pandemic
Medical	Inclusion of persons with hereditary predisposition to neuroses in the risk group and their early preventive examination	Identification of persons with weak and unstable types of nervous system	Diagnosis of neurosis; pharmacological and nonpharmacological intervention	Clinical diagnosis, administration of medical treatment, prevention of complications	Control of the somatic state; adequate medical therapy	Treatment of physical and mental SFD complications
Psychological	Identification of persons brought up in neurosogenic family and their inclusion in the risk group	Correction of premorbid personality characteristics, escalation of stress resistance	Correction of psychosomatic reactions, psychotherapy	Correction of somatoform disorders, psychotherapy, psycho-pharmacotherapy	Correction of psychosomatic disorders, psychotherapy, psycho-pharmacotherapy	Psychological rehabilitation
Social	Identification and correction of disharmonies in family relationships	Correction of family relations and harmonization of personality socialization	Harmonisation of significant social relations	Adaptation to the disease, correction of interpersonal problems	Professional and family adaptation	Social rehabilitation
Spiritual and moral	Screening and correction of the moral climate in family	Correction of formation and development of the moral feelings	Correction of the moral image formation	Reconstruction of a moral position	Reconstruction of moral behavior	Spiritual and moral rehabilitation

Early recognition and adequate diagnostics of the SFD is of fundamental importance for a successful therapy and a favorable prognosis for the disease long before the *fractals of chronization and outcome.*

That is why further integration of the system of psychotherapeutic care into primary health care departments, the opening of psychosomatic departments in clinics and the arrangement of multidisciplinary services for mental health seem quite reasonable.

The medical block of the program. Pharmacological therapy of the SFD includes the use of a wide range of psychoactive drugs – antidepressants and anxiolytics, nootropics and neuroleptics. However, the use of psychoactive drugs in treating the SFD has its peculiarities. Prescribing a medication, it makes sense to choose monotherapy and use the drugs that are convenient to take. Taking into account a possible idiosyncrasy and side-effects, the psychoactive drugs are prescribed in small doses (compared to those, used in "senior" psychiatry). The other requirements for such therapy are a minimum influence on somatic functions, person's weight, minimum behavioral toxicity and teratogenic effects of the drugs, the possibility to take them in lactation period, low chances of interactions with somatotropic drugs.

The organization of SFD treatment must be strictly individual as they are quite resistive to therapy, and there is no uniform and well-proven strategy. The careful prescription of drugs to such group of patients is essential.

Nowadays the most convincing result in treating the SFD is given by antidepressants and antipsychotics. The anticonvulsant group shows effectiveness only in treating the somatoform pain syndromes (Pribytkov et al. 2014).

The psychological block of the program. Therapy of somatoform disorders includes a great variety of medical and preventive measures, requiring the participation of not only a general practitioner but also of a psychiatrist and a psychotherapist.

The fact that a patient may not realize or dissimulate the corresponding mental disorders is of tremendous importance. The patients usually resist every attempt to discuss the probable psychological nature of the symptoms, even if the signs of depression and anxiety are perfectly obvious. As the result of that, the basic direction of treating the SFD patients is psychotherapy, using its almost entire spectrum of contemporary forms and methods. The following are widely used: rational therapy, autogenic training, hypnotherapy, analytical, behavioral, positive, client-centered therapy and others. Despite being a priority, psychotherapeutic correction cannot be used without drug therapy, due to prevailing somato-vegetative components in the clinical picture. Even the strict directive methods in the initial period do not allow getting a quick and desirable result, which, in the end, compromises psychotherapy as a method (Allen, Woolfolk 2010).

The review of foreign studies on psychotherapeutic approaches to treating SFD (Pribytkov et al. 2014) points out a promising result of psychodynamic therapy and hypnotherapy, together with the necessity to further specify the effectiveness of these methods.

The social block of the program. Sociotherapy for SFD patients includes measures focused on explaining the nature of the disease and, accordingly, the unreasonable medical examinations and procedures, as well as on the organization of treatment and labor rehabilitation.

The socialization of the patients with a polymorphous type of disorder admits short-term presence in a day-and-night clinic to avoid the manifestation or aggravation of the signs of hypochondria developing and hospitalism. The reduction of the workload is not needed, provided that an entire set of measures for creating calm and permissive atmosphere in the family and at work be implemented.

The measures of social rehabilitation of SFD patients of the isomorphous type includes a lasting treatment in a day-and-night clinic (not less than 1,5-2 months, taking into account treatment resistance). And also a reduction of workload – cut working hours and a permission not to participate in the working process that is associated with a certain physical activity.

It is reasonable to provide healthcare to SFD patients in special departments on the basis of a clinical network, due to the necessity to differentiate these kinds of pathologies from the somatic diseases, which requires a certain qualification of the staff and laboratory equipment. Taking into consideration the borderline nature of these mental disorders, high labour and social adaptation, there is no need to follow up this category of patients in the psychiatric clinics.

The spiritual and moral block of the program is implemented through a common algorithm for all mental epidemics (chapter 7.3).

Thus, the SFD patients appear to be a quite complicated category and need a full-scale program of medico-psychosociospiritual care.

Chapter 17

Induced Neuropsychiatric Disorders: History and Hystero-Demonical Renaissance

17.1. Ethnoecology and History of Mental Epidemics

One of the fastest-growing scientific fields, existing at the junction where natural sciences and humanities meet, is mental ethnoecology. A synergistic biopsychosociospiritual approach allows for mental ethnoecology to be classified as a field involving the cooperation of ethnography and folklore, religious studies and sociology, psychology and psychotherapy, psychiatry and narcology, mental ecology and mental medicine. Historically, the earliest mental ethnoecology subjects were mental illnesses, which were named "hysterodemonic" in the 19th century. These are shamanic illness, Arctic hysteria, piblokto, hiccups, sheva hex, lishinka hex and keela hex, and others, referred to in psychiatry as induced neuropsychiatric disorders, underpinning the development of psychic epidemics (PE).

The separation of social and psychological mechanisms in the emergence of PE is only possible by analyzing historical forms of "hysterodemonic" disorders closely associated with specific forms of traditional spiritual culture.

The connection of *shamanism and shamanic illness* with nervous and mental disorders among different peoples of Northern Russia and Siberia has been marked in the works of many ethnographers (Ksenofontova 1928; Mitskevitch 1929; Popov 1947). N. A. Alekseev (1984) has analyzed the role of shamanic illness in the development of the concept of "being chosen" in one of the Turkic Speaking peoples of Siberia. He showed that the future shaman suffered from mental problems, although torments of individuals fated to become shamans were interpreted by the Siberian Turkic peoples in different ways.

Particularly, S. P. Davidenko (1947) described the role of mental disorders that influenced the formation of animistic magic visualizations as follows: "As soon as animistic ideas spread and strengthened, any direct relation with spirits became inevitable; such qualities of high nervous activity as the ability to fall into a more or less deep hypnoid state with partial wakefulness in some parts of the cortex, with dream-like wakefulness, with self-induced hallucinations, etc., i.e. all that characterizing hysteria, became of special value. As we know, "practicing" hysteria in a negative sense, can lead further to its significant deterioration."

We do not think it possible to whittle down such a complicated and diverse complex as shamanism, to the "cult of hysteria». However, "shamanology", that studies the complex phenomena associated with "professionally" classified individuals in traditional societies, who provide these societies with psychological balance in conditions of living in a world full of dangers, requires the development of a mental ethnoecological approach to shamanism.

The existence of a large number of individuals with hyper-suggestibility created a special psychological climate that enhanced the social significance of shamanism in traditional societies of the north of Russia and Siberia. It is no coincidence that death of a shaman often led to psychogenic illness outbreaks. The belief in vulnerability of human souls that resulted from shaman's death in the world of hostile forces used to turn into to mental impairment epidemics. The epidemics stopped when one of the diseased became a shaman. The universe balance, damaged by the shaman's death, was restored by the appearance of a new mediator between the world of human souls and the world of spirits. It is noteworthy that the word "shaman" which became an international scientific term, means an "excited, ecstatic person" (Tokarev 1976). It is no coincidence that L. V. Khomych (1956), one of the leading researchers of the traditional culture of the Nenets people, wrote: "Without considering nervous disorder as a cause of shamanism (shamanism is an ideological and partially social phenomenon), we shall still note that the formation of individuals engaged in shamanism, is strongly influenced by the unbalanced and easily excitable mind."

Strange behavior of the future shaman is usually mentioned along with other features that determine the predilection towards becoming a shaman. According to the Nenets people, close to the age of puberty, such individual "went a little bit crazy": used to sing or sleep for days on end, then strolled around without noticing anybody, etc. It was believed that tadebtse – spirits that had helped the shaman's ancestors – turned up and tormented him, forcing to start a shamanistic activity. Then the affected himself or his family would request the shaman to assist in his recovery. Only another shaman could alleviate to some extent the mental disorder of the "aspirant" to the place of the shaman.

We can assume that as "healers-psychiatrists" shamans were probably fairly well versed in their kind of "diagnosis" of mental illness. We get more prove of this conclusion when first, seeing psycho hygienic and psychotherapeutic function of the shaman as one of the most important of his activities, and secondly, the fact that the bulk of patients who turned to shaman were people with neuropsychiatric disorders.

During the shamanistic ritual, which, according to the Nenets, was a way of communication with spirits, the shaman would bring himself to an ecstatic state. Such trance technique played an enormous role in shamanism. Mastering the shamanic profession required much time. L. V. Khomich (1956) writes that, although one night was sufficient to teach the basic patterns to the future shaman, it took about two decades to become janumpa or inutana, i.e. a "top-qualified" shaman. During this time, the shaman received special knowledge and constantly exercised in the art of self-inducing into a state of trance or ecstasy. The mental instability that showed up in the shamanic illness was skillfully cultivated by the practice of shamanic activity. Perhaps it was such practice that led to the discovery of the archaic techniques of ecstasy and primitive methods of psychotherapy. It is also important to consider that probably the attempts to understand not the outside world, but changes in internal mental states stand behind shamanic concepts of the plurality of souls.

The shaman is an intermediary between the world of humans (human souls) and the world of spirits.Most likely, the majority of shamans believed both in spirits and in their extraordinary abilities. Moreover, shamans probably could see and feel the images of spirits, being in a state of ecstasy and self-hypnosis. The ecstatic state is a necessary condition to visit the world of spirits. "Ecstasy is a blissful frenzy, a religious form of communication with God; I would say, more effective than epiphanal contemplating of gods. It is more specific and more physical than the later revelation. God is ideated to have entered the person and acting through that person. A person in ecstasy is not responsible for their actions», - O. M. Freidenberg (1978) writes.

The ecstasy technique has social significance for the psychology of traditional societies. Self-hypnosis and ritual, which are, in fact, an archaic technique to achieve the ecstatic state, in some cases might be accompanied by the phenomena of auditory and visual hallucinations, derealization, depersonalization and delusions. The collectivity of the action itself was of major importance. The mechanisms of mutual hypnosis and self-hypnosis determined to the great extent the "speed" and "depth" of achieving the mental state necessary for communicating with spirits during the ritual.

The variety of psychogenic states, arising from the ritual, significantly broadened the limits of the normal mental condition. The system of shamanic concepts considered the dream-state soul that left the body for the contact with spirits, to be a normal but special form of existence, making it possible to influence the processes and phenomena that lie outside of the real-life experience. The same explanation existed for a spontaneous type of mental disorders such as shamanic illness; the descriptions made by different ethnographers reveal the analog onset and development of endogenous psychoses of the indigenous small-numbered peoples of the North. On the one hand, training for the person who suffered an attack of shamanic illness to become a shaman, allows the shaman to correct his mental state independently during the practice of archaic psychotherapy, and on the other hand, to carry out medical and psycho-prophylactic functions in his tribe. Shamanism accumulates almost all registers of active psychotic reaction, which regarding content corresponds to a particular specialization and qualification of the shaman. The shaman ritual can be considered as the earliest historical evidence of the subclinical nature of human creativity.

The most well-known forms of mental disorders in traditional societies of the North of Russia and Siberia were *arctic hysteria and piblokto*. They were thoroughly investigated in the works of S. I. Mitskevich (1929). Arctic hysteria is a disease presented in "severe headaches with delusions, obsessions and imitation of shamanic action». If a sick person had well-known shamans among relatives, the disease would be perceived by others as the beginning of "shamanic illness», a manifestation of unusual qualities of the future shaman, "call to serve the spirits." The Yakuts, Evenks and Yukagirs considered Arctic hysteria patients to be possessed and full of spirits. In addition, it is not coincidental that the main patients of Yakut, Yukagir and Evenk shamans were "people with mental disorders" (Gurvich et al. 1978).

Another common type of mental disorder was *piblokto*, characterized by increased fear susceptibility while shout, chock, or other acts unexpected for the persons. S. I. Mitskevich (1929), investigating and describing in detail the cases of Arctic hysteria and piblokto, showed that piblokto was spread throughout Siberia. It was mostly typical for females. It is noteworthy that the Yakut, Evenk and Yukagir people did not consider piblokto to be an illness. This affliction was thought as a funny inherent trait, reason for non-malice merry-making and scoff.

Probably, one of the first descriptions of "Arctic hysteria», as it was called in South Dauria, belongs to A. A. Kashin (1886). It presented in various forms of "abnormal imitation" such as hysterical echolalia, echomimia and echopraxia.

It is worth emphasizing, that this increased hysterical commitment, acquired in childhood, could be accomplished apart from the usual cultural environment, but definitely in a group of fellow countrymen, facilitating the expression of self- and mutual inductance. A. A. Kashin (1886) describes an interesting experience: during the training of one of the Transbaikal regiment of the Imperial Army, everyone in the subdivision, consisting of the natives of one village, began to repeat in chorus the command words. The angry officer started to swear, and the whole subdivision began to repeat his invectives.

In the European North of Russia, the interest in the field of mental ethnoecology is focused on such hysterodemonic forms as *hiccups* among the Russian population of the Pinega and Mezen river basins, *sheva hex* among the Komi people and *lishinka hex* among the Russian population in Izhmo-Pechersk region.

Hiccups are marked by cenesthopathy and autonomic disorders, hypersensitivity and irritability. Typical symptoms were a headache, loss of appetite, general weakness and hysterical strokes. The reason for a stroke could be almost any emotional irritant: smell (cases of attacks as a result of the smell of frankincense and tobacco were very frequent in the 19th century), color, sound, meeting with unknown person. The old-time Russian resident population of the Pinega and Mezen river basins separate the following forms of hiccups: "nemochischa», "nemukha" – silent hiccups with the most frequent and painful seizures when the patients could only emit jerky muffled sounds; "krikukha" or "revukha" – when the seizures less frequent, not so strong and during the seizures patients were able to pronounce words and snatchy phrases (often incoherent); "govorukha" when during the attack patients reached the state close to ecstasy, but retained the "ability to keep in touch with other people, responding to their questions."

Attack of hiccups lasted from a few minutes to a day or more. At the beginning of the attack, patients usually felt physical weakness, itching or numbness in different parts of body, stomach cramps, esophagus and throat. Then breath and heart rate and blood pressure increased. The beginning of the attack could be accompanied by yawning, lacrimation, sudden sweating, skin colour changes (redness or paleness). The main part of the attack was a kind of hyperkinesis of respiratory and phonatory types, incoherent speech turning into a cry and then into dull snappish sounds (in the case of "nemukha"). Shouts and conversation had an intrusive and forced nature; patients could not stop them on their own. The attack would end with a sense of weakness, weariness, depression and anxiety.

The Russian population of the Pinega, Mezen and Pechora river basins traditionally associated the hiccups illness with hexes and malicious magic. The Pinega and Mezen residents thought that the hiccups were "placed" into the human body by a sorcerer called "chaka." The "hiccups" penetrated into the body through the mouth. A female would feel as if she had swallowed something, assuming that it was the hiccups. And the "hiccups" were regarded as an independent spiritual substance. The suffering woman could even talk to the "hiccups" that were tormenting her from within. There could be several "hiccups», then they "were able" to converse with each other. The main concern of the patient woman and of her family was to prevent the hiccups attack and the desire to "appease" the hiccups, which may request a variety of things, such as beer, wine and sweets. During such conversation, people around usually could clearly distinguish the patient's voice and the voice of the "hiccups."

The "chaka," (the person who knew how to introduce the hiccups or who was suspected of placing them inside the body), was ostracized by the population. In the 19th century, there was a belief that only blood of the chaka could remove the "hiccups" from the patient.

Mentioning the existence of hiccups among the northern Russian peoples of the Pinega and Mezen river basins in the 19th century, we must pay attention to the ubiquity of the hiccups among the Komi people of the Pechorsk Region. The Russian word "ikota" (a hiccup in English) was not of Russian origin and came to the Russian language from Komi. Both the Russians and the Komi people have similar diseases attributed to the evil eye or hex. The hiccups were considered one of the manifestations of sheva hex by the Komi people. "Sheva" is a hex, disease, and evil spirit, personified in the form of butterflies, beetles, bees, flies, worms, threads and nodules (Sidorov 1928). The Russian peoples inhabiting the Pinega and Mezen river basins personalized hiccups exactly in the same way. According to the beliefs of the Komi people, during the attack an evil spirit – the "sheva" – spoke from within of the hysterodemonic patient. The seizures of the sheva patients among the Komi people were identical to attacks of hiccups among the Russian people in the area of the Komi-Russian ethnographic border area.

It is interesting to compare the phraseological locution recorded in the Pechora area "yersha spustit" (literally "send a ruffe fish") (i.e., send a disease with a sorcery spell). O. A. Cherepanov expressed an entertaining suggestion that the Russian word "yorsh" (literally "ruffe fish") with the meaning of "disease" was involved in the circle of mythological semantics by external identity with the Finno-Ugric word "yerekh" or "yorysh, yorsh" (nodule, patch, piece).

An important detail should be pointed out: hex in the Komi language means "vomida" (derived from the word "vom" – mouth). According to the ideas of the Komi and Russian peoples of the Pinega, Mezen and Pechorsk Regions, the hiccup spirit is ingested through the mouth and in the majority of cases is located in the stomach of patients. The notion of "sheva" that is common among the Komi as the term "hiccup" means both a disease and its cause, i.e. a certain independent spiritual substance.

Analyzing the process of "mastering" the ability to introduce or place hiccups inside a person, we observe a striking similarity in techniques of the Komi and the Northern Russians. According to the peoples of the Pinega, Mezen and Pechorsk regions, the following shall be done. "According to the Mezen people, a dog shall be taken into a bath-house, when it vomits, vomit shall be eaten; then one needs to refer to the "black book" (Bogolenov 1904). Among the Komi people, the apprentice of the sorcerer had to eat the vomit of either red or white dog in a bath-house, with the prompting of the sorcerer to learn the "black book" and carry out a number of magic acts (Sidorov 1928). The "black book" was, of course, a later phenomenon, which was included into the earlier ritual of the transfer of sacred knowledge, arising from an animistic set of concepts.

Many researchers write about the existence of an ancient Komi- understratum in the culture of the peoples of Pechorsk, Pinega Districts and Porechan people from the Mezen District. For example, in the lower reache of the Mezen river (among the Mezen-Pomor people) water plays the purifying force in hexes, and in the Leshukonsk district (among the Mezen-Porech people) this role is played by fire. Among the Komi people sheva hex can be destroyed only by fire. The Komi-cultural understratum is found in many elements of the culture of the Pinega and Mezen-Porech peoples, in particular, reflected in patterns of weaving and embroidery, in the semantics of images in Mezen paintings and in the language. So, in the Pinega region, non-Slavic names prevail in the names of rivers (about 85 percent), streams (50 percent), bogs and forest tracts (about 60 percent), and there is a high percentage of non-Russian words in the names of settlements (36 percent).

Among various reasons causing massive hiccups in the 19th century, the doctors mentioned poverty, starvation, dark, musty rooms, rough food, lack of heat, energy demanding labor, separated and subordinate position of women in the family and long polar winters. However, in these terms, the psychiatrists themselves reach a dead end, since it was impossible to explain why under the same specific conditions, there was a complete lack of hiccups in the western districts of the Arkhangelsk region and a ubiquity of hiccups among the Pinega and Mezen population (Shteinberg 1870).

Apparently, the hiccups in the population of northern basins of the Pinega, Mezen and Pechora should be historically regarded as a phenomenon of the Komi-cultural understate, the migration of which was facilitated by the induced nature of the neuro-psychiatric disorders. Demonological expansion among the Pinega and Mezen population was facilitated by the fact that "the Russians considered the representatives of foreign tribes (Komi, Finns, Karelians, Mordvinians) as more powerful sorcerers (Tokarev 1976). In the 19th century sheva-hiccups struck most of the adult female Komi population. Cases of hiccups among men were also known.

The evidence of M. B. Edemskii (1931) on cases of hiccups in the Kanin Peninsula is of interest for us. According to the stories of the Russian inhabitants of a village in the Kanin Peninsula, it was the Nenets people who had the ability to "place hiccups." "There is a Samoed person in the Kanin Peninsula who can do anything: send afflictions, hiccups, demons…." M. B. Edemsky himself noted that the beliefs connected with "magic", "sorcery", "nonconscience" were widespread in the Kanin Peninsula and were equally frequent among both the Russian and the Samoed people. The conclusions of M. B. Edenskii on the origin of hiccups have something in common with the point of view of P. S. Efimenko: "The local peasants were infected with hiccups from their Samoed neighbors." P. S. Efimenko found confirmation to his opinion in the fact that in the last century peasants from the Mezen district attributed hiccups "namely to Samoed sorcery." The similarities among the whole group of hysterodemonic diseases – hiccups, Arctic hysteria and piblokto – should be noted. The similarity of the symptoms of hiccups and piblokto was observed both in the groups of patients (mostly women) and in the nature of disease's development, seizures and the causes for them. Similarities were evident to some extent in the terms used. A woman suffering from hiccups was called "ikotnitsa" among the Pinega, Mezen and Pechora, and men sick with hiccups were called "miryak." The similarity of the words "miryak" and "emiryacheniye", (piblokto in English), does not seem to be accidental.

Due to the features of the spiritual culture, the ideas on mental health and pathology among the Pinega people had their own specific character. Hiccups were deemed within demonology as an "abnormal norm», i.e., a state in which the seizure provided contact between the patient and the spirit. In this context, the disease and the seizure played an important social role. It is important to note that in case of sheva, as well as of menerik (Arctic hysteria), emiryacheniye (piblokto), and shamanic illness, people would approach the "demons," which were inside the patients, treating them as oracles, asking about the future, asking for help in finding lost or stolen items etc. (Efimenko 1864).

For a better understanding of the nature of hysterodemonic diseases, it is important to pay attention to the socio-cultural hysterodemonic context in the Komi and the Nenets-Russian ethnographic border areas. Here, under unified geographical conditions different ethnicities of different economic-cultural types met and interacted with each other: the Komi hunters and fishermen from the northern taiga (Northern coniferous forest), Nenets cattle-herders and Russian farmers. There were also strong linguistic differences at the level of language family (Finno-Ugric – Komi, Eastern Slavic – Russian, Samoed-Nenets) between the ethnicities that were in contact. These populations had different belief systems. By the time of the contacts with the Russians, the Komi possessed the complex ideas associated with the use of magic, related to hunting and fishing. They retained animistic beliefs and totemic elements. At the same time the Nenets were shamanists and the Russians in relation to the above mentioned ethnic groups were the representatives of a developed class society (first, feudal and then capitalist), the developing state structures and the bearers of an Orthodox state ideology. All of these differences in the ethnic and cultural "genotypes" referring to these ethnic groups that used to contact with one another, were reflected in the forms of hysterodemony.

The question of Christianization of the Komi and Nenets has been deeply elaborated in the literature (Zaitsev 1983). However, the specific features of the social development of the Russian northern areas influenced the attitude towards Orthodoxy among the population of the Northern Russia. The clash of the monastic brotherhood with the peasant world during the exploration of the northern lands, forests, seas and rivers created a fertile ground for a very tepid "work-like" attitude towards Orthodoxy among the peasants. That contributed to the preservation and existence in the Russian north, not only the Orthodox heresies (primarily various dissent of the Old Believers), but also the more ancient pre-Christian beliefs of a demonological character.

Moreover, influenced by contact with populations possessing magical and animistic concepts, a kind of "renaissance" of hysterodemony and demonology occurred in the ethnographic border areas. As an example, the phenomenon of hiccups among the Russian population of Pinega and the Mezen basins can be used. In addition to hiccups, in the Pinega territory, other forms of malignant suggestion developed, for example, keela hexes.

Keela hex referred to boils appearing on the face of the affected person as a result of magic, hexes, coming from sorcerers or chaka.

17.2. Modern Mental Epidemics

The development of different techniques of suggestion and ways of influencing the human psyche among the Russian population of the Pinega district, probably explains to some extent the phenomenon of St. John of Kronstadt. He is a native of the village of Sura, who demonstrated the high efficiency of the Christian (Orthodox) approach in confronting collective obsession psychosis. Sura was one of the largest centers of hysterodemonic diseases in the North of Russia. According to the villagers, several generations of witches and priests had been among the ancestors of St. John of Kronstadt.

It is no mere chance that the last major collective psychosis outbreak of hiccups was in 1970, precisely in the village of Sura and affected almost the entire indigenous female population.

The locals sent a letter to the regional party committee of the city of Arkhangelsk asking to handle the problems and take action concerning persons "placing hiccups." With the instructions of public health administrators, a psychiatrist, neurologist and lecturer from the educational society "Knowledge" flew to Sura. The employers of children's centers, schools, hospitals, shops, and other establishments were involved in combating against the epidemics. It was discovered that the outbreak of hiccups epidemic arose when during the attacks several patients pronounced the names of women who allegedly had "placed the hiccups." Residents used various repressive actions against these women: one of them was strangled, stabbed with an awl, her house was set on fire, and she was forced to leave home and change her dwelling place. Court actions began. For centuries it was believed in this area that "hiccups speak" on behalf of a "hex placer" and only the blood of a "chaka" (person capable of "placing the hiccups") could save them from the disease. The patients demanded public confessions and breaking a hex spell, and after getting "refusal" patients dealt with chakas at their discretion.

Such archaic ideas about the nature of the disease, in particular, the possibility placing it upon someone, have been existing for ages, are strongly popular with the indigenous population and were a factor in chronic mental traumatization. The work of Associate Professor V. V. Medvedeva who was a member of the team working on the elimination of this outbreak has become the beginning of our long-term studies on induced neuropsychiatric disorders with symptoms of "hiccups" in the Pinega district of the Arkhangelsk region.

Over nine years (1970-1979) 146 neurosis patients with symptoms of "hiccups" had been studied. The major part of the patients was examined in their ordinary working and living conditions; some of the patients underwent outpatient and in-patient examination and treatment in the city of Arkhangelsk (in the Arkhangelsk Regional Clinical Psychiatric Hospital № 1). Catamnesis – for 5 to 9 years.

In addition to a clinical psychopathological method of research, experimental psychological method, EEG and laboratory (biochemical) methods were introduced; patients were also subjected to a thorough therapeutic, neurological examination and consultation with other specialists. The leading etiopathogenetic characteristics of neuropsychiatric disorders with symptoms of hiccups are presented in Table 17.1.

All examined patients were women, the majority (34.2 percent) were middle aged (40-49 years old). In the case of 73.7 percent of the patients, their relatives suffered from various forms of hiccups. We had records on the whole families whose members suffered from "hiccups." The hereditary burden of other mental and nervous diseases was not identified.

74 percent of the patients got primary education, 19.1 percent were illiterate. Experimental psychological methods revealed a low intellectual level, poorly developed abstract thinking, limited interests and needs in 97.9 percent of patients. All patients and their parents – natives of the Pinega district of the Arkhangelsk region – lived all their lives in one place, without traveling anywhere. In premorbid state hysterical and asthenic traits of character prevailed for the majority of patients.

The professions of the patients were associated with extensive contacts with children and adults. There was a constant contact between "hiccups" patients and a frequent possibility to see "hiccups" attacks.

Past medical history of the patients or their current state contained chronic somatic diseases, endocrine disorders in the form of menstrual disorders and decreased sexual desire. All patients were found to have autonomic disorders in the pre-onset period that deteriorated during attacks. Examination revealed the inversion of autonomic nervous reflexes.

Table 17.1. Etiopathogenetic characteristics of induced neuropsychiatric disorders with hiccups symptoms

Biogenesis	Psychogenesis	Sociogenesis	Animogenesis
• The frequency of closely related marriages with the accumulation of somatic and mental pathology • Hereditary burden of nervous and mental disorders (74 percent of relatives have suffered hiccups) • Onset coincided with altered reactivity during abortion, childbirth, pregnancy, menopause • The frequency of somatic diseases and endocrine disorders (menstrual disorders, decreased sexual desire) • Therapeutic resistance, high risk of recurrence	• Low intellectual level • Hysterical and asthenic temperamental attribute in the premorbid state • Familial forms of alcoholism and alcoholic husbands • Early exposure children to the sick person, frequency of observation of "hiccups" attacks • Perception of "hiccups" as a defensive strategy of avoidance • Low levels of resistance to stress • Internalized personal conflict • Neurotic personality development • Pathological personality development	• Onset coincided with the social stress disorder • Defective upbringing • Low level of education (74 percent possess primary level education, 19 percent are illiterate) • Sensory deprivation • Permanent (lifelong) residency in one place • Authoritarian parenting style in family • Social-class homogeneity • Rudimentary socioeconomic and political life • Low professional level	• Limited interests and needs • Troubled morale climate in the family • The prevalence of alcohol associated practices • Early formation of alcohol environment • Low level of culture • Ambivalent and unformed spiritual and moral sphere • Prevalence of syncretism and pagan beliefs • Prevalence of superstitious ideas about hexes and "placement of hiccups"

84.9 percent of the patients associated the start of the disease with a specific external factor, 54.7 percent indicated trauma as the cause of the disease (death of beloved ones, family troubles, quarrels and accusations of the "hiccups placing"). For 30.2 percent of the cases, the beginning of the disease coincided with delivery, abortion, pregnancy or the beginning of menopause. Only in 16.1 percent of the cases, the disease began with no obvious reason. Three forms of the disease were distinguished. Names of the forms were taken from the terminology that was currently used among the local population: "nemochischa" (literary mute), "revushchaia" (roaring) hiccups and "govoriaschaia" (talking) hiccups. Each form has its own clinical features, but at the same time, all the forms have several common characteristics (Table. 17.2).

Attacks can be triggered by anxiety, negative and positive emotions, unsatisfied desires, strong odors and sounds, the presence of strangers or seizures of any present person. Some patients have a kind of aversion or addiction to certain types of food or smells. This applies to the memories, associations connected with these objects or situations. Thus, a female used to get attacks in connection with a drinking husband (psycho-traumatic situation); the attacks could be caused by seeing a drunk person or smell of wine. Other female patients' hiccups were caused by the smell of tobacco or benzine. One patient said: "Mine [the hiccups] is modest, gentle, as it was placed inside me in girlhood. It likes warm wine, doesn't want to catch a cold; I find drinking warm wine disgusting, but I am afraid to disobey – immediately the attack starts." Another female patient said that she had three types of hiccups: "One of them does not like oil, the second one – sugar, and the third likes alcohol. I am completely exhausted; I don't know how to please them."

Table 17.2. Common clinical signs of "hiccups"

№	Clinical signs
1	The attack is provoked by excitement and strong emotions, unpleasant smells and sounds, unsatisfied desires and problems
2	The attack begins with signal symptoms: weakness, numbness, discomfort, yawning, watery eyes, increased heart rate and breathing, chills, fever, tremor
3	Hyperkinesis (ticks) of respiratory phonation type – voiced and verbal, obsessive and violent
4	Duration of the seizure – from several minutes to several days
5	After the attack – weakness and weariness, anxiety and depression
6	Patients' conviction that the hiccups are a material entity that enters the body through the ears, eyes, nose, skin
7	Forms of hiccups: roaring (63 percent), mute (25 percent), talking (12 percent)

All patients had the attack started with precursors (signal symptoms): weakness, discomfort in different parts of body, numbness, creeping sensation, globus sensation in throat, esophagus and stomach, irresistible yawning, tears, redness or paleness of skin, increased breathing and heart rate, palpitations, chills, fever, rash, hand and eyelid tremors or high blood pressure.

In all patients, the primary radical of hiccups attack is a kind of hyperkinesis (ticks) of respiratory or phonation type – voiced and verbal (genuine hiccups). They are of an involuntary, compulsive, obsessive-violent or violent nature. Patients cannot stop them voluntarily.

The duration of seizure is from several minutes to several days. At the end of the attack, patients feel weakness, fatigue, muscle relaxation, depressed mood, anxiety, and sometimes a sense of shame or embarrassment.

Among the examined patients, especially among the older age group, it is revealed that for centuries there is a belief (interpretation) that hiccups is a material creature that can enter the human body through ears, eyes, nose or skin. In humans, it may take the form of hair, fly, cockroach, worms or other living creature. It rules the body: "Where the hiccup lives, it beats like a heart, if it is in the spine, I cannot bend. If it is in the pit of the stomach or comes up to the throat, then it clamps down so that it is difficult to breathe, or if it moves to the hand and foot it looks as if mice are twitching. They say that it is nerves, but I do not believe." Patients attribute their specific addictions, painful sensations in the body and so on, to the influence of hiccups. According to them, hiccups can be obtained by direct contact with "hiccuper female», or through some kinds of objects or animals. In other words, patients have explanatory, interpretive, archaic ideas of possession, acquisition, witchcraft and "hexes" at a superstitious level.

Among our observations, the most common form of hiccups (63.7 percent) was the "roaring" form followed by the "mute" form (24.7 percent) and the "talking" form (11.6 percent). All of these forms can be considered as a single flow of stages of the same disease, as it is often started with a "mute" form, subsequently replaced by the "roaring" and then by the "talking" hiccups.

The mute form of hiccups is characterized by the following symptoms. Patients, suddenly, after some psychogenic influence, and sometimes without any reason, start to feel uncontrollable yawning, tears, redness or paleness of skin, chills or fever, there is an increased pulse rate, increased heart rate, blood pressure increased by 20-40 mm Hg, hyperhidrosis is observed as well as tremor of the hands and eyelids. Patients pronounce deep, sharp sounds, accompanied by a loud hiccup ("the hiccup fyikaet, khlykchet"). This form of the disease is called "nemochischa." The emotional state of patients during attacks varies (irritability, maliciousness, restlessness, tearfulness, anxiety, depression or adynamic state). Patients strive to be alone and need to lie down. During the attack the patient always remains conscious: patients are aware of their surrounding and are self-aware, answer questions in the periods between the hiccups and continue to converse or work until another attack starts. Seizures often occur in public places, but also may happen in private, and patients cannot stop it on their own.

The roaring form of the hiccups has the following clinical manifestations: more often after some unpleasant occurrence, and sometimes for no reason, patients suddenly start to suffer from yawning, lacrimation, rapid breathing, redness or paleness of bone covers, increased heart rate and blood pressure. The throat muscles and the diaphragm contract involuntarily, the patients' voice completely changes, they make yawling sounds, which people refer to as a "dog barking, bird singing, screaming rooster," etc. All this is accompanied by violent hiccups with crying or laughing. During attacks, patients complain of severe weakness, inability to work and go to bed. Other patients find it physically easy to tolerate these attacks and continue work or conversation. Patients, with the mute form also, always remain in conscience. During this time, as a rule, irritability, depressed mood, unfounded melancholy or anxiety arise. Patients strive to be alone, not to attract the attention of others. Some patients with characteristically emitted sounds declare that they have a hiccup in the form of a dog, bird or mouse in their body and the attacks express their displeasure or pleasure.

The next clinical form of hiccups is "talking" one. As for other forms of hiccups, the attack usually begins with unpleasant sensations in different parts of the body, numbness, creeping sensation, fever, globus sensation in the throat, esophagus or stomach, tears and uncontrollable yawning. At the same time, there are increased heart rate and blood pressure. Strong plangent hiccups are accompanied by the shouting of single words or phrases, which are often disarticulated. Patients shout out the names of those people who, in their opinion, hexed them. During the attacks, they let out information that in a normal state they would have never told anyone. Occasionally bouts of "govorukha" ("talking" hiccups) come up in the form of shouting of obscene words (coprolalia), echolalia or echopraxia. Other women suffering from hiccups always gather around the patient and persistently, over and over, repeat the question, asking the name of the woman who "placed" the hiccups. And the patients shout out the names. If a name is pronounced, the surrounding people strongly insist that the patient female dispose of the hexer. Patients can automatically submit and against their will instigate violence. Also automatically, "against their will», they assault the surrounding them people or smash everything within their reach. During the attack, the patients do not respond to questions, their conscience changes, narrows, they remember the conversations of others, automatically perform different requests of doctors, but this is despite their will (automatic obedience). They may respond to the wishes or orders of strangers that they regret after the bout (fight, smash surrounding items, undress, walk off somewhere else). The presence of delusional and hallucinatory experiences has not been determined. The duration of attacks varies: from several minutes to several hours or rarely days, with short interruptions. After the attack, for several days, many patients continue to experience weakness, fatigue, depressed mood, depression, and anxiety. Many patients are afraid of their "talking" hiccup attacks, because they understand that they pronounce the names of innocent people, friends or relatives, and the locals always start to take revenge on mentioned people and their family. This often leads to fights, attempts to murder and legal trials.

The mute form manifests with simpler, more elementary hysterical disorders. Roaring and talking forms are more complex, with a peculiar alteration of conscience (narrowing of conscience, hypnoid state) with increasing pathological obedience and suggestibility.

The developed and implemented preventive, corrective and therapeutic rehabilitation program consisted of four units: medical, psychological/psychotherapeutic, social and spiritual/moral.

The psychological/psychotherapeutic block. A series of workshops was held for all physicians in the endemic area; they were introduced to etiopathogenesis and the clinical overview of the disease, and the particularities of conducting psychotherapy for patients. Psychotherapy was conducted individually and collectively, in the latter case the sessions included patients with the same forms of the disease and gave them an opportunity to be grouped with those whom they wished to be with and whom they trusted. The psychotherapy consisted of seven to nine sessions of 30 minutes each. Before the first session, the patients were told in simple terms the essence of the disease. Seriously ill patients went through a course of hypnotherapy.

Rational psychotherapy was available to all doctors working in the neighborhood and district hospitals. In the form of conversation, the patient was explained the reasons of her hiccups, their development and ways of elimination. Psychotherapy was individually provided concerning the patient's personality characteristics, her relationship with the social environment and traumatic factors. Patients were helped to rationalize conflict situations. Mediation was conducted, and they were taught to give constructive responses to stress and were rid of their fear to have hiccups "planted" upon them. Psychotherapy was the core of the treatment and rehabilitation programs.

The medical block included remediation of neuropsychiatric basis and treatment of psychosomatic diseases, the use of general health promoting methods and vitamin therapy. To remove the affective and autonomic disorders, tranquilizers, nootropics, antidepressants and psychostimulants were used. Neuroleptics were used only for the relief of big attacks of hiccups. Treatment of patients with severe "talking" forms of hiccups began with hospitalization, and patients with "mute" and "roaring" forms were treated in the outpatient department. Supportive therapy with the use of psychopharmacological agents was carried out over the course of a few months.

The social block of care was aimed to improve the quality of life of the population of the endemic area, increase in production efficiency and work safety, social monitoring of risk factors and correction of the social and economic development of the area, leisure-time activities and assistance in solving social problems.

The spiritual and moral block of care was aimed at correcting of the moral and psychological climate in the endemic area, the early detection and prevention of mobbing degradation of ethics and dehumanization of relations, prevention of demoralization syndromes and destructive professiogenesis of society, training the ethics in business communication and providing constructive spiritual and moral guidance against superstition, conducting educational and awareness programs among youngsters, correction of morale climate in families with hereditary forms of hiccups, the correction and reconstruction of moral character and position of patients.

The implementation of a comprehensive program of care made possible the improvement and recovery of 82.2 percent of patients within five years. There were no further outbreaks of "hiccups" in the Pinega area. A young priest of the Sura parish, a participant of the 9th St. John Readings at the Northern State Medical University (2013), had not come across the "obsession with hiccups», replacing the modality in the mentality of the population in the endemic area with vicarious and other electronic forms of dependency, filling the psychological emptiness.

In conclusion, the following basic branches of research on mental ethnoecology and ethnomedicine in the European North of Russia can be defined: 1) transcultural mental ethnoecology studying mental health and mental illnesses in connection with socio-psychological and ethno-cultural factors; the literature describes the clinical picture of schizophrenia, neurosis, alcoholism among ethnic minorities; 2) cross-cultural mental ethnoecology that studies comparable aspects of mental health and mental disorders in different cultures. In this publication focused on a set of induced neuropsychiatric disorders among the Nenets, Komi and Russian peoples, we have tried to show the productivity of integrated studies in ethnographic border areas; 3) studies of culturally connected endogenous and psychogenic disorders, occurring within a particular ethnic group (shaman disease, Arctic hysteria, piblokto and others.); 4) "folk mental medicine" ("folk psychotherapy, psychiatry and relaxation") as a section of narrative ethnography and history of medicine; 5) ethnonarcology that studies traditional drugs of different nations, the recipes for their preparation and use patterns in different rituals and customs (ethnoecology mental and ethnomedicine section), for example, the use of of red fly agaric tincture by shamans during rituals; 6) interdisciplinary synergy research within mental ethnoecology and ethnomedicine framework, requiring cooperative efforts of psychiatrists and general practitioners, narcologists and psychologists, sociologists, and historians, ethnographers and philologists; 7) mental ecology of culture –study of social role of particular forms of mental illnesses in traditional culture, religious rituals, magic, shamanism and occultism, establishing of interrelationship forms of biomedical, ethno-social, ethical-psychological aspects of the spiritual culture of ethnic people and the world of art, psychology, international relations, and so on.

The separation of these areas helps to outline the subject of mental ethnoecology research and map out new horizons in traditional ethnography and innovative mental medicine.

Chapter 18

Destructive Professiogenesis

18.1. The Concept of Adaptive and Destructive Professiogenesis

Professional development or professiogenesis is a dynamic phenomenon, which includes not only the growth and improvement but the exhaustion and disruption, deformation and destruction, which affects the dynamics and trajectory of professional destiny.

Occupation affects the personality and gradually changes its behavior in general. *Professional deformation* - the destruction or modification of existing psychological structure of the individual in the production process. The emergence and development of professional deformation negatively affect the motivation and socialization.

Professional deformations are developped under the influence of working conditions and age, they distort the configuration of the personal profile and have a negative impact on labor productivity (Beznosov 2004). The socionomy professions, such as "man-man" are the most subjected to deformations.

The psychological determinants of the development of professionally associated deformations are the conflicts of professional self-determination, the crises of professional development and professional disadaptation, features of thought and action, social patterns of behavior, some form of psychological defense.

In Japan in the 1980s, the term "karoshi," which means "death from workaholism," was born. The word entered the lexicon after some prominent Japanese officials died during several years. The indirect cause of their deaths was the chronic fatigue at work and the stress, caused by lack of relaxation (Widlin, Kuntshe 2012).

The medical clearance of negative impact of the profession on the personality was the occupational burnout syndrome (OBS). For the first time, this term was presented in 1974 by American psychologist Herbert Freidenberg. Over 70 years before this the disorder clinic was described by Russian physician and writer V. Veresaev in the "Memoirs of a Physician" (1902): "For seven years now I have been a doctor. Every year you more than ever change into a wreck-neurotic: you lose the joy of life and adoration for it; lose, even worse, responsiveness and ability to feel the warmth ... The heart is vague and terribly empty. With horror, I feel that I am ill, seriously ill. For the last two years already I have been witnessing, how I am getting more and more exhausted, but only now I clearly realize what I have become." In the parlance of our time, Vikentiy Vikentievich was able to compensate his neurotic growth with therapies of creative expression, becoming a writer.

OBS is a long-term stress response or a syndrome, arising from the prolonged occupational stress of medium intensity. OBS is a process of gradual loss of emotional, cognitive and physical energy, which manifests itself in symptoms of emotional, mental exhaustion, physical fatigue, personal detachment and reduction of work performance satisfaction (Vodopiyanova 2011).

OBS is generated by personality the psychological defense mechanism in the form of full or partial exclusion of emotions in response to the chosen psycho-traumatic, stressful impacts. It is the acquired stereotype of emotional, mostly professional, behavior. The "Burnout" - is a partly functional stereotype, because it allows using the energy resources economically. At the same time, there may be its dysfunctional actions, when the "burnout" has a negative impact on the performance of professional activities (Ronginskaya 2002)

OBS is a multifaceted combination of stress disorders mainly with psycho-social manifestations. They insensibly destroy normal communication and human interaction. The main cause of these disorders - is the social characteristics of the society, which does not meet the natural human needs for the harmony of happy life, in joy and love, in the variety of worthy events (Kitayev-Smyk 2009).

OBS is the example of the interdisciplinary integration of psychiatry and occupational medicine because it is based on the clinical picture of neurasthenia, defined by American psychiatrist George Byrd in 1868.

We (Sidorov, Rodygina 2008; Sidorov, Novikova 2012) have developed the synergetic concept of a *destructive professiogenesis* (DP) - biopsychosociospiritual disorders, caused by a negative influence of occupational factors (on the medical workers model). The following *mental components* were indentified: social stressful and post-traumatic disorders (PTSD), depressive and anxiety-phobic, neurasthenia and related disorders (workaholism, alcohol and drug addiction, etc.), mobbing and deformation of the individual. *Somatic component* includes somatoform disorders and psychosomatic illnesses, occupational diseases. *Social component:* the violation of socialization, social dysfunction, disadaptation and degradation. *Spiritual and moral component,* which is manifested primarily in de-ethization and dehumanization of professional conscience and the development of the demoralization syndrome: the impoverishment of the inner world of the doctor; the loss of self-awareness and the spiritual personality of the patient; the perception of patient as a set of analyses; the utilitarian-consumer attitude to the patient; the deformation of a doctor's clinical thinking (feldsherism, psychology, biologism); leveling of psychotherapeutic impact and syntonia; substitution of communication with technical manipulations; clinical characteristics of a disease replaces the identity of the patient from the doctor's conscience; the reduction of the ethics in business communication with the patient to the professional patterns and stamps; "hystero-demonic renaissance" with the rejection of traditional medicine in favor of the occult and parapsychological studies; formation of economic dependence on the aggressive expansion of the pharmaceutical industry; the transformation of medical practices into the cynical business.

Considering, that a key symptom complex of any professional deformations is neurasthenia, we can say that over the past 145 years under the influence of interdisciplinary and methodological (synergistic) integration there was the evolution of its diagnostic dispersion from the classical neurasthenia to the OBS and then to symptom complex of destructive professiogenesis. It is crucial to note that the synergetics allows making a system diagnostic inversion, highlighting the *adaptive professiogenesis* - a regulatory biopsychosociospiritual professional development of the individual.

18.2. Prevalence of destructive professiogenesis

Medical activities are very diverse and not confined only to the treatment, as it is considered to be in the non-medical surrounding. A variety of types of medical activity creates different ways of its implementation, but it raises the problem of the specificity of the effect of different types of medical practice on the professional identity of the doctor and his value orientation.

The doctor's activity takes place in the conditions of elevated spiritual and moral and social-psychological needs and is associated with high intellectual and psycho-emotional stress.

Analysis of the literature showed that the OBS prevalence among health workers (table 18.1) is from 15 to 100%. According to average estimates, the most frequently observed OBS is among dentists, followed by psychiatrists and critical care physicians. Every second employee of oncological and somatic institutes, university professors has the OBS signs. Noteworthy is the following fact that every fifth employee of the rehabilitation institutes has the OBS, despite the fact that the working conditions in these institutions are less intense and stressful. The OBS is observed among doctors and nurses. Most researchers say about the higher incidence of OBS among nursing staff.

An important consequence of the OBS is mental morbidity among doctors. The data of a large sample of British doctors of different specialties shows a high prevalence of mental disorders among gastroenterologists, radiologists, oncologists and surgeons-oncologists, equal to 27% (18% of the population) (Levin, Kissane 2007).

Table 18.1. Prevalence of occupational burnout syndrome

Specialty profile	Author, year	Prevalence (averages)
Dentistry	Vragina 2007; Fokina 2009; Larentsova et al. 2010; Petrov, Gaidar 2012	72%-90% *81%*
Psychiatry, narcology, psychotherapy	Yuryeva 2004; Makarova 2006; Maligin et al. 2006; Lukyanov 2007; Gafarova 2008; Plotkin 2010	29%-100% *66.0%*
Intensive care	Mironov, Astafieva 2007; Nazarov 2008; Gafarova 2008; Belov et al. 2012	48,0% - 82,3% *65.2%*
Oncology	Soboleva, Globenko 2006; Kosimovskaya 2008; Olennikova 2010; Sidorov, Novikova 2012; Stiefel, Krenz 2013	28% - 96% *54.6%*
General somatic medicine	Kryachkova et al. 2006; Parpaley, Volodiy 2007; Zolotukhina, Shadrina 2007; Parfyonov 2012	30% - 80% *53.2%*
University professors	Berebin 1996; Kutuzova 2006; Kurapova 2009; Ivanova et al. 2011; Sidorov, Novikova 2012	32,0% - 72,1% *48.6%*
Surgery	Gafarova 2008; Gubin, Evdokimov 2009	15,0% - 45,0% *30.0%*

F. B. Plotkin (2014) rightly calls for more careful attitude to overdiagnosis of OBS in psycho-drug treatment community and do not forget the principles of evidence-based medicine. The irony of the author about the researchers, who detected 100% of its revelation among the doctors and their patients, is understood: "In this situation, the OBS, along with plague, cholera and anthrax should be recognized as the highly infectious disease (HID)." However, it is not excluded that the tomorrow's development of mental epidemiology will require the answers to no less dramatic challenges.

18.3. Etiopathogenesis of Destructive Professiogenesis

Among the occupational stressors, which contribute to burnout syndrome, the need to work in a strictly defined mode and emotional richness of the act of interaction are noted. The stressful interaction occurs because communication takes place hour after hour, day after day, for many years, and the recipients are the sick people, with severe fate, disadvantaged children and young people, criminals and victims of disasters, who tell them about the most intimate.

When analyzing the OBS as a one-dimensional structure, this phenomenon is seen as a state of physical and mental exhaustion, caused by a prolonged stay in the emotionally overloaded situations.

The OBS key component is the workplace stress: the discrepancy between the individual and specified requirements. The *organizational factors*, which contribute to the burnout, include: high workload; the absence or lack of social support from colleagues and superiors; inadequate remuneration for the work, both moral and material; inability to influence important decisions; equivocal, ambiguous requirements to the job; constant risk of penalties (reprimand, dismissal, prosecution); drab, monotonous and hopeless activity; the need for external showing of emotions, which do not meet the real (e.g., the need to be empathetic); no weekends, holidays and interests outside of work (Skugarevskaya 2002).

The *occupational risk factors* include: "helping," altruistic professions, where the work itself requires helping people (doctors, nurses, social workers, psychologists, teachers and even priests). The work with "difficult" clients is predisposing to burnout too. In medicine, they are geriatric, oncological patients, aggressive and suicidal patients, patients with addiction. Recently, the concept of a burnout syndrome has spread to the specialties, for which the contact with people is not common at all (programmers) (Makarova 2003).

Among psychotherapists and consulting psychologists the OBS is exposed to people with a low level of professional security, such as the lack of professional education and systematic skill improvement, inability to participate or irregular participation in Balint and Supervising groups; young age with a lack of life and practical experience. The emotional burnout syndrome may be provoked by illness, weakness after illness, experiencing severe stress, psychological trauma (divorce, death of a loved person or patient) (Lukyanov, Igumnov 2007).

The researchers from Vanderbilt University (Teaford et al. 2012) analyzed the reaction of the two teams of volunteers to perform the tasks of increasing difficulty. It was found that the "workaholics," who are ready to work more for the greater reward, have a high level of dopamine in the striatum of the brain and its ventromedial share - areas, responsible for reward and motivation. The "slackers" have increased dopamine level in the areas, responsible for risk and emotions assessment. The attempts at forcing such employee to work hard are virtually useless.

Among the factors of destructive professiogenesis in the cycle of our research we highlight the following:

- *social*: the lack of remuneration; "helping" professions; the need for externally emoting, is not really; activities, coupled with the responsibility for the lives of people; high degree of uncertainty in the assessment of the work performed; emotional richness of interpersonal interaction;
- *personal*: a high level of emotional lability; high self-control; idealistic orientation of the person; increased susceptibility to anxiety and depressive reactions; high empathy; sensitiveness; rigid personality structure; low resistance to stressors; disorientation of values of the individual;
- *professional*: high workload; monotonous, intense psycho-emotional activity; lack of understanding in the team; strictly regulated mode of operation; access to medicines; low material and technical basis of hospitals; frequent night shifts; no weekends, holidays (Sidorov, Novikova 2012).

18.4. Synergetics of Destructive Professiogenesis

In the synergetic methodology of the development of destructive professiogenesis, there are four vectors (Table 18.2), which determine a multidisciplinary and integrated approach to the investigation of pathokinesis of professional deformations.

Sociogenesis involves the development of social roles and relationships. The *disharmonious family* acts as a predisposition of the sociogenesis of destructive professional person development. Among the first signs of such a family is the presence among its members of some addiction, including its variants, associated with dependence on work. From the standpoint of synergetics, human desire to evade the stable states is clearly represented exactly in the need-motivational sphere of the psyche, and the last option of the stability of the system is a stop or loss of any system. Minor fluctuations in the stability of the positive and negative development of the subject of work, in all appearances, determine the professiogenesis destruction.

The logical process of following fractal dynamics is a *violation of personal socialization*, while in the age and professional aspects this process coincides with the period of occupational choice and entering into the independent professional life. With the increase in work experience and frequently repetitive negative emotional states, there is a *decrease in frustration tolerance* of the specialist. The person cannot devote himself to the work as before, feels the rapid depletion after professional activity, and to some extent, this is the economic, professional position and protective personal attitude. The following fractal of sociogenesis is the *workaholism.*

Table 18.2. Fractal dynamics of development of destructive professiogenesis mental epidemic

Ontogenesis vector	Prenosological fractals			Nosological fractals		
	Predisposition: family dysontogenesis	Latent: diatheses	Initial: functional disorders	Full-scale clinical picture/mental epidemic	Chronization: types and forms of the course/destructive mental epidemic	Outcome: /pandemic
Somatogenesis	Hereditary burden	Disorders of neuro processes	Somatoform dysfunctions	Somatization disorder	Psychosomatic disease	Professional pathology
Psychogenesis	Neurosogenic family	Personality accentuations	Psychopathization of personality	Personal decompensation	Deviant behavior	Personal defect
Sociogenesis	Disharmonious family	Personal socialization disorders	Decrease of frustration tolerance	Workaholism	Professional deformation	Social disadaptation
Animogenesis	Spiritual and moral family deficiency	Violation of moral feelings formation	Deformation of moral image	Destruction of spiritual and moral position	Probability of immoral behavior	Probability of unlawful behavior

Workaholism is manifested in the perception of the work as the only (or the most significant) means of self-realization, achieving of recognition, receiving the subjective satisfaction from life.

These symptoms constitute the basic framework for the possibilities of following *professional deformation*. The field of professional deformation of the person covers different by the nature phenomena. These phenomena, determined by a professional activity, should be distinguished from neurotic personality development, as well as mixed forms of not always effective tools to work, developing in the period of significant decrease in the inner resources of an employee under the influence of age and diseases.

The result of sociogenesis of destructive professional development is the *social disadaptation*, understood as a partial or complete loss of the ability to adapt to the conditions of the social environment.

Psychogenesis in its predisposition is determined by the length of professional activity performance, influence on the singularity of the individual development of the work subject. The important role is played by disorders of family relationships, as most of the socialization from birth takes place in the family. In particular, the neurogenic family is the first fractal in the formation of professional deformation and its outcome. As a result of an interaction of the broken family relationships and long-term performance of the same activity, the *personality accentuation* is professionalized, woven into the fabric of individual style and transformed eventually into professional deformations. *Personality psychopathization* in the "edge" version, is born under the influence of chronic psychogenic trauma, unfavorable social and psychological factors. Emerged pathological and characterological shift often "comes off" from the underlying cause and the pathological character's "self-development" begins (the psychogenic reason disappears, and the pathological changes of the person continue to grow). *Personality decompensation* is manifested in the expressed social dysfunction, leading to serious conflicts of interpersonal and intrapersonal characters.

Deviant behavior of a person is designated as a system of actions or individual actions, which are contrary to the accepted norms of society and manifest in the form of imbalance of psychic processes, non-adaptivity, and failure of self-actualization process or a deviation from the moral and aesthetic control over their behavior. In addition, the possible outcome of this process is *personal and psychic defects* in mild features of negative changes, expressed in psychic astenisation, excessive fatigue, the phenomena of irritable weakness, narrowing the range of interests and the gradual leveling of the individual properties of the character.

Somatogenesis of professional deformation at the beginning of its formation is possible with unfavorable *hereditary loading*. Under the influence of the negative factors of the social environment, as well as of the constitutional predisposition of the body in the form of imbalance of neural processes, firstly, the initiation of *functional disorders* and *somatization disorders* is possible. Then, in the process of increasing the intensity of factors of social impact, as well as the duration of this exposure, the *psychosomatic illness* is generated. The outcome of this process is the *occupational pathology,* caused by a psychosomatic illness, with all its multi-variant development.

Animogenesis is a central part of the proposed somato-psychosociospiritual ontogenetic model and with the various modalities of the mentality of the subject is integrated into all three considered vectors, filling them with a unique personality. Formation of mentality starts with family upbringing. The worst starting positions are *spiritual and moral deficits* and family anomie, with a high probability of marginalizing the younger generation. It appears in imperfection or violation of *moral sentiments formation* - duty and conscience, faith and responsibility, which may prejudge future violations of moral socialization and personality development, which has low adaptive capacity.

The school, with all the problems of general education, often becomes a testing ground of "Training fixing" of *disharmonious and deformed moral character*, with rudimentary or unformed social attitudes and ideas of humanism, mercy and tolerance. It lays the groundwork for the possible future development of the syndrome of demoralization.

Vocational training at university now has no official ideology for relaying of the spiritual and moral ideals. The traditional basis of professional education and training are replaced by "more modern" Western:

- christian virtues – by blurred universal values of freedom without responsibility;
- respect for elders and the joint work – by the development of the selfish individual and total consumerism;
- chastity, self-control and self-restraint – by permissiveness and intolerance;
- love and self-sacrifice – by the psychology of self-affirmation "at any price";
- interest for native culture – by an exceptional interest in foreign languages and foreign traditions.

All this leads to the increase of *dehumanization and de-ethization of professional conscience*, leading to deformation and *destruction of a moral position* - the ability to distinguish between definitions of good and evil, manifestations of selfless love and willingness to overcome the trials of life, culminating in the development of the syndrome of demoralization.

In the future professional activity, the *basis for moral conduct and ethics may devalue and destroy,* prejudicing the immoral behavior.

In the outcome fractal, the readiness for *unlawful behavior is formed.*

Thus, the synergetic methodology of mental medicine allows systematically consider all biopsychosociospiritual factors of development of destructive professiogenesis, which makes it possible to form comprehensively preventive-corrective and treatment-rehabilitation services in the framework of a multi-disciplinary program.

18.5. Features of Destructive Professiogenesis among Medical Workers of Oncological Institutes

In the literature, the professional work of oncologists refers to the risk group for the OBS development. Thus, the main frustrating factor is the necessity to deal with patients, who suffer from chronic little curable disease (Lozinskaya 2006).

Patients in the departments of oncology are the "risk factors" in the OBS formation, social disadaptation of health care workers according to their medical and social characteristics, diseases, treatments, operations and outcomes (Kasimovskaya 2008).

Patients with malignant neoplasms have a high prevalence of borderline mental disorders. Particularly, the nosogenic reactions in oncologic patients are found in 20-100% of cases

(Smulevich 2011). The presence of mental health disorders causes additional problems during the work with such patients.

Employees in the departments of oncology are constantly experiencing a state of chronic stress, associated with negative mental experiences, intense interpersonal interaction, tension, the complexity of work, etc. Gradually formed as a result of it, the OBS reduces the quality of medical care, creates a negative and even cynical attitude to patients, mental and physical fatigue, indifference to the job.

We (Sidorov et al. 2011) examined 40 employees in the Arkhangelsk Regional Oncology Center: 15 doctors and 25 nurses. The average age of the doctors was – 31.50 ± 1.79 years, and among nurses – 39.54 ± 2.03 years. The experience of professional doctors activities was – 6.70 ± 1.67 years, and nurses – 18.76 ± 2.45 years.

The comparison group was 20 police officers (Internal Affairs Agencies) of the Arkhangelsk region and 90 mentally healthy university students. The average age of the police officer was 32.30 ± 1.11 years; total work experience in law enforcement – 8.41 ± 0.78 years and the average age of students – 21.1 ± 0.34 years.

We have assessed the presence of the alleged 21 mental disorders: stress disorders; posttraumatic stress disorder (PTSD); social stress disorders; somatoform disorders; dissociative disorders; anxiety and phobic disorders; neurasthenia; depression; psychosomatic diseases; organic mental disorders; schizophrenia and delusional disorders; affective bipolar disorders; mental and behavioral disorders, associated with alcohol dependence, drugs, tobacco and other addictions; sexual dysfunction; eating disorders; sleep disorders of inorganic nature; personality disorders and behavior in adulthood; emotional burnout syndrome. As a result of responses, we defined the alleged mental disorder. For each of the disorders, the indicator values ranged from 0 to 18 points. Lower values indicated a greater likelihood of having a mental disorder.

Analysis of the results of the survey of health workers in the Oncology Center as described in the "Index of the mental ecology of personality" (Figure 18.1) showed the satisfactory levels of mental health in the majority of examined. At the same time, the index of the mental ecology of the personality among doctors and nurses was significantly lower compared to the police officers ($p < 0.05$) and students ($p < 0.05$).

Nurses had even lower IMEP values, that is in many respects related to the more frequent occurrence of mental disorders, probably, caused by the three times longer experience of their professional activities. The received data confirm the results of other authors, which refer to a more frequent occurrence of OBS among nurses compared to doctors (Soboleva, Globenko 2006).

The analysis of the components of the personality mental ecology (Figure 18.2) showed that oncologists and nurses had significantly lower values of psychogenesis in comparison with police officers ($p < 0.05$) and students ($p < 0.05$), that means they have a higher incidence of mental health problems. According to somatogenesis, the nurses had the lowest values in comparison with police officers ($p < 0.05$) and students ($p < 0.05$), that indicates on the somatization of the occupational stress symptoms among nurses and their possible manifestations of psychosomatic or somatoform symptoms.

The sociogenesis values among nurses were lower compared to students ($p<0.05$), indicating their dissatisfaction with the material situation, living conditions and interpersonal relations with others.

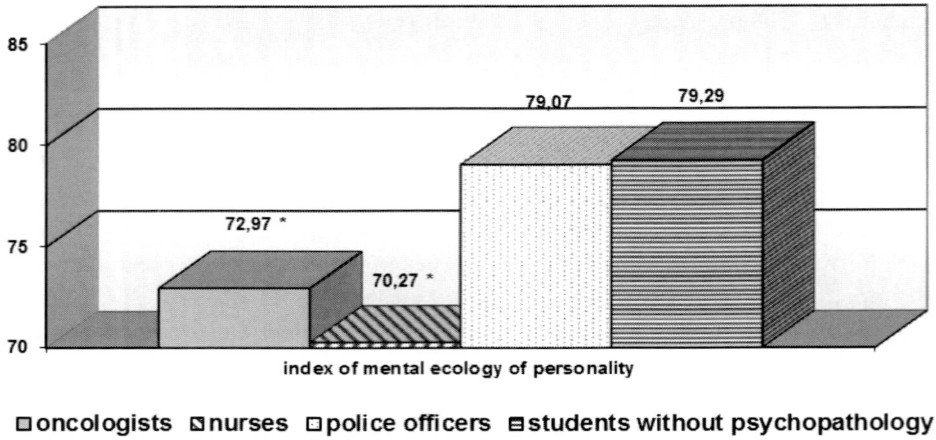

Note: The differences are significant at $^*p < 0.05$.

Figure 18.1. The index rates of the mental ecology of the person in different categories of the examined (M ± m; points).

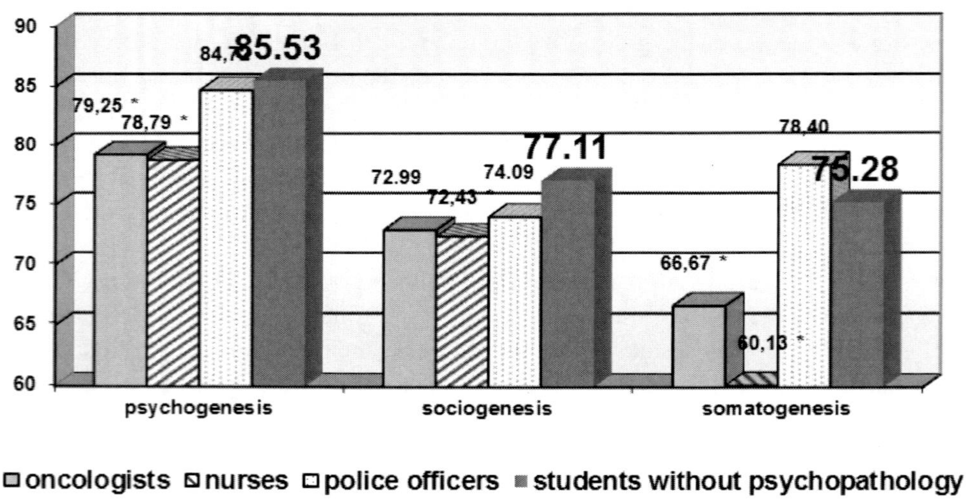

Note: The differences are significant at $^*p < 0.05$.

Figure 18.2. Component rates of the mental ecology of the person at different categories of examined (M ± m; points).

The screening of the borderline mental disorders among oncologists (Figure 18.3) showed that more than half had a tendency to the formation of social stress disorders and other addictions (tobacco dependence); nearly 40% had signs of depressive disorders, 1/3 had neurasthenia, stress and anxiety-phobic disorders. Every tenth doctor had signs of PTSD and alcohol dependence.

Nearly 2/3 of the nurses had signs of social stress disorders, among ½ - anxiety-phobic and stress disorders, every fourth - neurasthenia and dissociative disorders.

We can say that the medical staff of the department of oncology tends to have a frequent presence of psychiatric disorders of a neurotic level, which can be combined into one group -

post-stress disorders (socio-stress, stressful, anxiety-phobic). Doctors are distinguished with a large tendency to the addiction to tobacco and alcohol. Every tenth medical attendant had the signs of PTSD.

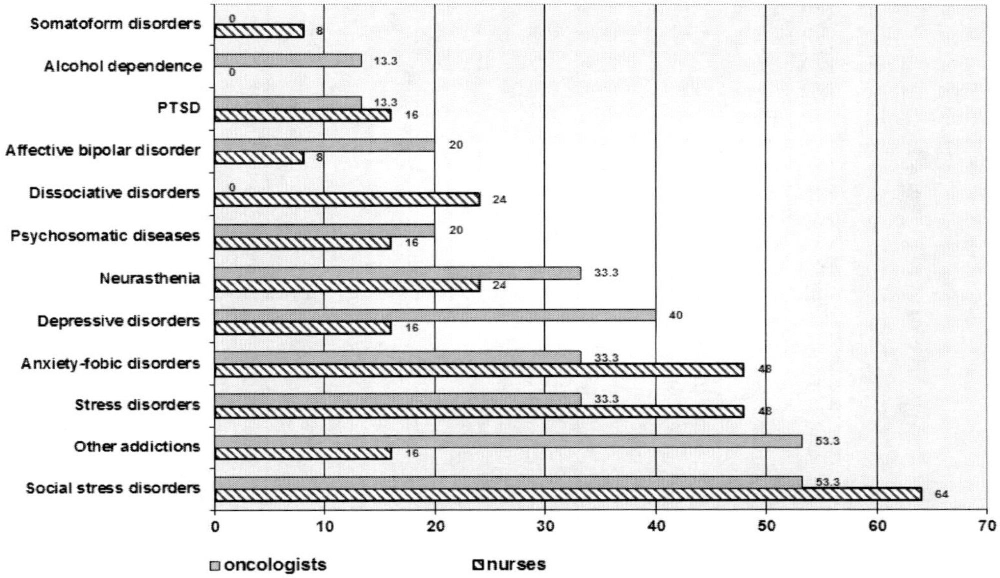

Figure 18.3. The screening of the borderline mental disorders among employees in the Arkhangelsk Oncology Center according to the questionnaire "Index of the mental ecology of personality" (%).

Our information is consistent with the studies of other authors, who noted the worsening of oncologists' mental state. Thus, the psychic disease incidence, according to T. Levin and W. D. Kissane (2007), is equal to 32%, and the frequency of OBS - up to 41%.

Thus, the health workers are exposed to the development of destructive professiogenesis, which confirms the need to examine the factors, contributing to its development and organization of preventive measures.

18.6. Medico-Psychosociospiritual Care

The synergetic concept of development of social epidemics of dependent disorders formed the basis for a program for preventive-correctional and treatment-rehabilitation help, which is a single multi-disciplinary protocol, implemented by a team of specialists. This program includes four blocks: medical, psychological, morally-spiritual and social (Table 18.3).

Primary preventive measures must be taken in predisposition fractal, where they can be aimed at determining hereditary and psychological predisposition, and socio-psychological and morally-spiritual harmonization of family relationships.

In the latent fractal, actions should be aimed at detecting people inclined to develop organ neurosis, on correcting moral socialization of the personality, psychopathic personal qualities.

Table 18.3. Program of medico-psychosociospiritual care in destructive professiogenesis

Blocks	Prenosological fractals			Nosological fractals		
	Predisposition: family dysontogenesis	Latent: diathesis	Initial: functional disorders	Full-scale clinical picture/mental epidemic	Chronization: types and forms of the course/destructive mental epidemic	Outcome: pandemic
Medical	Inclusion of persons with hereditary predisposition to neurosis in the risk group and their early preventive screening	Identification of persons with weak and unstable types of nervous system	Diagnostics of neurosis; pharmacological and nonpharmacological intervention	Clinical diagnosis, administration of medical therapy, prevention of complications	Control of the somatic state; adequate medical therapy	Treatment of somatic and psychic complications of SFD
Psychological	Identification of persons from neurosogenic families and their inclusion in the risk group	Correction of premorbid personality characteristics, escalation of stress resistance	Correction of psychosomatic reactions, psychotherapy	Correction of somatoform disorders, psychotherapy, psycho-pharmacotherapy	Correction of psychosomatic disorders, psychotherapy, psycho-pharmacotherapy	Psychological rehabilitation
Social	Identification and correction of disharmonies in family relationships	Correction of family relationships and harmonization of personality socialization	Harmonisation of significant social relations	Adaptation to the disease, correction of interpersonal problems	Professional and family adaptation	Social rehabilitation
Spiritual and moral	Screening and correction of the moral climate in family	Correction of formation and development of the moral feelings	Correction of the moral image formation	Reconstruction of a moral position	Reconstruction of moral behavior	Spiritual and moral rehabilitation

In the initial fractal in the case of functional disorders, the medicated and drug-free measures are assumed, hindering the development of destructive professiogenesis.

In the fractal of a full-scale clinical picture the early professional medical, psychological, social, spiritual and moral assistance is required. Timely detection and adequate diagnosis of destructive professiogenesis are crucial for successful treatment and a favorable prognosis. In the *chronicity and outcome* of the destructive professiogenesis, the most important are the socio-psychological and spiritual and moral occupational rehabilitation. Our experience shows that the effectiveness of aid will depend on the speedy institutionalization of the multidisciplinary and synergetic mental health services.

Of course, Confucius was right, saying: "Choose a job you love, and you will never have to work a day in your life." However, the path to such harmony for each person is own, and it is available only for creative souls, who do not get tired to refine oneself.

Section IV. Mental Epidemics of Dependent Personality Disorders

Chapter 19

Dependent Personality Disorders

Human society is dependent and manipulative in nature. Successful behavioral strategies in the environmental fate are possible only with the adequate assessment of all the variety of influences and relationships. Any behavior is predetermined by something and dependent from something. In a literal sense, there is no independent behavior; there is a variety of modalities and vectors, degree and levels of dependency.

The subject of clinical psychology and psychiatry becomes the dependent behavior, as deviant version, with the following characteristics:

- irresistible subordination of foreign interests;
- excessive fixation of attention on certain subjects or activities;
- reduced ability to choose and control their behavior;
- increasing of tolerance;
- loss of alternative interests; neglecting of complications and harmful consequences;
- an appearance of abstinence syndrome.

The addictive behavior includes:

1. "chemical dependency," or dependence on psychoactive substances – alcohol and drugs, sedatives and sleeping pills, stimulants and hallucinogens, tobacco and volatile solvents;
2. eating disorders – anorexia and bulimia;
3. sexual deviations and perversions (paraphilia);
4. psychostimulant non-chemical addiction – the extreme sports activity, gambling, kleptomania, pyromania, serial murders;
5. vicar (occupying the psychological void) addiction – hoarding, workaholism, secular entertainment, codependency, "binge reading," fanaticism as the dependence on the reference group or leader;
6. electronic forms and versions of dependencies – film and television, computer games, excessive use of computers and the Internet.

19.1. Prevalence of Dependent Behavior

Over the past half-century, the level of alcohol consumption in Russia increased by several times. According to official statistics, in Russia, the number of patients, who abuse alcohol, is more than 2.7 million people. This includes patients with alcoholism, alcoholic psychosis and alcohol abuse with severe consequences. According to experts, the real number of patients may exceed the official statistics in 5 times, reaching the index of 13.5 million. The important economic component is the abuse of alcohol among persons of working age. In the Russian Federation, about 2% of men and 1% of women, aged from 18 to 60 years, suffer from alcoholism. Moreover, almost one-third of working-age men regularly drink alcohol in hazardous doses, and their somatic diseases are associated with alcohol intoxication. According to the Health Ministry of Russian Federation, the level of alcohol per capita is 18 liters a year. In Russia, 75,000 people die each year from the effects of alcohol.

According to UN statistics, the highest number of drug addicts is in Iran and Afghanistan, the third in the list is Russia. Today in Russia 6.99 million people regularly use drugs. Official statistics on the drug abuse gives the number of 650 thousand, but it only appeals to those, who willingly are registered in the medical records. The number of deaths from drug use in recent years has increased in 12 times, and among children - in 42 times. In recent years, drug abuse is becoming a major cause of the increasing incidence of AIDS.

Currently, the world leaders in the number of gamers are Hong Kong, the US and Canada. In Russia, from 1 to 2% of the population are gamblers.

The Table 19.1 shows the prevalence of dependent disorders and comorbid diseases.

The records in Table 19.1 clearly show that Russia is characterized by a high prevalence of various forms of addictive behavior and comorbid disorders.

The common types of modern dependencies include *sexaholism and shopaholism, dependence on drugs and manipulation, dependence on exercises and suntan.* All this is the evidence of the growing prevalence of dependent personality disorders, many times changing during the life modality dependence. Growing manipulativeness and marginalizing of modern society facilitates the organization of any attachment for motivated TV or Internet producer.

Epidemiological studies show a prevalence of *game addiction* from 1 to 10% of the population: USA - 5%, Estonia - 3.5%, Ukraine - 8.3%, Russia - 4.8%. Herewith the game addiction among adolescents and young adults meets in 2-4 times more frequently than among adults (Chambers, Poteuza 2003). For each female-gamer there are about three men.

The prevalence of gaming in Russia is growing steadily, combining all forms of dependency. Not surprisingly, 3 of 4 patients had suicidal thoughts, and 10% committed suicide (Kekelidze, Shemchuk 2008). 34.2% of gamers were punished for criminal offenses, 60.5% admitted to committing them (Avtonomov 2010).

Russia is among the countries with the very high level of tobacco consumption. Up to 70% of men and 30% of women aged 18-49 years, smoke in Russia. The number of deaths from smoking has increased in 20 years by 1.5 times and is equal for the year to 400 thousand people. Still experts note the lowest cure of addiction and high volatility of remission with a large number of drugs and complex treatment and rehabilitation approaches. It is obvious that there is a need to build a fundamentally different system approach for the understanding of the pathogenesis and treatment of addictive diseases (Babanov 2002).

Table 19.1. Prevalence of dependent disorders and comorbid pathologies

Social ailments	Official statistics	Expert evaluation	Comorbid and associated disorders
Alcoholism	Approximately 1.7% of the total population	Eight-ten times higher (up to 15% of the population)	2/3 of the sufferers are unemployed (Yanko 2004)
Drug addiction	According to Ministry of Health – 0.3% of the population; State drug control agency – 3%; Ministry of Science and Education – 4.5%.	Real figures are 10-30 times higher; up to 12% of the population.	Between 17 and 73% are unemployed. In 2006 70,000 HIV- infected in St. Petersburg (Kozlov 2006)
Gambling addiction	In developed countries – 3-10% of the population; in Russia – 2 mln. people	In Moscow 300,000 (3%), in St Petersburg some 50,000 (Ministry of Health).	In men three times higher than in women; in teenagers 2-4 times higher than in adults
Smoking	60% of men and more than 15% of women; two times higher than in Europe (WHO)	Up to 65% of the population (Manvelov 2004)	Annually causes 1.2 million deaths or 14% of all lethal cases in European countries (WHO)
Crime	In January-November 2012 – 2136.1 million crimes were registered; in 2011 755,6 thousands of people were imprisoned	2-2.5 times higher than official statistics – 9-12 million crimes per year (Sitkovskyi 2004; MSRI MIA RF)	1/3 of road accidents occur under the influence of alcohol; every 6th crime is committed under the influence of alcohol; 80-90% of murders are committed under the influence of alcohol; every 10th person is registered in psycho-neurological clinic (Sedov 2004); among those sentenced, about half (400.000) have mental disorders; 86.000, have tuberculosis; 37.000 are HIV-infected (Federal Penitentiary Service)
Prostitution	There is no official statistics; the country has about 1 million people working in this sphere; in Moscow the number is about 150,000 people.	Several times higher (figures are not available)	47-71% abuse psychotropic substances; in St Petersburg 50.000 working in this sphere have HIV (Kozlov 2006); in 2005 – 1039 crimes involving into prostitution were registered
Unemployment	1.7 million; 6.1% registered	4.5 million (International Labour Organisation)	59% of those committed a crime do not have stable income (MIA, 2007)
HIV-infection	By 31.10.2012 – 703.8 thousands of Russian people are infected	five times higher (MH RF)	94% take drugs; 43% are unemployed; 20% of drug addicted who are accused of crime have HIV;
Tuberculosis	83,8 of diseased out of 100000 people (MH RF); annually 120.000 new cases and 30.000 die	Several times higher (figures are not available)	60-78% are unemployed; 60-80% have narcological problems (Tsoy 2004); 1/3 –in prisons
Sexually transmitted diseases	1041-1321of cases out of 100.000 of population	Several times higher (figures not available)	70-90% of cases of syphilis infecting are alcohol induced

The system concept of the different mechanisms of psychoactive substances (PS), and nicotine addiction, in particular, comes from the fact that the biological mechanisms of the dependence syndrome are identical, regardless of chemical substances supplies and are related to the specific dysfunctions of the dopamine neurotransmitter system, increasing with repeated and regular intakes of substances.

The prediction of the patient's condition with PS dependence and success of its treatment are impossible not only without the knowledge of prehistory (family and clinical anamnesis) and his personal identity but also without representations about the trajectory of the development of man as a biopsychosociospiritual self-organizing system in all transient and clinically executed states.

Summary data of many epidemiological studies show that 10% of smokers become ill and subsequently die from malignant swellings. Smokers get sick from myocardial infarction in 2-8 times more likely than non-smokers.

Almost half of children regularly breathe the air, polluted by tobacco smoke, and more than 40% of children have at least one parent, who smokes.

In human organism, there are no organs and systems, which can avoid the fate of becoming the target of smoking. So, in the course of many years of research, the connection between smoking and the intensity of pain even in the back has been shown (Behreud et al. 2012).

According to the WHO estimates by 2030 the tobacco dependence directly or indirectly causes 8 million deaths worldwide each year. More about 600 thousand lives are taken by passive smoking.

19.2. Etiopathogenesis of Dependent Personality Disorders

Currently, the mechanisms of etiopathogenesis and clinical phenomenology of dependencies differ with a great disputing. The following evolution of views can be built briefly and generally in historical dynamics on the concepts of addictive behavior.

Socio-hygienic concept explains the nature of the dependencies and relationships of living conditions of people, the nature of the customs of the social microsphere, production and economic relations.

Socio-psychological concept treats the dependencies as nonspecific indicators of socio-psychological personality insolvency, its undeveloped moral value sphere, person's non-involvement into socially active life.

The genetic concept, based on clinical-genealogical and twin research methods, convincingly shows the role of genetic predisposition. Molecular biological studies have shown that individual predisposition to alcoholism and drug addiction is genetically determined by the peculiarities of the function of "reinforcement system" of the brain, various organization of activities of the catecholamine system and its control by the genetic apparatus.

Genetotrophic concept tries to explain the dependent behavior by the hereditary metabolic disorders, which are based on the unusually high demand for some necessary food components (vitamins of group B, unsaturated fatty acids, trace elements, etc.).

The ethanol (narcotics) concept sees the main cause of alcoholism and drug addiction in the specific effect of alcohol and drugs on the body. According to this concept, people are divided into “alcohol-resistant” and “drug-resistant,” “alcohol non-resistant” and “drug non-resistant.”

Adrenochrome concept explains the addiction by disorders of catecholamine metabolism, resulting in permanent psychic tension. Psychic tension depends on the ratio of adrenaline in the body and its decay products - adrenochrome and adrenolutin, their precursors: the more adrenalin is in the body and less its metabolites, the more tension is expressed, removed by one or another addiction.

Endocrinopathy concept is confined to the fact, that dependent persons have the primary weakness of the endocrine system and for the appropriate emotional responses, the permanent artificial stimulation must be, especially in extreme conditions. Alcohol and drugs, other forms of addictive behavior activate the endocrine system and thus facilitate the exit of the person from psycho-traumatic situations.

Psychopathologic concept emphasizes the role of psychic, mainly of character, personality traits in the etiology of addiction. The trouth is that it is not always possible to clearly assess - these features are primary or secondary.

Bioenergy concept comes from the fact that alcohol and toxicants act primarily on the water-ionic structure of the body, disrupting its stability. The pathological architectonic of water-ion systems with a resonant spectrum memory occurs in the case of chronic intoxication. The resonance setting of bioenergy systems requires the constant use of alcohol and drugs, which leads to loss of stability of bioenergy structures of the human body and physical dependence.

System concept of the mechanisms of psychoactive different psychoactive substances (PS) comes from the fact that the biological mechanisms of the dependence syndrome are identical, regardless of chemical substances supplies, causing it development and related to the specific dysfunctions of the dopamine neurotransmitter system, increasing with repeated and regular intakes of psychoactive substances.

Synergetic concept is based on the developed by us (Sidorov 2004) biopsychosociospiritual methodology of mental (integrative) medicine, which takes into account all the etiopathogenetic diversity of mechanisms and trajectories of the disease development. The multidisciplinary methodology allows in the block-modular mode to design personified programs and routes of care.

The variety of views mentioned above underlines the need of multidisciplinary research of addictive behavior.

19.3. Synergetics of Dependent Disorders

It is possible to present the synergy concept of social epidemics of dependency disorders in a general and somewhat symbolic way (Table 19.2). For the ease of perception, the model is presented in a flat projection, even though it is multi-dimensional and nonlinear, unstable and non-closed loop, the trajectories of development are set and corrected at the bifurcation points, achieving spiral-like qualities and multi-options. Instead of the linear nosocentric dynamics with traditional stages and benchmarks, there are nonlinear discretion and fractality. The illustration shows only the progredient option of epidemic addiction development in four multi-dimensional interconnected planes: sociogenesis, psychogenesis, somatogenesis and animogenesis. The epidemicity of the disorder and its individual development trajectory are defined by a unique combination of various bio-psycho-socio- spiritual and adaptive mechanisms, predetermining the quality of remission, the risk of exacerbations and complications.

Sociogenesis is in some way predetermined by violations of the structure and function of parental family, disorders of maturation and socialisation of the personality in a disharmonic millisocial environment. Such personality has no psychosocial resources for productive self-realisation in studies or work activity, communicative environment and family relations. In many ways, it is the reason why non-pathological dependent behavior develops via compensatory mechanisms, characterised by obsessive fantasies, expressed in obsessive-compulsive actions regarding animals, governance of personal interests to paraphilia, long-term fixation of attention and lowered ability to control immersion in addiction, dependence and passivity in choosing a behavior strategy. Pathologically dependent behavior is defined by presence of episodes of changed conscience when submitting to the psychological and physical addiction, overwhelming and compulsive nature of addiction, stereotyping of a criminal way of life, withdrawal syndrome. In the end – total social disadaptation.

The trajectory of epidemic development can change in bifurcation points when mobilising adaptation resources, compensation or defence. In this case, the object or style of addiction may change. Remission in the synergy context means switching the dependent person to a different modality and behavioral trajectory while retaining the dependency patter (Figure 19.1).

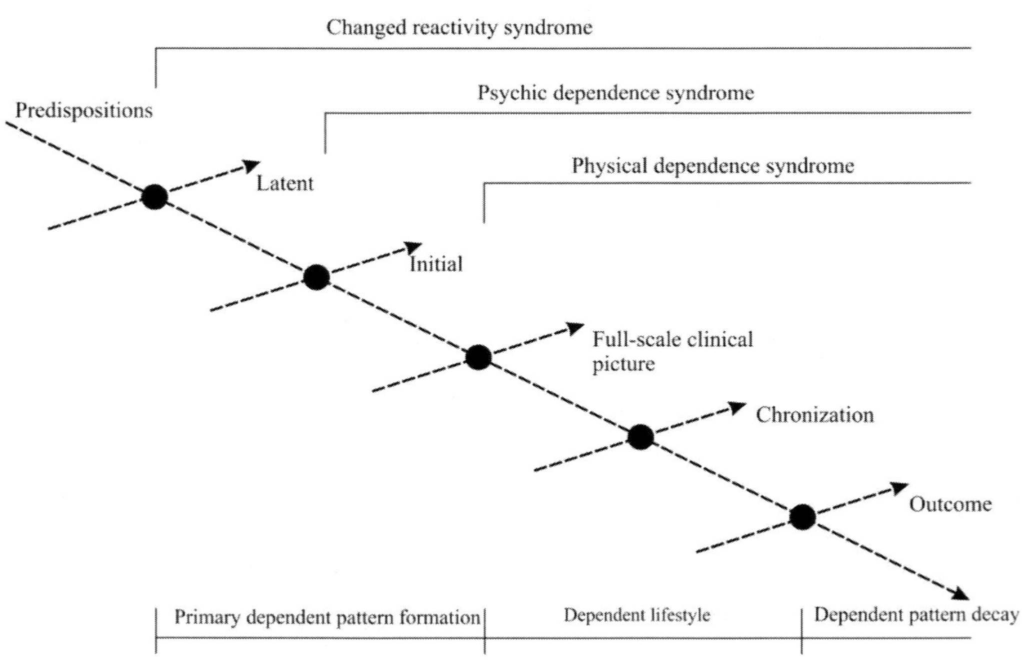

Figure 19.1. Fractal trajectory of dependent disorder development. ● - bifurcation points.

Psychogenesis is in a significant way predetermined by the premorbid psychopathological load, different from emotional and communicative defectiveness, which are later displayed as the addictive radical of psychopatisation and personality deformation. Such personality, even when encountering banal living difficulties, can exhibit various social-stress disorders that start the process of the primary dependent pattern forming. The dependent personality, outside the personality disorder, exhibits bright realistic reminiscences and fantasies with background infantilism and suggestibility, naivety, sensual spontaneity, curiosity or high search activity, maximalism and egocentrism, impressionability and impatience, tendency to risk and invite danger. Dependent personal disorders are characterised by a depletion of normative sociality, deformation of the personality and emotional burnout, inability to make decisions independently outside a criminal way of life, combination of schizoid personality traits with poor tolerance to loneliness, which supports the development of anxious depression and pushes towards committing delict, offering a temporary psycho-emotional release.

Dependent personality disorders in ICD-10 include inability to make decisions without advice from other people; readiness to let others make important decisions; readiness to agree with others out of fear of being rejected, even when realising that they are wrong; difficulty in starting something independently; readiness to voluntarily do demeaning and unpleasant jobs with the aim of gaining support and love of people; poor tolerance of loneliness – readiness to undertake significant efforts to evade it; feeling of void or helplessness when a close connection is broken; fear of rejection; easy vulnerability, amenability at the slightest critique and disapproval from outside.

As a result, one can expect a psychological defect, significantly differing with various types of addiction: from emotional burnout syndrome for workaholism to psycho-organic syndrome with chemical addictions.

Somatogenesis is one of the least researched aspects of this problem. An important role is played by non-specific hereditary load, unfavourable intra- and perinatal influences. The response to various challenges and difficulties may be various normative psychosomatic reactions, which later turn into psychosomatic disorders (organic neuroses) and somatoform disorders, clinically defining the individual peculiarities of the developed "withdrawal syndrome." The severity of possible comorbid psychosomatic diseases is predetermined by the duration of the "withdrawal syndrome," inability of the deformed personality to achieve a psychological release within the adaptive behavior. The illusion of release is only achieved via delict and dependent behavior. With all forms of dependent behavior, there is a lack of parallelism in expression of mental, neurological and somato-vegetative disorders. If chemical addictions reach in somatogenesis an evolution of disorders, significantly connected to the toxic agent, then non-chemical addictions have comorbid psychosomatic diseases as compensatory option of development. It can be called the somatisation mechanism of addiction. In the end, one can expect somato- neurological complications. The notion of comorbidity is based not so much on the traditional understanding of compatibility of pathology but on the etiopathogenetic unity of the majority of forms of dependent behavior. In the most progredient option the fractals are replaced: pre-disposition – changed biopsychosociospiritual "ground"; latent – memories – obtrusive reminiscences; initial – obsessive fantasies – obsessive-compulsive actions (premonitory sign of detailed clinical findings); detailed clinical presentation – behavior with dependency traits; chronization – forms and types of disease course; outcome – reverse pathokinesis.

Table 19.2. Fractal dynamics of mental epidemics of addictive disorders

Ontogenesis vectors	Prenosological fractals			Nosological fractals		
	Predispositions: addictogenic family	Latent: addictogenic diatheses	Initial: functional disorders	Full-scale clinical picture/mental epidemic	Chronization: types and forms of the course/destructive mental epidemic	Outcome: somato-neurological complications /pandemic
Somatogenesis	Hereditary burden	Disorders of neuro processes	Somatoform dysfunctions	Comorbid psychic diseases	Psychoorganic stigmatization	Somato-neurological complications
Psychogenesis	Psychological burden	Psychopathisation of personality	Dependent personality beyond personality disorder	Persistent personality disorders	Dependent personality disorder	Mental defect
Sociogenesis	Family structure and function violations	Personality socialisation violations	Non-pathological dependent behavior	Pathologically addictive behavior	Social decompensation	Social disadaptation
Animogenesis	Moral and spiritual family deficiency	Violation of moral feelings	Deformation of moral image	Destruction of spiritual and moral position	Demoralization syndrome	Unlawful behavior

The non-episodic dynamic of epidemic forms of dependent behavior is expressed in the growing emotional burnout and deforming of the personality, development of comorbid psychosomatic disorders.

Animogenesis starts in the fractal of predisposition – addictogenic family, with a moral and spiritual deficit and a high possibility of dependent disorders in the parents and closest relatives. This is expressed in "addictogenic sensibilisation" of the child's internal world. Such a family is anomic in its nature and is highly likely to marginalise the growing generation to begin with, not leaving any chances for normal formation of moral feelings and moral portrait, predetermining moral socialisation disorders in teen years and deforming personality development.

Street company often becomes the testing area for the "training reinforcement" of the deformed moral portrait, with rudimentary or unformed social settings and ideas on humanism, mercy, and tolerance. This sets the basis for the future development of demoralisation syndrome.

Epidemic development of addiction leads to deformation and destruction of the moral position of the personality, dehumanisation and de-ethisation of conscience, loss of the ability to define good and evil, expressions of friendship and love, readiness to overcome life's obstacles. All this accumulates in the demoralisation syndrome development.

As the addiction epidemic develops, the very core of moral behavior and ethics is devalued and destroyed, predetermining amoral and illegal behavior.

The synergetic approach allows implementing a single methodology for analysing all epidemic forms of dependent disorders – from alcoholism and drug addiction to fanaticism and terrorism, corresponding to priority directions for development of mental medicine.

19.4. Medico-Psychosociospiritual Care

Synergetic approach supposes significant reconsideration of preventive and treatment-rehabilitation strategies for helping dependent personalities, changing the ideology and methodology of traditional narcology service. A dependent personality demands non-stop and interactive sanitation and correction that can only change the vector and modality of the addiction.

The task of therapy for such person consists in maximally early replacement of modality from the destructive onto constructive, from maladaptive onto adaptive, from asocial onto prosocial, from autoaggressive onto self-perpetuating. Preventive strategy for dependent subpopulations requires the adequate and regular load of *adaptive psychosocial and spiritual and moral content.*

Traditional approaches to the consideration of the effectiveness of therapy for the duration of remission need to be complemented with the assessment of comorbid psychosomatic diseases. The self-perpetuating way of life and its decent quality become the main priority for rehabilitation. Bio-socio-psycho-spiritual synergetic model of addictive behavior requires the introduction of multi-disciplinary brigade organization forms of psychoprophylaxis and correction. The subject of preventive activities should be a new class of preventology professionals, professionally engaged in the self-preserving behavior.

Table 19.3. Program for medico-psychosociospiritual care in addictive disorders

Blocks	Prenosological fractals			Nosological fractals		
	Predisposition: addictogenic family	Latent: addictogenic diatheses	Initial: functional disorders	Full-scale clinical picture/mental epidemic	Chronization: forms and types of the disease course/destructive mental epidemic	Outcome: complications/ pandemic
Medical	Detection of people with hereditary predisposition, including them in the group of risk, early preventive screening	Detection of people with organ neurosis	Diagnostic of somatoform dysfunctions; medication-assisted and drug-free treatment	Detection of comorbid psychiatric diseases, prescribing medications, prevention of complications	Proper medication therapy of psycho- organic stigmatisation	Treatment for somato-neurological complications
Psychological	Detection of people with psychological burden and taking preventive measures with them	Sanitation of psychopathisation of the personality	Detecting the dependent personality beyond personal disorder and correction	Correction of persistent personality disorders, psychotherapy	Psychotherapy and psychopharmacotherapy of dependent personality disorder	Psychological rehabilitation of personality defect
Social	Detection and correction of violations of family structure and function	Correction of personality socialisation	Correction of non-pathological dependent behavior	Complex treatment of pathologically-dependent behavior	Correction of social decompensation	Social rehabilitation
Spiritual and moral	Screening and correction of the family "moral climate"	Correction of formation and development of moral feelings	Correction of formation and development of moral image	Reconstruction of moral position	Reconstruction of moral behavior	Spiritual and moral rehabilitation

Questions of medical and psychosociospiritual care for dependent disorders are discussed in detail in the two editions of "Addiction medicine preventology" (2005, 2006), so here they are stored only for the importance of demonstration of the methodological unity of the approaches to all variants of mental (social, asocial) epidemics.

On the basis of the synergetic concept of the formation of addictive behavior, we have developed a program of preventive-corrective and treatment-rehabilitation care, which is a single multidisciplinary protocol, implemented by a team of specialists. The program consists of four parts: medical, psychological, spiritual and moral and social (Table 19.3).

Primary preventive measures must be taken in predisposition fractal, where they can be aimed at determining hereditary and psychological predisposition, and socio-psychological and morally-spiritual harmonisation of family relationships.

In the latent fractal, actions should be aimed at detecting people inclined to develop organ neurosis, on correcting moral socialisation of the personality, psychopathic personal characteristics.

In the initial fractal when the non-pathological dependent behavior occurs, the medication-assisted and psychotherapeutic action is prescribed, stopping the development of dependent behavior and correction of the moral portrait. In the fractal of detailed clinical findings early qualified narcological and psychotherapeutic, psychological and social, spiritual and moral care is required. At the chronisation stage, experts provide adequate medication-assisted therapy, psychotherapeutic treatment of the dependent disorder, socio-psychological and spiritual and moral correction of demoralisation syndrome.

When psychiatric defect and social disadaptation occur, psychological and social, medical and spiritual and moral rehabilitation based on multi-disciplinary mental health service have to be organized.

All preventive-corrective and therapeutic-rehabilitation routes of the biopsycho - sociospiritual program are imbued with the ideology of correction and change of pessimistic, catastrophic paradigms of perception of the world for the resource and creative life strategy, which predetermines adaptive professiogenesis, sustainable development and the freedom to choose the path of their destiny.

Chapter 20

Mobbing Syndrome: Mental Terrorism of "Office Wars"

20.1. Definition and Classifications

In a German reference book "Psychiatry and Psychotherapy" (2010) mobbing is separated as an independent psychiatric syndrome, including harassment and insulting an employee at the working place to make him/her quit the job voluntarily.

Mobbing (mobbing – from English to "mob" – to be rude to someone, to crowd around someone in an unruly way) – is a form of psychological violence, when a staff mobs its employee in order to make him/her quit the job. Mobbing is manifested in a long-term nagging, intimidation and harassment of a staff towards its employee. Mobbing includes negative statements, unfair criticism, social isolation and distribution of misleading information, moral pressing and even physical coercion (Druzhilov 2011; Sidorov 2013).

The concept of "mobbing" was introduced in 1958 by biologist Konrad Lorenz (1963), who described the phenomenon of a small animals' group attack on a bigger enemy. The term was coined in psychology and medicine in the 1960s by a Swedish doctor P. Heinemann, published the book "Mobbing - Group Violence among Infants and Adults," where he compared the behavior of children towards their peers with the aggressive behavior of animals. Another Swedish researcher H. Leymann (1996) on the basis of human behavior in a staff, characterized mobbing as "psychological terrorism," including systematically repeating hostility of a person or several people to another one.

There are two types of mobbing: *vertical* - "bossing" (from English "boss"), when the psychological terror is originated from the boss, and *horizontal* - when the harassment is performed by the colleagues. Mobbing may be manifested latently (inwardly) or openly.

The literature (Skavitin 2004; Kolodey 2007) provides numerous varieties of mobbing: silent treatment, nagging, mockery, misleading information (gossips), whistle-blowing and slanders, personal injuries, pilferage, damage to personal belongings. The situations of multi-layered and network harassment are called sandwich-mobbing while short-term actions via the internet or mobile phone are called flesh-mobbing. Dramatic variants of psychological terrorism with aggression and cruelty are called bullying (Rekosh 2002).

There are the following main forms of mobbing (Malkina-Pykh 2006; Solovyev 2009):

- *verbal aggression* towards an employee (provocative questions; false statements; expression of doubts in the level of professionalism and competence; emotional assaults and intimidation; distrust of the made arguments; reasonless accusations of something etc.);
- *constant discussion* with the employee in order to talk him/ her down (rude and arrogant interruption of a subordinate; expression of disagreement before he/she is able to express his/her opinion, explain a viewpoint or make an argument; perception only of the information, which may be somehow used against the employee; neglect of objective and valid arguments etc.);
- *bursts of anger,* accompanied by rude statements, humiliating the employee's personality, instigating him/her to make mistakes or inducing to disparage;
- *ostentatious refusal* to continue discussing problems with the employee or in his/her presence;
- *reduction of terms for assignments* or deliberate procrastination in decision-making, related to the tasks performed by the employee;
- *intentional failure to provide the employee with comprehensible and reliable information,* necessary for the performance of a committed task;
- *unwarranted change in wage rate* of the employee;
- *displacement of the workplace* to suppress the employee morally;
- *intentional dissemination of false information* and gossips about the employee;
- *illegal participatory consideration of the behavior* of the employee;
- *paying attention to faked complaints and denunciations;*
- progressive *social deprivation and isolation* in the staff, ostentatious exclusion of the victim;
- *dramatization of the situation* – the aggravation by the harassment participants of the employee's frustration;
- *mockery and abuse* of the victim.

V. Skavitin (2004) highlighted four main types of a mobbing-terrorist:

- "*Two-Headed Snake*" – people, manipulating the social mind of a staff, generating rumors and gossips behind the back of a victim, damaging reputation (37%);
- *"Screaming Mimi"* – defiantly outrageous behavior of an abuser, instigating the "victim" (13%);
- *"Gate-Keeper"* – a person, trying to set up total control over all kinds of resources and to limit the access to them for the "victim" (20%);
- "*Permanent Critic"* - a person, assaulting and nagging at the victim on a daily basis, leading the "victim" into the inferiority complex (3%).

The most dangerous are serial bullies, distinguishing by masterful deceit and the ability to improvise. They easily act like Mr. Nice Guy, hiding ungenerous rancor behind it. They are amiable in the presence of their boss, but behave disgustingly and even sadistically with their subordinated. They pay great attention to their external image, trying to imitate erudition and successful management. They are prone to self-admiration, arrogance, narcissism and hysterical personality disorder. They easily adjust their words depending on the task. After another victim has quitted the job, the serial bully finds a new object for mobbing.

Mobbing is a syndrome of *destructive professiogenesis* – psychosomatic and socio-spiritual disorders, caused by a negative influence of occupational factors. Mobbing is characterized by the focus on a socially harmful result. A person is oriented to destructive professional values and results. Consequently, he/she sets socially unacceptable goals and uses destructive means for the staff to reach them (Druzhilov 2011; Sidorov 2013). The examples of self-destructing activities are acquisitiveness and egocentrism, vehement recusancy and manipulation.

20.2. Prevalence of Mobbing

Evaluation of mobbing incidence discovers a large variety of different gender and age, occupational and social groups. According to generalized estimates, the prevalence of the disorder in the western industrial countries is from 1 to 10% (Laux, Meller 2010; Hokhlova 2010).

According to the results of a survey of 4500 employees working in different business spheres in Germany (Solovyev 2013), almost two-thirds of the Germans (61%) experienced mobbing at the workplace. Moreover, in 34% of the cases it was originated by "dear colleagues," and in the rest of the cases - by the boss. Only a quarter of the respondents assured they had not experienced mobbing personally, and 12% confessed, that they had taken part in the harassment of their colleagues.

By order of German Federal Office of Labor Protection and Healthcare a special research was conducted, having indicated the "mobbing quota" for Germany equal to 2, 7% (an average rate for Europe). It reflects the percent of people experienced harassment in their companies against the total number of the employed. By calculation of this rate concerning the average time of active working life of a person, it appeared that every ninth German of the working age experienced mobbing at least once. The risk group includes people under 25 ("mobbing-quota" – 3,7) and over 55 (2,9%), employed in social professions (preschool, school and university teachers) and those, who work in the service sector. Women's chances to become a "mobbing-target" are higher by 60%.

In the sphere of education of France (Rekosh 2002) mobbing incidence (30-50%) twice as large as in other spheres of activities; the duration of moral bulling is from one to five years and in 90% of all cases it is originated from the boss.

In the USA there is a special organization, studying the problem of bullying of employees in the workplace - The Workplace Bullying &Trauma Institute (WBTI). According to the survey of 1000 respondents (Solovyev 2009), the mobbing of women (50%) and men (30%) prevails towards female employees; harassment of male employees by men (12%) and women (8%) is less prevalent. In the vast majority of cases (71%) the mobbing is originated from the boss, while in 17% - from colleagues of the same status and in 12% of the cases, the harassment is performed by the subordinates.

3–4% of new-hired people find themselves in the situation of direct or indirect psychological pressing because a new employee always influences the relationship existing in a staff. Among the employees, who have already been working in an organization for a long time, 30-50% of them become the victims of mobbing (Bazarov 2006).

The survey of 17-22-year-old students of a technical college in the city of Apatity, Russia (Legotina 2006) discovered that 98,5% were the witnesses of mobbing, 66% were the "mobbing-terrorists," 20,8% count themselves "mobbing-targets."

20.3. Etiopathogenesis of Mobbing

Biological and genetic origins of mobbing are described in ethnological researches when an organized group of animals attacks single species to expel them. In developmental psychology and pedagogics, harsh group behavior of infants is described towards their peers having special mental features and not meeting age, personal or social standards. Later, the acquired stereotypes of "maladaptive socialization" are transferred to the adult educational and professional environment. Nonetheless, the roles can multiply change. Later on, an infant's social and psychological experience of being a mobbing target can be transformed into the image of mobbing-terrorist by compensatory mechanisms. It goes much faster in the army when after two years of the draft a young soldier acquires the skills of humiliating the juniors (Sidorov 2013).

A modern stressful by its nature labor market in the epoch of global crisis dramatizes the problems of destructive professiogenesis.

A key predictor of mobbing is a stress at the workplace: inconsistency between a person and the requirements imposed upon him/her. There are the following non-specific organizational mobbing-factors: high workload; lack or deficiency of social support from colleagues and boss; inadequate reward for the job both, moral and material; inability to influence important decision-making; ambiguous, unclear requirements to work; constant risk of fine sanctions (reprimand, dismissal, legal prosecution); monotonous and unpromising activities; necessity to express the emotions, which are not real (e.g., necessity for a doctor or teacher to be empathic); lack of holidays, vacations and interests outside work.

The non-specific professional risk factors include: "helping" and altruistic professions, where the work itself obliges to help people (doctors, trained nurses, social workers, teachers and even clericals). Work with "difficult" clients also predisposes to mobbing. In medicine, these are gerantological, ontological, aggressive, suicidal, and addictive patients. The destructive professiogenesis has currently begun to spread to the specialties, which are not characterized by contact with people (programmers) and there the mobbing fightings are started in the internet ("virtual mobbing").

Among psychotherapists and consulting psychologists there are people exposed to mobbing, who have a low level of professional security, for example, people with absence of professional education and systematic advance training, inability to participate or non-regular participation in balint and supervising groups; young people without life and work experience. Mobbing can be provoked by disorders, severe emotional stress and psychological traumas.

General conditions of origination of mobbing in a staff are low corporate culture and inefficient management:

- prevalence of parental and (or) sexual relationship;
- mature employees, who are afraid of losing their position;
- duplicating positions and diffuse responsibility;
- tolerance towards intrigues and gossips;
- diffuse limits of employment duties;
- the inconsistency of a workload – one person has to work hard, another one relaxes;
- lack of opportunity to advance in career;
- weak and coward boss, considering quarrels in his staff to be a mechanism of manipulative management.

The risk group of mobbing-targets includes:

- unusual people;
- emotionally opened simpletons;
- arrogant individualists;
- chronic complainers;
- breachers of corporate morals and unspoken rules;
- ambitious newcomers;
- bosses, who are prone to favoritism and their “whisperers”;
- abruptly promoted or demoted employees;
- new bosses, generating innovations;
- colleagues to share the work with;
- “don juans” and “messalinas,” overplaying with the opposite sex;
- vicious jokers knowing no measure;
- too sensible people with subnormal stress and frustration tolerance.

There are the reasons of mobbing origination, indirectly connected with the victim’s behavior:

- external crisis for the staff;
- competition for a vacant position;
- envy as a latent aggression;
- fear of losing position;
- fear of corporate frauds discovery;
- rejection of “others” (former countrymen, dissidents, foreigners, etc.)
- political and social preferences;
- lack of feedback;
- poor management of information flows.

S. A. Druzhilov (2011) highlights three main personal reasons of bossing.

1. *Bossing as a lifestyle.* The boss sacrifices not only valuable employees but also the interests of the organization for his/her ambitions. Play with subordinates as pawns is one of the oldest, the most amoral and, unfortunately, the most engrossing one.

Dominating, causing dissension and working up the employees against each other are the matters of life for such boss.

2. *Bossing as a compensation for personal complexes.* Lack of self-confidence and pathologic suspiciousness makes the boss see "enemies" in everybody; he/she is used to assert him/herself by means of the subordinates. In this case his/her pressing becomes the reason for the horizontal mobbing.
3. *Incompetence in the sphere of management,* particularly, poorly-adjusted mechanism of communication with employees, lack of competent conflict management, deficiency in skills of professional task setting and correct evaluation of their performance.

The general reasons of bossing are inferiority complex and intolerance to others, fear of rivalries, envy, boredom and inaction.

20.4. Synergetics of Mobbing

Synergetic model of mobbing development may be notionally represented in four vectors (Table 18.2), which reflect the multidisciplinary and integral approach to the consideration of all manifestations of pathokinesis of destructive professiogenesis.

Sociogenesis supposes development of social roles and relationship. Disharmonious family serves as a predisposition of mobbing sociogenesis. Among the first indicators of such family there is any addiction of any member, including its variety, connected with addiction to work or behavioral mobbing-stereotypes of reactions.

A mobbing background may be the unsolved conflicts at the workplace, disbalancing the social relationship and psychological climate, actualizing early infant practice of resistance with behavioral mobbing scenario in the family and the school. The most popular and simple mobbing-model of response to emotional tension is the search of "offender," initiating harassment and giving the deformed staff the illusion of cohesiveness. The group aggressive insults and nagging become systematic and independent of real actions and results of the "victim's" activity. In any action of the victim the others find only negative moments, that is why the mobbing-target persistently feels like an animal at bay, having the symptoms of psychosomatic malfunctions and acute exacerbation of chronic diseases.

A. V. Skavitin (2004) in the course of a sociological study highlighted the most widespread reactions, accompanying pressing: stress (76%), "paranoia" (60%), headaches (55%), feeling of rejection (41%) and guilt (38%), nightmares (49%), insomnia (71%), absent-mindedness (71%), eating disorder (35%), and abusive alcoholic behavior (28%). Every fourth mobbing-target begins to suffer from suicidal thoughts and harbor plans of revenge to the mobbers. Having faced with the pressing at the workplace once, the employee remembers the negative experience for life even after he/she has changed his/her place of employment.

These symptoms become the base of the future social decompensation and isolation, covering naturally various phenomena. So these phenomena, determined by the conflicts in the professional activities, should be apparently distinguished from neurotic or paranoiac development of personality of mobbing-terrorist or mobbing-target as well as from mixed forms of adaptation to a staff which is not always effective, developing in the period of significant decrease in the employee's internal resources influenced by age and disorders. Full or partial social isolation is a protective response, minimizing pressing of mobbers: "victim" avoids team building and corporate events, minimizes the interaction in the process of work. All the more mobbing targets are not invited to celebrations, colleagues' birthdays, tea-parties, etc. Finding him/herself in social isolation and information vacuum, the employee loses reference points and becomes more and more helpless and unconfident in his/her professional activities. Occasionally frequent incapacity increases the risk of triggering the "defence by illness."

Psychogenesis in its predisposition is associated with disturbance of family relationship, because the main part of socialization from the moment of a human birth arises from the family. It is the neurogenesis family with mobbing-like stereotypes of behavior and reactions, which is the first fractal in the formation of the future matrix of professional deformation and its consequence. As a result of the interaction of disturbed family relationship with long-term realization of psychological defense, the accentuations of personality are formed, entwining the individual style of activities and finally transforming into professional deformations and mobbing. Psychopatization of personality, in "boundary" variant, occurs under the influence of chronic mobbing psychogenic traumatization and effect of many negative sociopsychological factors. The emerging pathocharacterological shift often "releases from" original cause and then the pathological "self-development" of character is initiated (the psychogenic cause disappears while the pathological personal changes continue developing). A multivariant personality disorder is manifested in a significant disturbance of social functioning, leading to serious interpersonal and intrapersonal conflicts. Styles of behavior and thinking are formed with rigid excessively expressed responses.

Further neurotic (mobbing target) or paranoiac (mobbing terrorist) developments are manifested as imbalanced psychic processes, maladaptiveness, and disturbances of self-actualization process or as avoidance of ethic and aesthetic control under the person's behavior. In this case, the possible consequence of the process is a mental defect manifesting in benign of negative changes: psychic asthenization, undue fatiguability, phenomena of irritable weakness, curbing of interests, and gradual amputation of individual characterological peculiarities.

Somatogenesis and *animogenesis* of mobbing do not differ much from the described fractal dynamics of development of destructive professiogenesis syndromes (chapter 18.4).

Mobbing conflicts, organized by professionally deformed bosses or colleagues seriously problematize the "victim's" professional worth, making him/her think of mental and physical health preservation. The practice shows that it is better to change the place of employment than to continue the self-destructive fight.

20.5. Prevention of Mobbing

We have developed the program of preventive and correctional as well as treatment and rehabilitation care based on the synergetic concept of mobbing formation. The program includes four blocks: medical, psychological, spiritual and moral as well as social (Table 18.3), unified for all the forms of destructive professiogenesis.

In severe clinical cases, the syndrome of mobbing reveals traditional symptoms of induced neuropsychic disorder. Mobbing terrorist is characterized by paranoid personality disorder while mobbing target has avoidant personality disorder. Thus, the main mobbers and their victims in a staff require medico-psychosociospiritual therapy, while the induced groups of followers require psychological and psychotherapeutic help.

There are special recommendations for the management of an organization to prevent mobbing (Plastinina 2012; Sidorov 2013):

- to form a healthy corporate culture;
- to support a healthy social and psychological climate;
- to improve management skills of senior executives;
- to support the feedback mechanisms;
- to precisely define the boundaries of individual responsibility and employment duties;
- to provide division of labor and avoid the duplication of duties;
- to stimulate the system of professional development;
- to provide information availability and transparency of management decisions;
- to eliminate parental and sexual relationship between management and subordinates;
- to scotch gossips and intrigues;
- to eliminate favoritism and manipulations;
- efficiently respond to the threads of mobbing, nipping the conflicts in the bud.

In case the boss found him/herself involved in mobbing, it is important not to make hasty decisions and not to lose the psychological balance, choosing evolutional ways for future improvements instead of revolutionary.

Behavioral strategies for avoiding mobbing at the workplace may be narrowed to the list of recommendations (Druzhilov 2011; Sidorov 2013):

- be kind and appealing;
- do not gossip, avoid intrigues;
- compliment on real achievements;
- stay yourself without showing up;
- don't allow humiliating yourself and don't humiliate others;
- keep up traditions and rules;
- remember: people offend those, who can be offended;
- do not fraternize with the boss;
- fulfill your duties in good faith;
- be patient and tactful.

In several countries (Germany, France, Sweden) the laws on moral bullying at the workplace are passed, which prevent the appearance of this phenomenon, protecting and ensuring the safety of the employees, including an emotional component of health at work. The evidence of the legal claim sufficiency is the mobbing diary of a "victim."

In conclusion, we would like to note, that synergetic model of mobbing allows organizing preventive measures against it as early as at prenozological level and establishing individual preventive and correctional as well as treatment and rehabilitation routes. The offered level-structured multidisciplinary provision system of adaptive professiogenesis should become a priority for social protection in any professional community, the basis for better performance and innovative development.

Chapter 21

Terrorism as a Polymodal Dependent Disorder

The pandemic of terrorism undermines civilizational fundamentals of the contemporary world. Fear and anxiety, which deform social conscience, are becoming an everyday reality. Many countries have developed and implemented special technologies to provide special psychological and psychiatric help in case of emergency, disaster, terror, or violence. However, the questions of efficient resource provisions for the early and systematic prevention of destructive social epidemics remain unsolved.

The relevant task is to present a conceptual and methodological explanation of terrorism and its forms and to demonstrate its place in the classification of destructive social epidemics. It is also very important to single out mechanisms of manipulation with a human conscience in extremist organizations and to show characteristics of the mental paradigm of national security. Grounding of the effective defense synergetics in the frames of the mental medicine and mental epidemiology methods present a very significant issue.

21.1. Syndrome of Terroristic Demoralization

The terrorist attack in Volgograd (December 2013) and its following media coverage "exploded" Russian public conscience and demonstrated exhaustiveness of traditional obstructive strategies used to counteract suicidal terrorism. The experience of other countries demonstrates that one must not respond to terror with terror – as it only spurs violence and the spiral of terror unwinds even further. That is why the announced formation of a new antiterrorist unit in the city of Volgograd (07.01.2014) was perceived by terrorists as an official recognition of defeat from Russian authorities and a call for expanding the geography of violence. The serial murders in Stavropol (January 2014) became a continuation of this antiterrorist scenario. Psychologists have spent many years discussing the phenomenon of terrorism and compared it to a flood when antiterrorist measures are an attempt to scoop out water with a teaspoon: "Personally addressed counterterrorism only procreates terrorists" (Medvedev 2004).

The escalation of terror and state counterterrorism represents the best way to eliminate countries and peoples. Every day we can find the confirmation of this fact in our "mental TV sewerage," it is present even on family and history channels. Thus, hundreds of millions of TV viewers all around the world enjoy a wonderful TV serial "The Magnificent Century." It draws a bright and convincing picture that shows how the awe of unmotivated death, terrorism and state counterterrorism created the great Ottoman Empire. The same terror, having reached its apogee and worldwide protest reaction (that was caused by the barbarian genocide of Armenians) destroyed the Empire and made it possible for Atatürk to create a secular republic. This republic has recently undergone the difficult times of "Islamic reformation."

Since time immemorial, terror has been the most archaic way of governing people and societies. In the contemporary technological-virtual world it is acquiring new epidemic features that symbolize the completion of another global civilizational cycle. The point here is that *terror itself has become the universal form of war prosecution*; it has radically changed the concept of warfare and armed forces. There is no front line, and there can be no battle line in the contemporary world, that functional and organizational army infrastructure is a thing of the past, it has lost its efficiency with the parity of military space forces.

Ten years ago it was possible to try and compare terrorism and guerrilla warfare, terrorism and revolutionary violence, terrorism and struggle for national liberation. In the past, this comparison could be based on the subject's position and differential diagnostic evaluations. Today there are practically no alternatives – it is more and more evident that terrorism is becoming a new universal form of war prosecution. In this new quality, terrorism demonstrates independent epidemic mechanisms of self-development and has nothing to do with the traditional reasons and factors that used to provoke it in the past. Terrorism is becoming an independent tool for solving political problems: "The future picture of the world is no longer possible without terror and violence" (Gilinskyi 2004).

The notion of civil population is disappearing from our lexicon, and what we have left is *already dead and still alive, everyone is confused by the informational explosion waves brought by the pandemic of terrorism.*

The special feature of the Volgograd tragedy is the fact that, for the first time, Russian mass media stopped spreading explosive informational waves of this attack and damage the public conscience of the country. To intimidate and demoralize society – is the objective of terrorists, it is not the objective of mass media. Russian leading psychologists have been discussing the necessity of censoring reports on terrorist attacks for ten years.

It is possible to try and link the tragedies in Volgograd and Stavropol with the preventive intimidation of Russia before the Olympic Games in Sochi. However, it is much more important to see and hear another communicative message from terrorists – "Russia is destroying itself," and it happens because more and more frequently terrorists are of Slavic origin.

Sorrowful information about civilian casualties and the consequences of yesterday's failed "Volgograd battle" are known, with the active phase of the antiterrorist war only beginning. It is important to learn the lesson promptly and make adequate conclusions by building a system of effective defense.

Long before becoming suicide bombers terrorists themselves became victims of *mental terrorism* – destructive manipulation with their conscience in extremist camps, gangs, and armies. As a result of this "brain wash," they developed a fanatic belief in their messianic and self-sacrificing role of fighters against the "infidels." The outcome of *terrorist demoralization syndrome* manifests itself in the deranged formation and deranged development of moral feelings, cast of mind, social position, and behavior, which are responsible for personal moral socialization.

The ontogenetic approach forms the foundation of this definition. Derangements in the formation of *primary moral feelings* (conscience, duty, faith and responsibility) are most often predetermined by spiritual and moral deficit as well as by family ambivalence. Such derangements develop even above orthodox and pious backgrounds as well as above patriarchal characters. During adolescence derangements in moral socialization cause a delay and disharmony in the development of *moral make-up fundamentals* – such as patience, tolerance, mercy, humanism, honor, and dignity. At the same time, manipulative characteristics of conscience and susceptibility to nationalistic provocations with xenophobia begin their formations.

Derangements in the formation and development of the spiritual and moral position, accumulated in the personality's motivational and mindset complex, manifest themselves by the decreased ability to differentiate between right and wrong. It is hard to distinguish friendship and love, amorphous personal position and low level of self-criticism in everything that does not include the categories of "infidels" and "strangers." Inability to see life perspectives, the presence of the pessimistic and catastrophic perceptions of the world, capitulation before encountering difficulties sublimated in the sacrificial struggle, failure to realize the value of human life - these all are the manifestations.

As a result of the terrorist (fanatic, extremist) demoralization syndrome, a complete loss of the socially accepted moral norms of behavior occurs, as well as demonstrative neglect of traditional concepts concerning what is due and what is unallowable. A person rejects any moral duties and moral self-control, it is impossible for him or her to act independently and, thus, responsibility for one's actions weakens. Increased suggestibility and dependence, complete devaluation of legal awareness and law-abidance, loss of social and personal identity - all these are the manifestations of the demoralization syndrome. All this allows a militant-manipulator to easily "create" new generations of suicidal terrorists. The recruitment of suicide terrorists looks even more tragic and dramatic when it comes to women, aged people, mentally ill and disabled individuals, teenagers and children. On January 08, 2014 the 1st Russian channel reported a story of a ten-year-old Afghan girl whose father and elder brother were forcing the child to become a suicide attacker. It was a miracle that she managed to escape and reach the police station that she was supposed to explode by the order of her relatives. This story reflects the monstrous *family variant of the terrorist demoralization syndrome* when parents are ready to send children to their death. In this case, it is not so important whether they do it for money or fighting for an "idea." Any form of terrorism inevitably destroys and eliminates individual human lives of terrorists as well as the lives of family members who support it. That is why from the psychiatric point of view terrorism represents the most destructive form of the *epidemic suicidal behavior*. To launch and support such destructive social epidemics of suicidal terrorism three conditions are sufficient and must be met: the religious culture of martyrdom, the decision of a terrorist organization, possibility of compulsory but made to appear as voluntary recruitment of future suicide attackers.

The development of demoralization syndrome has multiple variants in the ethnocultural environment. It has a minimum dependence on the intellectual potential and quality of education. Terrorism, like alcoholism and drug addiction, can derive from rich and poor backgrounds. There is no coincidence that the number one and most mythologized terrorist of the world Ben Laden came from a well-educated and wealthy family.

21.2. Asocial Epidemic of Terrorism

Demoralization syndrome – is a moral and psychological foundation of any social epidemic regardless of its form: drug addiction, fanaticism, extremism, terrorism and many others.

Epidemiological recognition of the threats and challenges posed by terrorism and extremism is not another myth or banal abuse of psychiatric terminology. It is not what happened in the case of trappidomania diagnosis or so the called pathological craving for freedom among American slaves, delirium of reformation, and criminal prosecution of homosexualism in the USSR. Today clinical psychiatry makes diagnoses, which yesterday were viewed as a purely social phenomenon. For example, the Mobbing syndrome evolved from banal "office wars." Today it is a form of non-lethal mental terrorism that destroys the mental health of its "Mobbing targets" and corporate society.

In the etiopathogenesis of religious fanaticism and terrorism, several social and psychological complex causes are identified:

1. disgrace and humiliation, experienced in the past or taking place now;
2. division of the world, based on the inability to tolerate ambivalent attitude and ambiguity, into two opinions: the good and the demonic;
3. submission, based on the fear of loneliness, to dehumanizing religious or pseudo-religious organizations;
4. threats to the ideals, causing the narcissistic rage;
5. the demand for perfection and purification, including in the form of suicide terrorism;
6. perceived uncritically, as a doctrine, the link between violence and purification;
7. suppression of sexual desire;
8. manipulation of religious heritage texts;
9. maintenance of intolerance due to the shift of religious meanings and values onto the irreligious and different from the spiritual, targets and models of intolerant behavior;
10. religious disguise of eased access to vulnerable populations in their destructive purposes (Bushman et al. 2007; Jones 2008; Abu Raiya et al. 2008; Sidorov 2014).

It is of fundamental importance to note the unity and universality of the social epidemic base. Drug and alcohol addictions, crime and violence, extremism and terrorism unite the subpopulations of people "exiled" from the normative social systems.

The following (Moshchelkov et al. 2007) groups of conditions initiate the epidemiological spread of terrorism:

1. *formation of the information society*, that indefinitely spreads the potential effect of terrorism;

2. *vulnerability of the technological environment* that is responsible for human existence it makes the pinpoint destruction of the technological environment's social, natural, and technological foundations possible;
3. *smearing of the traditional society* with modernization and liberal values: concept of the social contract, ideas that proclaim state authorities responsible before their society, ideas promoting the value of law and human life;
4. *crisis stages of social development* accompanied by the ideas of separatism, religious, ethnic, and ideological conflicts.

Terrorism is one of the most multimodal and multilevel variation of asocial epidemics. At the primary level of mental epidemics, it is represented by mobbingogenic mental terrorism, which threatens the collective public conscience or the inhabited locality. The mental epidemic of mobbing becomes destructive when it begins to threaten the social conscience of the whole country, using this or that nationalist or religious ideology. Then mental epidemic evolves into a social - threatening the public health in the region and destructive social epidemics when the threat extends to the entire country. It is presented phenomenologically by syndromes of bullying and crowding. From now on the epidemic develops into asocial, presented actually by terrorism. Depending on the degree and extent of threats to the national security of the country as a whole, it can become destructive. The final form is the pandemic of terrorism, spanning the countries and continents. Today, the most famous of such pandemics is the "Islamic State" (IS) - the international Islamic terrorist organization, operating mainly in Syria and Iraq since 2013 as Islamic unrecognized quasi-state with the Sharia form of government. The IS formation was preceded by the union in 2006 of 11 radical Islamist groups, led by the local unit of "Al-Qaeda." By 2016, in the IS ranks, there were tens of thousands of followers from nearly 100 countries.

Terrorism is an exceptionally polymorph phenomenon with different types and classes of usable aggressive agents. That is why it is present in all four groups of the suggested classification. Thus, the arsenal of bioterrorism includes 13 types of viruses, 7 – bacteria, 3 – rickettsiae that cause dangerous infectious diseases, 12 microbial toxins. Long ago special methods of diagnostics and therapy have been developed to counter these threats.

The situation with *mental terrorism* appears to be much more dramatic. This form of terrorism affects mental health together with ideological, spiritual, and moral bases of culture, society, and statehood. Furthermore, it is followed by the stirring of national hatred, depreciation of spiritual and moral values with their ideals, marginalization and criminalization of social conscience. This is an everyday reality for Russia while it keeps on sinking in the "waterfalls of mental TV sewage." As a result of this phenomenon increased uncertainty about tomorrow develops and hesitancy about the state as well, also a profound sense of anxiety, aggression and emotional instability, suggestibility and trustfulness, distrust to official information with preference given to rumors, decreased criticality.

Such peculiarities of the public conscience are characteristic of emergencies. It turns out that in Russia the state of emergency, caused by mental terrorism, exists de facto, but de jure the society is yet unable to perceive it adequately. Furthermore, public conscience and the Russian state itself are undergoing painless destruction under the anesthesia of the «mental TV-sewage». This image has a serious associative and medical interpretation. The psychiatric practice has encountered and described cases of cloacae gas poisoning that had led to the instant death of the cerebral cortex and visualized in the form of profound encephalopathy.

Hydrogen sulfide intoxication can take place in natural environments: areas of natural gas release, around sulfurous mineral waters, in deep wells and pits, with rotting organic substances that contain sulfur. During my 40-years clinical practice, there have been only several cases of such intoxication. For example, when construction workers opened airtight pits half of them died, and the remaining half acquired dementia.

It is the decrease of the stress-resistance threshold using the infantile reverberatory tuning of public conscience through electronic mass media that allows exploding the public conscience with the informational shock waves of any terrorist attack or any emergency. The chain reactions of anxiety and fear are multiplied and doubled. Their cumulative effects are amplified as they provoke different kinds of induced socially stressful and somatoform neuropsychic disorders. Today's mass media policy significantly favors this harmful influence. It relies on the "sinister charm of violence and fear" and is guided by the principles like "corpses make our picture more alive" (Nazaretyan 2011). This is how mass media imprints the image of our contemporary society on the public conscience. It is the society of utter and unpredictable violence. Due to perverted professional ethics and esthetics, the media coverage of any terrorist attack or tragedy turns into a "satanic necrophilic feast" that creates epidemic waves of induced disorders.

The world epidemics of drug addiction and terrorism are closely interconnected. According to the American Drug Enforcement Administration, 39% of terrorist organizations are associated with drug dealing. The global volume of drug traffic, according to different estimations, makes up from 400 to 1 000 billion dollars every year. There is no coincidence that the former president of Columbia M. Pastrana called drug dealing "the main financier of terrorism and death in the world" (Moshchelkov et al. 2007). One can easily add here the total corruption that systematically embraces the entire civilized infrastructure and creates premises for *planetary suicide.*

Social epidemics become *generalized* as a significant percentage of the dependent subpopulation (population suffering from dependent personality disorders) gets involved. According to our data, it makes up 30% of the whole population.

The first generalized social epidemic in the Russian history was "Smutnoe vremya" (the Time of Troubles) that ended 400 years ago. It was accompanied by large scale hysteria-demonic and infectious epidemics, plunder, robberies and demolitions, burning of witches and magicians, the appearance of various impostors, summoned and recognized by the corrupt elite. The whole country and its population have remembered this lesson for 300 years, and it was only in 1917 when the October revolution demonstrated its blood "red" results and dramatic scenarios.

The student disturbances in Paris (1968) are an example of a *bloodless color revolution* in the contemporary European history. The organizers of this coup d'etat who overthrew President Charles de Gaulle gave young people a possibility to "let off some fume" on barricades. That protesting youth was sincerely engrossed with the ideas of Sartre and was held captive by the romantic illusions of Anarchism and Trotskyism.

Today the mental design of the technological-virtual world (which is composed of numerous ideas and illusions) quickly changes its arrangement of the public conscience, and it happens as if somebody unnoticed swings his mighty wand to conduct the show. One way or another, the newest generations of "color" revolutions industrialized the strategies, tactics, forms and techniques of destroying traditional, natural, cultural and socioeconomic structures of countries and people for the benefit of the financing party. That is why it is extremely difficult to develop *mental immunity to all kinds of social epidemics, and the development of such immunity has become one of the major priorities of the state.* Spiritual immunity is composed of moral and value-based potential of a personality realizing its unity with countrymen and motherland. It is the spiritual culture that happens to be the first target of the contemporary aggressor.

Anomia forms the foundation of any destructive social epidemics; it becomes apparent when fundamental moral values of a system get corrupted. Contradictions typically develop between the announced objectives and the impossibility for the majority of citizens to achieve them using traditional methods. It results in the personality's isolation from society and depressive disillusionment in life. Anomia favors the spread of *permissivity* – destabilization and the abolishment of socially accepted prohibitions that are structural and ethical elements of society. In such conditions, any person can lose his supporting point and be left without his system of moral values as well as the support of traditional public morals. All this creates basic conditions for the recruitment of individuals from the dependent subpopulation and their further participation in different forms of destructive social epidemics. The most tragic form of these epidemics is terrorism.

21.3. Forms of Terrorism and Mechanisms of Personality Deformation

Terrorism (from Latin terror) – is a weapon of mass destruction, that combines direct physical damage to the victims with the significant damage done to the biopsychosociospiritual resources of a society. The meaningful content of terror is restricted to three characteristics: act of intimidation, request of submission, meaningful content.

Generalized psychological portrait of a terrorist most often includes the following characteristics:

- young people around 20 (+/– 5);
- patriarchal or highly religious family culture;
- dominant view about some historic injury of his nation;
- deep emotional connections with his ethnos;
- anxiety about pinched national pride;
- distorted and mythologized views about some historical insulters and need for revenge;
- psychological traumatization, often is caused by the death of relatives in front of the future terrorist;
- early deprivation of parental care and attention;
- deficit of emotional connections during childhood;
- high level of pretentions that showed up since childhood, overrated self-esteem, tendency to fantasize and demand of increased attention;
- as a rule "black sheep," an outsider among his peers;
- disposition towards aggression and vandalism;
- often has obvious or hidden physical defects;
- traumatogenic youth with privations, humiliations, bereavement;

- disturbance of moral socialization;
- settlement of conflicts only through violence;
- difficulties with adaptation to social principles and regulations;
- seeking recognition and self-assured;
- prevalence of hysteric explosive traits of personality;
- high level of neurosis and frustration;
- personality disorders with high level of aggression and self-actualization;
- submission of one's individuality to group identity;
- high impulsivity, inclination to immediate actions.

Among the most characteristic *mental peculiarities of terrorists* it is possible to single out the following features:

- displacement of time perception (present includes past);
- archaic and a binary picture of the world;
- the disappearance of borders between reality and fantasy;
- infantilism and naivety, high suggestibility;
- the primitiveness of cognitive styles;
- the presence of apocalyptic feelings and fantasies;
- ideas of messianism, the unique purport of life and sacrificial service;
- ambivalent sadomasochist position;
- identification with aggressor;
- no receptiveness to counterarguments and dissuasion;
- loss of pragmatism and rationality;
- the religious arrangement of ideas promoting struggle and revenge;
- cultivation of concepts about death and life after death;
- glorification of sacrificial death and the heroic deeds of martyrs;
- the absence of fear and repentance;
- derangements in the formation and development of moral feelings (conscience and duty, faith and responsibility), character (patience and tolerance, mercy and humanism, honor and dignity), position (ability to differentiate between good and evil, expression of friendship and love), behavioral ethics and communication;
- a predilection for an illusory-compensatory way of satisfying one's needs instead of active and creative;
- a tendency to quick, final and easy solutions;
- primitive mythologizing and sign-symbolic mediation of one's primary activity with compulsory emphasis made on the list of enemies;
- utmost, terminal and artificial dramatization of the situation;
- loss of tactical prognostication resources and vision of strategic perspectives in life.

Contemporary terrorism is characterized by the galloping tempos of its cruelty growth, usage of newest lethal and non-lethal weapons, cyber and nanotechnologies, expanded reproduction of terrorist movements' quantity, generalization and globalization of their activity scale, high level of organization and professionalism, sacrificial fanaticism and shocking corruption. A long time ago Israeli psychologists came to the conclusion that it is impossible to reconstruct or reform the personality of convicted terrorists. This conclusion might be connected with the fact that quite recently special antiterrorist units all over the world began to liquidate terrorists rather than detain them. However, attempts to find corrective methods have not been stopped. Thus, neurobiologists from the Oxford University made an announcement about the development of a pilot technology for treating Islamic fundamentalists. This announcement was made two weeks after a shocking public murder in London (2013) when two Nigerians cruelly killed a soldier of the British army (Lee Rigby). The technology includes both biological methods and psychotherapeutic sanitization of extremist beliefs. Moreover, the scientists have suggested that "radical attitudes" should be classified as psychic disorders. It was revealed that the British security service MI5 had attempted to hire one of those Nigerians six month before the terrifying murder took place. It means that one cannot rely solely on special services in the struggle against terrorism. They simply cannot have all necessary information to prevent such acts of terrorism. These tragedies have demonstrated that the approach towards terrorism requires a systematic synergetic review. It goes without saying that special operations and systematic monitoring of the information field are necessary antiterrorist activities. However, fighting against destructive social epidemics of terrorism requires, figuratively speaking, *a dyke of spiritual immunity that is structured by the moral and value-based potential of the population and cemented with the energy of creative and rallied nation.*

The classification of terrorism forms includes ideological and religious, political and ecological, chemical and physical, nuclear and biological, psychological and suicidal, spiritual and mental forms. According to its territorial scale, terrorism can be classified as corporative (including the syndrome of mobbing-terrorism in "office wars"), municipal (provincial, regional (republics of the Northern Caucasus), federal, international.

We have singled out (Sidorov 2005) the following mechanisms of exposing influence on personality in extremist and terrorist organizations. These mechanisms lead to the practically irreversible deformation of one's personality.

1. *Monolog* – unidirectional impact that excludes alternative sources of information.
2. *Mythological* – use of tested mythological schemes that inspire to die for some idea.
3. *Emotional* – compensation of emotional feelings and care that were not received in society.
4. *Collectivism* – use of group forms self- and mutual induction: training "referent group" prepares a suicide terrorist and leads him to the very end.
5. *Counter argumentation* – suggestion of counter arguments to anticipated doubts and contradictions that is done in advance.
6. *Intolerance* – stimulation of suggestibility in the background of psychophysical exhaustion, especially in field conditions and underground.
7. *Selectivity*– recruitment of suicidal terrorist among the most non-adapted and deficient people.
8. *Manipulative* – use of an extensive psycho-technological arsenal of suggestion.
9. *Paranormal* – use of fictional achievements based on supersensory experience.
10. *Controllability* –ensuring total control of personality and his behavior.
11. *Ritualistic*– creation and nailing down of behavioral habits and models of killing and committing a suicide.

Teaching hatred and brainwashing have three objectives:

1. to deny a positive emotional evaluation of the enemy;
2. to cultivate malice and fear, (a classical example of it can be found in the novel of D.Orwell “1984” «five-minute periods of hatred»);
3. generation of decisions based on mistaken cognitive conclusions and faulty critical thinking (Steinberg 2003).

The model of psychology of hatred developed by Robert Sternberg (2003) has three components and the following blocks:

1. *Disgust* or rejection of closeness with the enemy. Its source can be found in the peculiarities of the subject’s personality, his own actions or propaganda.
2. *Passion* as a measure of emotional energy, connected with the dynamics of hatred, described in the terms of fear emotions, malice and rage.
3. *Obligation* that consists of two components: cognitive aberration to decrease the value and significance of the hated group of people: individuals who compose it are viewed as not quite human and very often as “subhuman.” Its second component is behavioral; it is a decision to struggle, use violence and even die.

Interaction between these three elements allowed the author to single out six types of hatred:

1. Hatred expressed in the form of «*disgust*» towards a hated group (for example a nation).The subject does not want to have anything in common with them because they, from his point of view, have very little in common with people.
2. «*Furious*» hate is expressed in extreme emotional manifestations of malice and fear and it can lead to violence or attempt to avoid the threat that is (in the view of the hatred subjects) posed by the hostile group.
3. «*Cold*» hate that is characterized by the perception of a hostile group as low and mean.
4. «*Boiling*» hate that combines disgust towards a hated group with the need to illuminate the threat that this group poses.
5. «*Hardly restrained*» hate is characterized by the feeling of constant disgust and fear; at the same time, the hostile group is perceived as a gathering of “supermen.”
6. «*Burning hate*» This type of hate is associated with a feeling of necessity to exterminate the hated enemy physically. In this case, all three elements of hate are present, and this type of hate most often becomes the subject of study in frames of terrorism research and studies.

This is how *–through brainwashing and teaching hatred–* the personality of a future suicidal terrorist gets destroyed to turn him into a simple “means of transportation.” Only the organizers get the greater part of the client’s reward. There is nothing personal here. Some action appears on TV screens, and a sum of money is transferred to someone’s bank account. *A terrorist war* is a business of its organizers and bloody politics of the ordering party.

21.4. Synergetics of Terrorism Pandemic

The conventional and generalized synergetic concept that demonstrates the development of social epidemics of terrorism is presented in Table 21.1. The illustration of this table shows only the basic markers of this dynamic disorder which has a great polyvalence and multivariance; those markers are connected with the clinical psychopathological and somato-neurologic, socio-psychological, spiritual and moral personal topologies as well as the forms and trajectories of epidemic development.

Animogenesis begins in the fractal of *predisposition* (mobbing family and/or environment). It is distinguished by *spiritual and moral deficiency* and ambivalence, high frequency of asocial and dependent disorders of parents and close relatives, various forms of violence, harassments, cavils, intimidations, insults, mockery, rudeness, deception, moral pressing and isolation.

Early imposition of the "mobbing target" image on children and adolescents leads to "mobbing sensibilization" of the inner world, the formation of perverted and simplified mental models of interpersonal interaction and behavior. This family and millisocial environment have anomic and permissive nature; they are very likely to marginalize and dehumanize the moral values of a personality.

During the *latent fractal of bullying diathesis* defensive and compensatory, spiteful and aggressive protest reactions of behavioral nature develop for self-assertion; they increase the polarization of relationship and isolation.

The deformation of spiritual development shows itself in the form of distorted self-esteem and failure to understand the purport of life, unreadiness to act independently as a full-grown individual, undeveloped moral self-conscience and moral responsibility.

In the initial fractal of crowding mass outbreaks (mass forms of sadistic aggression and vandalism), a deformed moral image becomes fixated. It happens through training and behavioral practice in street teenage gangs and groups, various legal and illegal fan movements, radical and extremist movements. It lays the corner stone to the development of the demoralization syndrome. Delay and disharmony of the development of the moral image foundations show themselves as the absence of tolerance, patience, mercy, humanism, honor, and dignity. Deficiency and disharmony of creative potential in spiritual, figural and productive activities are present. Unreadiness and inability to be professionally and socially labile, as well as failure to maintain continuous development and education characterize this condition. The manipulative capability of conscience and susceptibility to nationalistic provocations reveal. Painful emotional stress caused by strangulated national pride and xenophobia and exceptional stereotypical reactions to challenges and difficulties (aggression and vandalism) are present.

In the debut fractal of the social epidemic of terrorism, the pro-social spiritual and moral position of personality is lost, and the syndrome of terrorist demoralization is formed; at the same time the abilities to differentiate good and evil, friendship and love decrease. An affected personality becomes amorphous and deficient; low self-criticism develops together with the personality's impairment. The vision of life becomes stereotyped with the only purport of life being the struggle for the right and the inability to realize the value of human life. Crowding terrorists are distinguished by the archaic and binary ethical picture of the world that has blurred borders between reality and fantasy. They are fixated on dominant ideas of the nation's historical trauma and perverted mythologized image of the enemy. Crowding terrorists remain prisoners of their obsessions with messianic ideas and believe in a special meaning of life that infers selfless service in the name of justice and historical revenge. They distinguish themselves with easy perception and neglect of multiple adaptation difficulties to social conventions and moral rules. Inclination to "solve problems" only with the help of quick and easy solutions based on violence, preferably primitive styles of mental representation, and armed aggression is typical for them. Their struggle for the right has religious, ritual coverage; they heroically cultivate ideas about martyr death and redemptive life after death.

The fractal of chronization of the destructive social epidemic of terrorism is characterized by different forms and types of immoral and illegal behavior development; this behavior threatens the national security of a country. The syndrome of terrorist demoralization shows itself as a complete loss of the socially accepted mediated moral behavior that is based on the concepts of good and evil, indebted and unacceptable. Such persons demonstratively disregard any moral duties and reject moral self-control. They depend on and are irresponsible of personal actions, unable to carry out moral self-evaluation of one's behavior and respect the ethical norms of business communication. There is a loss of personal and social identity, devaluation of legal awareness and law-obedience, avoidance of personal moral choice in such people. The anonymity of cyber-terrorists and facemasks on participants of terroristic civil wars demonstrates it.

The fractal of outcome is characterized by the maximum epidemic level of pandemic, terminal complications and consequences for the society and terrorists. The ethical component of personality's difficult asocial development makes terrorists insensitive to counterarguments and dissuasion. Together with comorbid and associated disorders, it leads to mental defects, results in the loss of pragmatism and rationality, the absence of fear and repentance, super- the glorification of sacrificial death and heroic martyrdom in the terrorist civil war.

All this allows militant manipulators to "create" new generations of suicidal terrorists easily. In fact, they are engaged in *mental terrorism – individual, distractive and mercenary creation of adherents.* The only difference of mental terrorism from traditional forms of propaganda and agitation is in the population format of the public conscience; that is "being attacked" by mass media. The growing network interactivity of the global world is making the information front line the primary battlefield in the war on terrorism. The *population form of mental terrorism* realized in the Media, is represented by the "carpet slanderous bombing and burning-out with falseness napalm" of the social conscience of countries and peoples. A quarter of a century ago, it was still possible to discuss the characteristics of destructive conscience control, features of recruiter and stages of interaction with psycho-manipulator, forms and types of victimity, mechanisms and strategies of influence on the person. Today the need for personification and mediation of the destructive manipulation of public conscience is reducing. All this is effectively managed with network and system media and the Internet, through which the culturally-specific forms of management of public conscience are implemented.

Serial and deadly equifinal terroristic wars develop according to the mechanism of a dependent disorder when only an injurious act of terrorism can provide a psycho-emotional relief and fill a desperate and inescapable existential situation with illusionary meanings. These illusionary meanings are covered with the masks of "unknown soldiers."

Table 21.1. Fractal dynamics of epidemic development of terrorism

Ontogenesis vectors	Prenosological fractals			Nosological fractals		
	Predisposition: mobbingogenic family and/or environment	Latent: bullyingogenic diathesis	Initial: mass crowding	Debut: asocial epidemic	Chronization: destructive asocial epidemic	Outcome: pandemic and terminal complications
Somatogenesis	Hereditary somatic burden	Neuroprocess disorders	Somatoform dysfunctions	Somatized disorder	Comorbid psychosomatic illness	Somato-neurological complications and degradation of public health
Psychogenesis	Psychopathological burden	Polymodal psychopatization of personality	Asocial and/or dependent personality beyond the personality disorder	Asocial and /or dependent personality disorder	Asocial and/ or dependent personality development	Psychic defect and destruction of public conscience
Sociogenesis	Family structure and function violations	Personality socialization violations	Non-pathological dependent behavior	Pathologically addictive and/or asocial behavior	Social decompensation	Disadaptation and dehumanization of society
Animogenesis	Moral and spiritual family deficiency	Moral feelings formation disorder	Moral image deformation	Loss of moral position	Amoral and unlawful behavior	Serial criminality and suicidal terrorism, demoralization of public conscience

The development of the terrorist demoralization syndrome is exceptionally multivariate; it is predetermined by the initial ethical topology of personality, ethnocultural and socio-economic, religious and political factors of the environment. The latter factors are turning into a dehumanized and demoralized *"terroristic world" that is undermining the civilizational foundations of humanity.*

Sociogenesis in the *fractal of predisposition* is characterized by the high frequency of various disorders in the structure and functions of the mobbing family. They substantially predetermine the mental representation of destructive cognitive models of disharmonious interpersonal relations: the cult of strength and aggression, humiliations and insults, social deprivations and isolations, negativism and protest.

In the latent fractal of bullying diathesis the dispersion and inversion of the "mobbing target" and "mobbing terrorist" take place as a result of the personality's maturation and socialization disorders. These disorders develop in a disharmonious millisocial environment and are later followed by the "bullying terrorist" whose distinctive features are hyper-compensatory cruelty and aggression. Such personalities do not have psychosocial resources for productive self-realization through their professional and educational activities, inside their families and social networks. To a significant extent, that is the exact reason *why non-pathological dependent behavior* develops through compensatory mechanisms. It is characterized by perverted obsessive fantasies that are realized through sadistic and cruel compulsive group tortures of defenseless animals and vulnerable peers. Personal interests are subordinated to some kind of paraphilia, attention is longly fixated, and the ability to control is decreased. The immersion into asocial dependence is very usual, as well as dependency and passivity when choosing behavioral strategies and verbal response strategies, self — and mutual induction during *mass outbreaks of crowding terrorism in the initial fractal.*

In the fractal of the social terrorism epidemic debut, the reference nucleus of the epidemic hotbed and its leaders display pathologic dependent and asocial behavior; it is notable for the episodes when changed conditions of conscience are present at the moment of psychological and physical dependence realization, irresistibility and compulsivity of the asocial activity, stereotypization of the terroristic lifestyle, cancelation syndrome between delicts and acts of terrorism.

In the chronization fractal, a destructive social epidemic of terrorism unfolds; it has different instruments and mechanisms depending on the type and form of terrorism. However, it inevitably leads the participants of an epidemic process to *social decompensation* and threatens the national security of a country as a whole.

In the outcome fractal, a total social disadaptation is formed at liberty; in the case of lifetime imprisonment a forced adaptation to the prison conditions develops. The development of terroristic pandemic is accompanied by and matched with various social markers of the global dehumanization crisis and civilization degradation: famine, unemployment, migration, etc.

Psychogenesis in the fractal of predisposition. To a significant degree psychogenesis is predetermined by the premorbid psychopathological burden of the mobbing family, it is distinguished by non-motivated psycho-emotional instability and communicative deficiency. Children who grow in such families, even those with orthodox and patriarchal backgrounds, experience an acute shortage of emotional connections, and painfully go through the early loss of parental care. Trying to compensate for them they develop an aptitude to fantasize and demand increased attention. Very often an early psychological trauma is related to a glorified martyr death of a relative or another close acquaintance that was witnessed by the future terrorist. This death becomes a matrix of mental representation for tomorrow's terroristic lifestyle and death.

In the latent fractal of bullying diathesis, addictive radicals of an early psychopathic disorder and personal deformation are formed and fixated. They show themselves as anticipating malicious and aggressive verbal reactions to all challenges and difficulties. They stereotype aggressive and auto-aggressive styles of behavior, launch the mechanism of hypercompensation "asocial hysteria" and polymodal asocial dependent disorder. Such a personality can demonstrate various socially stressful disorders even in the situation when it encounters banal life difficulties. All this speeds up the formation of a primary dependent pattern that will be able to change its modality later as well as the form of dependence. However, the asocial radical of this dependence will be steadily preserved engrossing the personality's nucleus.

In the initial fractal of crowding terrorism mass outbreaks, behavioral realization of previously learned mental schemes and scenarios of asocial self-assertion takes place, this is the only outcome based on the cognitive and cultural, personal resources. An *asocial and dependent personality* demonstrates vivid, realistic reminiscences and fantasies glorifying terrorism *outside personality disorder*. It happens above the background of infantilism and suggestibility, openheartedness and sensory spontaneity, curiosity and high searching activity, minimalism and egocentrism, impressionability and impatience, aptitude to taking risks and provoking dangerous situations, generalized aggression and vandalism. This personality gets a chance to overcome the inferiority complex of an individual rejected in his prosocial environment and get rid of the "black sheep" label only in street gangs, extremist and fanatic groups. The extrusion and disactualization of such obsessive reminiscences about one's traumatic youth that had multiple humiliations and losses are accompanied by the hyper-compensatory necessity to revenge not only some particular offenders but the whole cruel and unjust world, revenge for one's nation. This is how the psychological mechanisms of epidemic terrorism generalization demonstrate themselves.

All ten types of personality disorders, described in ICD 10, can take place among terrorists and extremists. However, the most significant role in launching epidemic processes belongs to mutually reinforcing asocial and dependent disorders with their radicals. They easily create a TV image that shows the unity of people and their leaders. An epidemic develops according to self and mutual induction mechanisms as it adds complications to the existing personality disorder.

Borderline personality disorder — is a severe emotional instability and impulsive aggression, disturbance of interpersonal relations and self-destructing behavior. Prevalence among the population is 1.5-2%.

Personality disorders - are deep-rooted styles of behavior and thinking with rigid response reactions in excessively expressed forms. Prevalence is 6-18% (Laux, Meller 2010).

At the time of K. Schneider (1959), not only the afflicted person suffered from this disorder, but also the whole society was affected as well. Today the epidemic spread of extremism and terrorism mobilizes the mechanisms of induction and generalization; it turns them into a global populational mutation and poses the threat of civilization suicide. Moreover, it is necessary to take into account the fact that up to 30% of the population suffer from various forms of dependencies, the controlled social switching of their modality can quickly lead to the emergence of social epidemics.

The debut fractal of the social epidemic of terrorism is most often represented by asocial and dependent personality disorders of the epidemic hotbed referent nucleus. It induces the fellow-fighters who make part of the polymodal subpopulation. Dependent personality disorders are characterized by the deficiency of normative sociality and widening of the asocial manifestation's specter, personality deformation and emotional burnout, inability to make decisions independently outside one's terroristic lifestyle, frequent combinations of schizoid personality features with a bad tolerance of loneliness. It facilitates the development of anxious depression, urging an individual to commit excesses, delicts and acts of terrorism that provide a temporary psycho-emotional relief.

The fractal of chronization of the destructive social epidemic of terrorism is represented by multivariate *asocial and dependent personality developments*; terrorism begins to take the leading position in their constellation, and it turns into a dominant dependence. A changing personal and social identity, new cognitive schemes and mental models of business interaction allow moderators to find suitable euphemisms easily ("red brigades," "right sector," etc.), and complimentary-compensatory labels (commandant, centurion, national guardsman, etc.). Although, all this is not able to change a developed terroristic nucleus of a paraphilic personality.

In April 2014, all Russian TV channels showed the recording of Alexander M. (one of the leaders of Kiev Maidan) when he expressed his sadistic threats to the deputies of the regional council. In this video, he appeared dressed in camouflage and was holding an assault rifle as if it was a phallus like a prosthesis. In a different video he experiences a masochistic ecstasy from the strikes of female heels against the head. Undoubtedly, internet screening and TV pictures can let us express only a supposition about sadomasochism or multiple disorders of sexual preferences that are usually represented by a combination of such paraphilias as fetishism, transvestism and sadomasochism. The producers of tragedy could not allow this militant (who sincerely believed in his messianic role of a fighter) to continue his vivid illustration of this clinical case of paraphilia. This "TV hero" was doomed to failure from the moment of his TV screen debut. *Terror inside a terroristic community is a law of moral anomia in a legion of assassins.* The classification of paraphilia as a dependent disorder, the same refers to mobbing, bullying and crowding, makes it possible to *view terrorism as a peculiar polymodal and polymorphic dependent disorder.*

There is no doubt that the participants of mass murders and sexual violence in Odessa's Hatyn, (those that were registered by audio and video devices) will never be found by any international commission.

The weapons of terrorists, besides their direct purposes, serve as a *hypercompensatory attribute* that masks the inability to make decisions without advice of their senior leaders and financing mentors; readiness to delegate them rights without demur when it comes to making decisions of critical importance; anticipating preparedness to agree with their masters caused by the fear to be rejected (even when knowing that they are wrong); difficulties when starting something independently; readiness of one's own free will to carry out risky and dangerous orders in order to get a reward or appraisal from the principle; bad tolerance of loneliness and readiness to undertake any efforts in order to avoid it; feeling of being drained or being helpless when falling out of one's "national guard"; easy susceptibility and vulnerability to manipulability, enchainment with anxiety and fear to be rejected that pushes to commit new and new delicts and acts of terrorism.

In the outcome fractal, one can expect a psychic defect – it differs considerably depending on various forms of terroristic asocial dependencies that range from the syndrome of emotional burn out and destructive professiongenesis with mobbing-, bullying- and crowding –terrorism to the psychoorganic syndrome with traumatic lesion of the brain or chemical dependences.

The escalation of a terroristic civil war inevitably leads to the augmented *destruction of the public conscience as an integral quality of the nation's mental health.*

Somatogenesis refers to the least studied aspects. It is generally accepted that nonspecific hereditary burden *(fractal of predisposition),* unfavorable intra- perinatal exposures play an important role in it. Different normative psychosomatic reactions can be response reactions to challenges and difficulties; later they transform into functional psychosomatic disorders — organ neuroses *(latent fractal)* and somatoform disorders, they provide a clinical description of an individual with forming "withdrawal syndrome" *(initial fractal).* The severity of possible somatization disorders *(debut fractal)* and comorbid psychomotor disorders is defined by the duration of the "withdrawal syndrome," unwillingness and inability of a deformed personality to attain psycho-emotional relief in frames of his adaptive and prosocial behavior *(chronization fractal).*

All forms of social epidemics are characterized by the absence of parallelism in the expression of mental and somato- neurological, moral and spiritual, social and psychological disorders. While chemical dependences during their somatogenesis result in the evolution of the given disorders and are strongly connected to the toxic agent, the non-chemical ones (as a compensatory variant of development) more often lead to comorbid psychosomatic disorders. The accepted name of this mechanism is somatization of dependence. In the outcome fractal one can expect different somato-neurological complications; as for the level of social health – regress and degradation can be expected. The notion of comorbidity is not so much based on traditional views about the compatibility of pathologies but on the etiopathogenic unity of all dependent behavior forms.

Dependency signs may stipulate dangerous aggressive actions in frames of self- and mutual induction of social terrorism epidemics; they become evident with the following classic syndromes:

1. *syndrome of changed reactivity* is represented by an increase of delicts and acts of terrorism, growth of multimodal tolerance and sadistic aggressiveness, impoverishment and exhaustion of the out of normative episode sociality;
2. *syndrome of psychic dependence* is represented by an obsessive attraction, mental comfort condition during a deviant and criminal situation, changed and perverted form of emotional experience towards delict or act of terrorism;
3. *syndrome of physical dependence* is represented by a compulsive attraction, composed of physical comfort during a deviant or criminogenic situation; changed and perverted forms of delict and terrorist act manifestation, "withdrawal syndrome."

The syndromes of psychic and physical dependence determine the multi-episodic and compulsory nature of the epidemic generalization with asocial dependent behavior as well as the involuntariness of its appearance and difficulty in overcoming the anomalous attraction of the commenced episode. They influence the degree of freedom when it comes to choosing a behavioral pattern. That is how they act as a psychopathologic foundation of possible dangerous serial actions. Unfortunately, "Odessa's Hatyn," is just the beginning…

The growth of tolerance acts as a psychopathological foundation for the increased amount of aggressiveness and autoagression, severity of repeated and serial delicts, acts of terrorism.

The out of episode dynamics of social terrorism epidemic shows itself in the form of growing destructive professiongenesis, emotional burnout and personality deformation, development of associated and comorbid psychosomatic disorders.

It is of principle importance to emphasize, that the model of "synergetic individual" allows obtaining a unified biopsychosociospiritual methodology of analysis for all epidemic forms of dependent disorders — ranging from alcoholism and drug abuse to fanaticism and terrorism, it corresponds to the high-priority directions of the mental medicine and mental safety development.

21.5. Civilizational Terroristic Suicidal Blackmail

The XX century ended with artificial birth in the social and technological centers of the leading world powers of *simulacrum "terroristic world" - dehumanized and demoralized, intolerant and aggressive.* The formal-inertial existence of the institution of the international law reveals the utter helplessness in the practice of mediation of ethnic and religious, civil and military conflicts. The position of the UN Security Council becomes increasingly interesting only to the Council. As the irony of history is perceived the International Hague Tribunal of the victors over defeated, showing only the cyclic age to the archaic law of the strong over the weak.

An important characteristic of the evolution of the terroristic world is increasingly accelerating blurring and the destruction of the spiritual and moral foundations of traditional societies - latent mental terrorism. The striking evidence is the convincing victory in the Eurovision Song Contest (May 2014) of the elegant bearded Austrian "singer," becoming a collective shot on brundeshaft in the culture and spirituality of the Old World. The fact that target was precisely multicultural and demoralized, Europe is shown in the bearded form. If this "mental terroristic bomb" would dare to come up with a beard in the "style of bin Laden," it had little chances to survive to the finals. This call to the Islamic fundamentalism could blow not only to the Eurovision but the whole of Europe.

A kind of pathetic symbol of blurring the boundaries between the terroristic war and terroristic attack became the armed helicopters with the symbols of the United Nations (UN), involved in the "anti-terrorist operation" of Kiev authorities in the southeast of Ukraine (May 14, 2014).

It is widely practiced in recent decades, *to legitimize the political terrorism in the form of system and echelon sanctions,* aimed at the destruction of the countries and peoples of the economic and geopolitical interests of the transnational oligarchy that is essentially a non-contact and formally non-military tool of mass destruction in today's "terroristic world." Moreover, the ethics of international relations is still formally observed in verbal and virtual partnerships appeals. In this regard, a unique psychological illustration is the press conference by the USA President Barack Obama in South Korea (January 25, 2014), when he declared his readiness to continue cooperation with Russia in the fight against terrorism. Against the background of more and more sanctions (the United States applied sanctions to 97 countries out of 242), the partnership looks pathetic and Hollywood interaction of target and bullets, flying into it. The very same rhetoric speaks of a deep mental inertia, categorically denying the multivariate and multidimensional picture of the world perception.

Even more clearly it was evident in the first round of debate of contenders for the post of President of the European Commission (April 29, 2014) when participants almost unanimously recognized the *unprecedented growth and political legitimization of extremism and neo-fascism.* At the same time, they could not or did not want to see in the events in Ukraine a prototype of tomorrow's blazing Europe. The psychological and political mechanisms of repression and denial are there.

A special feature of any epidemic is that they do not stop at the customs and categorically do not comply the diplomatic protocol. Well-known are incubation periods of especially dangerous infections of bioterrorism. The "Ukrainian model" of starting social epidemics of mobbing-, bullying-, crowding-terrorism allows in the framework of synergetic methodology to calculate and predict the chain reactions of explosions of social conscience and the trajectories of chaos development literally from the moment of "mental infection" to "mental representation." Particularly impressed is the speed of evolution of pro-fascist "right sector", first into the National Guard, and then de facto into the police and punitive terroristic forces, in which their founding fathers started its activities. Their "Odessa Khatyn" was the monstrous prolog of Slavic terrorist civil war. The producers and directors of the Ukrainian tragedy are well aware that artificial mutations of "mental viruses" do not only enhance their contagiousness but do unpredictably dangerous for the whole world, even though the production of "terrorist factory of stars" was planned exclusively for Russia. Only time can show the speed of development and the quality of *mental immunity of countries and peoples to new mutations and new mutations of destructive social epidemics.* The tremendous success of nationalist parties in elections to the European Parliament (May 25, 2014) - is a clear confirmation of it.

Russia's opponents have a dream to repeat a unique historical experience of the Soviet Union self-destruction because of the old man's mental rigidity of the Politburo. Now folk and ritual, but tomorrow is probably a dramatic spiral of global sanctions could create serious social and economic problems. The domestic "mental TV-drain" in the details showed the forms and methods of responding to this kind of problems, by preparing potential scenarios of possible universal representation "peaceful demonstrations" in the style of crowding-terrorism, preparation and use of patriotic Molotov cocktails, capture and administration of warehouses with arms, etc. It is very specific and very serious.

In the meantime, continuous and daily "terrorist attacks and counter-terrorist operations", alternating and intertwined in the unwinding spiral of terrorist civil war destroyed the Little Russia. At the time, N. Machiavelli said: "If you want peace – prepare for war!." Today, this classic formula may sound different: "If you want to retain control of illusory virtual global world – blow up the moral and valuable fundamentals of the real human world." Rapidly growing pandemic of terrorism forms the *terrorist-suicide mentality of post-postmodern society,* creating a real threat to run the script of civilizational suicide.

Information phantoms called "war on terrorism", "anti-terrorist operation", "anti-terrorist retaliation" – is one of the main strategic myths of the modern world, through which a quarter of a century its active geopolitical repartition is going. The mental arrangement of information front of the terrorist war is given by producing it with geopolitical centers. The scale and the apparent accumulation of inconsistencies with information and horrific scale "anti-terrorist operations" (Afghanistan, Iraq, etc.) led to a rise of ethical tolerance of social conscience that manifests in escalating of more and more monstrous violence: Odessa Khatyn, kidnapping by terrorists of 240 schoolgirls in Nigeria, and others. It is not just a reflection of the dehumanization of modern "terror world," but the evidence of its growing perverse and pathologic moral anomia and paraphilia.

The pandemic of terrorism radically changes the basic idea of the civilization foundations of modern society. The reality recognition of paradoxical "terrorist world" requires the organization of life on the principle "in war as in war», but whether such existence can be called a life? This rhetorical question, of course, has the affirmative answer of fighters in actively growing armies of guards and mercenaries, laborers of arms market and electronic security systems, armored doors and windows, bullet-proof vests and armored cars, etc. – all those, who exploits the fear and capitalizes the illusion of protection and security. The fire in the Ukraine showed the absolute illusory nature and vulnerability of the post-Soviet social and political institutions, the latest social engineering "color" constructors and concepts.

The singularity of the modern era, when in the geometrical progression there is the growing speed and complexity of scientific and technical progress, in proportion to the severity and dramatic nature of new civilizational challenges, including as a destructive social epidemics, requires utmost to improve the mental resilience of livelihoods, to take the *"Mental ecology doctrine of national security" and to create a mental health service* for a synergistic biopsychosociospiritual methodology of mental medicine. The time of simple and linear compartmentalized strategies to protect public health and social conscience is irretrievably gone.

The first steps in this direction could be the development and adoption of the *"Concept of mental security of the population,"* including the forms and safety rules of interpersonal interaction, intellectual work and social service; reducing the impact of mental illnesses and strengthening of the mental health of the population; reducing the prevalence of epidemic social illnesses from alcoholism and addiction to extremism and terrorism; reducing the high levels of mortality and disability, aggression and violence in society; reducing social vulnerability and victimization of sick and disabled people; overcoming of anomie and permissiveness, distortion of public conscience and social identity; the formation of multiple strategies of adaptive professiogenesis and effective self-management.

It is necessary to create a system of the spiritual and moral upbringing of the younger generation, designed to improve the quality of multicultural "mental vaccinations" radically, strengthening the *Nation's mental immunity to all kinds of epidemic social illnesses.* It is possible to cope with this task only when basing on the system resources of the mental health service.

The mental health service methodologically and technologically utilizes the resources of mental medicine, it creates a synergetic foundation that integrates classical clinical psychiatry, mental preventology (see table), makes it possible to organize a *system monitoring of mental health* and cardinally increases the efficiency of social protection from destructive social epidemics. It is necessary to reevaluate the mission of the prophylactic medical examination (that are currently undergoing reforms) and conceptualize the systematic monitoring of the nation's social and mental health, expand the spectrum of its activity from narrow-specialized tactical tasks (infections, customer oriented, and others) to strategic objectives that would create a social platform of national security.

V. A. Medvedev (2004) singled out the levels of motivation that give birth to terror and arranged them in a regressive sequence. This sequence shows the regression of generic and sociocultural nature and progression of individual personality components: biological (population), historical and cultural (mythological), ethnopsychological, group, individual psychopathology and sociopathy. The mirror reflection of these levels structures the echelon system of antiterrorist defense. All contemporary humanitarian counterterrorism models are based on the system spiritual and ideological construction of national security that is founded on the life-forming meanings and moral values.

The mental paradigm of national security includes abatement of mental ailments consequences, strengthening the nation's mental health; reduction of the spread of social destructive epidemics, self-destructive and dependent behavior, decrease in high mortality rates and social violence; lessening the social stratification, poverty and unemployment; elimination of social vulnerability of seriously ill people and individuals with disabilities; overcoming of anomia and permissivity, deformation of social and individual conscience, social isolation of an individual; formation of multivariant strategies of adaptive professiogenesis and effective self-management.

Terrorism is, figuratively speaking, a pillar of fire and ash, erupting from the crater of the volcano-pyramid of modern civilization. We are not the first and not the last on Earth. The skeletons of the pyramids of previous civilizations became the tourist wonders of the world, but they are also a reminder of how dramatically their historical cycle ended. The modern world is pyramidal and in all senses. Ahead is a long and difficult phase transition to a new quality of after the post-industrial society, which is inevitably doomed to revise the previous basic priorities and values, radically strengthening the humanistic component of a new civilizational paradigm. The unique mission of Russia may be in this humanitarian construction.

Chapter 22

Mental Terrorism of Hybrid Wars and Synergetics of Protection

One of the advance storming parties triggering serial "color revolutions" was Scientology – an umbrella structure of secret services professionally changing public conscience of target countries, carrying out the mission of mental terrorism in hybrid wars that escalate into *a civilizational war* in our eyes. That is why a conceptual-methodological grounding of an increasingly larger role in mental terrorism and mental weapons in the civilizational war is necessary. As well as a description of fractal dynamics of a Scientological pandemic development, evaluation of possibilities of hybrid neuro-bionic defense systems using the synergetic biopsychosociospiritual methodology of mental ecology and mental medicine, isolation of the key dispersion and inversion tendencies of the global security paradigm in the contemporary hybrid world.

Neocults refer to polymodal vicarious dependent disorders filling the moral-psychological vacuum. Scientilogy is one of the variants of *mental terrorism* – destructive mercantile manipulation of conscience.

According to V. I. Vernadsky, the *noosphere* is a sphere of society and nature interaction and within its boundaries, the human brain or conscience become the leading developmental factor. To determine the chapter goal, we just mention one of the deep psychoanalytic motives of the "noospheric doctrine" founder, and that sounds obviously in the externally too pretentious and reverently politically correct "Marxist-Leninist" refrain. In the parlance of our time, it is a message to "comrades-Bolsheviks" that manipulation of individual conscience and public conscience has limits, and it is self-destroying to go beyond the limits even for "the Marxist-Leninist sectarianism." The XX century history has convincingly confirmed this, showed how seemingly tactically perfect scenarios of political technologies resulted in a strategic equifinal collapse. Ever since information manipulations developed into mental terrorism, an analysis of its reflection in the "noospheric mirror" requires the involvement of the mental ecology synergetic methodology.

22.1. From the Information Weapon of "Cold War" to the Mental Weapon of Hybrid War

The principal characteristic of the "cold war" period was the nuclear confrontation represented by the warheads and delivery means parity. 45 years ago together with the Internet appearance, the mankind had ensured a new qualitative technological breakthrough, "having split" the noosphere or the global conscience into the virtual and real worlds, what spurred a singular "chain reaction" of self-development and self-destruction. Figuratively speaking, it was an anthropogenic mirror reflection of technogenic atom smashing associated even with the name of the cerebral cortex *mirror neurons* that are possible receptor matrices of mental Internet-virology initializing induction mechanisms and social epidemiology "chain reactions." In fact, info-communication instruments are the principal characteristics of the modern singular world, in which both scientific and technical progress and epidemic social diseases are developed exponentially. For example, the radio required forty years to cover fifty mln people, the television – hardly ten years and the Internet – three years. If in 1993, in "the global web," there were not more than fifty sites, then at present, their number exceeds one billion! The Internet has become a neuro-bionic instrument of global public conscience and personal mental health. The information war conduct experience in the "pre-internet" period was radically transformed with an account of new technological opportunities.

If atomic weapon tactical employment was completed by bombardments of Hiroshima (90-166 thou. deceased) and Nagasaki (60-80 thou. deceased), then it is just impossible to find correct or, at least, approximate statistical data on multimillion mental weapon victims and casualties, because casualties are recognized as secondary and cumulative destructive effects – *it is anonymous weapon that does not allow even to identify an aggressor.*

The irony of history is in the fact that self-developmental singular mechanisms in local "nuclear noospheric explosions" so far can be managed or compensated though with obvious severe and permanent consequences. However, prediction of approach to the point of no return of "a thermonuclear noospheric explosion" is still an open problem. And here, the mental ecology synergetic methodology allows to at least improving the quality of research models.

Many predictions and scenarios of global disasters exist. Practical understanding of global disasters exclusiveness and non-repeatability manifests itself in new generations of "Noah's arks" in the shape of Mistral-like yachts built by few enthusiasts, but even millions of nuclear bomb shelters (China, America, etc.) can hardly become something else than a necropolis service. Only integral synergetic characteristics of *noospheric resilience* (Sidorov 2014) measured by mental ecology can bring nearer to the realistic assessment of life support civilizational resources.

One can compare the "critical mass" image of deformed public conscience with *"the virulent simulacrum"* of the virtual world stimulating mental representation (or replication according to R. Doukinson) and spurring reverberatory-coherent "chain reactions" of epidemic behavioral self-destruction of the real world subjectness. However, each country and each nation have its "critical mass." The civilizational war overture developing before our eyes is already establishing on the map of the world a new "*decivilizational rating*" *of countries and nations exploded by terrorism*. The cliche media image of "hot zones" was long ago left only in children's fairy tales and the Funnies teleadventures…

Any relevant reason can fulfill the mission of a detonator of a public conscience explosion "chain reaction," but only info-communication netware of the process initiating social epidemic generalization is decisive.

The set "nuclear-noospheric" associative array can be extended by an *air blast* of protest actions and bashing; *penetrating information radiation* of new radical and extremist movements; *cumulative charges* of multilevel mentality deformation resulting in permissiveness and anomia; *independently targetable warheads* of multipurpose destruction of traditional society's values and meanings; *late effects* in the form of the post-traumatic stress disorder and the social stress disorder, noogenic neuroses etc.

Contemporary "chain reactions" of public conscience splitting and deformation are manifested in galloping development of destructive social epidemics of radicalism and extremism, fanaticism and terrorism. At this background, "the cold war" has changed into the *hybrid war* totally using all kinds of weapons (nuclear and physical, biological and chemical, information weapons and terrorism) in strong and echeloned attacks taking into account versatile and complicated dynamics of battlespace on the scale of the global world that requires quick and targeted adaptive and effective reactions.

The biggest American victory in the new generation of hybrid wars was the USSR destruction, concerning which the USA President B. Clinton said at one of the Headquarters Directors meeting: "Using the Soviet diplomacy's misses, Gorbachev's exceeding arrogance and his retinue including those who took up a direct pro-American position, by means of the ably applied electronic-information impact, we have managed to do what President Truman was going to do with the Soviet Union by means of a nuclear bomb" (Vorontsova, Frolov 2006).

One can call this practice *a strategic mental trap* reduced to efforts made in order not to allow a naive opponent to see the primary neocolonialism forest behind the liberal-democratic trees. A mental trap is a scientece euphemism specifying banal human stupidity that becomes strategic when performed by a statesman. The priority task of information wars was always a web-based inspiration of such traps with a pompous liberal-democratic arrangement.

In the nuclear arms race history, *the critical period* of unilateral American technological dominance continued for four years since the first atom test in New-Mexico in July 1945 till the first Soviet atom test in August 1949. At present, there is a similar critical period, when the American scientific-technological advance is determined by the Internet system administration and producing, quality of the satellite constellation and global monitoring, etc. Ten years ago, we explained the necessity and proposed pilot models of rocket-and-space activity system monitoring and system ecological monitoring, mental health system monitoring and mental health service, showed the importance of these instruments for national security protection. In 2007, the multidisciplinary team of researchers got the prize of the RF Government in the Area of Science and Technology for "Development and introduction of system ecological monitoring as a component of strategic security." Unfortunately in the years of 2000 – 2009, the urgency of perception of innovation perspectives of some priority security problems came close to zero.

In the contemporary situation of avalanche-type sanctions and their consequences, the nation's leadership has made operative decisions about a new defense doctrine and system information security, the launching of a new generation of communications satellites and adaptive defense of public conscience as an integral property of the nation's mental health.

The newest turn of the arms race has changed practically all resources of life support to hybrid weapons and made the Hybrid World a total theater of operations.

The attempt of involvement of Russia and the Orthodox world into a self-destructing hybrid civil war in Ukraine next to the Islamic world already flaring and exploded by terrorism, turns such war into a *civilizational* war that destroys countries and nations, stops development and poses a civilizational suicide threat.

During the recent quarter of a century, the biggest weight in hybrid weapons carries *mental terrorism* – explosive mercantile manipulation of conscience or a total of ways and methods of goal-oriented destructive impact on human mentality with the purpose to realize manipulators' interests. *A mental terrorist war* as a large-scale use of mental terrorism forms is described by:

- galloping increase in total cruelty and unmotivated violence;
- public conscience dehumanization and demoralization;
- generalization of all forms of social epidemics;
- increased anomia and permissiveness creating panic and chaos;
- the web-based inspiration of conflicts and provocations, mass disturbances and civil wars;
- destabilization of the social-political situation;
- intensive and unilateral misinformation of population;
- stirring of national-religious cleavages.

The global web is increasingly becoming a battleground. *Mental cyber terrorism* is aggressive manipulation of the Internet users' conscience that triggers web panic and social-stressful reactions allowing to mobilize huge heaps of people. "Assignment" of Alaa Fathi for a role of "the web Egyptian Moses" is to a great degree only legitimation of the nationwide protest, which system administrators and producers were very far in reality, and virtually – inside Tahrir public conscience constructed materially by mental virology.

Mental viruses are simulacra able to change conscience, reshape and deform mentality, to wash out and to destroy unique identity nano environment. The concept of simulacra as virtual copies absent in reality is largely a digital evolution of classical thought forms.

The terms "mental cyberterrorism" and "mental viruses" have been totally discredited in respect of science purposefully and successively in the Internet by enormous spam. It is possible to suggest that it is done for disactualization and mental weapon anonymity camouflage. Not by accident at the meeting of the RF Security Council in November 2014, the President of Russia V. V. Putin urged to refer to the Internet as to mass destruction weapons.

In the working classification of destructive social epidemics that we have proposed, mental terrorism is present in all forms of terrorism either as an independent phenomenon (vicarious and co-dependent) or as a fractal of the development of more socially dangerous forms.

Epidemic of mental terrorism is generalized, extended and uncontrolled reproduction of destructive psychic dependence in the shape of:

- expansive financial pyramids;
- pseudo-religious neocults;
- totalitarian sects;
- extremist organizations;
- fanaticism and radicalism;
- terrorist organizations etc.

The uniqueness of Scientology as a financial-cultic pyramid allows referring it to any of the listed groups and Scientological "auditors" – to the universal mental war soldiers.

One can say that mental (cognitive) weapon means new quality of "the cold war" information-psychological armament transition to contemporary hybrid neuro-bionic combat systems providing global and epidemic, multipurpose and echeloned mentality deformation and identity diffusion, sniper "outbreaks" of individual and public conscience spurring of "chain reactions" of destructive chaos and panic. At the fronts of new hybrid wars, priority targets are professional journalists, whose deaths can be seen everywhere.

In contemporary hybrid wars, tactical, mental weapons become increasingly important compared to strategic nuclear weapons that developed from a deterrence instrument into an attribute of *civilizational suicide*, practically excluding a pinpoint response or a preventive strike. Hybrid wars have actualized new classes of non-lethal and anonymous mental weapons that have a direct and targeted access to the individual and public conscience of social networks' subpopulations.

22.2. Mental Terrorism of Scientology

Scientology is an international movement consisting of a system of compiled religious ideas and pseudoscientific practices oriented at individuals being anxious to succeed. Such quite complementary definition is widely represented in many sources and reflects the international sect's ambition for an image of a quite prosocial civic movement.

In the terminology and methodology of mental ecology, *Scientology* is a form of mental terrorism from the hybrid war arsenal resulting in individual and public conscience deformation, destructive social epidemic progress, society demoralization and dehumanization. *Mental terrorism is a non-lethal mass destruction weapon in contemporary hybrid wars.*

During the recent quarter of a century in Ukraine, there was organized just "a sectarian Sabbath" with official registration of "the Church of Satan" in August as a peak. Scientology as other international sects played an important role in public conscience deformation in Ukraine during *the latent phase of preparation for a contemporary hybrid war* aimed at Russia and the whole Orthodox World.

The international neocults' mission particularly that of Scientology, includes hand sorting and filtration, manipulation and exploitation of dependent and asocial, marginal and renegade subpopulations. In the global web era, the ways both of adaptive and disadaptive manipulation of individual and public conscience shift more and more to the Internet making it possible to industrialize and intensify in continuous mode goal-oriented testing and screening both of individual users and social networks' subpopulations.

The rate and scale of Scientology spreading to a great degree are predetermined by the financial-cultic pyramids' marketing strategy when involvement and exploitation of more and more new adepts are stimulated by very concrete dividends. The other feature of the pyramidic marketing is much more dramatic: adepts outdated for "the Church of Scientology" should release it in time from excess social responsibility that is to die quietly: *any pyramid eats up its constructors*. Basically, it is a controlled self-destructive mental, behavioral and physical ("ritual R2-45") euthanasia well-kept from public eyes, what is not difficult to do for the Global Network producers patronizing Scientologists.

Presence or positioning of some of media personages in "the Church of Scientology" appears to be just a banal advertising transaction.

In practice, "the Church of Scientology" gives *universal indulgence* to its adepts for any abusive practices and unlimited rights and freedom without looking back to legislated citizens' social and state commitments and responsibility. This explains to a great extent the unprecedented periodicity of legal proceedings with "the Church of Scientology" that uses them for scandalous-advertising marketing campaigns yielding beneficial dividends regardless concrete court judgments.

Indeed, if a court sentences Scientologists, it is presented as civil righters' prosecution and creates glory of sectarians as "martyrs of conscience." If Scientologists win in the court, it is "a triumph of liberal democratic freedoms." Such *beneficial versatility is one of the symptoms of mental terrorism* deforming and destructing public conscience, a traditional lifestyle and culture.

American Scientologists appeared in the USSR in the early Gorbachev's period, then in the early Yeltsin's period, they were joined by American sectologists that provided additional scandalous publicity. After all, one of the priority tasks of mental terrorism (as of any other terrorism form) is "an outbreak" of public conscience using mass media, TV and the Internet. It is time to think about combat actions adequateness in the world mental terrorist war, one of the results of which is *the subpopulation of "believers without religion" ("none," "poor belief")*. Its appearance was predicted a quarter of a century ago by Viktor Frankl (1990) in his interview to the American journal "Times": "... there is a tendency to move away not from religion, but from those beliefs that just steal believers from each other. We go not to universal, but to personal and deeply personalized religionism."

It is confirmed by many peculiarities of the mental phenomenon of "believers without religion" being notable for the high level of education and professionalism, autonomy and independence, and most significantly – accessibility for real contacts exclusively or primarily in the virtual world. «Nones» generally prefer to say "no." Even considering the whole convention of the associative model, it is practical to refer public conscience of this actively growing subpopulation to the basic factor of accumulated "new critical mass" of "the thermonuclear noospheric charge." If local "nuclear noospheric blasts" became a commonplace of serial "color revolutions," then the critical mass and the mechanisms of "thermonuclear noospheric disintegration" can be a new civilizational problem with unobvious scenarios of the very possibility of life support.

The inspired by the USA impassioned debate between Scientology and sectology of official confessions also persecuted a deeper task *in the destruction of basic structures of the state national security that can be termed a cumulative strategy of international mental terrorism.* For example, drawing of the Ukrainian Security Council in externally convenient and simple forms of "hand field work" of the international sect's "auditors" has turned into a regular mental trap, which name was developed from the Russian formula "Simplicity is worse than thieving" into the newest Ukrainian model "Common thieving." In fact, the classics of intelligence psychology is a thesis that "a double agent is always a foreign agent." Moreover, international religious-financial pyramids have huge experience of quite simple buying of representatives of any government entities ready to provide them additional preferences. Official government and political figures' pretentious self-positioning as "pastors" or "auditors" is a *phenomenon of legitimated recruitment* that can be understood without actuality only by a marginalized society. The fact that some Ukrainian leaders are "national underbosses" of their hosts – the international sects that have recruited them tells about the critical demoralization of the country's public conscience and real destruction of both the national security structures and the traditional official confessions.

The main distinction of neocults (including Scientology) from Orthodoxy lies in their inchoateness and fragmented nature, exteriority and commercialism of the God's image symbols and meanings exploitation. Contemporary "clip conscience" imposed by marginal pop culture is based exactly on the inchoate and fragmented virtual reality that splits up real identity and deforms mentality in a mirror-rebounding way.

The population form of mental terrorism being realized by Scientologists in mass media is represented by "carpet slanderous bombing and lie burning with napalm" in public conscience of countries and nations. If a quarter of a century ago, it was possible to discuss characteristics of conscience destructive control, recruiters' signs and stages of interaction with psycho manipulators, forms and types of victimhood, mechanisms and strategies of impact on personalities, then at present, even the necessity of personification and mediation of public conscience destructive manipulation lowers. All this is effectively managed by the web and system mass media and the Internet, through which are realized cultural-specific forms of public conscience management that are produced by American Scientologists as well.

An explicitly marketing ploy of the Church of Scientology was the establishment of "*the Human Rights Civil Commission*" in 1969 – a non-governmental organization investigating and giving publicity to human rights abuses in the area of psychiatry. *Scientologists' radical anti-psychiatric movement* is just a form of self-promotion and legitimation in a huge front of civil righters in the spirit of political correctness that shyly forgets about commitments and responsibility. Mental medicine that we have created is system synthesis of the clinical psychiatry thesis and the antipsychiatry antithesis. It accumulates and positively transforms all argumentation of antipsychiatry in the new synergetic biopsychosociospiritual methodology. Health-oriented mental medicine has become a new paradigm of psychiatry development. The whole antipsychiatry was held in place only by the existing reductionism crisis of descriptive psychiatry. The synergetic integrity of the new mental medicine methodology creates real prerequisites for termination of the antipsychiatry period; it proposes new technologies of mental health promotion and treatment of mental diseases.

22.3. Development of Scientology Pandemic

The synergetic concept of the Scientological pandemic development has been presented in a generalized sense and a little conventionally in Table 22.1. The figure shows only the main markers of the dynamic disorder that is characterized by huge polyvalency and multivariance connected with clinical-psychopathologic and somato-neurologic, social-psychological and spiritual and moral personal typology as well as with the forms and trajectories of epidemic development in 154 countries of the world.

For perception convenience, the synergetic epidemic model has been given in the plane projection, though it is multidimensional and non-linear, unstable and open. The development trajectories are set and corrected at the bifurcation points, acquiring spiral-shapedness and multivariance. Linear nosocentric dynamics with traditional stages is changed by non-linear discreteness and fractality. A fractal is a projection on the wide scientific field of quantum concepts. A fractal is an interval of dissipative system's development with its internal mechanisms of self-organization and self-development, multivariant motion trajectories in multidimensional space. In Table 22.1, there has been given only the progredient variant of the neocults' epidemic development in four interdependent planes of sociogenesis and psychogenesis, somatogenesis and animogenesis. The disorder epidemicity and its individual development trajectories are specified by a unique combination of various biopsychosociospiritual factors, the effectiveness of protective-compensatory and adaptation mechanisms.

Animogenesis begins in the *predisposition* fractal – *an addictogenic family* (and/or environment) notable for *spiritual and moral deficiency and ambivalency*, high frequency of asocial and dependent disorders in parents and close relatives, various forms of violence and harassment, cavils and intimidation.

Early imposition in childhood and adolescence of the role and image of a moral outcast results in formation of perverted and simplified mentality models of interpersonal interaction and behavior. Such families and millisocial environments have anomic and permissive nature. They are very likely to marginalize and dehumanize moral values of a personality.

In *the latent fractal of addictogenic diatheses,* protecting and compensatory and protest behavioral self-assertion reactions appear exasperating relationships' polarization and isolation. *Formation of primary moral senses is disturbed*: good conscience and duty, faith and responsibility.

Deformation of spiritual development shows itself in deformed self-esteem and bad understanding of the meaning of life, unpreparedness and avoiding full-rate individual responsible behavior, the immaturity of moral self-conscience and moral responsibility.

In the initial fractal of adepts' conversion and recruitment in the course of mass bombings with attention and love of "auditing" and "clearing," training and practical behavioral encoding of a *deformed moral image* takes place, when feelings of love and loyalty exist only regarding Scientology and personally Ron Hubbard. All this gives grounding to the future development of the *syndrome of Scientological demoralization.*

In the fractal of Scientological mental epidemic debut, a personality prosocial spiritual and moral stand is lost. The syndrome of demoralization with a low ability of distinction of the good and the bad is formed, as well as personality amorphism and deficiency, low self-criticism and an identity disorder, stereotypization of life prospect seeing solely in fighting for the Church of Scientology ideals, a loss of understanding of value of human life ("ritual R2-45" with a Colt). Scientologists are notable for the archaic and binary ethic world view with a blurred distinction between reality and fantasy. They are fixed on dominating ideas about their messianic role and the perversely confabulated image of an enemy (particularly, of psychiatrists and psychiatry), being in thrall to compulsive and predominant ideas, the special meaning and high mission of life with behavioral and not very selfless service to their Church and the pyramidic business corporation.

The fractal of chronization of the destructive Scientological mental epidemic is presented by different types and forms of development of amoral and illegal behavior threatening public conscience and countries' national security. The syndrome of Scientological demoralization is manifested in a selecting and lacunar loss of moral-guided behavior accepted in society and based on the concepts of the good and the bad, the proper and inadmissible, demonstrative disregard of any moral commitments and refused moral self-control, dependency of actions and behavior irresponsibility, inability of moral self-assessment of behavior and observance of ethic standards of business communication, loss of personal and social identity, devaluation of legal conscience and law-obedience, avoiding of personal moral choice and any responsibility manifested in actions under the banners of the Church of Scientology.

The outcome fractal is characterized by the maximum epidemic level of the pandemic, terminal complications and consequences for public conscience. The ethic component of personality's severe asocial development reaching the mental defect level together with the comorbid and associated disorders makes adepts absolutely insensitive to counterarguments and dissuasion, results in lost pragmatism and rationality, the absence of fear and repentance.

All this allows "auditors"-manipulators to "create" new generations of adepts easily. In fact, they are engaged in *mental terrorism – individual, destructive and mercenary manipulation of adepts' conscience*. The only difference of mental terrorism from traditional forms of propaganda and agitation is in the population format of public conscience "attacked" by mass media in the framework of the information wars. The growing network interactivity and resonance of the global world make the information front line not just the leading one in any terrorist war but turn the war itself into the world mental war: against the Orthodox World, the Islamic World, etc. The Russian Orthodox Church confrontation with Scientologists and other neocults is one of the fronts of *the mental terrorist war* for the public conscience of the Orthodox Church. It is very complicated to win in such a war with traditional tools, so, its outcome is the increased subpopulation of "believers without religion" (up to 30% in Russia).

The Scientological demoralization syndrome development is entirely multivariant and is predetermined by the personality initial ethic typology, ethnic-cultural and social-economic, religious and political factors of the environment that is more and more turning into a "dehumanized and demoralized *"terrorist world" undermining the civilizational and humanistic foundations of the humanity.*

Sociogenesis in the predisposition fractal is characterized by the high frequency of various disorders in the structure and functions of marginal families. They substantially predetermine mental representation of destructive cognitive models of disharmonious interpersonal relationships: a cult of strength and aggression, humiliations and insults, social deprivations and isolations, negativism and protest. Such behavioral stereotype just needs legal prosecution, scandals and conflicts, antipsychiatric actions and protest marches only in order to come to notice.

Table 22.1. Fractal Dynamics of Scientological Pandemic Development

Vectors of ontogenesis	Prenosological fractals			Nosological fractals		
	Predispositions: Addictogenic and/or marginal family and/or environment	Latent: Addictogenic diathesis	Initial: Conversion - recruitment	Debut: mental epidemic	Chronization: destructive mental epidemic	Outcome: pandemic and terminal complications
Somatogenesis	Hereditary somatic burden	Disorders of neuro-processes	Somatoform dysfunctions	Somatized disorder	Comorbid psycho-somatic disease	Somato-neurological complications and public health deterioration
Psychogenesis	Psychopathological burden	Personality polymodal psycho-pathization	Asocial and/or dependent personality outside personality disorder	Asocial and/or dependent personality disorder	Asocial and/or dependent personality development	Personality defect and public conscience destruction
Sociogenesis	Family structure and function disorders	Disorders of personality socialization	Non-pathologic dependent and/or asocial behavior	Pathologic dependent and /or asocial behavior	Social decompensation	Social disadaptation and society dehumanization
Animogenesis	Family spiritual and moral deficiency	Disorders of moral senses formation	Moral image deformation	Loss of moral position	Immoral and unlawful behavior	Serial criminality and public conscience demoralization

In the latent fractal of addictogenic diathesis, dispersion and inversion of "addictogenic targets" into "mental terrorists" take place as a result of personalities' maturation and socialization disorders in a disharmonious millisocial environment. Such personalities do not have full-rate psychosocial resources for productive self-realization through their professional and educational activities, inside their families and communication environment. To a significant extent, that is the exact reason why *non-pathologic dependent and asocial behavior* develops through compensatory mechanisms. It is characterized by perverted obsessive fantasies that are realized through sadistic and cruel compulsive group tortures of defenseless animals and vulnerable peers. Personal interests are subordinated to some kind of paraphilia, attention is longly fixated, and the ability to control is decreased. The immersion into asocial dependence is very usual, as well as dependency and passivity when choosing behavioral strategies and verbal response strategies, self — and mutual induction during Scientological conversion and recruitment *in the initial fractal.*

In the debut fractal of the Scientological mental epidemic, the referent nucleus of the epidemic hotbed and its leaders display *pathologic dependent and asocial behavior.* It is characterized by altered states of conscience in psychological and physical dependence realization, irresistibility and compulsivity of asocial activity, stereotypization of the sectarian lifestyle, the cancelation syndrome between delicts and acts of mental terrorism, "clearing" and "auditing" of cleptomaniacs' network marketing.

In the chronization fractal, a Scientological destructive mental epidemic unfolds. It has different instruments and mechanisms depending on the type and forms of mental terrorism. However, it inevitably brings participants of an epidemic process to social decompensation and threatens a country's national security on the whole.

In the outcome fractal, total social disadaptation is formed or adjustment of deformed personalities to conditions of conscience strict control. Scientological pandemic development is accompanied by and matched with various social markers of *the global dehumanization crisis and civilization degradation*: business failures and unemployment, suicides and criminality, migration, etc.

Psychogenesis in the predisposition fractal is predetermined to a significant degree by a premorbid psychopathological burden of marginal families; it is notable for non-motivated psycho-emotional instability and communicative deficiency. Children who grow in such families, even those with the Orthodox and patriarchal backgrounds, experience an acute shortage of emotional connections, and painfully go through an early loss of parental care and family warmth. Trying to compensate that, they develop a proclivity to fantasy formation and require increased attention. Frequent early mental traumas often become a matrix of mental representation for tomorrow's style of self-destructive life.

In the latent fractal of addictogenic diathesis, addictive radicals of early psychopathization and early personality deformation are formed and fixated. They show themselves as anticipating malicious and aggressive verbal reactions and impulsive deeds concerning all challenges and difficulties. They stereotype aggressive and auto-aggressive styles of behavior, launch mechanisms of hypercompensation "asocial hysteria" and the polymodal asocial dependent disorder. Even when they encounter banal life difficulties, such individuals can demonstrate various socially stressful disorders, accelerating the formation of a primary dependent pattern that will be later able to change its modality or a dependence form, but steadily will preserve the asocial radical assimilating a personality's nucleus.

In the initial fractal of "Scientological communion" and recruitment (adepts are mental targets themselves), the behavioral realization of previously learned mental schemes and scenarios of asocial self-assertion takes place, this is the only outcome based on cognitive and cultural personal resources. *Asocial and dependent individuals outside the personality disorder,* demonstrate vivid, realistic reminiscences and fantasies heroizing Scientology against infantilism and suggestibility, openheartedness and sensory spontaneity, curiosity and high searching activity, maximalism and egocentrism, impressionability and impatience, a proclivity for taking risks and provoking dangerous situations. Only in criminal gangs and totalitarian sects, extremist and terrorist groups, such individuals get a chance to overcome the inferiority complex of an outcast in the prosocial environment and get rid of their humiliating tail of "an odd fish." The extrusion and disactualization of such obsessive reminiscences about one's traumatic youth that had multiple humiliations and losses are accompanied by a hyper-compensatory necessity to revenge not only some particular offenders but the whole cruel and unfair world. This is how the psychological mechanisms of generalization of the Scientological epidemic of mental terrorism are manifested.

Epidemic spread of mental terrorism mobilizes the mechanisms of induction and generalization and turns them into a global population mutation. Besides, it is necessary to take into account the fact that up to 30% of the population suffer from various forms of dependencies (Sidorov 2006), controlled social switching of their modality can quickly result in the emergence of social epidemics. In that context, Scientologists as other neocults fulfill the mission of "sectarian sensibilization" and screening of public conscience of target countries, allowing correcting budgets of a regular "reloading-overload."

The known theologian Jon Atack (1990) wrote: "The problem is that most of the people requesting help from Scientologists are in a crisis state. The Scientological recruitment technique untruly promising solution of all problems is oriented at manipulation of people and development of their suggestibility. From the very beginning, artificial manipulations cause a sensation of euphoria in a newly convert. Often, striving to such euphoric state purely comparable with drug dependence deprives members of any critical thinking concerning the organization. Very quickly, the sect gets overall control of its members and prohibits them to contact all people that regard it critically and suggests its members' thoughts about the global conspiracy for Scientology elimination. A fanatic's distinctive feature is his/her immunity to any evidence. Unfortunately, most Scientologists coming in contact with criticism of their movement plainly close their eyes and ears."

According to F. V. Kondratyev (2000), psychic state of an individual exposed to an "auditing" procedure should be determined as "temporary state of conscience described by its narrowed volume and sharp focusing on suggestion content that is connected with a changed function of individual control and self-conscience." In other words, it coincides literally with the definition of the concept "hypnosis" given in the dictionary "Psychology" (1990) and in other sources.

In support of the opinion about the possibility of considering "auditing" as a variant of hypnotic influence besides the mentioned narrowed volume of conscience, in which a client is during an "auditing" session, one should point out a rapport state typical of the hypnotherapy method. It is a contact between a hypnotized person and a hypnotizing person during a hypnosis session." (Conclusion of the Complex Medical Expertise of the Hubbard Humanitarian Center of the Serbsky State Science Center of Social and Forensic Psychiatry of 30 June 1999//Iriney Lionsky Center).

As a result of "auditing" sessions, euphoric states can appear similar to drug-induced states that make clients address Scientologists again and again. Using the "clearing" system, Scientologists attain fanatic loyalty of tens of thousands people. According to the American psychiatrist J. G. Clark (2002), Scientological interviews or "auditings" are a carefully designed method of bringing a person into a controlled trance state: "The goal is to make a person fully identify himself/herself with the doctrine until the full refusal to recognize other modes of thinking and to disconnecting with any external cultural influences."

The fractal of the mental Scientological epidemic debut is most often represented by the asocial and dependent personality disorders of the epidemic hotbed referent nucleus of the Church of Scientology inducing fellow-fighters who are included in the polymodal dependent subpopulation. The dependent personality disorders are characterized by a deficiency of normative sociality and a wider asocial manifestations' spectrum, personality deformation and emotional burnout, inability to make decisions independently outside one's sectarian lifestyle, the frequent combination of schizoid personality features with a bad tolerance of loneliness. This facilitates the development of anxious depression, urging an individual to commit delicts and new recruitments that provide a temporary psycho-emotional relief and replenish a budget.

The fractal of chronization of the destructive mental Scientological epidemic is represented by multivariant *asocial and dependent personality developments*, mental terrorism begins to take the leading position in their constellation and turns into a predominant dependence. A changing personal and social identity, new cognitive schemes and mental models of business interaction allow moderators to find easily suitable euphemisms ("clearing" etc.), and complimentary-compensatory rank labels ("auditor" etc.). All this accelerates the formation of a nucleus of a paraphilic personality deriving satisfaction of mercantile manipulations of conscience of many new adepts. Referral of paraphilias to dependent disorders, as well as mobbing, bullying and crowding allows also considering *mental terrorism a peculiar type of the polymodal and polymorphic dependent behavioral disorder.*

For Scientologists, the ritual arms (Colt) and tools ("stress-test," "E-meter" etc.), besides their direct purposes, serve also as a *hypercompensation attribute legitimating fraudulent activity.* This activity usually masks the inability to make decisions without advice of their senior mentors; readiness to delegate them inviolately the rights for making most important decisions; forward-looking readiness to agree with their masters caused by their fear to be rejected, even when knowing that they are wrong; difficulties when starting something independently; readiness of one's own free will to carry out risky and dangerous orders in order to get a reward or appraisal; low tolerance of loneliness and readiness to undertake any efforts in order to avoid it; feeling of voidness or being helpless when falling out of one's own "church"; easy vulnerability and manipulative sensitivity, enchainment with anxiety and fear to be rejected that pushes to commit more and more new "deeds."

In the outcome fractal, one can expect a psychic defect that differs considerably in various forms of sectarian asocial dependence: from the emotional burnout syndrome and destructive professiogenesis to the psychoorganic syndrome in the brain traumatic lesions or chemical dependencies.

Escalation of various mental terrorism social epidemics results inevitably in an *augmented destruction of public conscience as an integral property of nation's mental health.*

Somatogenesis refers to the least studied aspects. Nonspecific hereditary burdens (*the predisposition fractal*), unfavorable intra- and perinatal exposures play a generally recognized important role in it. Different normative psychosomatic reactions can be response reactions to challenges and difficulties; later they transform into functional psychosomatic disorders – organ neuroses (*the latent fractal*) and somatoform disorders providing a clinical description of individual features of the formed "withdrawal syndrome" (*the initial fractal*). The severity of possible somatization disorders (*the debut fractal*) and comorbid psychosomatic diseases is predetermined by the "withdrawal syndrome" duration, unwillingness and inability of a deformed individual to attain psycho-emotional relief in the framework of adaptive and prosocial behavior (*the chronization fractal*).

All forms of mental epidemics are characterized by the absence of parallelism in the expression of mental and somato-neurological, moral and spiritual, social and psychological disorders. While chemical dependencies during their somatogenesis result in the evolution of disorders strongly connected with toxic agents, then the non-chemical dependencies as a compensatory variant of development more often lead to comorbid psychosomatic disorders. The accepted name of this mechanism is dependence somatization. *In the outcome fractal*, one can expect different somato-neurological complications, and at the level of public health – regress and degradation. The notion of comorbidity is not so much based on traditional views on the compatibility of pathologies, but on the etiopathogenic unity of all dependent behavior forms.

It is important to emphasize that the model of a "synergetic individual" that we have developed makes it possible to obtain a unified biopsychosociospiritual methodology for analysis of all epidemic forms of dependent disorders – from alcoholism and drug abuse to sectarianism and terrorism.

22.4. Synergetics of Protection from Destructive Mental Epidemics

Contemporary psychiatry having quite limited medical-social resources in principle cannot and should not try to resist alone polymodal international religious-commercial corporations. *The anti-psychiatric trick of Scientological activity is only an echo of the classic totalitarian strategy "divide and rule"* when country's public conscience and its national security are attacked in the most vulnerable part. The increasing crisis of descriptive psychiatry reductionism confirms it obviously.

However, any other departmental strategies of neocultic social epidemics control are equally inefficient. Frontal counterattacks of Scientology at best only "tail the dragon" once again, the tail always grows again providing renovation and reproduction. This neocult has wonderfully learned to transform the energy of fight against it into sociogenic and modified forms of destructive activity skillfully, providing outgrowth of more and more new "tentacles of the many-headed serpent." For example, a neocultic mental epidemic evolves into a destructive one and becomes a pandemic in future.

It is obvious that new strategies of fight built on the synergetic biopsychosociospiritual methodology of mental ecology and mental medicine are necessary.

The synergetic approach that forms the foundation of the mental medicine methodology presupposes a significant review of preventive and medical rehabilitation strategies of care to dependent individuals, a change in the ideology and methodology of traditional socio- and psychotherapeutic, psychological-psychiatric and addiction relief services. A dependent individual requires constant and interactive sanitation and correction that can change only the vector and modality of dependence. When treating a dependent individual, the main task is as early as possible to change his/her dependence modality from destructive to constructive, from non-adaptive to adaptive, from asocial to prosocial, from autoaggressive to self-preserving modality. The preventive strategy for treating a dependent subpopulation requires adequate and regular loading of adaptive socio-psychological and spiritual and moral content.

On the basis of the synergetic concept of destructive social epidemics, we have elaborated a program of preventive-correctional and medical rehabilitation care that represents a *unified multidisciplinary protocol* realized by a brigade of specialists. The program includes four blocks: medical and psychological, spiritual and moral, and social (Table 22.2). The blocks are based on four interdependent ontogenesis planes (sociogenesis and psychogenesis, somatogenesis and animogenesis) representing the synergetic methodology of mental medicine.

It allows formulating a synergetic functional diagnosis including clinical and psychological, social and ethic diagnoses, as well as comorbid and associated disorders. On the ground of functional diagnoses, individual preventive-correctional or medical rehabilitation patterns of clients or patients are established. A mission and efforts volume of each specialist are entered in multiprofessional brigade protocols. Only such approach allows ground and realizing individual multidisciplinary programs of preventive-correctional and medical-rehabilitation care on the basis of the biopsychosociospiritual methodology.

The key part of a mental health service is a brigade or a team allowing starting resonant and cumulative sociogenetic and animogenetic, psychotherapeutic and biogenetic mechanisms accumulated in sanogenetic therapy by means of efforts' parallelism and polymodality.

Sanogenetic therapy is adaptive biopsychosociospiritual control of patient/client conscience destabilizing stable pathologic states, activating body resources and personality resources, restoring and harmonizing structural-functional systems of vital activity.

The same as 70 years ago, when nuclear-weapon technologies made the creation of conversion nuclear power industry and radiation medicine possible, at present, mental weapons create neoconversion technologies of mental medicine and mental ecology. One of the examples of such technologies is sanogenetic therapy realizing instrumentally the national security paradigm that is actively and on a daily basis tested with the hybrid war sophisticated and latent methods. Truly speaking, in the case with a mental cognitive weapon, it would be more reasonable to name it *inversion weapon* that developed from the militant perversion of psychotherapy and psycho-correction techniques. This fits in the civilizational dehumanization trend of the *contemporary hybrid epoch*.

The Internet's mental virology has been described in many guides, but only the synergetic biopsychosociospiritual methodology of mental ecology allows to monitor and predict in the four-dimensional space all epidemic variety of clinically and behaviorally significant phenomenology. Upon that, the fourth spiritual and moral dimension of animogenesis is increasingly the leading marker of adaptiveness and destructiveness of the virtual world content; it is in interactive line with peculiarities of identity and mentality both of separate individuals and public conscience of social networks' subpopulations.

It is crucially important to note that exactly the synergetic methodology of mental ecology makes it possible to turn confabulated cyber weapons into inversion preventive correctional and medical rehabilitation technologies of mental medicine and mental preventology.

Mental preventology of social epidemics has a huge arsenal of ways and methods. It would be odd even to try to mention hundreds of kinds of psychocorrection and psychotherapy. I merely point out the popular semi-folk "dishes" of our daily "mental TV-kitchen" from the nutritional therapy of the "Ural Snack-bar" to the ironist Zadornov's laugh-therapeutic circular marathons. In addition to that, healthy irony and self-irony of the nation continue to be the most important sanogenetic resource of public conscience resilience. Mental preventology itself increasingly turns into *civil self-protection* against destructive mental virology. Such seemingly too pompous change of accents in recently quite banal psychoprevention is excused by today.

The start by the English secret services on the Internet of a global mental counterterrorist operation "Not in my name" was a regular turn of the development of the world terrorist self-destruction. *Individualized and authorized anti-terror is "a brotherhood duel"* ensuring a guaranteed suicide. Not by coincidence, yet Grigory Pomerants said: "The devil begins from foam on the lips of the angel that has entered the battle for the right holy cause. All turns into dust: both people and systems."

The flywheel of political and mental inertness appeared in taking a decision by the UN Security Council (24.09.14) on the establishment of a world antiterrorism protection system though all newest experience of such fight was reduced literally to "firefighting with kerosene." And indeed, is it possible to expect the effective fight, when all the world system is built on a practically *terrorist ideology*: sanctions, threats, blackmail etc. All this is more like delusory-imitation activity destined to mask *the global depopulation strategy* that stimulates the processes of civilizational self-destruction comprehensively.

Usama Bin Laden was fostered by America against the USSR on the Afghan operational theater, but made a momentary non-disarming attack exactly against the USA. The Islamic State militants armed by America against B. al-Assad have become an independent global threat requiring massed NATO bombings. The IS militants "were famed" for public executions of foreign hostages, their kidnapings and getting a ransom is the principal article of income. Among the hostages executed in spring 2014, there was one Russian Sergey Gorbunov. At present, several thousands of hostages (27.10.14.; 9tv.co.il) are captured. There can be very many examples like this, but it is important to ask a principal question – who and what, where and when will be the next destructive social epidemic born according to the dispersion and inversion mechanisms of the Global Security Paradigm? To our opinion, the psycho-technologically and cyber-terroristically armed, politically expansive and economically effective financial-cultic pyramid of scientology can tomorrow, as a minimum, surprise very much its producers, and as a maximum, develop a real threat to the Global Security.

This position was supported by the Resolution of the VII International Conference of the Orthodox Centers for Research of New Religious Movements in Saint-Petersburg in September 2014, concerned with the Church of Scientology and chaired by the Ecumenical Patriarch Archbishop of Crete Irenaeus. Specialists in sectology from 14 countries gathered at the Research Forum; they represented eleven Local Orthodox Churches. In a special Conference statement, it was noted that: "Several years ago, sect-protecting organizations began a campaign for discredit of the personality and activity of the Psychiatrist, Academician of RAS P. I. Sidorov unmasking the destructive nature of sects in his works" (www.missiaspb.ru/ newspoint125.html).

All that is left to do is to recall a long-standing "commonplace" – the sorceries about a new humanization world order, which after all can approximate the reality, but only in the case of an obvious global threat. Figuratively speaking, "the world pregnancy" with the civilization war becomes more visible. Though the Founding Fathers of the market reality, according to age-old inertness, see only "snivel" of a regular form of the "bird flu" that attacks the humanity again along the beaten African track and demands a new multi-billion dollar mobilization from the budget of the global community... One can name it a mental trap of "the blurred public eye" though it is more accurate to define it within the frame of semiotics of mental medicine as *the secondary mental immunodeficiency syndrome*. Unfortunately, this phenomenon is so far perceived unilaterally as an absolute achievement of international "mental virology" produced from the richest budget. And for this reason, Russia lost all information wars from the start.

However, cycles fetch not a circuit, but a spiral. As well, just as the horse cavalry after the First World War was preserved only in the sport-esthetic format at hippodromes and in circuses, so at present, armored iron acquires new esthetics in ballet and corps de ballet of self-propelled guns. Tomorrow, space and suborbital tourism will enter upon a new phase of passenger "high-cost airlines." So far, approaching the task of *adaptive noospheric management* takes place only in the improvement of the anthropogenic block of the Global monitoring and virologic simulation on the Internet, in developments of artificial intelligence systems and hybrid neurobionics. The growing danger of the civilizational war full-scale development requires beginning of the adequate *International Scientific Program "Mental Ecology of Global Security."*

At the meeting for development of the Project "State Arms Program for 2016-2025" (10.09.2014), the RF President V. V. Putin mentioned that there have long ago been "... developed theories of a global disarming strike" in the contemporary world. One of the possible principles of an asymmetric response to such kind of danger is development of *hybrid neurobionic defense systems* – inversion technologies uniting electronic-information and biomedical, social-psychological and spiritual and moral resources of mental ecology and mental medicine. The synergetic biopsychosociospiritual methodology allows settling this problem in an instrumental-technological way, as well as to measure and predict trajectories of individual and public conscience development in the four-dimensional space of the real and virtual world realizing the national security priorities.

The American "war hawks" still lament the fact that President Truman allowed the USSR to catch America in the sprint nuclear race. The USSR lost the 'cold war" long distance run. At present literally, "a death march" is started, but it will not be possible to decide its winner in principle, as "the hybrid world" has overvalued and perverted all views of the rules and standards. The loss of basic civilizational matrices turns into a critical approximation of the point of no return. Tomorrow, there will be nobody to recall that yesterday a war was expected. *Indeed, the civilizational war can be only the first and the last war.*

Table 22.2. Program for medico-psychosociospiritual protection against neocult mental epidemics

Blocks	Prenosological fractals			Nosological fractals		
	Predisposition: marginal and/or addictogenic family	Latent: addictogenic diatheses	Initial: recruitment, functional disorders	Debut: mental epidemic	Chronization: destructive mental epidemic	Outcome: pandemic and terminal complications
Medical	Detection of people with hereditary predisposition, including them in the group of risk, early preventive screening	Detection of people with organ neurosis	Diagnostics of somatoform dysfunctions; medication-assisted and drug-free therapy	Detection of comorbid psychiatric diseases, prescribing medical therapy, prevention of complications	Proper medication-assisted therapy of psycho-organic stigmatization and psychosomatic diseases	Treatment for somato-neurological complications
Psychological	Detection of people with psychological burden and taking preventive measures with them	Sanitation of psychopathisation of the personality	Detecting the dependent personality beyond personal disorder and correction of disorders	Correction of persistent personality disorders, psychotherapy	Psychotherapy and psycho-pharmacotherapy of dependent personality disorder	Psychological rehabilitation of personality defect
Social	Detection and correction of violations of family structure and function	Correction of personality socialization	Correction of non-pathological dependent behavior	Complex treatment of pathologically-dependent behavior	Correction of social decompensation	Social rehabilitation
Spiritual and moral	Screening and correction of the family “moral climate”	Correction of formation and development of moral feelings	Correction of formation and development of moral image	Reconstruction of moral position	Reconstruction of moral behavior	Spiritual and moral rehabilitation

Section V. Mental Epidemics of Endoecological Mental Disorders

Chapter 23

Schizophrenia

Within synergic methodology and terminology, schizophrenia is a polymorphous resonantly-coherent mental illness. This illness is one of the most widely spread mental illnesses characterized by a combination of positive symptoms (hallucinatory-delusional, catatono-heberphrenic, emotional, etc.) with deficit symptoms (insensibility, abulia, emotional and social stangeness, etc.) behavioral and cognitive abnormality (of memory, attention, thinking) and which leads to the unfavorable social-economic consequences.

23.1. Prevalence of Schizophrenia

Data on the prevalence of schizophrenia in the world range within wide limits (from 1.9 to 10 per 1000 of the population), so far as the diagnosis in different countries is diagnosed on the basis of different understanding of this disease's limits. Prevalence of schizophrenia among men and women is much the same, although some people note more big prevalence among men, other – among women. The first spurt often occurs at 20 or so, by age 30 most patients have a strong indication of the disease and in early growing age while studying retrospective analysis characteristics of aggression and anti-sociality can be found. The first spurt among women often occurs at 25 or so.

23.2. Etiopathogenesis of Schizophrenia

Schizophrenia is a complex development disorder of the axion, full variety of which unlikely responds to the abnormality of some control action of the neurotransmitter.

Research of the most risks (environmental and genetic) can find out points of convergence, which are taking part in manifestation such as neuroinflammation, stress and folacin deficit. These environmental factors, in the presence of genetic disposition, can interrupt normal enlargement of the brain, inducing cognitive deficiency and deficit symptoms (Goff 2013).

Two main theory groups of etiology and nosogenesis of schizophrenia (psychological and biological theories) can be established. The psychodynamic model can be ranked to *psychological schizophrenia theories*, where a deep abnormality of interpersonal intercourse and also phenomenologically existential, which supposes a change of a patient's "existence," his inward (schizophrenia is a "special" form of the personality's existence) are established to be the causative factor.

Among *psychological theories of schizophrenia* a Gregory Baetson's (2000) concept of "double bind" can be noted. A child gets from a parent two logically incompatible orders (e.g. "if you do this I'll punish you" and "If you don't do this, I'll punish you"). The only thing left for him is to go mad. Catastrophic thought process disorder and view of life in a patient can be explained only if "double bind" is considered to excite a deepest emotional conflict.

N. D. Linde (2014) reduces causes of schizophrenia to three main factors:

1. self-management with a help of absolute violence, freedom from spontaneity and immediacy;
2. self-loathing and personal hatred of incredible power;
3. suppression of all feelings and sensual contact with reality.

The author finds confirmation of his theory in G. M. Nazloyan's maskotherapy (2012), who thinks that diagnosis "schizophrenia" is totally artificial and finds only self-identity abnormality in the so-called patients. The identity disorder rebuilds itself through cathartic while communicating with a mask – whether with personality's prosthesis or with its new image.

Among *biological theories of schizophrenia* the following are known nowadays:

- *the genetical hypothesis* (results of the genetic burden in cases of schizophrenia study, which showed accumulation of illness's cases in schizophrenic families and data on probandwise concordance for schizophrenia are the basis for this hypothesis);
- *the neurotransmitter hypothesis:*
  - dopamine (dopaminergic system dysfunction);
  - serotonin (serotonergic neurotransmission insufficiency);
  - noradrenergic(noradrenergic neurons degeneracy);
  - glutaminergic (glutaminergic brain's system dysfunction);
- *the immunologic hypothesis* (they are based on notions about autoimmune processes, i.e. body's ability to produce antibodies to antigens of its brain tissue);
- *the dysontogenetic theory* (pathology can occur under the influence of genetic, toxic, viral and other factors in prenatal period. The supposition that deviances in enlargement of encephalic structures at the cellular and subcellular level are the basis for risk for schizophrenia and enlargement of clinical pathognomy, i.e. clinical disease, takes place under the influence of stress factors which induce decompensation of the function corresponding to «ill structures»).

All recited theories are not independent, and most of them concede rendering from the perspective of other theoretical models and awareness of brain's function. A variety of views upon schizophrenia underlines the actuality of the development of new theories of this disease's origin.

23.3. Synergetics of Schizophrenia

Enlargement of schizophrenia and its path are found with the help of various combinations of biopsychosociospiritual factors, the effectiveness of endogenic, adaptative, compensatory, defense mechanisms and exogenetic influences. A variety of views upon the schizophrenia actualizes the necessity of its multidisciplinary investigations and the usage of new strategies for new medical rehabilitation programs.

Regarding the concept of schizophrenia from the perspectives of the synergetics, it is wise to take into account the cooperation of all interrelated vectors, for which lays of the synergetics will be isomorphic and extrapolated on all concerned spaces. These vectors will function in different proportions (depending on the fractal of enlargement of schizophrenia), successing destructive sympathy (desynchronizing the system, causing it's decoherence) or optimizing body's functioning (timing its rates coherently).

These vectors regard the problem of schizophrenia in different aspects: 1) dissipative system of family and society – sociogenetic aspect; 2) dissipative body system – biogenetic aspect; 3) dissipative personality system – psychogenetic aspect; 4) dissipative moral and spiritual system – anymogenetic aspect.

Monitoring of the functioning in one integrative stylistics and with inclusive of the cross-cultural language of these systems, which estimate not isolated phenomena of separate directions but the dynamics of energetic exchanges of the dissipative system with the environment and with each other, can be accomplished by polymodal mental medicine. Here interests of biological trend are realized by clinical medicine, of the psychic trend -by clinical psychology and psychiatry, of a social trend - by a complex of social disciplines, of moral and spiritual trend by biomedical ethics. By these dissipative systems systematic monitoring, ability in effective correctional influences all the areas of person's life and activities is formed.

Synergetic paradigm has a potential in discovering new mechanisms of psychokinesis. Functional (balanced, coherent) and non-functional (imbalanced, decoherent) dissipative system differentiations are listed in the Table 23.1.

Table 23.1. Criteria of approximation to the bifurcation point and changes of fractal

Criteria of differentiation	Dissipative system	
	Functional	Non-functional
Influence of environmental factors on the dynamics of dissipative structures	Very few factors can change the development scenario and path	Environmental factors can easily change the development scenario and path
Role of environmental factors in the fixity of dissipative structures	Balanced providing of self-oscillatory motion	Abundance of factors which strengthen the oscillatory amplitude
Range of oscillative motion	Small (fluctuations)	High
Condition of autoregulation	Can keep energetic balance	Energetically imbalanced

Sanological and compensatory protective resources of the body are represented on different stages by mechanisms of restitution, neoformation, immunomodulation, adaptation, compensation, decompensation, chronization, misadaptation (Sidorov 2014). The main tendency of psychological life corresponds to the unentropic process which is not easy to be reversed; that is why many people do not go beyond guideline (Bakusev 1994). These mechanisms can be as independent for each separate fractal as change each other infractionally, determining self-path of enlargement of schizophrenia, which takes into account not only the condition of a biological trend but also psychological status and social niche compensation adequateness in each concrete case. Schizophrenia is a dissipative system which is determined by the sum of corresponding fractals of this disorder, influencing the whole body transforming it globally as well as transforming the surrounding socium.

Two effects are possible in the work of these mechanisms: 1) increasing of the work of outer system maximum by means of neoformation processes' energetic supply reduction; 2) reduction in the work of outer system maximum by means of energetic supply reducing and relocation of energy currents for processes of neoformation (Kaznacheev 1971).

Domination of the first type processes leads to the system's resources reduction and its misadaptation in the broad sense of the word and of the second type allows the system to neoformate acceptable functioning condition. Adaptation to the changed body's living conditions is viable only if there is a strong stimulant which threatens its existence. In this case, optimizing self-organization of dissipative body's system occurs, switching to another level of functioning is realized, which is accompanied by change over bifurcation into next fractal. If the dissipative system which is in the situation at risk continues functioning normally in some time and corresponds to the formal criteria of mental health, it cannot be the basis for refusal of further monitoring: resources of a system are not boundless. Such construction of a dissipative structure in the process of a long critical condition can be a chart which successes further development of schizophrenia.

Schizophrenia as an example of a dynamic disease (Glass, Mackey 1991) is a model of dissipative system behavior in the conditions of influencing environmental factors on it along with changing internal and constant hereditary factor. Main features of dynamic disease are:

1. The onset of regular oscillation of high amplitude, which exceeds amplitude of oscillation in the normal physiological system that correlates such mechanism with a systaltic *desynchronized* (decoherent) functioning of a dissipative system which loses its stability. In the case of schizophrenia, this situation can occur by means of frank affective phren tantrum and also by means of properly mental illness manifestation and recrudescence.
2. Occurrence in the already existing periodicity of an attribute of new subperidiocity, causing analogies with fractal dynamic and bifurcate transitions which are caused by adhesion of fractal attractors. This situation generates resonant multilevel adaptations of the polymodal dissipative system, *which determine clinical polymorphism of mental illness.* In the case of schizophrenia it can manifest in the symptoms' coexistence. These symptoms can have different levels of actuality for the patient when during the treatment asymmetric syndromokinesis occurs and the elements of criticism can be present. Given position also means lop-sided autochthonous enlargement of clinic of schizophrenia when along with syndromes which are usual for early stages, typical clusters of its enlargement period (exodus) ("the islets of

epilogue in the prologue," which become strange attractor attracting trends of schizophrenia in the next fractals), which generates clinical polymorphism of schizophrenia.

3. Occurrence of quasi-periodic dynamic which generates the formation of clinic of schizophrenia outside linear stylistics and categories of causalgic necessism, which is unable to solve many problems of this pathology. In the case of schizophrenia this is total disharmony of psychophysical enlargement in the shape of fractional and disproportionate (asynchronous) changes of subject's rates of development on the back of its general dispalacticity of a psyche; *decoherent mismatch of psychic processes* and its inner contradictory which form schism – a supra-syndrome-based characteristic of schizophrenia.

All attributes of dynamic disease are representative for evidence of schizophrenia which make it easier to use the synergetic instrumentation in its study. Fractal dynamics of schizophrenia is presented in Table 23.2, and its syndrome-based filling by fractals is shown in Table 23.3.

Selection of the number of fractal sets is historically traditional. Pythagor considered six to be "the first perfect number." Perfect numbers in his philosophy are "beautiful image of virtue" and represents an optimum between extravagance and deficiency. They are caused by "perfect order" but "veritable" and "imperfect" numbers are not regulated, and they are not caused by a defined goal, so they are similar to blurs which are equally numerous, anarchical, and indefinite.

There was a special attitude towards number 6 in alchemy: «Number «6» is fit in the best possible way for brood: it is both even and odd, implicated to the dynamic nature as an even and to the material nature as odd that is why the ancients called it marriage and harmony. This is the only number which is perfect in all parts of which is composed» (Jung 1997).

Duration of the first *fractal of predisposition* is nine months. During this period biological trend predominates in functioning of a body and pre-sickliness condition of schizophrenia, axion and cerebral cortex are laid and formed. The genetical theory of schizophrenia is not confirmed nowadays, but nevertheless statistical confidence of inheritance of this mental illness is well-known.

The somatogenesis of schizophrenia does not start at once, in spite of the potential hereditary load (as against Down's syndrome), doesn't determinate obligate mortal fate. However, biological factor stays as notional through this fractal: stresses, which pregnant women have leads to the expulsion of catecholamines which influence the fetus diaplacently. It can have an excessive activation of a sympathoadrenal system which leads to the rising of fusion of cortisol, of adrenocorticotropic hormones and of catecholamine of glucagon, low level of serotonin which lead to the protection of fate from hyperactivity and forced helplessness. DNA receptors of a fetus percept this information which can become habitual influencing the algorithm of further individual's enlargement thereby triggering the mechanism of hormone neurotransmitter imprinting of brain.

The sociogenesis of schizophrenia and body in this fractal also influences its further enlargement: a fate responds to the sensory cues which are generated by its surrounding particularly to mother's voice (14-18 weeks), showing in connection with it certain emotions, differentiating and remembering information.

Table 23.2. Fractal dynamics of epidemical development of schizophrenia

Vectors of ontogenesis	Prenosological fractals			Nosological fractals		
	Predisposition: schizogenic family	Latent: schizotypical diathesis	Initial: schizoid state	Full-scale clinical picture /mental epidemic	Chronization: forms and types of schizophrenia course/ destructive mental epidemic	Outcome: somato-neurological complications /pandemic
Somatogenesis	Dysontogenesis	Displasticity of psychosomatics	Psychosomatic responses	Psychosomatic disorders	Psychoorganic stigmatization	Encephalopathy
Psychogenesis	Disharmony in diad: mother-fetus	Schizotypic diathesis	Schizoid state	Full-scale picture of schizophrenia	Postschizophrenical developments	Schizophrenical defect
Sociogenesis	Schizogenic family	Disharmony in family relations	Social desintegration	Social decompensation	Social desadaptation	Disability
Animogenesis	Spiritual and moral deficiency or ambivalence of the family	Disharmony of moral senses formation	Deformation of moral image	Destruction of spiritual and moral position	Probability of immoral actions	Probability of unlawful behavior

Table 23.3. Syndromal content of fractal dynamics of schizophrenia

Psychokinesis parameters	Prenosological fractals			Nosological fractals		
	Predisposition:	Latent:	Initial:	Full-scale clinical picture	Chronization	Outcome
Status	Dysontogenesis	Psychovegetative diathesis	Premorbid period	Psychopathology		
Syndrome	Changes of activity. Presyndromal neuromediator imprinting	Asthenical, similar to neurosis, depressive-hypochondrical	Paranoic mood	Paranoic, paranoid, Kandinsky-Clerambault	Paraphrenic	Apatho-abulic
Disorder level	Functional, prenosological			Full-scale clinical picture, nosological		
Compensatory resource	Adaptation	Compensation	Protection	Decompensation	Chronization	Desadaptation
Epidemiology	Public conscience			Mental epidemic	Destructive mental epidemic	Pandemic

The dissipative system of dyad "the mother and the fate" functions because of synchronizing activity of each part of this bimodal chart or causing its desynchronization which is connected with deviations from optimal trend. At this stage a brand, new interfamilial system connections are formed which can be as a factor of coherent synchronization of dissipative structure functioning so the case of its desynchronization. Hereafter interfamilial connections will transmute into parenting.

The psychogenesis of a fate is almost tabula rasa, even regarding influence of Jungian archetypes which have typical universalism of a myth and retrieve exclusive personality of an epos only in case of inclusion in this observing system. A subject with his individual psychological peculiarities which form in the deployment process of latter fractals of body functioning (with the establishing of higher nervous activity which undergoes constant modifications): "Reality is high-individualized experience" (Jung 1939). However, fate's mother's attitude towards pregnancy, her thoughts and disposition which are included in the subject's own memory at the level of cellular memory (its bearer is DNA) which can be kept for years, leaves steady trace in its psyche as for the bit about involvement of hundreds of cellulars.

At the level of intuitive, sensual experience, a child achieves emotional accent of relationship with the world. Children who were emotionally affected in wombs occur to be sensitive to stress, avoiding which can influence their further life. "While a child is in the womb, many its actions and rhythms are consonant with his mother's. It occurs because of the variety of rhythmical influences: mother's "sleep-awakeness" cycle, the circadian rhythm of her hormones, daily routine, regular heartbeat, etc." (Grojsman 2002). These rythms can influence a fate as coherently so decoherently. *The gestational dominant* influences the formation and content of the interfamilial systematic connections, particularly its psychological component which allows determining behavioral stereotypes and variants of experience of identification of pregnancy most of which are originally colored with negative emotions which shows the immensity of woman's psychological alteration. Parenting relationships which are formed in future also can be marked by the same negative emotions which were transformed by the real context of the situation.

The animogenesis of a fate in this fractal appears by means of unbalanced harmonic relationships in the dyad "the mother and the fate" when emotional coldness or ambivalence within schizogenic family lay changed psychoemotional and interactional ground for future shizotic abnormalities of the interpersonal relationship ethics.

Bifurcation point is the child's birth which opens *latent fractal.* Synergectics of this moment determines new priorities and pathes for the individual and his family's enlargement. The appearance of a child in family means the formation of new dissipative system which implies complex reorganization of spousal entirety which sometimes endangers existence of the whole system. The further the system stands up for the norm, the less protection of a body against schizophrenia is shown.

Trend mainly depends on the *somatogenesis*, which was noted as yet by P. Gunnushkin and E. Crachmer (individual's habitude; actualization of genetic factors; newborn's health; compensation abilities of its axion which continues developing; timely and relevant delivery of health; interfamilial phenotypic polymorphism, etc.). Moment of birth disturbs habitual rhythms of a newborn. It must reorganize its biorhythm and behavior to correspond to the extrauterine environment and particularly sensory stimuli on the part of the mother (touches, voice, warmth, conversation, eye contact) help to do it. Sound stimuli have definite undular characteristics which influence child's condition through resonating with it in the particular sense and changing rhythms of its functioning (high-pitched and arrhythmic cause qualm by generating the tachyrhythmia and tachypnea, low-frequency and rhythmical – calm, generating bradyrhythmia). The natural circular rhythm of prelum – ecstasia, strain-relaxation which is the basis for each manifestation of organic life, occurs in sucking reflex.

The psychogenesis is largely caused by social circumstances. "A person does not realize that relatives with direct influence on him engender in him an *image* partly true to its model and partly using the subject's own psychic material. Imago is born out as a result of a meeting of parental influence and the child's particular reactions" (Jung 1994). A mother's lifestyle can determine her child's further style of life, enlargement of its intellectual, communicative, emotional abilities. It is from the mother that an infant learns its first abstraction, copies the first semantic gesture – "no," taking it and learning to demonstrate society its aggression. The father joins "the mother - child" dyad, turning it into a triad, some time after the first 18 months, usually when breastfeeding stops. This separation is a great emotional shock for the child before he is unable to perceive himself separately from the mother. Psychological approaches determine mother's behavior as complementary about the child's behavior. When the habitual dyad breaks, new factors must come in to adapt the system, variegate its rep of synchronicities, adding new polystylistic arrangements of the biological, psychic, social, spiritual context for a positive change of the situation.

At this time vector of *sociogenesis* is accented: paternity is a mainly social factor, and as against maternal, more invariantly, undergoes rampant oscillations of variants which have wide amplitude. Society in the family is formed taking into account structural and destructive dogmata and child's parent's priorities, denoting deep roots of the true genesis of the possible problem of the mental illness which was formed not at the moment of birth and not even at the moment of the family's creation by his parents. «Communication deviances in parents, which are more subtle measure than pathognomy, are more reliable factors of abnormality in children than the presence of any symptoms in parents» (Semichev 1977).

Specific features of some families can interrupt child's sociogenesis. Such features are:

- schizogony – emotional coldness which comes to deprivation, hyper protection, excessive criticalness, formalization of relations, suppression; ambivalence of parent's behavior, the antipathy of their dogmata, domination of rigid mother;
- psycho-somatology – restless or hyper-protective, hypohondrically - oriented mother; relatives' comorbid diseases;
- affectogenic – high emotional expression, unsteadiness of relations, parent's affective pathology;
- addictogenic– absence of primary values and traditions, upbringing in emotional denial, which leads to the lack of emotions;
- nervosity – parent's orientation to career and their hypersociality chronic fatigue, low father's status, high level of mother's mental stress, malaise, family conflicts (Zakharov 1988).

These charts can form the basis for further family dysontogenesis. Systems of upbringing which are formed into pathological constructions ("schizogenic mother," "concerned mother," etc.) and neurosogenic psychopedagocial "systems" ("idol of the family," "cinderella," etc.) can become a part of further evolution of mental illnesses. Disharmonic family mostly supposes a possible enlargement of psychovegetative diathesis (neuropathy) in a child. In the process of child's upbringing neurosogenics of the family can increase: "inadequate notion about the environment is an assimilation of a complex" (Jung 1939).

In psychiatric literature the concept of "shcizofrenogenic mother" is widely spread. According to the V. D. Mendelevich's (2014) point of view such mother assigns child's style of reality understanding or mental representation by means of inserting in his mind pathogenic formers of life logic which in future easily transform from belief to delusion under the influence of endo-, exo-, or psychogenic moments.

In Russian medicine, there is the concept of "phychic diathesis" (pre-illness) - predisposition to mental disorders. Already at this stage, the child may have symptomatology, relatively harmless in terms of psychiatric diagnosis, based on the basis of psychophysical disharmony. This may be mismatch of biological age with actual one, both at the level of systems, and in general - decoherence; irregularity of development (coexistence of mental functions attributable to different periods of development -dissynchronization) and its dissociation (elements of paradoxical ambivalence in respect to stimuli); occurrence of deficiency of mental life.

The central place in the structure of psychovegetative diathesis is taken by psychomotor and affective excitability; tearfulness; eating disorders; speech disorders; instability of vegetative functions combined with hyperesthesia and subfebrility, not associated with somatics; hypochondria; exhaustion which responds poorly to the influence of traditional sanitizing action; pronounced features of behavior retardation (timidity, fear of the new) with a loss of naturalness and ease, decrease of emotional response.

Clinical appearance of defense mechanisms of the body in this fractal takes the shape of *personality* epiphenomena affecting the source radical and modifying it in the direction of a clinically neutral status in an attempt to synchronize processes. Despite the non-specificity the majority of abnormalities of this period are among the most universal manifestations of phrenic misadaptation (Romashkevich 2005), and the blurring of the clinical picture, the body requires attention and appropriate corrective manipulations involving biological and psychological, social and spiritual and moral resources. Social and environmental factors become a stress on the nervous system of the child.

Period of early child's upbringing (up to three years) forms the basis of personality provides their relation to the world, forms readiness to overcome difficulties in further paths of enlargement, giving an opportunity for adaptation to more difficult levels of functioning. Psychological component of gestational dominant can continue influencing family's situation as a system, desynchronizing its functions and rhythms. At the same time adequate (synchronizing) socio-psychological amendments of dissipative system can potentialize the positive dynamics by normalizing the condition of children and parents.

Abnormalities of the *animogenesis* show themselves by dyschronose, deficiency and disharmony of moral feelings and intrafamilial relations. A negative attitude to a mother or ambivalent symbiotic connection with her is present, as well as the phenomenon of protodiacrisis and fear of people with the total indifference to them at the same time.

In abnormalities of communication function disorders of speech take a big place: true or pseudo mutism, elective aglossia, echolalia, speech stereotypies, neologisms, "stumblings," and disorders of "stammering" type. Contact skills are not formed and are destroyed by autistc behavior, which can be seen since the first month of life, and by the age of one year and older it becomes more evident by reaching "pseudobindless" and "pseudodeafness" degree. Henceforth moral socialization is slowing down.

In this fractal external influences can form *extra faint fluctuations* as body and family's regulation and optimization functioning so influencing them destructively that pushes the evolution of schizophrenia (patrimonial catharsis, imprinting, egalitarian family, dogmata of inadaptive social aims, etc.).

Several scenarios of schizotypic diathesis are possible. Firstly, full compensation of psychological diathesis right up to full recovery can happen. Secondly, schizoid features of different intensity from accentuation to psychopathy gradually form. Thirdly, by going through fractals and bifurcations, from symptom formation to unfolding of the clinical image of early child autism or schizophrenia.

The point of next bifurcation will be a crisis of the 7th life year, which influences all the family and is accompanied by emotional tension and high level of restlessness: parental orientation appears; the level of family claims often without regard to child's activities and interests. The crisis will be determined by a phase of dangerous decreasing of stability of a dissipative system when under the changed circumstances preformed life stereotypes can lead it to self-destruction. The scenario of crisis recovery can lead to brand-new adaptational changes which happen on higher levels. While overcoming the crisis the ontogenetic development of body systems at all levels does not lead to the emergence of functional mental disorders. Dysfunction of any of the evolutionary vectors forms a breeding ground for a variety of mental illnesses in the future. Psychovegetative diathesis caused by desynchronization influences from outside and combined with reduced resource abilities, predispones neurotic and psychosomatic disorders. It can develop on different paths (in the direction of progredient of pathology or the direction of subject's recovery), depending on the accidents near the bifurcation points and, in the worst desynchronizing influences they find themselves as a new stage in the evolution of schizophrenia.

The next is initial pathology fractal, which bears more clear marks of mental disorder, characterized by the strengthening of the influence and the increase of relevance of sociogenesis and animogenesis, which determine the compliance of human behavior with social and ethical norms. Fractal is accompanied by a reduction of degrees of freedom in self-regulating accustomization, caused by social taboos. The functioning of adaptation barriers is increasingly disrupted, due to the influence of not only biological vector but also of social disintegration of an individual that affects the state of his body. "Maladjusted personality functioning is the basis of the formation of psychopathological manifestations, typical for border forms of mental disorders" (Bazhin, Korneva 1989). Border psychic disorders are functional, representing epiphenomena – additional structures that are corrected relatively efficiently without causing deep bio and psycho and socio and mental destructions.

Incipient deformations of morale deflection become discernible in the *animogenesis*, presented by the inefficiency of endurance and patience, humanity and mercy, modesty and tact. This creates prerequisites for the possible enlargement of demoralization syndrome, the clinical picture of which is formed and added by comorbid and associated disorders in somato-, psycho- and sociogenesis.

There are negative changes in the *psychogenesis* also. Characterological changes, a tendency to obsessions and rituals, bizarre thinking, strange interests, emotional coldness (hyperesthesias-anesthetic proportion by E. Kretschmer) begin to form in person. Micro catatonic phenomena, episodes of derealization, a sense of self-alteration, confusion, anxiety, intrapsychic ataxia, formed in the result of perversion of channels of information, "abaissement du niveau mental" with their narrowness and difficulty of judgment and weakness of will, and erased forms (formes frustes) and subclinical paranoic pathognomy ("abortive debuts" (Kutsenok 1989), which during this fractal can be invisible, staying at the level of subpathalogic suspicion, distrust, pessimistic teenage skepticism with nihilistic tinge to authority and social canons, one-sided perception of reality (although the clinical polymorphism here already has a fairly distinct sound), which reduces the intensity of the incoming information flows, reducing the number of degrees of freedom for optimizing the timing self-organization of dissipative structures can occur.

Pathological inlays of this kind indicate the display contents of the attractor of *the next* fractal, to which will be attracted paths of the system, forming a more distinct clinical picture in the future. The problems of awkward age become actual that masks the true clinical content of a fractal, creating mixed subclinical phenomena, which formally are within frames of the competence of pedagogical correction, which sanative intervention often are limited to.

A frequent precursor (satellite) of this fractal are the problems of puberty and somatic pathology, indicating the activation of *somatogenesis*, which intensely connected to the functioning of the body and possibly potentiating the enlargement of schizophrenia, influencing system decoherently. Biological problems can be a trigger for further enlargement of schizophrenia, emphasizing the relevance of this trend in the correction of the patient's status. "Neurosis never crosses a dangerous line, but then suddenly it happens that the patient steps over it and obviously turns into a real psychotic" (Jung 1939). Somatic and pseudo somatic complaints step forward, masking mental deviations (Sukiasyan 1996). The main feature of these conditions is that they stem from mental disturbance, leaving the true nature of the problems not identified. Polymorphism of embodied sensations, lack of parallel between subjective and objective clinical images, mismatch of the innervation to complaints, a nosological uncertainty of pathognomy can describe the true content of these problems (Sukiasyan et al. 2001).

This fractal from the position of synergetics can be considered as premorbid of schizophrenia. Further nonlinear enlargement paths of mental illnesses can continue in the next fractal, which defines the shapes and types of the course of schizophrenia, its outcome, where steady psychobiological changes are formed, growing social misadaptation and deformation of a moral portrait.

Future events in a synergistic model of schizophrenia and new scenarios of enlargement fall on prepared by the previous fractals ground, schizogenic basis, which includes: pathobiological matrix, individual subject's psychological characteristics, adverse social circumstances and a reduction of morale in their inharmonious, destructive, decoherent interaction. It is not improbable that versions of the accents of proportions of these four vectors determine forms of schizophrenia. Biological trend will predispose the enlargement of malignant variants of schizophrenia, schizophrenia tardae, and catatonic and hypertoxic schizophrenia. Psychological - the formation of a moderately progredient types of current schizophrenia. Social trend will predispose the enlargement of the recurrent type of schizophrenia. And animogenic - of defensive-continuous sluggish schizophrenia.

The next *fractal is clinical*. In the *psychogenesis* radical changes are happening. The disease has posted, after passing bifurcation of "crystallization of delusion", the precipitation of symptomatics. "Instead of a puzzled look comes alert one, staying on the details, trying to understand their special meaning" (Jung 1939). At first psychopathology refers itself as paranoic; then unsystematized paranoic pathognomy ("indicators of schizophrenic mental illness" (Maher 1983) - neologisms, mentizm, sperrungs, symptoms of the I-st rank by K. Schneider). Characteristics of mental decay processes, dissociation of the personality-motivational and operational and procedural areas of thinking (tangentiality, schematism, symbolism, paralogism, diversity with the actualization of latent attributes of subjects and objects) are seen. This is the Manifesto of schizophrenia, which can hardly be called debut: visiting a doctor is often delayed; in addition, it is incorrect to call a "debut" a process that began earlier, as was indicated by the symptoms-"lightning" (which took place during the previous fractals), foreboding a negative (or questionable) clinical perspectives.

The *somatogenesis* is also undergoing noticeable changes. Metabolic abnormalities, the frequency of which, according to CATIE, is 40%, indicates a link between metabolic abnormalities and the leading cause of deaths in patients with schizophrenia (pathology of the cardiovascular sphere becomes the cause of death in 6-7 pathologies, pathology of the respiratory system is 2-6 times more frequently than in the General population; high death-rate in connection with consequences of obesity, diabetes, infectious pathology (Harris, Barraclough 1998). Oncopathology is also on the list of causes of schizophrenes' deaths (Burlakov 2006, 2007). K. Jaspers (1997) identified a group of symptoms that are the source of psychopathology or are in a certain connection with it. In schizophrenes he identified the following somatic symptoms: changes in the pupils, edemata, cyanosis of hands and feet, increased transpiration with odor, seborrheic dermatitis on the face, pigmentation, trophic abnormalities, and weight changes. Menstrual irregularities are observed in 60% of patients with schizophrenia paranoica and in 93% of patients with catatonic schizophrenia.

The sociogenesis and *the animogenesis* are largely determined by the narrowing and loss of social contacts due to the increasing negative pathognamy: autisation, apathy, abulia, and also peculiarities of subject's delusional structures. Possible invalidization also limits social potency of the subject. The transformation of the ethics of social communication in the style of minimalism defines the social status of the subject, limiting the degrees of freedom of its dissipative system, losing opportunities for optimal self-organization.

In the *animogenesis***,** destruction of the moral, spiritual position distinctly appears: ability to distinguish between good and evil reduces, as well as tolerance to ethico-psychological stresses; signs of destructive professiogenesis appear.

Fractals of chronization and outcome of schizophrenia in the sphere of the *psychogenesis* are accompanied by respectively paraphrenic and apathoabulic pathognomy, interweaving with each other in various proportions; considered to be low curable conditions. Emotional emasculation, apathy, abulia, autism severely limit the number of degrees of freedom for dissipative structures. At these stages productive pathognomy of schizophrenia fades, giving way to the negative pathognomy, indicating the extinction of DSSH's energetics, its involution and entropy, which was reflected in the definition of K. Conrad "reduction of energy potential." The energy potential of schizophrenia has exhausted, its dissipative structure ceases its further enlargement.

The biogenesis develops in the direction determined in the previous fractal in the algorithm of comorbid pathology.

The sociogenesis is determined by the intensity of subject's negative symptoms and social losses.

The animogenesis appears as a result of demoralization syndrome with different forms of immoral and offending behavior.

Consequently, the synergetic methodology of mental medicine allows registering all inner and outer factors of pathoplastics and pathokinesis of schizophrenia systematically, giving an opportunity to prove and arrange compositely individual preventive-correctional and treatment and rehabilitation ways within the multi-disciplinary program.

23.4. Medico-Psychosociospiritual Care

Within the framework of the synergetic methodology of mental medicine we have developed preventive, corrective treatment and rehabilitation routes in case of schizophrenia (Table 23.4), which compose a single multidisciplinary protocol implemented by a team consisting of a psychiatrist, psychotherapist, clinical psychologist, specialists in social work and bioethics.

During the *predisposition* and *latent* fractals, the priority is to optimize sanitation of all vectors, but with different emphases depending on their phenomenological content. Correction and synchronization of systems activity "the pregnant and the fetus", "the mother and the child", "the mother and the father and the child", which significantly predetermine the formation and development of the moral feelings and in the general adaptability of moral socialization is of great importance.

Biological causes and characteristics of a family bringing up a child with emotional disorder state the relevance of ethical and psychological and psychiatric sanitation interventions, which micro psychiatry can carry out. Micro psychiatry is an area of medicine that studies the psychology and psychiatry of children of early age through the prism of dyads "the pregnant and the fetus", "the mother and the child" and the triad of "the mother and the father and the child."

In the given fractal, priority to the ethical-psychological trend may be given. A more effective correction can be done if parallel socio-psychological (and possibly biological) sanitation of all family members is conducted. Harmonizing (synchronizing) influence of social trend should also be considered and used: the relationship of these vectors is obvious. Adequate preventive effects on the body and family in the period before the next regular bifurcation could become an argument and a tool which allows changing (mitigating) of the further enlargement of schizophrenia. "Personal beddings" can neutralize biologically-determined pathogenic trends of the forming disease process, can be equal to the last by the force and are themselves have deeply founded representation in a biological substrate. However, desynchronizing influences on the subject in all components of a single biopsychosocial field are capable of changing its further development destructively, creating conditions for the evolution of schizophrenia. It is appropriate to recall M. Klein's concept (1928), who considered that a child of the first year of life passes through the oral phase, marked by two phases: depressive and paranoid-schizoid, because for him such an object, as the mother's breast, can be "good" - satisfying feeding, and "evil" - unsatisfactory, denoting, therefore, the conceptual splitting (schisis)of phren and matrix of pathology of affect in any child, which is partly confirmed by M. Mahler's researches (1975), who concluded that the behavior of children with infantile autism is a continuation of early childhood, and between the baby and child-psychotic there is a fundamental similarity: the first has not achieved what has not achieved a second - I-identity.

Table 23.4. Program of medico-psychosociospiritual care in schizophrenia

Blocks	Prenosological fractals			Nosological fractals		
	Predisposition	Latent	Initial	Clinical: mental epidemic	Chronization: destructive mental epidemic	Outcome: pandemic
Medical	Dysontogenesis prevention and correction (genetic counseling, women's health clinics, perinatal centers of fetal and neonatal medicine service, prevention of accidental pregnancy, perinatology demedicamentation	Pediatric service optimization (neonatal centers, breastfeeding, vaccine prophylaxis)	Medication-assisted treatment of psychosomatic direction (children's clinics and hospitals, psychosomatic departments)	Psycho-pharmaco-therapy, chronization prevention (various methods of biological therapy in psychiatric centers)	Psychotropic therapy, resistance and complications overcoming (biological therapy)	Psychotropic and metabolic therapy (biological therapy)
Psychological	Harmonisation of resonance relations in a dyad "mother-child" (perinatal psychotherapy)	Psychological correction of family relations (all kinds of family psycho-correction and psycho-prophylaxis)	Psychological correction and psychotherapy (psycho-educational and developing personal growth of the technique, psychological testing, psychotherapy, physical therapy rooms in children's clinics)	Psychotherapy (a wide range of psycho-techniques - from Gestalt therapy- to autogenic training)	Psychotherapy, psychological adaptation (psycho-educational modules for schizophrenic patients, the use of the available psycho-techiques)	Psychological correction of initial states (psycho-educational modules for patients with schizophrenia, available psychotherapy modules)
Social	Formation of the parental relationship before the child is born: social education programs, social support in accessible formats	Adaptive socialization of the child and his family; educational child care centres and development programs	Social microenvironment correction, integration of the subject into society: educational institutions and programs, clubs, classes, movements	Social rehabilitation: medical therapy, occupancy therapy, creative expression therapy	Social support and reintegration into society; social programs for patients dehospitalization, psycho-educational modules for their relatives, work therapy	Rehabilitation of the disabled: psycho-educational modules for relatives and patients, work therapy
Spiritual and moral	Screening and correction of "morale climate" of the family	Correction of the formation and development of moral feelings	Correction of the formation and development of moral character	Reconstruction of moral position	Reconstruction of moral behavior	Spiritual and moral rehabilitation

According to the concept of synergetics it is obvious that in the *initial fractal of pathology* a corrective influence as on surrounding society – upon 4 blocks so on the body will be current. It's not necessary to talk about finally formed schizophrenia, but the correction with biological drugs, including of psychotropic (not neuroleptic) register, in some cases seems appropriate inclusive of given subpatolothical symptoms. Resonant-coherent fluctuations and algorithms for the enlargement of schizophrenia has led to certain changes in the body, leading to a further operation of this system in the direction of the likelihood of further formation of mental illness, an actualizing algorithm of progression.

The synchronization of efforts has a particular importance, giving a synergetic effect on all the four blocks because new ethical and social, psychological and biological conditions become a significant stress factor. Among new conditions, we can distinguish load, related to requirements of society to learning; the social activity of a teenager or a young person who enters his individual life; his communication ethics and a large-scale restructuring of the functioning of biological systems of the body. These conditions require the body's large-scale self-regulatory changes, the maximum facilities and are accompanied by non-obvious in their potential result fluctuations.

In *the clinical fractal*, primary biological correction of the trend becomes obvious and urgent. But the traditional priority given to psychopharmacology, should not exclude correction effects on other trends which shape schizophrenia: "Its symptomatology indicates, on the one hand, on the underlying destructive process, possibly of toxic rock, and on the other hand – to the extent that psychogenic etiology is not excluded, and psychological treatment (where relevant) is effective, - with an equal degree of importance on the mental factor" (Jung 2000).

In recent years, this problem is paid more attention, but with a glance to traditional psychiatric paternalism and well-known rigidity of thinking supporters of clinical dogmata, social, mental and moral and spiritual trends are developing relatively slowly and not always in the right direction, becoming servile, optional to biological trend; whereas they should be of the same great importance in the correction of schizophrenia – indirectly through the society and the body. Traditionally, psychotherapy is considered to play a great supporting role in psychiatry. Hence the attitude to non-biological areas of patient's status correction, which transforms the social and psychological effect on him, and the more moral-sensitive, in a completely formalized "the event."

The polymodal set of possible remedial actions is often reduced to the monopoly of the biological trend. Work with family and closest environment rarely takes place, leaving his functioning at the same level. The released patient returns to his previous socio-psychological conditions and dives into the same spiritual and moral climate that once already had become one of the causes of his mental disorder. In some cases clinical psychologists and social workers are involved to conduct such patients (routine diagnostic tests not taken in consideration) without significantly affecting the situation. Four vectors of schizophrenia continue to function destructively, asynchronizing dissipative structure and exacerbating mental disorders, but only one of them is exposed to attempts of correcting. This fractal often becomes a long and stable stage in the course of schizophrenia, ending its further evolution, indicating preservation of mental disorders by a biological trend - even in the absence of serious corrective intervention of psychological, spiritual, moral and social vectors of a single dissipative structure.

The main method of schizophrenia therapy is the use of antipsychotic drugs (neuroleptics), affecting the so-called "productive" symptoms of psychosis and preventing its further enlargement, the impact of which is primarily due to the suppression of dopamine activity, in spite of their significant side effects.

At present, atypical antipsychotic drugs are the first-line treatment for schizophrenic patients. This is due to the fact that they affect a wide range of symptoms of the disease, including the effect on the positive and the negative symptoms, cognitive process disorders, fluctuations of mood, and level of aggression (Mosolov 2004; Mazaeva 2006; Ovsyannikov, Balanina 2010). The patients show a higher tolerance to the new atypical antipsychotic drugs, because the conventional neuroleptics (perphenazine, fluphenazine hydrochloride and haloperidol) have apparent neurologic and other adverse effects. They have a particularly negative effect on memory, attention and thinking.

The choice of antipsychotic drug depends on the severity of the condition, duration of illness, stage of therapy (acute episode, stabilization phase, maintenance, and phylactic therapy), structer and evidences of syndromes of schizophrenia, patient's personality trait.

Ratio of the first two parameters has a great importance while choosing a neuroleptic drug and determining its spectrum of psychotropic activity, i.e., the global antipsychotic and primary sedative effects. They are the basis for modern clinical classification of antipsychotics.

Modern antipsychotic drugs have the following effects: the antipsychotic effect, capable of removing various manifestations of psychosis; primary sedative (inhibitory) effect; selective effect, aimed at particular symptoms (delusion, hallucinations, thinking and behavioral disorders); activating effect, aimed at the negative symptomatology; cognitive effect, which helps to improve thinking, memory and attention.

Individual choice of antipsychotic and selection of effective dose depend on many factors, and primo on the tasks of therapy (relief of activation or aggression, reduction of hallucinatory-delusional symptoms, correction of abnormalities of behavior or diminished evidences, backset prevention and containment of the rate of progredient of a disease, improvement of patients' self-management and the creation of optimal conditions for conducting psychotherapy and socio-rehabilitation events) that are closely connected with the clinical features of the disease (clinical form of the disease, the type of flow, leading syndrome and its shades, the predominant symptoms).

Antipsychotic rescue and stabilizing antipsychotic therapy can be used when conducting antipsychotic therapy in schizophrenia patients in this fractal of disease.

Antipsychotic drugs rescue therapy. Therapy is focused on rapid rescue of psychotic patognamy (psychomotor agitation, aggressiveness, negativism, hallucinatory-delusional experiences and catatonic-hebephrenic disorders). It starts from the beginning moment of assault and ends with the establishment of clinical remission, i.e., substantial or complete reduction of psychosis. With adequate neuroleptic treatment its duration may range from 4 to 12 weeks (6-8 weeks are often required to reach full therapeutic condition monitoring).

In the acute phase it is better to consider monotherapy with one of the atypical antipsychotic drugs (risperidone, olanzapine, amisulpride); and the use of first aid neuroleptics (haloperidol, sultopride, zuclopentixol–acetate) should be limited by symptomatic tasks and minimum terms. Psychomotor agitation and severe affective-psychotic symptomatics usually go away in the first days of adequate antipsychotic therapy. Steady antipsychotic effect usually develops not earlier than through 3-6 weeks of treatment.

Stabilizing antipsychotic drug therapy. After stabilization of state, it is better to proceed to continue receiving of effective neuroleptic after reaching clinical (therapeutic) remission to the alleged spontaneous end of attack. The length of this treatment is from 3 to 9 months. Activities here should be directed to the suppression of residual positive symptoms, the gradual decreasing of the sedative effects and increase of the stimulatory effects of neuroleptics, the correction of deficit symptoms and restoration of the previous level of social and labor adaptation and the fight against pre-relapsed or early relapsing disorders.

With the prevalence of disorders in the negative status, special attention should be paid to the correction of deficit symptoms, with a reduction of which the restoration of the previous level of psychological, social and labor adaptation is associated. For correction of deficit symptoms drugs with activating and anti-autistic direction of action, i.e. disabscopal (sulpiride, carbidine) or atypical (risperidone, olanzapine, quetiapine or amisulpride) antipsychotics are being used.

In the case of therapy of negative disorders, it is important to distinguish primary (diminished) deficit symptoms associated with the passage of the schizophrenic process itself, and secondary, which was injected in the picture of disease by other different factors, such as depression, parkinsonism, productive (hallucinatory-delusional) disorders, or phenomena of hospitalism. Unlike secondary deficit symptoms modern pharmacotherapeutic possibilities of correction of the defect (of primary deficit symptoms and neurocognitive deficits) are represented much more limited and methodologically difficult to be proved correct. The only drug in respect of which there are such evidence, is amisulpride (soliane).

In recent years, especially due to the emergence of a new generation of antipsychotics, the possibility of pharmacological correction of neurocognitive deficit is also widely discussed in literature. Cognitive deficit is closely connected with the intensity of deficit symptoms and is part of the cruder psycho-organic defect.

It is known that 40-60% of patients with schizophrenia with a relapsing course in the case of a therapy interruption the recrudescence of insanity develops within the first six months. In patients with chronic schizophrenia the risk of relapse in the case of placebo is 10% per month, and in the case of anxiolytic medication - 1%.

The most suitable patients to use the atypical antipsychotics during all stages of treatment are newly diagnosed patients with schizophrenia (first episode psychosis).

Psychotherapy is also widely recommended and used in schizophrenia, although sometimes treatment options are limited by pharmacology because of problems with funding or inadequate staff training. In addition to treating the disease, it is also focused on social and professional rehabilitation of patients. Family and cognitive-behavioral psychotherapy are used.

Reconstruction of a moral position and behavior within the generated syndrome of demoralization requires the use of training resources of ethics in business communication, coaching and expressive therapy, spiritual and religious practices, which are especially effective in a case of defensive slow progressive schizophrenia.

In the fractal of chronization, the traditional correction of patients with paraphrenic and apathy abulia symptoms is reduced to a standard biological component ("maintenance therapy"). It happens despite the fact that numerous psychological and social programs allow affecting the quality and the content of patients' lives while changing the fluctuation of this dissipative structure. The difference of methodological approaches and semiotic nuances in different areas of science and practices at this stage raise up the highest interdisciplinary barrier between diverse specialists influencing the succession (the term itself implies some event relay when, as the implementation of narrow-profile problems, a patient is transferred from one specialist to another.

Mental medicine involves synchronous-integral correction of mental illness that combines a complex of effects that are not isolated from each other. Habitually traditional causal determinism, which builds a fatal construction of unfavorable clinical prognosis and is looking at complementary perspectives in relation to biological trend with a pessimistic skepticism, influences the situation essentially and negatively. If the implementation of non-biologists specialists in the patient's fate in a different semiotic system occurs, carrying almost optional character, it reduces the possibilities of a potentially achievable result.

Anti-relapse (maintenance) antipsychotic therapy will be demanded in this fractal. It is focused on prevention of the enlargement of new attacks and the slowing-down of the progredient rate of the disease. Anti-relapsing therapy is held indefinitely but not less than 1-2 years to assess its effectiveness. Thereat the dose of the antipsychotic is decreased to 20-30% of maximum in case of the acute episode.

Modern international standards of therapy recommended conducting continuous antipsychotic therapy within two years after the first episode, at least five years after the second and indefinitely long period (in most cases for life) after the third attack of schizophrenia. In the case of termination of treatment, relapse develops in 75% of patients within 1-2 years. The main indications for such therapy are paroxysmal and continuous forms of schizophrenia and firstly – paranoid. The use of prolonged forms of neuroleptics, which in recent years has received the greatest distribution, essentially facilitates the implementation of long-outpatient therapy. The modern alternative to prolonged neuroleptic during the prolonged anti-relapse therapy is the use of atypical antipsychotics. The number of exacerbations in the first and the second year of therapy with the use of atypical drugs is reduced by almost 2 times compared with patients who took out-patiently various traditional antipsychotics.

Other methods of schizophrenia treatment include electroconvulsive therapy (ECT) and insulin shock therapy. ECT is not considered when making the initial choice of therapy strategy, but may be prescribed if other methods fail. It is more effective if catatonia symptoms are present (Mashour et al. 2005). Insulin shock therapy was used for schizophrenia treatment in the West since its inception in the 30-ies years of the XX-th century and till the 50-ies when it was recognized that there is no evidence of its effectiveness.

The movements, organized by 'the clients of mental health services', have become an integral part of the recovery process in Europe and America; such groups as Hearing Voices Network and Paranoia Network have developed self-help techniques, aimed at providing support and assistance outside the traditional medical model adopted by most psychiatrists. Avoiding consideration of personal experience in terms of mental illness or mental health, they aim to destigmatize these experiences and inspire the person to take personal responsibility and choose a positive self-image. Increasingly partnerships are established between hospitals and patients ' communities, while doctors help return people to the society, develop their social skills and reduce the frequency of re-admissions (Goering et al. 2006).

Main directions of psychosocial and mental-spiritual care in schizophrenia are: individual compliance - therapy aimed at establishing optimum contact between the doctor and his patient; individual and group cognitive – behavioral therapy; education in the field of psychiatry and psychology (individual, group and family); vocational rehabilitation (individual and group); training of ethics in business communication and social skills (group therapy); cognitive rehabilitation (cognitive remediation) in individual and group forms; family therapy; therapeutic management in individual and group form. All of these forms and methods of work are important for the socio-psychological and moral and spiritual rehabilitation which is aiming at correction of pessimistic-catastrophic attitudes and maintenance of an optimistic- resource view of life.

Thus, *schizophrenia can be defined as a polymorphic resonant coherent mental illness.* Biological confirmations of the appropriateness of such a definition are studies of NMDA-receptors which are involved in many important brain processes. They modulate the production of dopamine by neurons of the ventral cortex, modulate low-frequency oscillations of the brain by inhibitory interneurons of the thalamus, and modulate neurons of the hippocampus and prefrontal cortex processes of neuroplasticity and memory (Zhang et al. 2009; Hillman et al. 2011; Goff 2013).

Synergetic terminology is not just a mechanical substitute for the textbook clinical categories (in particular, autism as a resonant disorder or defense mechanism and schisis as a coherent disorder), but discovers a fundamentally new conceptual and methodological resources which allow combining different trends in their not arithmetic, but integrative interaction.

The concept of synergetics allows to explain the recurrent form of schizophrenia and "to break" effect of shock techniques in the course of this mental illness: through the chaos of the disorder adapting self-organizing of dissipative systems is realized, which reaches order through simulated with external circumstances fluctuations. Adequate complex correction prevents further progredient movement of schizophrenia, refuting its fatalistic determinism, assigning the subject's body adaptive level of functioning.

In the current system of interpretation of schizophrenia, it is unclear why there may be a spontaneous improvement in schizophrenic patients (preagonal remissions; remission caused by somatic pathology). The concept of synergetics implies that a significant change in the biological vector in a schizophrene changes the path of the enlargement of mental illness by redirecting the emphasis of priorities and turning the patient to another level (in another fractal) of the functioning of the psyche, while his body is developing in the algorithm of comorbid pathology. H. Baruk's concept (1920) receives confirmation about the somatopsychic balancing, which is explained by the energy deficit of bimodal chart of psyche-somatic. G. Nazloyan's results, who dealt with patients which were deemed uncurable, become understandable. Updating of adequate corrective influence on the part of socio-psychological and moral and spiritual vectors of multimodal scheme for the patient, including additional resonances in his dissipative system, becomes an effective remedy which allows in combination with action of biological vector to optimize body function, successfully opposing progression of schizophrenia.

"To make the correct diagnosis and to stop in confusion before a poor prognosis is not a too significant contribution to the art of medicine" (Jung 1939). Psychiatry deals with the whole man and must take into account all confounding factors that may participate in the formation of mental illnesses. Mental medicine is more consistent with precisely integrative, holistic understanding of mental illnesses, armed with a methodology of synergetics, revealing the regularities of enlargement of mental illnesses with new perspective, taking into account the interaction of vectors anima-, socio-, psycho - and biogenesis, giving the rationale for multidisciplinary trends in psychological prevention and correction of schizophrenia, defining new technological tools for adaptive bio-, psycho-, socio- and spiritual management of developmental pathways of schizophrenia.

On the basis of a multi-disciplinary methodology, synergetics allows separating priority directions of preventive work of professionals (doctors, psychologists, speech-language pathologists, specialists in social work and bioethics, teachers, etc.) in all fractals of schizophrenia enlargement, by developing for patients, appropriate preventive-corrective and treatment and rehabilitation routes, which include integrative functioning methods and programs.

Synergetics is a constructive basis, which does not contradict current diagnostic criteria and therapy of mental illness, which can be overlapped by any clinical data which extend the level of comprehension of the essence of mental illnesses, which adopt as the development of psychopharmacology and techniques of examination, socio and psychological, moral and spiritual diagnosis and correction. The development of prenosological categories in psychiatry reduces diagnostic and prognostic uncertainty in schizophrenia.

Thus, medico-psychosociospiritual care for schizophrenic patients within synergetic methodology of mental medicine can significantly improve the effectiveness of the preventive-corrective and treatment and rehabilitation programs, and also activate the work in the prenosological area.

Chapter 24

Depressive Disorders

Depressive disorder is characterized by a low mood together with a pessimistic evaluation of the situation, reality and self-evaluation, intellectual and psychomotor retardation, lack of impulses and somatovegetative disorders.

24.1. Prevalence of Depressive Disorders

According to the WHO data depressive disorders (DD) are one of the most common psychopathologic disorders among mental illnesses. The number of people suffering from this illness is steadily increasing. Nearly 350 million people around the world experience depression according to epidemiological studies and the WHO data. The probability of unipolar depression development during a person's life is about 20%. Nearly 100 million people in the world report depressive symptoms annually (Krasnov 2014).

In primary care settings depression is the most commonly diagnosed mental illness among patients (Topchy 2005). According to clinical and epidemiological researches in general medical practice, depression is diagnosed in 20-40% of patients (Kornetov et al. 2010; Smulevich et al. 2014; Ilic 2011).

Accompanying DDs negatively influence the course and prognosis of somatic diseases. In general medical practice diagnosing of affective disorders is often a difficult task because the clinical picture can be abnormal and depression symptoms are sometimes "wrong" manifested as somatic pathology. Thereby many patients are not supervised by psychiatrists for a long time and thus, do not receive qualified medical care.

Women suffer from depression about twice as often (5,5%) as men (3,2%) (Ferrany et al. 2013). The risk of depression progression during a woman's life is 20% and 10% for men. Depression may occur at any age. However, 50% of patients have their first episodes of depressive disorders at the age from 20 to 50 years, thus the average age being 40 years (Yastrebov 2014). According to the WHO prognosis, depressions can occupy top positions among diseases interfering with the ability to work by 2020, and will be the first disease among most costly ones by 2030.

24.2. Etiopathogenesis of Depressive Disorders

Up to the present times, depression etiology is understudied similar to the majority of mental illnesses. However, it is possible to single out some risk factors causing depressive disorders:

- genetic factors presuppose the presence of emotional disorders in family anamnesis (the type of inheritance is unknown), lack of neurotransmitters in the brain (it concerns mainly noradrenaline and/or serotonin);
- psychosocial factors include psycho-traumatic situations, information overlearning, unfavorable family relationship, unsatisfactory living conditions, etc.);
- constitutive-psychological factors combined with personal development peculiarities.

Constitutive-psychological factors include the following aspects: gender (women suffer from depressions about twice as often as men); middle and elderly age; ectomorphy; alcohol and other psychoactive substance abuse; medications taking (amphetamines, other CNS stimulant, barbiturates, benzodiazepines, cimetidine, clonidine, β-adrenergic blocking agents, corticosteroids, indomethacin, methyldopa, oral contraceptives, estrogens, reserpine, guanethidine, sulfanilamide, interferon); pregnancy and delivery; perinatal infections; loss of mother in childhood (under 11 years); melancholic persons (pedantry, rigidity, desire to reach maximum result in everything, monotonous sthenicity, pettiness, inclination to hesitations and doubts).

The following diseases are considered to be connected with depressions (Topchy 2005; Ilic 2011): rheumatic (systemic lupus erythematosus, rheumatoid arthritis); cardiovascular (coronary artery disease, myocardial infarction, arterial hypertension); endocrine (hypo- and hyperthyroidism, diabetes, hypercalcemia, Cushing syndrome, postpartum disorders); gastrointestinal (liver cirrhosis, colitis, pancreatitis, diseases of the biliary passages); hematologic (sickle cell anemia); nutritional disorder (lack of Vitamin B12, folates, iron, thiamine, nicotinic acid); infections (encephalitis, hepatitis, influenza, infectious mononucleosis, pneumonia, tuberculosis); kidney diseases (uremia, kidney transplantation); tumors (leukemia, lymphoma, pancreatic cancer, intracranial tumor); nervous system diseases (subdural hemorrhage, multiple sclerosis, Parkinson's disease, uncontrolled epilepsy); psoriasis; sarcoidosis.

24.3. Synergetics of Depressive Disorders

Synergetic model of DD development is represented in Table 24.1.

Anhedonic family fractal is considered to be a primary one when DD is developing. It is a well-known fact that poor family relationship can trigger this pathology development. Such families are characterized by pessimistic views of life, loss of happiness and pleasure both in the context of the world around and interfamily relationship. In such a family a child's developing social behavior and response models lose their effective adaptation. Early and persistent "emotional depression" creates a foundation for an anhedonic core of a personality being formed.

Table 24.1. Fractal dynamics of the epidemic development of depressive disorders

Ontogenesis vector	Prenosological fractals			Nosological fractals		
	Predisposition: anhedonic family	Latent: anhedonic diathesis	Initial: primary asthenic-depressive neurosis	Full-scale clinical picture/mental epidemic	Chronization: Different types and forms of the disease/destructive mental epidemic	Outcome: somatopsychic complications of DD/pandemic
Somatogenesis	Hereditary burden	Violation of neuro-processes	Somatoform disorders	Depressive disorder	Forms and types of depressive disorder	Somatopsychic violation
Psychogenesis	Anhedonic family	Premorbid personality traits	Asthenic-depressive neuroticism of personality	Personality decompensation	Dependent personality disorder	Personal defect
Sociogenesis	Emotional-deprivation family relationships	Affect-genetic disharmony of personality socialization	Violations of meaningful social relationships	Transient social dysfunction	Social decompensation	Social disadaptation
Animogenesis	Spiritual and moral deficits of family	Disharmony of moral sentiments formation	Deformation of moral character	Destruction of the spiritual and moral position	Probability of immoral acts	Probability of illegal behavior

Current notions about neurotic depression etiopathogenesis point out significant role of troubles in relationships that are important to a person (Karvasarsky et al. 2012). Thus, a family is a direct source of mental health (Zakharov 2006). There is a real connection between dissatisfaction, tension and conflicts in the family on the one part and various neuropsychic disorders in children on the other part.

As a psychogenic disease in a forming personality astheno depressive neuroticization reflects many problems in human relations. First of all, these problems concern people's mutual understanding and communication, discovering one's own "Ego," optimal ways of self-actualization, self-affirmation, acceptance and love.

According to psychoanalytic tradition, poor emotional relations between a growing child and his/her parents play the leading role in neurosis development. Neurosis progression in children commonly occurs in families with obvious relationship asymmetry between parents, both parents' low self-respect, a wife's emotional reprobation of a dependent husband, love overestimation accompanied by sexual relations underestimation, both parents' emotional dependence on their mothers while a father's personality is poorly appreciated.

Neurosogenic and anhedonic family, in particular, is characterized by disharmonic family education as a result of parents' neuroticism (Schyogolev 2008). Defective interpersonal relations system, prevalence of negative values, dissocial attitudes, etc. are also peculiar to a neurosogenic family.

Thus, an anhedonic family as a type of a neurosogenic family is characterized by moral and spiritual deficiency, disharmonic family education as a result of unfavorable personality qualities of parents. All of this becomes apparent in emotional deprivation of a child and neurotization.

The next fractal is *anhedonic diathesis*. Diathesis (from Greek "diathesis" in the meaning of "inclination") is a constitutional organism susceptibility to a particular disease due to peculiarities of inborn metabolism, physiological reactions, etc.

Anhedonic diathesis is manifested by multiple-factor inherited and constitutional susceptibility to both mental (affective predominantly) and functional somatovegetative disorders. Moreover, regulatory disorders connected with emotional sphere are likely to be accompanied by constitutional (inborn) anomalies in organs. People with weak or unbalanced nervous system, high anxiety level, psychasthenic and astheno-depressive character accentuations are susceptible to anhedonic diathesis.

Anhedonic diathesis is represented by disharmony and monotony in basic moral senses formation and development, which can be further obvious in moral socialization and personality development disturbances with deficient adaptive potential.

A person with anhedonic diathesis can suffer from *primary astheno-depressive neurosis* under the influence of stressors.

Primary neurosis manifests in somatovegetative disorders and patient's complaints about somatic symptoms including headaches, heartache, tachycardia, high arterial blood pressure, changes in respiratory frequency and depth, abrupt muscular weakness, etc. Such conditions are short-term and not severe. Also, personality neurotization occurs, which can declare itself in the form of non-specific astheno depressive, disturbing and neurotic symptoms.

Primary astheno-depressive neurosis in animogenesis manifests as multivariate and personality dependent deformation of morale, which triggers further development of demoralization syndrome and destructive professiogenesis, the clinical picture of which is formed and supplemented with comorbid and associative disorders in somato-, psycho- and sociogenesis in every particular case.

Further mental traumatization presupposes transformation of somatovegetative disorders into *depressive disorder*. Such disorders are more persistent and are accompanied by repeated, multiple and clinically significant complaints. The clinical picture in a typical case is characterized by the main symptoms manifestation such as complete loss of interest, satisfaction and pleasure in any activity, appetite and sleep disorders, loss of strength, weakening of attentiveness and sexual dysfunction, inferiority and feeling guilt, recurrent thoughts of death and suicide.

Depression full-scale clinical picture in animogenesis declares itself in the destruction of a person's moral and spiritual position, which "breaks" and loses its emotional and energetic potential together with the ability to resist and struggle.

Forms and types of depressive disorder course must be considered within chronization fractal. The more likely depressive disorder can declare itself in such forms as disturbed, asthenic, apathetic, somatized one and others. A severe personal disorder, social, moral and spiritual compensation failure, which manifests in immoral behavior, occurs within this very fractal.

Further transition into chronic and irreversible *somatopsychic complications* is possible, which can impair a patient's ability to function at work.

Demoralization syndrome manifestations are increasing in animogenesis together with the risk of illegal behavior.

Thus, the synergetic methodology of mental medicine makes it possible to take into consideration all the internal and external factors of depression pathoplastics and pathokinetics, and fully organize individual preventive, correctional, treatment and rehabilitation measures in the framework of a multidisciplinary program.

24.4. Medico-Psychosociospiritual Care

We developed the multidisciplinary program of care for patients on the basis of the synergetic methodology of mental medicine. In consists of the following four units: medical, psychological, social, moral and spiritual (Table 24.2). Preventive and correction measures are realized within the framework of the first three prenosological fractals, while treatment and rehabilitation measures are undertaken within the next three nosological fractals. Together they constitute a multidisciplinary protocol carried out by a professional team including a psychiatrist, a psychotherapist, a clinical psychologist, specialists in the sphere of social work and bioethics.

Within the framework of somatogenesis, the *medical block* includes care by general practitioners, therapists or psychiatrists. Within the framework of psychogenesis, the *psychological block* presupposes involvement of specialists dealing with mental health such as psychotherapists, clinical psychologists, and psychiatrists. *Social care* is provided within the framework of sociogenesis when the involvement of social services specialists takes place (specialists in the sphere of social work, community workers).

Table 24.2. Program of medico-psychosociospiritual care for patients with depressive disorders

Blocks	Prenosological fractals			Nosological fractals		
	Predisposition: anhedonic family	Latent: anhedonic diathesis	Initial: primary asthenic-depressive neurosis	Full-scale clinical picture of the DD/ mental epidemic	Chronization: forms and types of DD course/destructive mental epidemic	Outcome: DD complications /pandemic
Medical	Inclusion of individuals with hereditary predisposition to neurosis into risk group and early screening	Identification of individuals with weak and unstable types of nervous system	Diagnosis of neurosis; medication-assisted and drug-free therapy	Establishing of clinical diagnosis of somatoform disorder, medication-assisted therapy,, prevention of complications	Control over the somatic condition; adequate drug therapy	Treatment of somatic and psychic complications of somatoform disorder
Psychological	Detection of persons, who are brought up in a neurosis-genetic family and their incorporation into the risk group	Correction of premorbid personality characteristics (accentuations), increase of resistance to stress	Detection of the dependent personality out of personality disorder and disorders correction	Disorders correction, psychotherapy, psycho-pharmacotherapy	Psychosomatic disorders correction, psychotherapy, psycho-pharmacotherapy	Psychological adjustment
Social	Disorders identification and correction of the structure and functions of the family	Correction of individual socialization disorders	Correction of non-pathological addictive behavior	Adapting to the disease, correction of interpersonal problems	Professional and family adaptation	Social rehabilitation
Spiritual and moral	Screening and correction of "morale climate" of the family	Correction of the formation and development of moral sentiments	Correction of the formation and development of moral character	Reconstruction of moral position	Reconstruction of moral behavior	Spiritual and moral rehabilitation

The moral and spiritual block in the framework of animogenesis is carried out with the help of family and relatives in micro social and work environment with the use of modern methods and forms of education and upbringing, coaching and ethical training. This unit also requires the involvement of experts and consultants of mental health services and ethical committees, especially when there is a threat of destructive professiogenesis occurrence (mobbing, conflicts etc.), which requires mediation measures implementation. Moreover, this unit realization requires involvement of spiritual advisers from official confessions while relatives and people suffering from depression are also taking part in public organizations' programs, as well as volunteer and social movements are. Participation of ethical-social services of veterans and labor union organizations is also required.

Primary preventive measures should be already carried out within the *predisposition fractal (anhedonic family)*, where they can be aimed at detection of inherited and psychophysiological susceptibility and at ethical psychological harmonization of family relationship.

Within the *latent fractal,* measures are aimed at detection of persons subject to depressive disorders progression (people with weak and unstable nervous system, high level of anxiety; psychoasthenic, astheno-neurotic and hysterical character peculiarities), at correction of moral personality socialization and preclinical features.

Initial fractal presupposes medication-assisted and drug-free therapies in cases of primary depressive neurosis to prevent depressive disorders progression.

Early quality medical, psychological, social, moral and spiritual care is needed *within the fractal of full-scale clinical picture* of depressive disorders.

Appropriate depressive disorders detection and diagnosis play a key role in therapy effectiveness and favorable prognosis for a disease.

The medical block of the program. First of all, depressive disorders treatment includes *psycho-pharmacotherapy*. The choice of psychopharmacological medications depends on the common clinical symptoms detection, understanding pathogenetic mechanisms of depression development. Moreover, age, gender and somatic condition of a patient should also be taken into consideration (Pilyagina 2003; James 2012).

Antidepressants are basic group of psychopharmacological medications which are used for depressive disorders treatment. Relatively mild neurosis-like cyclothymic, latent or situational depressions also serve as indications for prescribing antidepressants, though in reduced doses. It is necessary to choose an individual dose capable of causing antidepressive effect without obvious side effects in the shortest possible period of time to achieve a therapeutic effect.

It is reasonable to advise a patient to follow some basic rules of antidepressants taking:

- to use the new antidepressants;
- not to take antidepressants in doses exceeding prescribed one;
- to remember that clinical effect of the majority of antidepressants is not achieved immediately: antidepressive effect accumulates gradually and becomes sufficient only by the end of the first two weeks of treatment;
- to follow a recommended treatment course, which is not less than 1,5 months. In case of marked, recurrent and lingering depressive conditions this treatment course can be prolonged till 2-6 months and more depending on the patient's condition;

- to avoid particular combinations of psychotropic medications (because of increasing risk of side effects and possible psychotropic medications interaction).

Psycho-pharmacotherapy is the main treatment method of severe and moderately marked depressions. However, its effectiveness over the past 20 years is not more than 40-60%, while remissions are possible only in 20-40% of patients (Mosolov 1995, 2015). This situation requires searching for new multidisciplinary care resources and algorithms.

The psychological block of the program. Psychotherapy is the most significant part of depressive disorders treatment. In the cases of depressions, it helps patients to develop skills of emotional self-regulation and to cope with crisis situations more effectively in future. Various types of psychotherapy are used including rational, cognitive, meditative, hypnotherapy, family therapy and others.

According to psychodynamic model internal unintentional conflicts are considered to be the basis for psychological depression. Thus, the aim of the therapy is to recognize the conflict and help to solve it constructively, which means to learn how to find the balance between independence and proximity, develop the ability to express one's feelings constructively and maintain a relationship with people.

Behavioral psychotherapy is aimed at current patient's problems solving and removal of behavioral symptoms such as passiveness, giving up pleasures, monotonous life, isolation from society, impossibility of planning and involvement in purposeful activity.

Cognitive psychotherapy represents a combination of both approaches illustrated above and accumulates their advantages. It presupposes work with actual life difficulties and behavioral depression symptoms as well as work with their internal psychological resources (deep notions and convictions). A so-called negative style of thinking serves as a basic psychological depression mechanism in cognitive psychotherapy. It is characterized by inclinations of a depressive patient to regard everything happening to him or her in a negative context. Changing such style of thinking requires careful individual work aimed at developing more realistic and optimistic views of the world, future and a person him- or herself.

The social block of the program. Social assistance in case of depressive disorders includes correction of different social interactions. Group and family psychotherapy is used for this purpose.

Group psychotherapy is treatment in a group of people with similar problems. In such groups a psychotherapist manages the process of clearing up psychological reasons of interpersonal and intrapersonal conflicts, developing abilities to express one's feelings directly and perfecting skills of interpersonal interaction.

Family therapy is aimed at specific family problems detection and favors the improvement of the quality relationship.

To correct relationship training of social skills may be used by means of acquiring positive experience capable of altering self-perception, and changing a negative style of thinking. It is necessary to make a negative opinion about a person's self and future the opposite one.

In the framework of social rehabilitation, one can use social skills training, which is aimed at strengthening a patient's resistance to stressors (public demands, family conflicts). Its aim is also to form communication skills with different government institutions, skills of family budget allocation, housekeeping, shopping, leisure time organization and skills of interpersonal interaction (conversational skills, family and friend relations).

During such training, specialists discover problems, which patients are likely to face in their everyday life. Training objectives are established together with patients, and then there is a rehearsal in the form of role plays imitating real everyday life situations. After that real-time practice takes place which presupposes practicing acquired skills outside those made-up education conditions, while the therapist still controls the situation. The last step is a patent's independent employment of acquired skills in his or her everyday life.

The spiritual and moral block of the program. Screening and correction of anhedonic family moral climate are put into practice during family psycho- and sociotherapy, which fulfills the tasks of ethico-psychological harmonization of interpersonal relations as well as a moral and spiritual development of a family.

Correction of the main moral senses and portrait formation and development is fulfilled for all moral and spiritual personality modalities, because of which a demoralization syndrome and destructive professiogenesis complex of syndromes may develop. That is why within the framework of early interference and mediation strategies, specialists of ethical committee and mental health services provide adaptive professiogenesis maintenance and carry out training on ethics in business comunication to prevent mobbing and bossing, deethization and dehumanization of interpersonal interactions.

Moral position and behavior reconstruction within the framework of a formed demoralization syndrome requires coaching, therapy by means of creative self-expression and sanogenetic therapy, ethical training and behavioral psychotherapy as well as spiritual and religious practices.

Moral and spiritual rehabilitation is implemented within the framework of supporting therapy, which fulfills the tasks to correct pessimistic, catastrophic and suicidal attitudes and form optimistic and resourceful life strategy instead.

Thus organizational model of medical, psychological, social and spiritual care provision for patients experiencing depressions presupposes early preventive measures. In the case of disorder occurrence complex assistance should take place immediately.

Section VI. Preventive-Correctional and Treatment-Rehabilitational Resources of Mental Medicine

Chapter 25

Biological Resources of Mental Medicine

25.1. Sanogenetic Therapy

Sanogenetic therapy (ST) is an adaptive biopsychosociospiritual mind and health management and engineering, as a result of which the destabilization of sustainable pathosis, activation of body reserves and personality resources and recovery of structural-functional life support systems happens (Sidorov 1988, 2008).

This technique uses a unique author's arrangement of human brain's biorhythms which enables the activation of recovery mechanisms and harmonization of body functions. Sounds and encoded frequencies of binaural and monaural beats (frequency amplitude oscillations with varying characteristics on the right and left channels) on the audio disc directly interact with specific brain areas causing the rise in production of endorphins, enkephalins and serotonin – substances which increase working efficiency and improve mood.

To comprehend the essence of sanogenetic therapy, it is important to understand the existence of a complex and multilevel system of information and energy exchange which provides the multimode interface of body functional system and its joint integration.

Sanogenetic therapy is based on primary and secondary sanogenetic mechanisms (Figure 25.1)

Primary (physiological) mechanisms of sanogenesis exist in a strong constitution, are triggered by extreme stimulus and function as follows:

- adapt the body for normal functioning when interacting with the extreme stimulus;
- prevent the pathogenic agent from penetrating the body;
- recover the function altered by a pathogenic agent, therefore, prevent the progression of a pathogenic process.

Secondary sanogenetic mechanisms originate in the process of pathology progression; they are based on the resultant damage and function as follows:

- participate in localization of a pathological process, destruction or excretion of toxic substances, microbial products from the body;
- participate in functional compensation of a body's organs and systems;
- come into action in case of organ damage and tissue dysfunction.
- Sanogenetic therapy is aimed at a diverse range of *recovery mechanisms:*
  1. *immediate and unstable*, defensive-compensatory processes or reactions (seconds, minutes) representing defense reactions of reflex character with the help of which the body gets rid of hazardous substances and reactions focusing on preservation of such constants as arterial pressure, osmotic pressure of blood and tissues, blood sugar level, etc.;
  2. relatively stable defensive-compensatory mechanisms of *moderate duration* (days, weeks) which include:
- activation of spare capacities, or reserve stamina, of lesional and healthy organs under the conditions of a disease;
- activation of multiple regulatory systems and switching them to another level;
- processes of binding of poisons by blood and tissue proteins, their neutralization, activation of connective tissue cells.
  3. *Long-term and stable* protective-compensatory processes which last months and years. Those include compensatory hypertrophy, reparative regeneration, immune reactions (antibody response, proliferation of T and B lymphocytes), multiple plastic responses of central nervous system composed of the following mechanisms:
- defense plastic reaction of central nervous system;
- defensive inhibition in the central nervous system;
- protecting-defensive (unconditional and conditional) reflexes (Bazyan, Grigoryan 2006).

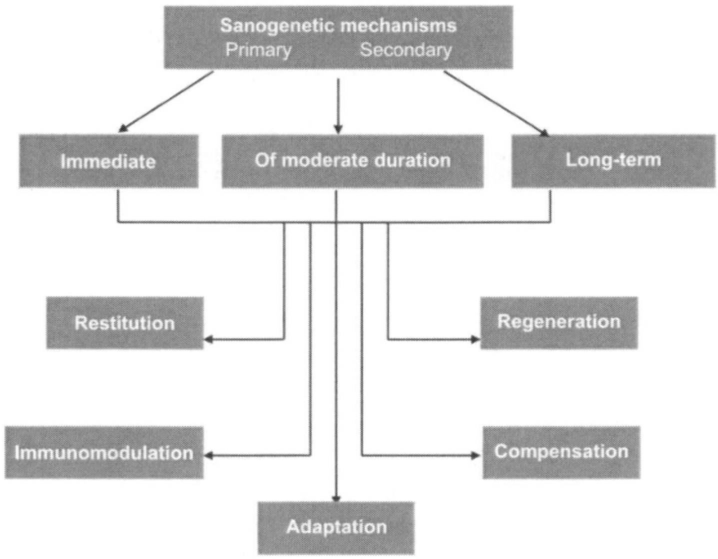

Figure 25.1. Primary and secondary sanogenetic mechanisms.

The first basis of sanogenesis is the process of formation of its mechanisms. Mechanisms of sanogenesis provide the control of regulatory, energy and structural homeostasis. Homeostasis is a dynamic balance state inside the body. Any living system is always unbalanced in relation to the environment. It is a universal characteristic of all living. Mechanisms of self-organization provide a dynamic stability of the system meaning maintaining itself in motion, in the process of exchange with the environment. On a somatic level the most elaborately studied mechanisms of sanogenesis are:

- *adaptation* – the adjustment of organs and systems to normal functioning when the body interacts with extreme stimulus to make compensatory-adaptive reactions of the human body work;
- *restitution* – the process of a recovery of the activity of reversibly lesional structures which occurs as a result of the normalization of bioenergetic processes in cell structures;
- *regeneration* – structural-functional recovery of the integrity of lesional tissues and organs as a result of growth and reproduction of specific tissue elements aimed to preserve the required level of functional activity;
- *compensation* – a process combining a variety of complex and diverse reactions on vicarious functioning or compensating of lost or deficient functions; compensatory reactions arise as a response to the signalizing of defect of functions, structures, exchange processes, and are reactions of a holistic body;
- *immunomodulation* – immune system is sensitive to the environmental changes and reconstructs its functioning.

On a psychological level, compensatory reactions present themselves in the mechanisms of repression of a psycho-traumatic situation in the subconscious, in the mechanisms of sublimation, regression and others, allowing the individual to stay adequate to the environment.

Regeneration, adaptation and compensation provide the individual's health mainly by influencing on the form-building process, by reshaping, by adjusting to stress under physiological conditions (adaptation) and in the course of the disease (compensation).

Because of the human's integrity, sanogenetic mechanisms of somatic and mental levels interact while the mental level remains leading.

The focus of a complex system of the sanogenetic therapy is a control of mental, neurological and somatovegetative disorders. The system includes components that activate physiological reactions of adaptation, stress limiting system and a system of antioxidant protection of a body.

For a development of a program of the sanogenetic therapy the following principles are of the most practical importance:

a) early start of the therapeutic intervention;
b) step therapy from the predisposition to the outcome;
c) continuity of treatment during all fractals;
d) integrative character of therapy;

e) individualization of treatment measures with consideration of adaptive potential and personal characteristics of a patient.

The understanding of sanogenetic capabilities of a body allows one to take into account the synergetic specificity of treatment implications and the special aspects of a body's own resources of spontaneous self-organization which ensures the success of remedial and rehabilitative measures carried out.

Sanogenetic therapy has to be aimed at all fractals of disease and its correction in bifurcation points in order to compensate the pathological state.

Sanogenetic correction in a bifurcation point of fractals of family dysontogenesis and diathesis involves a psychotherapeutic influence on the substrate, in other words - on psychogenesis simulation.

Correction in a bifurcation point of fractals of diathesis and functional disorders aside from psychotherapeutic influence includes a multimodal impact on sociogenesis.

Concerning bifurcation point of fractals of functional disorders and full-scale clinical picture, sanogenetic therapy consists of psychotherapy, medico-social work and correction of systems and functions of a body with a help of various methods which have an impact on biogenesis mechanisms.

Sanogenetic therapy has to be intensified to the maximum both in bifurcation points of fractals of a full-scale clinical picture and in chronization and outcome. It includes an integrated effect on psychogenesis and sociogenesis, biogenesis and animogenesis.

The use of the sanogenetic therapy is a harmonizing mean of influence on bioelectrical brain activity. This method is not addictive and doesn't have a pendulum effect. The longer the duration of treatment, the longer and more stable the effect is. And later, under the influence of the treatment, a stable autonomous realization of functions and characteristics of central nervous system is formed ("self-education" of brain structures). It allows achieving the required effect on its own without the use of sanogenetic therapy and ensures a long-term effect of the method. Binaural rhythms form a rhythmic activity of a brain in the required way and also form the kind of state of conscience to which self-preservative behavior strategy is inherent. Moreover, the binaural rhythms ensure a highly effective use of the method when treating psychosomatic deceases, addictions and when holding rehabilitation activities.

Sanogenetic therapy is used in almost all areas of healthcare and is considered to be a pathogenic and psychophysiological method of therapy of psychosomatic and mental disorders in all their diversity, as well as various addictions.

A self-preserving lifestyle, a decent quality of life and its moral meaning become the main rehabilitation priorities. The biopsychosociospiritual synergetic model demands an implementation of new multidisciplinary forms of organization of psychoprophylaxis and correction.

25.1.1. Sanogenetic Therapy of Nicotine Addiction

In a modern world, tobacco smoking is a bad habit dangerous to the individuals' health and leads to the development of mental and physical nicotine addiction. It is one of the main factors leading to genesis and development of a large number of non-communicable diseases.

There are more than 120 ways to treat nicotine addiction, and 40 of them are actively used in practice.

In order to study the influence of sanogenetic therapy on heart rate variability index when treating nicotine addiction, we (Sidorov et al. 2010) have conducted an experimental non-controlled study in which students of a medical university (18 people) participated as subjects. Respondents with nicotine addiction received a sanogenetic therapy as a part of individual preventive-correctional and medical, rehabilitative course.

"VNS-spectrum" software ("Neurosoft," Ivanovo) to record electrocardiography (ECG) and to analyze heart rate variability (HRV) was used. ECG had been recorded for 300 sec. before and after the sanogenetic therapy counseling.

The methods of analysis and physiological interpretation of HRV indexes were carried out in accordance with the recommendations of European Society of Cardiology and North American Society of Pacing and Electrophysiology.

Temporal (static) HRV rhythmogram analysis included studying of the heart rate (HR, 1/min); average duration of R-R interval between sinus cardiac cycles (RRNN, ms); mean-square deviation of duration of R-R interval between sinus contractions (SDNN, ms); coefficient of variation (CV, %); modes – predominant indexes of cardio intervals duration (Mo, sec); amplitude of modes – figures of indexes of intervals equal to Mo in percentage to the total number of recorded cardio cycles (AMo, %); index of vegetative balance (IVB, c.u.); regulatory processes adequacy index (RPAI, c.u.), index of regulatory systems tension (SI, c.u.).

Spectral analysis of HRV included the study of such indexes as: total spectrum power on all frequency ranges (Total power – TP, ms^2 x 1000, 0,015 – 0,5 Hz) characterizing heart rate variability altogether; spectrum power of high-frequency component (High frequency – HF, 0,15-0,5 Hz, ms^2, %) reflecting a relative activity level of parasympathetic regulation part; spectrum power of low-frequency component (Low frequency – LF, 0,05-0,15 Hz, ms^2, %) reflecting the activity of hypothalamus-pituitary system; spectrum power of very low-frequency component (Very low frequency – VLF, 0,015-0,05 Hz, ms^2, %) reflecting a relative activity level of cortico-limbic structures; balance of sympathetic and parasympathetic effects (LF/HF).

Statistical analysis was carried out with the use of application programs SPSS, version 19. The type of distribution was defined using the Shapiro-Wilk test; due to the fact that data did not follow the law of normal distribution the nonparametric method was used for two linked samples – Wilcoxon test. The critical level of statistical certainty for evaluation of rightness of null hypothesis was 0.05 and less. All indexes of heart rate variability are presented in a form of a median (Me) and 1st and 3rd quartiles (Q1-Q3).

25.1.2. Synergetics of Nicotine Addiction

Nicotine addiction as a special case of the addictive behavior represents a classical model of a dissipative structure. Addictive behavior is not an individual's, but a personality disorder; consequently, it is based on an anomalous development of mental individuality. Mental individuality is a complex entwinement of psychophysiological, psychological and socio-psychological characteristics. The core of which is a higher nervous activity (biological component of mental individuality) where the character formation is based (psychological component of mental individuality). And then a personality (social component of mental individuality) and its moral and spiritual potential are established (animogenetic component of mental individuality). Therefore, the fractal dynamic of nicotine addiction is closely intertwined with the stages of personality socialization.

The development of nicotine addiction has to be reviewed from the perspective of one fractal transitioning into another: predisposition – latent – initial – full-scale clinical picture – chronization – outcome (Table 25.1). The trajectory of progredient development of nicotine addiction can be altered in bifurcation points as a result of a change in anomalous ontogenetic personality development and, consequently, interpersonal relations.

Fractal of predisposition (prenatal development). Maternal smoking during pregnancy can lead to the development of nicotine addiction of her children. The mechanism of formation of the dependency is that nicotine and its metabolites crossing the placental barrier affect the central nervous system of a fetus and cause an impairment of a brain dopaminergic system. Therefore, the nicotine addiction of youngsters, who start smoking, is formed rapidly due to the fact that the substrate of development has already been formed.

Latent fractal (from the moment of birth to the age of preadolescence). The imprinting theory followers think of the child's early experience as a primary factor of formation of his/her attitude to others. The core of the theory is about transferring the imprinting mechanism on a child's behavior without any official grounds. According to the hypothesis, children of an early age "imprint" the characteristic of an adult taking care of them; they imprint not only appearance, voice, clothes, but also smell and habits (particularly, the cigarette manipulation and other smoking attributes).

As a result, an image is created, forming an addiction on the analogy of the image of a mother.

Initial fractal (age of preadolescence) – an initial period of smoking which is characterized not only by a positive perception but also by negative experiences: dyspeptic disorders (vertigo, nausea, vomiting). An adolescent experiences a cognitive dissonance between own smoking and what mother (or any other significant other) says; even more so if she herself smokes. This, in return, causes a psychological discomfort motivating the adolescent to try and reduce the extent of the dissonance and possibly reach a state of consonance. This fractal of socialization of the personality suggests various development trajectories which are designated in bifurcation points:

- the adolescent can change his/her behavior by giving up smoking and then his/her cognition of how harmful smoking is will reach consonance with the knowledge that smoking is a health hazard;
- the adolescent can change his/her cognition of the effects of smoking i. e. stop recognizing the fact that smoking is harmful by denying it (especially when his/her mother or close relative is a longtime smoker and it hasn't affected their health in any way).

In this initial phase it is important to develop a method and a type of activity which will ease a timely activation of preventive measures in an attempt to give up the addiction, find the necessary spirituality and feeling of safety.

Fractal of a full-scale clinical picture (adolescence) matches an initial stage of nicotine addiction and is characterized only by a psychological need and a lack of physical addiction.

On this stage, minor vegetative abnormalities can be observed if tobacco is used systematically. This fractal can develop on different trajectories. According to Harry Sullivan, founder of the interpersonal theory, in this age introduction to smoking is related to the presence of a smoking adolescent in his/her environment. After that, the family's behavior and reaction, being an institute of socialization, are fully responsible for whether the adolescent will continue smoking. Disharmonious interfamily relations lead to a progression of the process and formation of a physical nicotine addiction. Therefore, parents or relatives can alter the scenario development by acting through "reference groups" such as friends, coaches, etc.

Fractal of chronization (adulthood) is characterized by the appearance of factors of physical addiction: formation of an abstinent syndrome, rise in tolerance. The impulse to smoke becomes compulsive, is coupled with irritation, decrease in physical and brain activity, vertigo, headaches, disturbance of sleep. Psychosomatic ill-being shows as a morning cough, initial stomach diseases (heartburn, epigastrium discomfort, occasional pain), transient heart discomfort, fluctuations of arterial pressure.

Fractal of outcome (late adulthood or senescence) is congruent to the manifestation of nicotine syndrome and is characterized by a high tobacco tolerance (up to 30-50 cigarettes a day). Or, on the contrary, a decrease in the number of consumed cigarettes, severe abstinent syndrome, asthenoneurotic symptoms leading to the rise of a social maladjustment are present. Smoking becomes automatic. The fractal of outcome is characterized by a complication of the nicotine addiction: symptoms of disorders of various organs and systems, primarily respiratory and cardiovascular, are noted.

25.1.3. Medico-psychosociospiritual Care

A human body is a holistic and developing real information-energy system. In the light of a concept of information-energy exchange as a primary integrating body system, any therapeutic intervention can be considered as a direct correction of damaged structures. The aim of any treatment is a normalization of the relation between various body subsystems.

A complex structure of sanogenetic therapy is to fight mental, neurological and somatovegetative disorders of nicotine addiction. It includes components that activate physiological reactions of adaptation, a stress-limiting system and system of antioxidant body defense.

Taking into account the information-energy specificity of therapeutical intervention and aspects of body's own power resources to spontaneous regeneration, the sanogenetic therapy is a formula for success in taking remedial and rehabilitation measures.

Our developed and implemented sanogenetic therapy was ahead of Daniel Siegel's mindsight (2014) by a quarter of a century as an ability to perceive and recognize both one's own feelings and thoughts and thoughts and feelings of others due to the particularly focused and direct attention.

Sanogenetic therapy of the nicotine addiction has to be directed to all fractals of the development of an addictive behavior and its correction in the bifurcation points in order to compensate a pathological condition and the addictive behavior (Table 25.2). The given matrix allowed every client and patient to build and individual preventive-correctional or remedial-rehabilitative course.

Table 25.1. Fractal dynamics of mental epidemic of nicotine addiction

Ontogenesis vector	Prenosological fractals			Nosological fractals		
	Predisposition	Latent	Initial:	Full-scale clinical picture/mental epidemic	Chronization: types and forms of the course/ destructive mental epidemic	Outcome: somato-neurological complications/ pandemic
Somatogenesis	Hereditary loading, including the formation of the "fetal tobacco syndrome" (when the mother smokes)	Immune system disorders, respiratory diseases, disorders of neural processes as a result of passive smoking	Somatoform disorders as a result of active smoking	Transient psychosomatic disorders	High tolerance to nicotine, psychosomatic disorders	Low tolerance to nicotine. Somatic complications
Psychogenesis	Impact of tobacco on the neuropsychic development of the fetus and child	Development of codependent personality	Cognitive dissonance between proper smoking, and what relatives were reported about	Obsessive desire of dependent personality out of personality disorder	Dependent personality disorders	Personality deformation
Sociogenesis	Family disharmony, early dysontogenesis	Availability of smoking socializing family: parents, guardians. Smoking as a tool of pseudo personality socialization	Ambivalence of the current microsocial environment	Loss of the value of opposing microsocial environment	Transient social decompensation	Social disadaptation of personality
Animogenesis	Spiritual and moral disharmony of family	Disturbances of moral sentiments formation	Deformation of moral character	Loss of spiritual and moral position	Probability of unlawful acts	Probability of illegal behaviorr

Table 25.2. Program of medico-psychosociospiritual care for nicotine addiction

Blocks	Prenosological fractals			Nosological fractals		
	Predisposition	Latent	Initial	Full-scale clinical picture/mental epidemic	Chronization: forms and types of the addiction/destructive mental epidemic	Outcome: complications/ pandemic
Medical	Inclusion of children of mothers with nicotine dependence into the risk group	Identification of individuals, who are prone to psychoactive substance abuse	Identification of tobacco smoking by screening	Establishing of diagnosis, drug therapy indications, prevention of complications	Control over the somatic state; drug therapy, prevention of complications	Treatment of somatic-neurological and neurological complications of nicotine dependence
Psychological	Identification of individuals with specific psychological personality traits and their incorporation into the risk group	Correction of premorbid personality characteristics	Somatoform disorders correction, psychotherapy	Psychosomatic disorders correction, psychotherapy	Psychosomatic disorders correction, psychotherapy	Psychological adjustment
Social	Identification and correction of family relationships disharmony	Correction of family relations and harmonization of personality socialization	Harmonisation of important social relationships	Adapting to the disease, correction of interpersonal problems	Professional and family adaptation of the personality	Social rehabilitation
Spiritual and moral	Correction of the moral climate of the family	Correction of the formation and development of moral sentiments	Correction of the formation and development of moral character	Reconstruction of moral position	Reconstruction of moral behavior	Spiritual and moral rehabilitation

Sanogenetic correction in the bifurcation point of family dysontogenesis and diathesis involves a psychotherapeutic impact on a substrate meaning a psychogenesis modeling. A psychogenesis of the addictive behavior is characterized, all in all, by a formation of an addictive personality which traits are infantilism, suggestibility, high search activity, egocentrism. The only effective type of a correction of mental changes, in this case, is the psychotherapy, which possesses a large arsenal of methods (analytical, educational, developing, transforming, modeling, encouraging, etc.).

Correction in the bifurcation point of fractals of diathesis and functional disorders aside from psychotherapeutic intervention includes a multimodal influence on sociogenesis. Sociogenesis of the nicotine addiction leads to a disturbance of a moral socialization of a personality. Therefore, its correction is consequently based on medico-social and spiritual and moral activity, which fundamental principles are:

a. eco systematization – a measurement of the whole system of relations between a human and his environment in a given problem paradigm;
b. multimodality – combinations in the system of medico-social activity of various approaches by the mode of action that are functionally oriented to a certain aim.
c. continuity – wholeness of a dynamical and planning nature of the medico-psychosociospiritual activity.

As applied to the bifurcation points of fractals of functional disorders and full-scale clinical picture, sanogenetic therapy is based on psychotherapy, ethical-psychological and medico-social activity, correction of systems and functions of a body using various methods which influence pathogenesis mechanisms. Within the framework of sanogenetic therapy the following forms of medico-social activity can be noted:

1. preventive – focused on the prevention of a development of an addictive pattern;
2. medico-social activity with problem personalities, whose addictive pattern is formed, and their microsocial environment;
3. medico-rehabilitative activity with the patients whose nicotine addiction has been formed.

Sanogenetic therapy in bifurcation points of fractals of full-scale clinical picture and chronization and the outcome has to be intensified to the maximum; it includes psychogenesis, sociogenesis, biogenesis and animogenesis. To speed the process of restitution of somatogenesis, the following methods are successfully used: electrosleep, galvanization, electrophoresis of biostimulants, vasoactive drugs, antioxidants, diadynamic therapy, amplipulse therapy, darsonvalization. The restitution is widely influenced by phototherapy, centimeter and decimeter wave therapy, and ultrasound. To stimulate regeneration processes, it is effective to use a number of natural factors: peloids, balneotherapy, laser treatment, ultrasound, sonic phoresis of antioxidants and biostimulators, electrophoresis of proteolytic enzymes, vitamins, and magnetotherapy. The activation of compensatory reaction is possible as a result of conducting medicinal electrophoresis of tranquilizers and affecting central nervous system by rectangular current using methods of electrosleep. Balneo procedures (oxygen, nitrogen, carbon, hydrogen sulfide baths), various methods of oxygen therapy have a normalizing effect on cortical-visceral structures.

Currently, clinical and experimental data has been accumulated, which confirms a successful use of a sanogenetic method in therapeutical programs of various addictions (Sidorov 1988, 2011).

It emerged that after a sanogenetic therapy session when comparing to the initial data, statistically important changes of time-line analysis of heart rate variability were found in the experimental group, (Table 25.3).

In the course of treatment HR (p<0,001), AMo (p = 0,006), SI (p = 0,001), IVB (p = 0,001), RPAI (p = 0,001) have decreased and Mo (p = 0,001), RRNN (p<0,001), SDNN (p = 0,002) have increased. All in all, this is a sign of a decrease in a tonus of sympathetic part of autonomic division of nervous system and activation of parasympathetic regulation of heart rate.

Redistribution of tonus between divisions of the vegetative nervous system was followed up by statistically significant changes in spectrum function of heart rate (Table 25.4).

Table 25.3. Indexes of time-line analysis of heart rate variability in the course of sanogenetic therapy, Me (Q1-Q3)

Index of HRV	Before	After	p-level
HR, beats per minute	78,0 (71,0-86,0)	72,0 (65,0-78,0)	<0,001
RRNN, ms	774 (710-875)	849 (780-939)	<0,001
SDNN, ms	53,5 (37,3-83,5)	67,0 (47,7-80,7)	0,002
CV,%	7,03 (4,82-9,53)	7,66 (5,46-10,23)	0,058
Mo, c	0,77 (0,72-0,92)	0,83 (0,77-1,03)	0,001
AMo, %	35,2 (25,1-52,6)	28,6 (21,8-41,8)	0,006
IVB, c.u.	118 (57,0-244)	68,9 (34,8-158)	0,001
RPAI, c.u.	46,2 (26,3-69,9)	33,2 (25,8-48,3)	0,001
SI, c.u.	78,8 (29,0-159)	39,6 (21,3-91,2)	0,001

Table 25.4. Indexes of spectrum analysis of heart rate variability in the course of sanogenetic therapy, Me (Q1-Q3)

Index of HRV	Before	After	p-level
TP, ms^2	3601 (1718-9133)	4970 (2698-7952)	0,003
VLF, ms^2	1317 (741-2477)	1843 (1187-3325)	0,248
LF, ms^2	1373 (720-2979)	1867 (882-3535)	0,199
HF, ms^2	581 (249-1971)	1004 (498-2121)	0,011
LF/HF	2,42 (1,61-3,68)	1,71 (1,28-2,60)	0,001
%VLF	44,9 (23,1-54,6)	33,5 (27,1-56,9)	0,619
%LF	38,8 (28,6-48,8)	39,9 (24,6-46,4)	0,048
%HF	15,7 (11,4-21,7)	20,5 (13,0-26,5)	0,044

During the analysis of the wave structure, an increase of TP (p = 0,003) was noted. Changes in the high-frequency range (HF) were observed, with the spectrum capacity increasing (p = 0,011). Wave spectrum was restructured which is shown by a rise in a %LF (p = 0,048) and %HF (p = 0,044) levels. The correlation between sympathetic and parasympathetic influences (LF/HF) has declined (p = 0,001).

In general, the capacity has increased and neurohumoral influences in heart rate regulation with a rise of influence of parasympathetic system amid a prevailing regulatory influence of hypothalamus-pituitary system and a decline in a cortical-limbic complex's activity. The evaluation of HRV results from the perspective of a double-circuit model of heart rate regulation has showed that the influence of an autonomic circuit on a central one in heart activity regulation has risen. The growth in activity of intrasystem mechanisms of a cardiovascular system's self-regulation characterizes the adaptive changes without an intervention of intersystem control level. The balance of regulatory systems is restored, and psychoemotional tension is relieved (Baevsky 2006; Palkova et al. 2008).

Therefore, sanogenetic therapy influences a personality as a whole and indexes of heart rate variability as an indicator of adaptation-adjustment changes in particular.

The synergetic concept of the addictive behavior realizes prognosis scenarios of nicotine addiction formation as early as in antenatal and postnatal life; that, theoretically, can be changed. This concept shows the necessity of multidisciplinary development of antismoking programs with a consolidation of all main institutes of personality socialization (family, school, various specialists). The use of sanogenetic therapy specifically during the premorbid stage is the one pathogenetic treatment method that is capable of preventing the addiction formation.

25.2. Nutritional Therapy

The traditional cuisine of every nation was formed depending on the region and climate, customs and traditions. Any country's national cuisine is a historically developed and thought through balance of microelements and proteins, fats and carbohydrates. However, in recent decades, the leading positions in the food industry has been overtaken by "fast-food culture" which provoked a mental obesity epidemic all around the world.

Based on the results of an online survey conducted by the Ministry of Health of the Russian Federation (2012), about 25-30% of the population have overweight and about 15-20% suffer from obesity. Up to 10% of the respondents consume fast-food several times a month and 3.4% - once a week.

Upon that, mechanisms of fast-food addiction are similar to drug dependency. P. J. Kenny and P. M. Johnson (2010), American researchers, had been carrying out an experiment on rats for three years. They divided them into three groups. The first one ate leaves and grains, the second one's ration partly consisted of fatty foods and the third one received only supermarket products: cheesecakes, bacon, chocolate cookies filled with cream, sausages. Rats specifically from the third group gained weight very fast, but moreover – they did not wish to eat anything, but fast-food, and were even ready to go through painful current discharges in order to get the desired. After excluding all the junk food from their ration, the rats were starving for two weeks, which was a demonstration of a laboratory model of the rebound effect.

An analysis of MRI-images of the animal's brain showed that the pleasure center of the third group rats was excessively active, and the level of dopamine was below normal. Fast-food has become a severe addiction of the rats, followed by a tolerance growth and compulsion. The same addiction is the foundation of self-destructive lifestyle, and it explains the desire of the overweight to eat unhealthy foods.

The main nutritional trends of the modern world are:

1. *a reduction in energy consumption* (in the middle of the previous century – 3000-3500 kcal/day, now – 1900-2100 kcal/day) that has led to the decrease in the consumption of biologically active substances necessary to the body;
2. *a change in the nutrition structure*: insufficient consumption of fruits and vegetables, berries and greens in favor of fast-food, unvaried ration, consumption of a large amount of processed and tinned food, diet disturbance;
3. *a change in the quality of food*: impoverishment of soil, time-consuming transportation and storage, change in the processing technology, canning and refining that leads to an impoverishment of biologically active substances in food.

According to the Ministry of Health and Social Development (2009), Russians consume an excessive amount of fats and an insufficient amount of complete proteins, polyunsaturated fatty acids (omega-3 and omega-6), vitamins and mineral substances, fiber and biologically active food agents. An especially crucial problem is a deficit of a number of vitamins and microelements. All in all, the consumption deficiency is:

- vitamin C – 60-70%;
- folic acid – 70-80%;
- iron – 20-40%;
- calcium – 40-60%;
- iodine – up to 70%.

Nutritional therapy as a treatment by special products and diets can be used to treat all kinds of diseases including excess weight and obesity. It is based on a functional nutrition. Nutritional resource of mental preventology is about the functional ration being a part of a healthy lifestyle. The functionality of nutrition reflects the ability to improve functioning of all organs and systems of a human body.

Functional products have to include not only vitamins and fibers, minerals and polyunsaturated fatty acids, but also probiotics and prebiotics. Functional products are not BADS, but special-purpose products of a natural or artificial origin which purpose is to replenish a deficiency of a whole number of vital substances in a body. It serves the purpose of not only preserving health but also supporting brain activity.

Functional nutrition is based on *protein foods* consisting of amino acids, several of which are neurotransmitters or their precursors.

Meat, eggs and dairy products are packed with protein. Beans, green leafy vegetables, whole grains, nuts and seeds are the best protein sources of plant origin.

Walnuts, almonds and hazelnuts combined with powerful polyphenol of grapes can lift up the spirits and improve memory and thinking. This effect is achieved by resveratrol – a natural phytoalexin produced by several plants as a mean of a defense reaction from parasites. By a recovery of functions of neurons' mitochondria, this substance slows down the processes of brain aging that influences gene expression. Resveratrol also induces the serotonin production that eliminates depression and improves overall health (Estruch R. et al., 2013).

Antidepressant products are trout, laminaria, almond, blueberry and broccoli.

Apart from proteins, *carbohydrates* are also crucial for brain activity, because they produce insulin which not only modulates glucose uptake but preserves brain cells' health: their growth and normal functioning. A lack of insulin leads to diabetes and Alzheimer's decease development. Moreover, its excess – to a decrease in mental activity and sleepiness, fast exhaustion and rigidity. To preserve the balance nutritionists recommend eating carb-packed products along with protein food which neutralizes the negative effect of sugar.

The most effective product to increase brain working capacity and prevent depression development is dark chocolate. D. Kennedy (2009) has showed that it is easier to perform arithmetical problems in the head after drinking hot chocolate and cocoa. The long intellectual load did not tire people due to cacao-beans flavonoids. These substances are also present if citrus, green tea and red wine.

The functional ration is also impossible without fats that are essential for brain structures that are 60% fat tissue. Omega-3 and omega-6 fatty acids are especially important, and fish and seafood, walnuts and seeds (pumpkin, flax) are rich of them. Omega-3 not only helps the brain to function but also prevents mental debility.

Salmon bred on a fish farm is considered to be the most nutritious. They almost don't have any mercury salt, which is widely common among sea fish, and are packed with omega-3.

American research data demonstrated that (Bowman 2011) among the 104 people (62% women, average age – 87), the best results of mental speed and memory were shown by patients whose blood contained omega-3 acids and a high level of B, C, D and E vitamins. The worst results were of those people who regularly consumed trans-fats (bakery, chips, donuts etc.). The findings were verified by brain scans (MRI). Brain size of fast-food consumers turned out to be less that of those, who ate vitamins- and antioxidants packed foods.

Fruits and vegetables antioxidants protect intercellular membranes and brain cells from oxidants. Sufficient vegetables and fruit consumption improves cognitive abilities. Fruits of a dark shade and blueberries are richer with antioxidants.

Minor biologically active compounds – flavonoids, indoles, and isoflavones are important to functional nutrition; even though they are present in trace quantities in food, they. However, are essential as exogenous regulators of metabolism. They evoke the expression of genes that are in charge of synthesis of human defending enzymes. These are the enzymes of the first and the second metabolism phases of xenobiotics – foreign dangerous and toxic substances. Basically, this is a system of antioxidant defense which protects a body from active forms of oxygen that are the reason for premature aging and have a carcinogenic effect (Tutyelyan 2015).

A special role in nutritional resources of mental preventology is taken by vitamins, especially of a B group: B_6 and B_{12} that positively influence the nervous system condition. Spinach, broccoli and green beans are the natural resources of this vitamin.

Vitamin D is important for the regulation of fat tissue formation. Therefore, women deficient in vitamin D weight 8-9 kg more than their peers, who receive a substantial amount of it; they age earlier and have an increased risk of a heart attack or stroke (Watson 2012). In this context, back to 2008 in American "norms of physiological needs" it was said that children and people of a working age have to receive 10 mcg of the vitamin (400 ME) a day, pregnant and breastfeeding – 12.5 mcg (500 ME), people older than 60 – 15 mcg (600 ME).

The question of a healthy lifestyle is the question of knowledge of natural resources of vitamins and microelements and their daily requirement (Liflyandsky 2006).

Functional nutrition is not only about well-being and normative somatogenesis, but also about the conditions of maintaining mental health. Therefore, a balanced ration reduces a risk of a stroke by 58%, of depression by 52% and increases a chance to avoid dementia by 71% (Xu et al. 2011).

The dramatic problem of Russian health service remains the prevalence and mortality of a stroke. Every year 450 thousand people in Russia suffer from strokes. Stroke mortality in Russia is one of the highest in the world (175 to 100 thousand of the population). In the recent decade, the mortality of people of the working age in Russia has increased more than by one-third and is 41 to 100 thousand people in the population (Skvortsova 2014).

A proper ration defends from a stroke by 85%. To prevent an ischemic stroke, it is recommended to:

a) cut out:
   - fatty meat and dairy, liver and sausages;
   - crude water from the tap that has harmful substances and lime, chloride and salts that affect vessels negatively;
   - reduce salt and sugar intake.

b) enrich the menu with:
   - vegetables: radish, cabbage, beet, pumpkin, eggplant, greens;
   - beans;
   - apples;
   - berries: current (black and red), raspberry, cherry, chokeberry;
   - grains: oat and buckwheat porridge, bran bread from whole grains;
   - crude oil, preferably – olive oil;
   - fish (at least 1-2 times a week);
   - non-fat cottage cheese;
   - green tea;
   - dark chocolate.

In this context, it is important to know that chocolate does not only protect intellectual activity but also is a resource of a nutritional stroke preventive care. American researchers (Shaz et al. 2010) found out that dark chocolate (not milk or white) protects people from an ischemic stroke due to epicatechin content – flavonoid that stimulates nuclear factor-erythroid2-related factor 2 (Nrf2)/ heme oxygenase one pathway. Moreover, the effect of chocolate and cacao consumption is achieved by flavanoids – antioxidants that lower blood pressure and improve vessel condition in opposition to stroke development. Consumption of 60-65 g of chocolate a week for ten years lowers the risk of a stroke by 17-19% (Friedman et al. 2012).

The prime priority in weight loss is a healthy sleep. American six-month research (Alleyne et al. 2011) of 500 overweight people showed that the best results were achieved by those with low level of stress and who slept not less than 6-8 hours.

Functional nutrition provides the body with the necessary energy and nutrient materials in correct proportions:

- sufficient amount of calories and nutritional substances;
- physiological balance of various nutritional substances.

A lack of the functional nutrition leads to the following disturbances:

- metabolism decline;
- body resistance decline;
- organs and systems activity decline;
- symptoms of nutrition ration disturbance.

In the end, all this is accumulated in the development process of *alimentary-addictive disorders:*

- atherosclerosis;
- arterial hypertension;
- hyperlipidemia;
- obesity;
- diabetes;
- osteoporosis;
- gout.

Those diseases are also psychosomatic.

Functional nutrition, as a general, is based on the same principles as a healthy lifestyle: moderation and balance, rationality and harmony. The synergetic biopsychosociospiritual methodology of mental healthcare allows integrating a healthy lifestyle and a moral meaning of life into the high quality mental health.

25.3. Psychopharmacotherapy

Pharmacotherapy of mental disorders suggests that a wide range of psychotropic drugs are to be used, mainly anxiolytics and antidepressants, nootropics and neuroleptics.

The main aim of pharmacotherapy is to reduce psychopathological disorders, to decrease the risk of impairment, to improve social functioning of patients. A diverse spectrum of psychotropic activity and efficiency of antidepressants and anxiolytics is more and more widely applied not only in psychiatry.

The aim of pharmacotherapy of psychosomatic disorders is to solve the following problems:

1) elimination of emotional disorders typical to the neurotic disorder (emotional lability, irritable weakness, anxiety, concern, tension, etc.);

2) treatment of asthenic signs, coping with physical and intellectual exhaustion;
3) regulation of vegetative disorders;
4) treatment of obsessions and phobias;
5) correction of personal characteristics;
6) elimination of negative factors;
7) detection and elimination of somatic disorders.

Use of psychotropic drugs to treat psychosomatic disorders is associated with a number of complications. They are connected to the characteristics of psychopharmacological drugs and the peculiarities of their compatibility with somatotropic drugs, a somatic condition of a patient and changed tolerance to pharmacological drugs due to a dysfunction of internal organs.

Pharmacotherapy methods are usually simple, because medical help to patients with psychosomatic disorders often given in general hospitals. The prescription of psychotropic drugs is mostly limited to monotherapy with the easy to use medications (simplicity of therapeutic regimen and dosage). Taking into account the possibility of hypersensibility and side-effects, psychotropic drugs are prescribed in small (compared to drugs used in "big" psychiatry) doses.

In order to minimize behavioral toxicity, manifesting itself as apathy, sleepiness, a slowdown of cognitive and motion functions, a change of prescribed drugs can be done (replacing neuroleptics with tranquilizers, using antidepressants of different groups).

The choice of psychopharmacological drugs depends on the intensity of psychopathological symptoms. To treat mild neurotic, affective disorders as a part of psychosomatic one's monotherapy with tranquilizers is usually enough. The treatment of apparent psychopathological forms the choice of a drug depends on the structure of the clinical syndrome.

Most frequently, in the case of psychosomatic disorder tranquilizers with anxiolytic action are used. Among them benzodiazepine derivatives are more spread; they, connected to the specific benzodiazepine receptors, increase the sensibility of GABA-receptors in γ-aminobutyric acids. When treating chronic anxiety (generalized or fixed), 3-hydroxy- or 2-ketobenzodiaepam (lorazepam, phenazepam, and diazepam) are mostly used. At the moment among tranquilizers the anxiolytics of non-benzodiazepine range like aphobazol, tenoten, strezami have taken the center place. It is connected to the fact that these drugs have a favorable tolerability profile and a high level of safety.

Modern medications that combine a mild thymoleptic effect with a high tolerability acquire a special significance among antidepressants: selective serotonin reuptake inhibitors (prozac, zoloft, paxil, cipramil), selective noradrenaline reuptake inhibitors (ludiomil), reversible monoamine oxidase inhibitors A (pirazidol, aurorix), α2-adrenoceptor blocking agents (lerivon), atypical serotoninergic tricyclic antidepressants (coaxil). The data of numerous researches shows the effectiveness of these drugs in psychosomatic disorders treatment. Among nootropic medications nootropil (piracetam), picamilon, cerebrolysin, encephabol, etc. are widely used. Among neuroleptic drugs eglonil, etaperazin, theralene, sonapax are often applied.

Several effects of psychopharmacological medications of psychosomatic disorders treatment according to the data of various authors (Smulevich et al. 2005, 2015; Drobizhev, Makuh 2007) are given in Table 25.5.

Table 25.5. The use of psycho-pharmacological drugs of different groups among psychosomatic patients

Drug groups	Indications	Positive psychotropic effects	Levels of intake safety	Side effects
Tranquilizers (anxiolytics)	Organ neurosis, nosogenic reactions with the predominance of neurotic (anxiety-phobic and somatized) disorders and sleep disturbance; reaction by the type of symptomatic lability (psychogenically provoked angina, asthma); time-urgent states accompanied by vital fear, panic attacks (myocardial infarction, severe injuries etc.)	The decline of risk of a development of severe ventricular arrhythmia, ventricular fibrillation in case of an acute myocardial ischemia; antiemetic action, reduction of gastric secretion and impoverishment of pepsin and hydrochloric acid in gastric juice	A wide gap between therapeutic and lethal dosage; absence of negative effects on a number of functional body systems; interaction with somatotropic drugs; can be used during pregnancy and breastfeeding	"Behavioral toxicity" (sleepiness during day hours, myorelaxation, attention and motor coordination disturbances; rarely respiratory and heart-vascular systems disturbances, allergic reactions, haematological complications; drug dependance
Antidepressants (counter-depressants)	Nosogenic depressive reaction and somatized dysthymia with anxious asthenic somato-vegetative and hypochondriac disorders prevailing	None	Tricyclic antidepressants are not to be used by patients with acute liver, kidneys injury, hematopoietic organs disorder, apparent cardiovascular decompensation, cardiac conduction disease, infectious diseases, cerebrovascular accidents, atony of bladder, prostatic adenoma; possible negative consequences of interaction with somatotropic drugs	"Behavioral toxicity"; orthostatic hypotension, sinus tachycardia, heart conduction delay; allergic reactions; cholinolytic activity (dry mouth, accommodation disorder, urine retention)
Nootropics	Nosogenic reactions with asthenic disorders prevailing	Antihypoxic action (decreases the oxygen requirement of tissues and improves body's hypoxia stability; membrane-stabilizing action	High tolerability of a high dose, possibility of intravenous injection; absence of clinically important side-effects	Decrease of convulsion threshold; transient sleep disturbances
Neuroleptics	Nosogenic paranoic reactions of nosogeny with "euphoric pseudodementia"; chronic somatoform pain syndrome	Eglonil: influence on pathological processes of gastrointestinal tract (duodenal ulcer, Crohn's disease, dumping syndrome); ethaperazine: anti-emetic properties; theralene: hypotensive effect	Not to be used by patients with acute liver injuries, dysfunction of hematopoietic organs, apparent cardiovascular insufficiency, pregnancy	"Behavioral toxicity"; allergic reactions; extrapyramidal disorders (rarely because of a low dose of the drug)

According to Smulevich A. (2007), pharmacotherapy's effect is positive in 69% of cases and in estimating long-term results (3-year follow-up study) – 60%.

The use of psychopharmacological drugs should not be seen as a plainly biological therapy, because with a decline of anxiety levels and a transformation of intrapsychic adaptation mechanisms based on a feedback, an adaptive reorganization of micro-social interaction is taking place. It is followed up by an increase in realism of perception, situation and personality evaluation, an ability of conscious self-control, an establishment of an adequate relation between frustration tension and behavioral integration.

To help patients with psychosomatic disorders sedative and activating agents of natural origin and vitamin complexes that have a calming, tonic and adaptating effect are used.

Complexes of biologically active agents of the maral root, schisandra chinensis, devil's club and aralia have a general tonic effect. Medications from ginseng, eleuterococus, rhodiolla rosea and several others plants combine a tonic effect on adaptational properties. Extracts from crude drugs are used as tonic medications and adaptogenes.

Adaptogene drugs from plants have a slight psychostimulant impact. Immunostimulation and improvement of tolerance to outdoor environment hostility (high and low temperatures, intoxication, radiation exposure, etc.) have been noted.

Relying on theoretical suppositions, experimental researches and clinical trials, L. Kremleva et al. (2014) suggest using pharmacological drugs in *very low dose* rates, because of a more special and mild effect without adverse events.

Therefore, psycho-pharmacotherapy can be used by psychosomatic patients in general somatic network, but a somatic condition of a patient, occurrence of neurotic disorders, interaction with somatotropic drugs have to be taken onto account. A combination of psychopharmacotherapy and psychotherapy is also reasonable.

Chapter 26

Psychological Resources of Mental Medicine

Famous Polish psychiatrist A. Kempinski speaking of problems in modern medical science pointed out that human beings have an astonishing bent for eliminating those who are "different." Formation of the bounds is a general wildlife phenomenon. This is particularly topical for the formation of the bounds of a human being and a group.

Clinical psychologist overcomes two bounds: the first one separating him from a sick man, the second one separating a patient from a healthy man. To overcome these bounds professor A. Kempinski described one of the conditions as "approach with a sick man – the effort necessary for coming into the world of a sick man, accept his feelings, do not assume an attitude of condemnatory, provide care at the same time realizing that this care can be pointless. Rueful feelings of a sick man often come across with the problems of a psychiatrist; these problems are often insensible."

Psychology and psychotherapy in mental medicine are key resources individualizing preventive and correctional, treatment and rehabilitation directions acting both as mental health promotion, and mental illnesses treatment.

26.1. Psychosynergetic Methodology

Models of psycho-synergetic teamwork are developing and improving continually. Specific specialization of psychologist and methods of direct psychological curation form reflection of different psychological concepts about microcosm like, for example, technocratic, protective and educational model.

Psychologist-technocrat provides patient's and client's care management in directive style. Technocrat recognizes human being to be dependent subject devoid of signs and treats his patients from the perspective of his authority. Often he represents a highly positioned specialist in the field of certain technics, for example, hypnosis. He is in charge of his patient, gives him instructions and advice, and controls its fulfillment, manage patient's social environment, writes down potential program of encouragements and punishments for a patient. Often technocrat gives directive instructions to the relatives, thereby shifting on them a part of patient's problems and intensifying co-dependency in some measure.

The patronizing-oriented psychologist also above all recognizes human being as a weakling calling for help. He does not act like adviser simplifying decision-making and resolution of individual intrapersonal conflicts. He helps to find confidence and courage, eliminates (or trying to minimize) psychic traumas, or acting like a social protector, comes to patient's home, helps him in solving lots of domestic problems. There are two variations of this model – *patronizing and clinical, patronizing and social.* In the first model, psychologist takes care of the patient undergoing medical treatment or requiring psychotherapeutic help. The patronizing and social model assumes that psychologist takes care of the patients after hospitalization, as well as helps people who are in a hard reality situation.

Finally, a *psychologist working in educational model* discovers unlimited possibilities of activity and development of individual, which are realized in concert with other people and within a well-organized social environment. The goal of a psychologist is finding the best potential opportunities of a human, all that healthy, valued and capable of development qualities he has. The core principle, which underlies this model, is a belief that the best protection from problems is preventing their appearance. Synonym of this approach is partner model of psychologist's work. Educational or partner model are the most optimal for mental medicine in many parameters – economic, effectiveness, order of population covering.

Hence, the core factor of clinical psychology in mental medicine is acceptance an individual to be of appreciated value. It is a human being who possesses resources of development and potential of self-realization enabling to solve problems.

The major task of a clinical psychologist is establishing a *psychological diagnosis* as evaluation of individual psychological resources or "personality adaptative potential" (Posokova 2008). The leading characteristic of this potential is ego structure providing coordination of diverse mental functions, its regulation and keeping identity throughout the whole life (Ovchinnikov et al. 2010).

To analyze psychological resources the following aspects should be examined: personality structure features; availability and character of intrapsychic conflicts; specifics of personal adaptative and compensatory formations. These are forms of psychological defense, mechanisms of coping, inner aspect of a disease and others, which have a prevailing nature reflecting on phenomenology of clinical, social, as well as moral, and above all psychological diagnosis.

There are not so many clinical psychology researches in terms of synergetic methodology. First of all, it is caused by aiming of clinical psychologists at effective influence but not at a scientific reflection. Despite WHO recommendations, most of the clinical psychologists do not know the answer to the question what does mental health mean. Just as the notions of illness and happiness, the notion of health is very subjective.

In all variety of notions, it is obvious that mental health is closely related to a value system. Regardless of any culture, mental health is attributed to a positive value and postulate nature. Therefore, people from everywhere started to believe that there is a need for seeking health. This feature requires maintaining the accuracy of notions, moderation in goal-setting and tolerance to opinions from research people and psychological field practice.

Since the concept of mental health is related to the culture and social state standards, one can say about *model of healthy life field.* According to a representative of ecological psychology, D. Stokolsa (2005), a healthy environment is characterized by its ability to give individual maximum gratification of wants and realization of public purposes, i.e., possesses "maximum potential of humanism."

The essential condition combining the goals and psychological strategies of mental medicine is *competence* as the overall performance of human capital.

There is a tendency of mental health theoretical model replacement in some psychological models by a notion of vital competence comprising various skills. To some extent the notion of competence is neutral, but instrumental at the same time. Human activity is controlled by universal aspiration to improvement his influence over environment – the more achievements human has in concert with the environment, the higher feeling of his competence he has.

Further research of competence problem showed it as a capacity of having such behavior; by which human can maximally implement his goals equally to the situation. It is referred to the ability to apply learned behavior strategies for their effective use in surrounding world – learn to refuse using surface active agents, control alcohol ingestion, cope with hardships, etc. However, this simple and very pragmatic theory is simplification of the notions like development and human life. This unilaterality is lighten by the notions connected with competence, as for instance, *the notion of communication competence* involving empathy, need for sympathy, relaxation, aspiration for being together, aspiration for understanding the partner, business cooperation ethics.

The advantage of these concepts comprises significant subjectivity, recognition of activity as the key condition of mental health. On the basis of these approaches they create different forms of finished scenarios for training regarding healthy living and moral purpose of life.

Strategic priority of mental medicine is formation and augmentation of *human capital* characterizing by four fundamental psychological abilities (Burikova 2015):

1) *Viability* – keeping oneself and posterity in chime of healthy living and moral purpose of life.
2) *Capacity for work* – performance of certain work in required quantity and required quality. Capacity for work reflects the extent of human life energy in different fractals of professional genesis.
3) *Innovativeness* – human ability to adapt to innovations in different areas of life, changing his conscience and behavior.
4) *Learnability* – individual learning capability and self-development for the achievement of adequate goals.

The human capital state can be socially and psychometrically evaluated regarding quantity and quality with the help of dozens of various indexes in four basic abilities and individual mental ecology (Sidorov, Novikova 2014). Developing human capital requires multidisciplinary synergetic methodology and team forms of care organization.

26.2. Synergetic Psychotherapy

Huge variety of psychotherapy techniques and methods is represented in many fundamental manuals and needs no special discussion.

The multidisciplinary synergetic methodology of mental epidemiology requires reviewing of actively developing integrative psychotherapy, which is a branch of the world trend of integrative medicine.

J. C. Norcross, C. Newman (1992) singled out principal conditions promoting integrative processes in psychotherapy:

- reviewing numerous forms and methods of psychotherapy complicating selection and application;
- the inadequacy of a single method for all patients;
- the imperfection of theoretical pathogenetic paradigm;
- improvement of communication between clinicians and researchers, experimentation capabilities increase;
- psychotherapy general base processes and mechanisms search;
- the equal efficiency of treatment regardless of the method;
- the key role of relationship quality psychotherapist - patient (client) in any forms of psychotherapy;
- increasing the role of short-term and symptomatic psychotherapy;
- unification socio-economic processes;
- development of professional associations, standardization of specialist training and quality of psychotherapeutic services.

Reflection of the world integrative trend became creation in 1987 international Journal of Integrative and Eclectic Psychotherapy (JIEP), as well as numerous professional associations: International Society for the Exploration of Psychotherapy Integration (SEPI) and International Integrative Psychotherapy Association (IIPA).

Integration and combination of different ways and methods in integrative psychotherapy have been changed greatly in recent decades. If 40 years ago the most common combination was psychodynamic and behavioral, then since 90-s it is cognitive and behavioral, cognitive and humanistic, cognitive and psychoanalytic combinations. In integrative psychotherapy A. A. Aleksandrov (2009) points out the following most common forms: pathogenetic psychotherapy, Gestalt therapy, integration of cognitive, behavioral and group methods.

At the same time, according to G. L. Isurina (2012), integrative psychotherapy is a myth associated with unwillingness or impossibility of theoretical self-determination of psychotherapists and their lack of systematic training. Irving Yalom (2008) has similar point of view and he believes that psychotherapy should not be constructed on independent theories recognized for mutually exclusive diversity, but on relations, by which new psychotherapy for each new patient is creating. It appears to him that the mission of psychotherapist is that he must select personalized program for a certain patient among the huge variety of integrative psychotherapy resources.

In huge variety of therapeutic forms the modern psychotherapy cannot possibly dispose of “patrimonial damnation” concerning “equivalence paradox” - their practically equal effectiveness (Kholmogorova, 2001; Sosland 2006; Stiles et al. 1986). One of the hypotheses trying to explain this paradox is about the existence of general and nonspecific factors – a kind of "psychotherapeutic constants" responsible for health benefit (Orlov 2006; Grawe 1995). Using biofeedback tear (BFB) has confirmed that common factors of psychotherapy effectiveness are extended on any other constructive and ethical communicative context (Trunova, Orlov 2014). Thus, once again the question of psychotherapy institutionalization urgency as a scientific medical discipline was raised. In fact, the question is seen in other – in the generalization of psychological and psychotherapeutic resource on the broad interdisciplinary field of mental medicine. Modern psychotherapy has been "outgrown" from the narrow medicine or psychological bounds long ago and, having accumulated the efforts in integrative modalities, it is seeking for a new synergetic paradigm. Anything but "strange attractor" can be the multidisciplinary synergetic methodology of mental medicine establishing *synergetic psychotherapy*, which includes adaptive control of patient's or client's conscience triggering self-development mechanisms.

To all-pervading principles of synergetic psychotherapy and especially to a launching of individual self-development mechanisms in coaching one can refer Goethe's comment: "If we take people for who they are, we make them worse. If we do treat them as they are who they are meant to be, we help them to become anybody whom they can become."

26.3. Methods of Assistance to Mental Terrorism Victims and Targets

At present foreign psychologists developed some working procedures with forms of mental terrorism — cultic dependence. Since this direction of experimental psychology is extremely actualized by terrorism pandemic, it does make sense to report some of its guidelines.

26.3.1. Counseling on Mind Transformation (CMT)

This method developed by Carol and Noel Dzhiambalvo is one of the most popular and widely applied in the USA. In its character, it is a non-directive educational approach of family counseling.

Its purpose — assistance in informed decision making on the basis of supplying related information. In the course of practical application, this method showed a high degree of reliability: in 90% cases, adherent is determined to leave neo-cult, if he gives psychologists enough time for supplying information (about three days). In other cases, the result is obtained in about 60 %.

In order to conduct CMT, it is necessary for family members to keep good deep ties with the adherent. After establishing connection and team involving 3-4 psychologists and concerned family member, the procedure of CMT is taken place lasting for about three days by 12-16 hours per day. Consulting in mentality reformation includes certain stages.

Introduction of a specialist in CMT. At the very beginning of influence, family should present a psychologist to an adherent. Specialists in CMT explain to client his intentions underlying that their presence is caused by anxiety covering the whole family, which is arisen by a participation of this person in a cult.

At that, it is not denied that participation in a cult is truly a good thing. The chief goal of consultant is overview of available information resources about this sect together with adherent, but not a dispute or conviction. Client must decide by himself which influence on his life will have this information.

Hostility, denial, and dissociation. During the initial CMT phase, there is often a denial from the side of an adherent of certain facts and memories accompanied with a demonstration of obvious or latent hostility. By denial facts or memories are suppressed or reinterpreted leaving behind only unclear awareness, as long as defence mechanisms are activated.

At the moment of denial, adherents do not lie consciously — this is unconscious lies. Helping a client to acknowledge at least some insignificant lies can call in question his fundamental assumption that team members and its leader never tell lies. If adherent begins to question this assumption, he becomes capable of acknowledging other cases of lies, on which cultic culture is depending. Patience is the most effective way to get through denial. As long as adherent's understanding is increasing, his need for denial is decreasing. Perhaps, conscience control tactics established in a cult should be discussed.

Resistance. Demonstrative adherent's resistance to information provided by a specialist in CMT constitutes positive sign since by that human is just trying to escape from discussion the subject matter, but not deny it. The signs of denial usually include attempts to change the subject or nagging. By noting the presence of resistance, a consultant must continue to exert information influence.

Interest. When a client begins to ask questions regarding information being provided to him and additionally require it, this person shows interest, activates the change of relations quality: silent hostility changes to warmth, friendliness; documents are examined without compulsion, etc.

Participation. This stage is characterized by complex interest. Now adherent does not only equire but also provides information about destructive group activities. He might be still not agreeing with specialists in CMT, but now he does not spit at them.

At this stage client is already involved in searching for the truth, but not only answer to psychologists' information. He finds the ability to look at the events from different perspectives and conceives that cult position is only one of them. This change has crucial character.

Interconnection. When adherent starts to relate snippets of information — it is a reflection of the fact that CMT process is moving successfully and positively.

The client begins not only notice all pros and cons, but estimate and compare them, and begins to create logical, independently chosen and based on awareness point of view, which is a signal of success. The client starts to think independently. Adherents having long "standing" are disposed to react on information faster than specialists in CMT do because they have had some opportunities to see "the dark" sides of a cult. Individuals who joined an organization not long ago, often hardly identify reliability of the information provided for them because this seems incompatible with their experience.

The signs of interconnection include:

- literal perception of the outside world and presence and legality recognition of various opinions;

- understanding of destructive cult manipulative influence as the reason of desadaptive attitudes formation;
- spontaneous and voluntary examples provision of the mind control in a group;
- recognition and acceptance of the moments of denial, resistance and dissociation;
- perception of cultic groups alternatives in the capacity of real choice, which client can make.

When client demonstrates such understanding and behavior, leaving the cult becomes not improbable. Psychologists must respect any choice. If a person prefers to stay in a group, the psychologist shall remind him and his family, that now they have knowledge, which can be used for strengthening his autonomy and improvement of family relations. If, in contrast, a client has decided to leave the cultic group, which happens in most cases, specialist in CMT provides him information about the resources which can help him.

26.3.2. Strategic Cooperation Approach (SCA)

The author of this approach is American consulting psychologist Steven Hassan. SCA is a form of behaviorally oriented family counseling using neuro-linguistic programming methods, Erickson hypnosis and role-playing games, which is designed to help victims of destructive mind control to freedom from cultic dependence and fulfill correction of cultic traumas.

It is focused on the process of change since it is more important how people have come to this change than what or how they have changed. It stipulates lots of psycho-technics focused on encouragement of psychological changes in a client's mind. Along with active use of psycho-technics, S. Hassan uses widely supplying information about the theory and real activity of any cult. The basic principles of SCA are the following:

1. People need and want to develop.
2. Concentration on situation "right here, right now." The client is induced to focus his attention not on any erroneous actions in the past, but at what he can do in the present. The past is useful only when it provides information, which is useful in the present time.
3. A human being always chooses what he thinks is best at this moment. Cult members permit to be brainwashed because they believe in good intentions of the group.
4. Each client and each situation are unique in its way. Consultant's work involves human understanding: what he appreciates, what he needs, what he wants and how he thinks. Psychologist needs to empathically understand the client in order to help him to implement the will of his personality — leave manipulative, destructive cultic group.
5. Focusing on family. Family members and friends are essential for the most successful cases. They can be taught the ways of maximum effective communication with cult participant through the role-playing games acquiring additional leverage to achieve adherent's collaboration. When family members know how to engage

substantively, they do a lot of things to help individual get out of the group. During the influence this factor often turns out to be crucial.

According to S. Hassan (2001) psychologist's work involves assisting adherent to realize four things:

1. He is in a trap.
2. He did not choose to be trapped actually (i.e., didn not give informed consent to it).
3. Other people in cults are in the same situation.
4. He can get out of the trap.

Regarding the four listed items, psychologist applying SCA should not try to force adherent to get out of the group, his mission — help to see different choices.

SCA procedure. First of all, strategic cooperation team building is taken place there. Besides client's family members it must consist of former participants of the cult he participates in, priest of the confession his family belongs to if they are religious, and psychologist.

SCA is a quite structured process having a certain subject, beginning, middle and the end, which are its required elements. Team members are introduced to the client according to the plan, which can frequently be changed depending on the needs arising during the process. People participating in strategic cooperation team take a break at their work for the duration of influence putting aside the trivial round and give adherent to understand that he is a man of importance for them, and his problem needs immediate solving. It is of first importance for team members that at the time of carrying out SCA procedure they have already established a positive relationship with adherent achieved in the course of the former mini interactions.

The reason for SCA positive results is that cultic mind control never achieves complete success in deleting initial human ego dictating prevailing cultic personality, which always suppresses him. Successful communication establishment with personality center does allow psychologist achieve positive results. In most cases people decide to get out of the cults. However, it should be understood, that this will not solve all the problems since former adherents require long course of rehabilitation. They need vocational assistance of psychologists and acceptance on the part of relatives.

26.3.3 Behavioral Training in Extremal Situations

The training developed by a group of authors (Reshetnikov 1990, Mockshantsev 2001; Nikiphorov 2003) is designed for acquiring ability to act in an extremal situation, reveal constructive and destructive patterns of behavior, learn to solve problems, take responsibility, as well as learning to analyze his behavior and problems of group interaction.

Holding duration is 2 hours. The holding of this exercise must comply with all training rules.

"The Shipwreck" Game. The aim of the game is to form communication skills in extremal situations; reveal constructive and destructive patterns of behavior.

A host would inform that a party of tourists 15 strong, which went by sea, suffered a shipwreck and was on a boat at the moment. In about 15 min a storm would arise, and victims would be able to survive only in the case if there was one person left in a boat. If there were 2-3 persons left, they all would also die, because the remaining people would be not enough for rowing. Under the terms of the game nobody can swim after the boat holding on its side – in this case everybody will die. If there is a person who leaves the boat as the game progresses, he will step beyond the limits of the playing room and should not come back before the announcement of results.

The host would announce the start of the game. He would inform “the victims” about the time left before the storm arose from time to time. In 15 minutes sharp the host would announce results of the game — either everybody was saved except one person or everybody died.

Discussion: conducted by an exchange of impressions, opinions, experiences, feelings. Dominant strategies of victims’ behavior would be analyzed — constructive or destructive.

“The Wall” Game. The aim of the game: self-examination in extremal situation. The task: imagine that a person walks over the long road and suddenly bumps into the wall. Going round the wall is impossible: the wall is endless.

Try to render, jumping over it is impossible too, the wall is too high. What is to be done?

In the course of the discussion one should reply to the question: what would feel a person who turned out to be in an unsolvable extremal situation?

“The Desert Island” Game. The aim of the game is to learn to solve problems in the extremal situations, actualize constructive interaction facilities, take responsibility, use group support, and train ability to suffer misfortunes and loss, as well as to spur the process of self-development.

The host would announce that the group (10-15 persons) by virtue of emergency circumstances found itself planted on a desert island in the tropics. By that time people in distress would already have nothing left, even reliable life preservers. The participant would be given a broadsheet, a box of plasticine, felt-tip pens. He needs to draw landing on the island, and then sculpt “himself” from plasticine and shelter on specified integrated space of the island. The host explains that the next 20 year the group is not fated to meet other people or sail away the island, i.e., they need to start a new life. The host can supplement “the life” of the participant with events: heavy shower destroyed something, illnesses began, etc., adjusting team development indirectly.

Discussion: conducted using analysis adaptation in the most difficult, first days of life on the island.

For an estimate of training efficiency it must be taken a test “Ability to function in strained circumstances.”

Thus, psychological techniques and exercises covered by this section are focused on individual sensitivity reduction to those psycho-traumatic objects and situations, which cause different appellative reactions of individual.

Behavioral training, consulting in mentality reformation — a method developed by Carol and Noel Dzhiambalvo, and strategic cooperation approach, the author of which is American consulting psychologist S. Hassan — are the most popular and effective processing techniques for cultic dependence and behavior in extremal situations within the modern crisis reality.

Chapter 27

Social Resources of Mental Medicine

27.1. Sociosynergetic Methodology

Social work in Russia has a long history. In 1701, Peter I issued a decree on establishing almshouses for the poor, sick and elderly at the Holiest Patriarch premises. This decree regulated the provision of social care to the abovementioned population groups.

Social work represents professional activities directed at the people who are in need of social care, support and social services. It is provided by both state and non-state services and includes the combination of social services and various medicosocial, psychosocial, sociopedagogical, social welfare and legal individual, family, social group and community support in problematic, crisis, critical and stressful situations and conditions. The services provided to protect and recover citizens' welfare are defined as social and humanitarian services. Social care practice has been for a long time dominated by paternalist approaches focused on specific forms of aid and foster care (financial, organizational, medical, etc.) whose subject was benefiting by obtaining particular assistance.

Social work in mental medicine has a range of differences when compared to general social work. The additional requirements and features of providing social care to psychosomatic, mental and narcological patients are as follows:

- despite the principle of distancing oneself from the mental disorders of a patient/client the medicosocial work is related to the clinical picture of the disease and its sequelae;
- the content of the social care *varies* at *different* stages of the disease, and it depends on the patients' age, personal traits and individual reaction to the existing condition;
- social work bears particular therapeutic energy since it is directed at changing the patient himself as well as his relations with the surroundings;
- social work should encourage the development of such qualities as being responsible for one's life and destiny along with social competency among the patients.

Social work in mental medicine is part of the overall social work which understands, accepts and assists the client together with his surroundings.

The American social work practice includes the following system-based classification:

1. Such a complex approach allows accessing the overall problematic *The system of change conductors* – agency social workers who function as direct assistants for their clients providing changes in their conscience, behavior and relations with the microenvironment after a thorough analysis of the situation and its causes.
2. *The system of clientele* – people who addressed a social employee with a request to solve their problems and difficulties and made a contract or a verbal agreement with him to cooperate in the discussion and possible solution of the created situation.
3. *The system of targets* – people who are the target of the influence.
4. *The system of action* – people who joined to influence the system of targets.

Such a complex approach allows to assess the overall problematic situation extensionally, to identify the position of the client himself in this situation and the real targets of the influence directed at the positive dynamics of the situation, particular ways, types, methods and action procedures. A detailed action plan is created. “Short-range” and “long-range” work perspectives, direction and order of actions are determined, etc.

The main *methodological principles* of social work in mental medicine consider the following conceptual provisions:

- Mental diseases have different causes, onsets and sequelae. Thus, social work is an important component in the biopsychosociospiritual model of assistance.
- Diagnostics, treatment, rehabilitation and prevention of mental diseases are inseparably linked with the social context of the disease and the lifestyle.
- Social work is directed at the mobilization of human strengths to improve personal relations with the social network. The working place of the social work specialist is not just a hospital or a dispensary but a school, a family, a group of teenagers i.e., the society.

The complex approach which revealed a general perspective for the specialists who practice in various areas of specific social work was particularly implemented in the ecosystem method. The implementation of this approach in mental medicine suggests the consideration of human relations with the environment from socio-functional viewpoints. At the same time, the possibilities of human adaptation to the conditions of existence are precisely analyzed and forecast. The main task of applying the ecosystem method is to establish interlinks between individual variable elements whose combination creates a clinical situation. Such a system analysis is used as a basis for a plan of appropriate actions taken by a social worker, a client and all the interested parties.

The key task of a social worker in a multidisciplinary team is to form a *social diagnosis* which reflects personal social resources and social identity features. The social diagnosis includes characteristics of social competency and an individual’s external social resources (Kotsyubinsky et al. 2013). The concept of social competency includes the potential abilities of a person to effectively interact with the social setting (Schroder et al. 1978). Weakening or disorder of the social competency results in the exclusion of mentally ill people from the production field and their loss of social links. When defining a social diagnosis, it is necessary to consider the dynamics of social competency of the patients during the premorbid stage and at this moment as well as the presence and features of interpersonal conflicts in the family, at work, in partner relations and other activity fields. The social diagnosis should also reflect external social resources related to the characteristics of family's social potential and referential mesosocium.

"The social diagnosis" must reflect psychosocial and surroundings-related problems of patients and clients in the most detailed and comprehensive way: family and individually significant surroundings-related problems, problems related to education, vocational occupation, accommodation and law-enforcing bodies.

Differentiation of social work practicing specialists is also based on the "clinicians"/"generalists" dichotomy. "Clinicians" perform specific direct tasks while using a particular set of psychological and psychotherapeutic methods. "Generalists" deal with individuals, families and population groups but do not restrict themselves to specific fields of work. They constantly engage in analytical, administrative and scientific activities.

Social problems of mental medicine can be classified into problems that cause and form disorders at the preclinical and clinical stages as well as the secondary problems which are the result of main disease complications.

Social work in mental medicine must be particularly directed at the improvement of the psychosocial climate of the multidisciplinary medical team where a doctor, a nurse, a social worker, a psychologist and a bioethics specialist are working.

The introduction of synergetics into social work was developed as a *socio-synergetic approach* characterized by the following main conceptual provisions (Yaskevich et al. 2007; Kotelnikov, Rudychev 2012; Nikulina 2012; Sidorov 2015).

1. In the context of general sociological theory, the society is viewed in the dynamics of organic unity and coevolutional development with nature.
2. The effectiveness of theoretical and methodological synergetics principle extrapolation upon the society is recognized.
3. The analysis of dynamic social system conditions is supported by nonlinear thinking principles with the use of attractive and dissipative bifurcation and interactive processes and evolution models.
4. The procedures for sociometric and empirical testing of perspective ideas and hypotheses about social evolution and partnership are elaborated.
5. The entire system of indices, measurement scales and indicators based on the evaluation of the system, its reliability, nonlinearity and the prevalence of regularity or chaos in it is laid in the foundation of qualitatively new methods and means of social diagnostics and analysis as well as sociogenesis evaluation and forecasting.
6. It considers the multidimensional trajectory dynamics of the developing condition or disease, a social process or epidemic depending on the proximity to bifurcation points, location within or outside the attractor zone, the nature of fractality element dissipation and configuration.

The integrating synergetic paradigm of all the rehabilitation programs related to social work in mental medicine is the concept of social support.

The following functional types of social support are distinguished:

a. *based on the direction* – received support, perceived support and enacted support;

b. *based on the content* – emotional (esteem, emotional, expressive support), instrumental (instrumental, practical, tangible, material support), information and appraisal (appraisal support);
c. *based on the sources* – family, educational, friendly, social and state;
d. *based on the place and type of communication* – consultative, ambulatory, stationary and interactive.

The effectiveness appraisal of the social support is performed according to the following main parameters:

a. the level of adaptation in the social system, the development of social competency, educational and professional achievements, the formation of individual human and social capital;
b. quality of life and individual psychic well-being, the ability to handle stress and to cope with its consequences;
c. rate and an amount of personal development potential actualization (Lifintsev et al. 2014).

The perception of social support is determined as the difference between the recipient's self-appraisal of the received support and the appraisal of this support by others. It is particularly important that the individual be satisfied and confident about the compensation of the perceived lack of understanding, information, feedback and other resources required for development and recovery. Rapid formation of diseases occurs against the background of chronic and often difficult to predict stresses of today's life along with the poorly developed mechanisms of coping. According to the research, the socially supporting process for mentally ill patients is characterized by the functioning of disintegrated and breaking apart social networks of "family," "friends" and "other valuables" which does not secure the patient's need for social support. For this reason the primary task of social work in mental medicine is formed by the normalization of the socially supporting process, where possible, or the shaping of new socially supporting networks.

27.2. Risk Assessment in Sociogenesis

The objects of system mental health monitoring are the social factors and the conditions of mental disease development which play the leading role in the prenosological fractals and are available for early prevention and correction.

Four degrees of *causative complexes* can be distinguished at the maximum level of generalization of mental disease sociogenesis: macrosocial level including the features of social and economic situation in the country as well as the social politics of the state; mesosocial level including the features of professional activities, psychological and moral climate of occupational/educational team or an informal youth group; millisocial level including the features of customs, traditions and lifestyle of the family as a particularly significant institute of personal socialization; microsocial or individual level including the features of predominantly moral valuing and motivation setting fields.

Macrosocial level

- Normative anomy and permissiveness.
- Dehumanization and demoralization of the society.
- The deep socioeconomic crisis with growing unemployment, inflation, non-payments, homelessness and a wave of strikes.
- Constitutional breaches and the exhaustion of legal state regulation mechanisms.
- Loss of previous ideology which is not compensated by forming a new ideological concept of most postsocialistic country development.
- Loss of trust in the management among the population, alienation and impoverishment of the people, deformation of public relations.
- The rise of nationalism and separatism, aggravation of contradictions between national cultures and religions.
- "Hysterodemonic renaissance" with a broad expansion of totalitarian sects and asocial ideologies.
- Long interstate conflicts and local, regional wars which cause posttraumatic stress-related diseases among combatants, refugees and migrants.
- The growth of crime and corruption, prostitution and suicides, asocial and amoral behavior.
- Life urbanization and spreading of socio-stressful situations, collapse of agriculture.
- Aggravation of contradictions between social groups, an increasing gap between the rich and the poor (alcoholism and drug addiction "caused by poverty" and "caused by satiety"), a nominal presence of the middle class.
- Devaluation of traditional national values, the breakdown of the material base of culture, leisure, education and science.
- Non-effective state anti-alcoholic and anti-drug politics, the collapse of the narcological service, the wide availability of alcohol, drugs and toxicants, closing up anti-alcoholic and anti-drug propaganda.
- Aggressive pressure and extended reproduction of legal alcoholic and illegal drug industry.

Mesosocial level

- The atmosphere of tolerance and lenience towards alcoholization and narcotization; asocial behavioral stereotypes and a deviant lifestyle among the referential surroundings, drinking traditions and customs, alcohol-related stereotypes of everyday communication and pastime.
- Asocial environment and a shortage of social stimulation, fashion and behavior style within the environment of alcoholization and narcotization.
- Neglecting work and education, delinquency, situation dependence, conformal and passive behavior, conflicts with teachers and disadaptation at school, socialization breakdowns and difficulties in adaptation to the new social environment.
- Loss of the socializing military service role and non-regulated relations in the army.

- Hard manual labor lacking any creative intentions; introducing iatrogenic addiction mechanisms as a result of irresponsibility among doctors.
- The disproportion of free time between men and women which encourages dissociation of interests.
- Demographic imbalance of male and female population – particularly, in remote rural areas.

Millisocial level

- Breakdown of family structure and function.
- Low educational and cultural level of parents.
- Wrong upbringing, negative psychological climate and alienation within the family.
- Leaving home and vagrancy.
- Poor living conditions and low family incomes.
- Weak social control and low legal family culture.

Microsocial level

- Social deprivation, low level of general culture and personal social development, narrow scope and instability of interests, the absence of passions and spiritual demands.
- The uncertainty of professional orientation, the absence of socially significant aims including the ones related to working activities.
- Low degree of pretension and shortage of behavior motivation, breaking away from responsible situations and decisions.
- Loss of life perspective and the vision of personal development paths; introversion and low sustainability against negative emotions.
- Irresponsibility and immaturity, opposition and tension, concern and fear.
- Excess curiosity and unawareness of alcohol and drug-related harm.
- Susceptibility and petulance, selfishness and emotional-volitional instability.
- Hedonistic aspirations and a consumer attitude towards life.
- Inability to follow organized and consistent activities.
- Lack of moral sense development and instability of personal relations.
- Preferred orientation towards contemporaries rather than the family.
- Erosion of substantive human qualities – decency and honesty.
- The inclination to the non-recognition of authorities, opposition and aggressiveness. Sometimes, the expression of timidity, realizing one's inferiority and insufficiency, inability to cope with difficulties, a disposition to seclusion and solving one's problems in a "chemical way."
- Inadequate self-appraisal and immature mechanisms of defense.

The variety of factors and conditions in sociogenesis of mental diseases and addictive behavior is appropriate to appraise within the scope of *dialectics of casualty and necessity.* Of course, a casualty cannot change a many-sided and multiple-factor human destiny. However, even what seems to be occasional today may turn out to be the destiny tomorrow.

The mentioned nonspecific factors and conditions reduce the threshold of personal biopsychosociomental adaptation, enhancing his sensitivity to any pathogenic phenomena. They are the main characteristics of the "group of risk" which is the key subject of addiction and other epidemic mental disease sociogenesis.

27.3. Partnership in Social Therapy and Rehabilitation

During the mental outbreaks of psychosomatic and mental diseases social rehabilitation plays an important role. Correctly arranged actions determine both the patient's disablement prevention and the society's humanization. Rehabilitation work should take into account not only the changes in mentality caused by an epidemic disease but also the elements of moral and spiritual as well as emotionally personal life, social identity and intellectual activities which remain to be preserved.

The effectiveness of social rehabilitation of the ill to a great extent depends on their willingness to cooperate, their desire and abilities to accurately follow the recommendations of the attending physician and the social worker. It is impossible to plan the scope and nature of socio-preventive actions properly without considering the social-psychological characteristics of the ill and their attitude to the disease. The interaction between the team and the patient influences all the aspects of the patient's life – his social, somatic, psychological and moral health. Compliance and patients' motivation towards rehabilitation play a critical role.

In recent years, group forms of work are used more often. Among those the most popular ones are *groups on training and self-assistance.* The most well-known ones are the training groups for DM, AH, BA and CHD.

For those ill who had myocardial infarction functioning of the *"Coronary club"* can be of great benefit. Its way of operation includes lecturing/discussions with the purpose of informing the patients about the disease and the risk factors as well as the psychotherapeutic effect (auto training, hypno-suggestive therapy, art therapy).

Methodology of the *"School for the ill who had coronary artery bypass graft surgery"* is directed at the correction of patients' mindset resources and the enhancement of their motivation towards the fulfillment of the medical recommendations.

Creating social-psychological *"Asthma clubs"* turned out to be helpful. There patients and their family members are provided with necessary information as well as develop skills of self-control and the abilities to regulate one's medical treatment according to the plan elaborated together with the physician.

The educational *"School for AH patients"* program plan includes the following subjects: some aspects of anatomy and physiology of cardiovascular system; current knowledge about causes of AH development and progress; main principles of AH treatment; AH treatment specifics for people with concomitant pathology and at elderly age; AH prevention. The training is provided by a cardiologist and a psychotherapist.

The program of the Saint-Vincent declaration about the improvement of support offered to DM patients includes some socio-psychological aspects such as: improving the quality of communication with patients, protecting the patient's self-esteem, tracking individual needs, supporting motivation for self-control, controlling the psychological quality of life, assisting medical staff with the organization of the effective joint cooperation (Dedov, Shestakova 2011).

Using educational programs at *"School of diabetes"* alters the patients' life-purpose attitudes which later improves emotional criteria, encourages the preservation of carbohydrate metabolism compensation with DM1 and enhances the patients' compliance.

In recent years, great attention has been paid to elaborating new patient rehabilitation approaches based on self-assistance, rehabilitation concept and psychotherapeutic aspects. For example, new approaches developed for supporting and rehabilitating psychosomatic patients – such as *psychosomatic integrative support and psychosomatic rehabilitation.* These include a system of measures which consider socio-psychological features of psychosomatic patients (Schermann et al. 2002; Rother, Nickel 2002; Sivik, Schoenfeld 2002; Schulz, Koch 2002).

In the past psychiatric support users including the patients and their relatives were regarded as exclusively passive participants. Today the users are becoming a legitimate and an important partner of the professionals in the implementation of the holistic approach to psychiatric support. In the *USA*, for example, there are functioning groups and organizations that represent a large network of self-assistance and family support of those who suffer from schizophrenia, depression, alcoholism, drug abuse and other mental diseases. "National Mental Health Consumers Association" (NMHCA) which was formed by the social groups "Network Against Psychiatric Assault" (NAPA) and "Mental Patients Liberation Front" (MPLF). The largest social organization "National Alliance on Mental Illness" (NAMI) which comprises more than 1.5 thousands of subsidiaries and branches.

The functioning organizations in *Canada* include "Canadian Friends of Schizophrenics" (CFS), "Schizophrenia Society of Alberta" (CAS), "Mood Disorders Association of British Columbia" (MDABC) and dozens of others.

"The national association of schizophrenia patients" (NSE), and "The Association of schizophrenia patients in Ireland" (SAI) successfully function in *Great Britain*. In *Australia*, this is done by "Schizophrenia Fellowship" (SF).

Similar organizations function in most European countries – the WArK association of mental patients' relatives in *Germany*, the organization of users in *the Netherlands*; three large associations which unite families, friends and patients in *France* (UNAFAM, UNAPEI, ENAPPS). The European organization of users and ex-patients is the ENUSP – European Network of (ex-) Users and Survivors of Psychiatry.

The main areas of these organizations' activities are as follows (Saraceno 2004):

1. Information support and educational programs.
2. Assistance with employment, family and domestic issues.
3. Publishing magazines, newspapers and electronic resources.
4. Coping with stigmatization and stereotypes of public opinion.
5. Organizing conferences and seminars.
6. Efforts made to observe the rights of mentally ill people.
7. Psychiatric support quality control and monitoring.

An important element of social rehabilitation of the mentally ill are the “Club houses” created in the USA and all the European countries. These houses perform the following tasks:

1. Organizing joint leisure.
2. Social support.
3. Involving into active social life.
4. Renting accommodation.
5. Social skills training.
6. Providing services.
7. Occupational rehabilitation (Bauer et al. 2001)

The patients who participate in social rehabilitation programs of “Club houses” are hospitalized at psychiatric departments quite more rarely. They are distinguished by a large number of social contacts, successful employment and minimization of psychopathologic signs (Rappaport et al. 1985).

It is not random that the users attend every WHO international conference about the issues of psychiatric help improvement as equal participants (Sartorius N., 2004).

The movement for social integration into a community of people who are mentally disabled is based on the experience of a broader movement for the rights of the disabled. Such activities have the following effectiveness criteria:

1. Partnership and control on the part of the users.
2. Commitment to social reintegration.
3. Supporting social surrounding resources (Carling 2001).

Social forms of support and care provided to mentally ill people in Russia began to develop extensively from the beginning of the 90s. This was taking place at the same time as issuing the Federal Law of the Russian Federation about psychiatric support and guaranteeing citizens’ rights when providing such support. During this period the first organizations of patients and their relatives emerged in Moscow and Leningrad (“Trust and light,” “Compassion,” “NIMB,” etc.). Today scores of such organizations exist in every large city (Yastrebov 2014). In 2006, a Community Council of Russian psychiatry voluntary sector was created under the jurisdiction of the head mental specialist of the Russian Health Ministry. In 2001 the Russian society of mental specialists established the All-Russian public organization of mentally ill patients and their relatives named “New opportunities.”

Despite the declared principle of partnership, the professional attitude towards the activities of users’ public organizations remains reserved. For example, according to the results of the survey conducted by V. Y. Yastrebov and O. A. Mitina (2013) among the staff of psychiatric institutions in four territorial entities of the Russian Federation nearly 92% of the respondents expressed a skeptical opinion about the effectiveness of such organizations.

O. V. Limankin (2013) surveyed about 500 employees of psychiatric institutions in Saint Petersburg and 100 users regarding the condition of psychiatric support and its development perspectives. Most professionals (56%) named the partner model as the acceptable one. Another 15% chose the client model. However, 22 % confirmed their commitment to the paternalistic model and 7 % could not provide a reply. When questioned about the participation of patients and their relatives in psychiatric support monitoring 63% of the respondents answered positively, 25% answered negatively, and 12% could not provide a reply. The performance of users' public organizations was appraised positively by 13% of the professionals, 43 % provided a neutral appraisal, 22 % provided a negative appraisal, and 22 % could not provide a reply.

Unfortunately, the overwhelming majority of survey participants were virtually not informed about the performance of public organizations of the ill and their relatives. Informing and educating the professional community about such issues with a further repeated survey could demonstrate the quality of professional conscience resilience, coping with negative stereotypes and stigmatization rigidity.

Therefore, today the programs of medico-psychosociospiritual support provided to psychic and psychosomatic patients are actual and popular. These programs include diagnostic, treatment and rehabilitation stages. The clinical field of mental medicine and epidemiology is much broader. The techniques tested on groups of patients with various mental diseases are now actively applied to strengthen the clients' mental health.

Chapter 28

Spiritual and Moral Resources of Mental Medicine

28.1. Ethical Basis of Mental Health

The spiritual and moral component is presented in all definitions of the mental health (WHO) as the ethics in business communication, as well as civil-political and moral-patriotic appeal "to contribute to the development of society." That is why it is important to consider the ethical and psychological basis of mental health, requiring organizational and functional, operational and instrumental formatting of synergetic mental health service.

Psychology of morality until recently did not belong to the priority areas of psychological research. Its relevance started to increase in proportion to the importance of its subject - the ethical issues of modern society and the individual, which is traditionally associated with globalization and secularization, science, technology and the information revolution, pluralization and individualism. *The global crisis showed the exhaustion of the previous socio-economic model* of market development and demanded a radical review of the role and place of cultural-humanitarian, spiritual and moral foundations of modern civilization trends of postindustrial society.

The traditional role of morality consists in the regulation of human behavior. Modern Russian society is characterized by the coexistence and confrontation of different morality systems or morals. Discrepancies and contradictions are related to the estimates of the moral acceptability of the death penalty and abortion, euthanasia and cloning, a combination of individual freedom and its responsibility to society. At the maximum level of generalization it appears in the *sejunction (schisis) and the desire for isolation or autonomy (autism) of public conscience, creating a "clinical" picture of the self-destructive "schizophrenic society."* The spiritual and moral field has become a supplier of an entire generation of new syndromes: battered wives and child abuse, mobbing and demoralization, destructive professiogenesis and social stress disorders. Such a radical expansion of the nosocentric boundaries of traditional psychiatry led to the mobilization of a multidisciplinary synergetic methodology and to the birth of mental medicine as a unified theory to strengthen mental health and treatment of mental illnesses.

The multidisciplinary demand of ethical categories required distinguishing the concepts of moral and morality. Thus, V. V. Znakov (2011) notes that in foreign psychology a concept of "moral" essentially absorbed the concept of "morality": there is a research field as moral psychology, but morality psychology is practically missing.

As for the national psychology, V. V. Znakov highlights two points there. According to the first point, the interpretation of the category of "morality" includes the category of "moral." The second point takes moral to the form of public conscience and morality - to a specific subject. In other words, the *moral is "localized" at the level of society and morality is the product of its adoption and assimilation by personality.* In the synergetic methodology of mental medicine, it reveals animogenetic mechanisms for the development of mental and social epidemics, from alcoholism and drug addiction to fanaticism and terrorism.

As referred to A. L. Zhuravlev and A. V. Yurevich (2013), this is where the problems of *moral socialization*, dictating the urgent need to distinguish these categories, are clearly indicated. Modern society is pluralistic in moral relation and unlike traditional socium is characterized not by any single unambiguously dominant moral (Christian, Communist, etc.), but the coexistence of different morals, which is manifested in the mentality multimodal options. The so-called "universal" (Christian or Muslim) moral is also an abstraction, different personalities are focused on different moral standards, which are transferred at the level of individual morality, and it creates very diverse and poorly predictable results, creating the phenomenology of mental medicine.

The specific features of the Russian moral socialization differ greatly. If in the Western countries it manifests mainly through the imitation of socially accepted norms and laws (the second stage of moral socialization according to L. Kohlberg). Among our fellow citizens, there is a "jamming" at the first stage where obedience is mediated by fear of punishment or it "jumps" to the third stage, based on the highest ethical principles and conscience.

Russian researchers of psychological problems of moral and morality are looking for guidance, based on one of three conceptual bases: 1) *existential-humanistic psychology* (A. Maslow, G. Allport, C. Rogers, V. Frankl and others.); 2) the *Christian religion* and the surveys of national philosophers of the beginning of the XX century (V. S. Solovyov, I. A. Ilyin, N. A. Berdyaev, M. M. Bakhtin, N. O. Lossky, G. I. Gurdjieff and others); 3) *sociobiology* (D. S. Wilson, R. Dawkins). According to I. A. Mironenko (2010), "each of these three areas appeared in the Russian science as a kind of protest against the Marxist sociocentric paradigm that prevailed in the previous period," and "a common space, the intersection of ethics and psychology is relevant to the others as self-worth." No coincidence that this feature is a key to the syndrome of demoralization, which provides the basis of animogenesis of mental and social ailments (Sidorov 2014).

Close approaches to understanding the morality matrices of behavior are offered by the Protoiereus Vadim Leonov (2013), who considered ideas about the mental health of a person due to his morality state. In the Old Testament period, the health was understood "as compliance with the habitual norms, and human conditions." In the New Testament, human health is revealed as a spiritual and moral category. Jesus Christ says that the basis of human diseases is a sin, so the true striving to health is inextricably linked to the struggle against sin and desire for righteousness.

The author identified *three main approaches to understanding the moral foundations of human behavior,* prevailing in European philosophy and psychology. In the *first case,* the human morality has subjective grounds and is regarded as a "cultural and ethical experience, passed down from generation to generation, as a product of the social evolution of man." *In the second concept,* the moral behavior is derived from its nature: "Morality is genetically inherent in man, that is, there is a kind of morals organ." *In the third case*, morality - it is the law of life, which is as real as the principles of the physical world.

In Orthodoxy, the morality is understood as a manifestation of God's image, inherent in every human being. Because God is holy and every person strives for holiness, so that "virtuous life - is the natural state of man, and sinful life is undernatural." Striving to moral behavior is ontogenetic characteristics of any person. As far as the image of God in man can be darkened by sin, the moral aspirations can be suppressed, distorted, directed toward the false targets. It explains the difference between the ethical systems in the unity of human nature. From a theological point of view, the *first approach* is incomplete and creates the illusion that human morality is variable, following the culture and can be artificially incorporated into the context of certain socio-political goals. The *second approach* also has disadvantages. Assuming the existence of a moral organ in the human, it is difficult to resist the temptation and not learn how to manage, for example, to treat neuroses, often arising from the torment of conscience. A *third approach* focuses on the elucidation of the essence of the moral laws for the subsequent implementation of them for the true good of man. From a theological point, this approach seems the most promising and useful to strengthen mental health.

Virtually all researchers note the *need to distinguish and organize the relevant sections of psychology science - the ethic psychology, moral psychology, morality psychology, moral and spiritual psychology.* As part of this trend, the "Ethical psychiatry," passing on the synergistic biopsychosociospiritual methodology, becomes a chapter of mental medicine.

The moral state of the modern Russian society gets a depressing assessment. "The destruction of values and moral principles, traditions, existing common moral led to the moralization (or demoralization, auth.) of the society under the slogan of "enrichment" and "tolerance" (including imported vices relating to perestroika-like homosexuality, usury), "- V. E. Semenov (2011).

A. V. Yurevich and D. V. Ushakov (2010) demonstrate the *moral condition of Russia* with quantitative indicators such as the 1st place of our country in Europe and the CIS in the number of murders per 100 000 inhabitants; 2nd place in the number of street children; 1st place among the countries with economies in transition to the Gini index, which expresses the unequal distribution of income; 146th position in the world out of 180 on the index of corruption, and so on. Terrifying are the data that every year we have 2 thousand children, who become victims of murders and get serious body injury; 2 million children suffer from the cruelty of parents and 50 thousand run away from home; 25 thousand minors get lost; 5 thousand women die from beatings, inflicted by their husbands; violence against women, the elderly parents and children is fixed in one in four families; 12% of teenagers use drugs; more than 20% of child pornography, distributed worldwide, is filmed in our country; about 40 thousand school-age children do not attend school; child and adolescent "social bottom" covers at least 4 million people; the growth rate of juvenile crime is 15 times ahead of the overall rate of increase in crime; in modern Russia there are about 50 thousand juvenile prisoners, that is about 3 times more than it was in the Soviet Union in the early 1930s, and so on.

Not only the scale of these phenomena oppresses but also what is more important – controlled by nobody and nothing generalization and extremalization of evil and violence, aggression and terrorism, like epidemic swept our society. At the same time, the tolerance to them is growing, provided with the efforts of the media, displacing them to the periphery of the public conscience of mainstream pop and scandalous glorification of marginal politicians, pathetic ignition of new and supernova “stars,” symbolizing only an approximation to a collapse of the “black hole” of the moral-deformed society. The *scale of the prevalence of mental destructive epidemics* from ordinary alcoholism and drug addiction to fanaticism and terrorism *require literally “moral resuscitation” social conscience.*

Among the various social groups of the modern Russian society, in which the destruction of the moral foundations is the most dramatic, a special focus is on youth. Thus, S. K. Bondyreva, G. V. Bezyuleva and D. V. Sochivko (2010) note that instability in the society generates instability and uncertainty among youth. A significant part of today’s young people do not use the categories of good and evil, morally acceptable and unacceptable, preferring concepts such as profitable-unprofitable, “cool, not cool” and so on. And according to E. Y. Strizhova (2011), approximately 85% of our young people do not see anything wrong with fraud, considering it an acceptable way of earning money.

Deficiency of spiritual ideals and unattainable overvalued level of material aspirations rise in youth a mass feeling of the meaninglessness of existence, which leads to the prevalence of various addictions. At the same time the traditional institutions of socialization - family, school, vocational education institutions and other - are losing their influence, and the resulting gaps are filled with readily available carriers of electronic information products. As a result, the characteristics of the modern Russian youth are: social immaturity and unwillingness to take responsibility for their own life, family and failures; infantile, immature position on the institution of the family; using as television and the Internet a key source of information; low interest in politics; a high level of self-confidence and intolerance, etc. All of these characteristics refer to prenosological fractals of demoralization syndrome and require the mobilization of mental preventology resources. However, researchers have concluded that it is difficult to talk about young people as a homogeneous population group, “more likely the case is about fundamentally different types of modern Russian youth within one generation” (Bondyreva et al. 2010), and youth subculture is mainly characterized for megalopolises and big cities.

“The primary cause of negative social phenomena is a violation of moral mechanisms of regulation of behavior, which are designed to create education and training. At the same time, the media and television have become the major institutions and instruments of moral degradation, creating and cultivating the characters of permissiveness and promiscuity, promoting criminal heroics, physical violence and aggression, that promote immoral behavior and aspirations and so on” - according to A. L. Zhuravlev and A. B. Kupreychenko (2010).

The conversion of the media in one of the major socializing institutions of modern Russian society is noted by V. A. Sosnin (2010), who emphasizes that they in this guise ever more visibly replace the impact of books, family, and school teachers.

O. I. Makhovskaya and F. G. Marchenko (2010) find that if you do not expose the TV to limiting psychological examination, it contributes significantly to the growth of “existential vacuum,” “when transmitted from screens norms and values are at odds with the traditional, socially and culturally enshrined in the minds of viewers.”

This expansion of the “existential vacuum” becomes a causal complex of galloping growth of vicar dependent disorders where psychological and moral emptiness is filled by hoarding, social life and fanaticism. They all begin with the spiritual and moral destruction of individual and social conscience.

As V. E. Semenov (2011) points, *"the country's infrastructure blemish operates more efficiently than all other infrastructures."*

Most of our fellow citizens, preferring immoral television shows, nevertheless at the same time are in favor of the moral control of the TV, for which 85% of respondents, among asked by V. E. Semenov are in favor of. The answer to "libera gema" of "not want - do not look" is paradoxical, but only at first glance, the formula of social conscience: "we want to look, but do not show us." This can be seen as *traditional contradictory and fatalistic Russian mentality.* The researchers are trying to associate the last characteristic with a high unpredictable variability of external, and, in particular, the climatic, conditions. Thus, the value of the harvest in Russia may change 6-7 times, and in Europe only 1.5-2 times (Goltz 2000), as well as the probability of large fires (Kleiner 2000) without mentioning corruption and crime.

Absurd and impractical are other well-known "libera gema," such as "Everything is permissive if it is not forbidden," "Prohibitions are ineffective», etc. They also destroy the moral regulation of behavior and social conscience, depriving society of bearing his spiritual and moral skeleton.

As history and synergetic methodology shows, the transition from the moral chaos of individualism to a constructive social, moral construction is only possible after passing the mandatory bifurcation points in the form of the *national idea and ideology of resonance aspirations of the population.* Historic Russian experience shows that the mobilization and consolidation of social conscience take place only at the terminal threats and challenges of national identities, when literally "The Motherland Calls!"

28.2. Spiritual and Moral Education and Development of a Person

A natural question arises - what can be opposed to militant immorality in our society and how to restore the moral principles?

The main prospects of the revival of morality are seen by A. V. Yurevich and D. V. Ushakov (2012) in the macro-social plane, offering: 1) formation in our fellow citizens of the adequate understanding of freedom, which now many of them perceive as the complete absence of prohibitions and restrictions; 2) the revival of the institutions of moral control over citizens; 3) establishment of existing in all civilized countries, not being "undemocratic" public control over the media; 4) giving the most important moral standards of the status of laws and the introduction of appropriate sanctions for their violation; 5) the decriminalization of our society and its consumer culture; 6) broad involvement of psychologists, sociologists and representatives of other related professions to the development of laws, that are not just legal norms, but are *the most general rules of social interaction.*

The need for an active legislative activity "to rein in infrastructure and promotion of vice and violence," as well as broad public initiatives for the revival of morality, in particular in the form of the creation of appropriate mass organizations, is stated by V. E. Semenov (2011). He is convinced that "a systemically important factor for working with young people, pupils and students should be spiritual and moral education," and the main "national project" now in the country is to become the project "Spiritual and moral transformation of Russia." The author regrets that "in the 1990s, the concept of "education" almost disappeared from the scope of the national education, youth policies and the media."

It is symptomatic that the thesis of A. S. Makarenko about *education as the unity of training and education* is delivered to oblivion, now displaced by the concept of "educational services," which implies a significant change in the status of the teacher, his actual reduction to the status of a waiter. It is quite natural that, as shown by Polls, obscene language on the lessons is practiced in about half of our schools, and teachers beaten by students and their parents became a common thing (Zhuravlev, Yurevich 2013). It is appropriate to recall Ivan Ilyin, who wrote: *"Training without education is a false and dangerous matter.* It creates most poorly educated people, suspicious and arrogant, conceited wranglers, energetic and unscrupulous careerists; it equips anti-spiritual force; it unleashes and encourages "the wolf" in human" (Ilyin 1956).

Many researchers offer more special, properly psychological measures to revive morality. Thus, A. V. Sukharev (2010) cites the use of the developed by him ethnofunctional method of using the images of folklore and the natural environment in order to reduce the using by youth the psychoactive substance. O. I. Makhovskaya and F. O. Marchenko (2010) describe the positive experience of TV program "Sesame Street," aimed at improving the relationship of children audience of orphans and disabled children.

It is urgent to have the reconstruction of moral education system, including the formation and development:

- *moral senses*: conscience and duty, faith and responsibility;
- *moral character*: patience and tolerance, compassion and humanism, honor and dignity, freedom and independence;
- *moral position*: the ability to distinguish between good and evil, manifestations of selfless love and friendship, willingness to overcome life's difficulties and trials, finding the meaning of life and pictures of happiness;
- *moral behavior*: readiness of serving the people and homeland, making proper moral standards of adequate and unacceptable, the formation of moral obligations and acts according to its own conscience, commitment and perseverance in achieving results, a high sense of justice and law-obedience (Danyluk et al. 2009).

Historically, the first *national educational ideal* was proposed by first Russian Academician M. V. Lomonosov: "Every selfless service for the benefit and in the strength of the Motherland shall be a measure of the meaning of life." The same, but in verse, as if about him, in one of the odes, he says: "You tried life as a time of joy. He neglected the life to the republic of success."

It is symbolic that Lomonosov completed his higher education only at the Medical Faculty in University of Marburg, which he graduated with a diploma "Master of Medicine." His canonical poetic lines about "Own Platons" sound today as a hymn to the mental health and spiritual greatness of Russia.

A. Y. Danyluk, A. M. Kondakov, V. A. Tishkov (2009) state the modern national educational ideal as follows - it is highly moral, creative, competent citizen of Russia, taking the fate of the fatherland as their own, taking responsibility for the present and future of his country, rooted in the spiritual and cultural traditions of the multinational people of the Russian Federation.

The basic principles of spiritual and moral education and development are offered:

- moral example of the teacher;
- socio-pedagogical partnership;
- individual personality development;
- integrative program of spiritual and moral education;
- social demand for education.

Description of *moral development* as a sequence of steps, starting with the self-awareness "as the beginning and end of the whole" and leading to comprehensive ethical principles, was proposed more by J. Piaget (1965) and L. Kohlberg (1981).

Bearers of basic national values are:

- family;
- cultural and religious community;
- national cultures, which components are the traditional Russian religions;
- Russian civic nation;
- the world community.

An important integral and synergistic mission in the education, social and pedagogical support of establishment and development of a highly moral, responsible, creative, proactive, competent citizen of Russia should be performed by biopsychosociospiritual mental preventology as preclinical part of mental medicine.

The NSMU (Northern State Medical University) experience has shown that there is a need for a single *Set of ethical codes of the health care system*, with a common conceptual and methodological framework and the organizational and functional tool of ethics committees practice.

The same *Set of ethical codes* is necessary for all *social service professions* regulated not only by the labor legislation but also moral obligations: health and social workers, teachers and clergy. It must be based on common principles. For example, in the Code of Ethics of the European Federation of psychoanalytic psychotherapy the following main principles are:

1) *the value of respect* and fair treatment to the identity of the client or patient;
2) *a policy of equal opportunities* and non-discrimination;
3) *social responsibility* to the client or patient;
4) *professional competence* and protection of the professional community from incompetence;
5) *informed consent*;
6) *confidentiality*;
7) *the borders* and a prohibition of the exploitation of the patient;
8) *honesty*;
9) *scientific commitments.*

In any of the codes of ethics, there must be sanctions for violation of prescribed rules until the termination of rights to engage in professional activities

28.3. An Innovative Program of Clinical Medical Ethics

A prototype of SM3 in the NSMU was created in 2000. Experience has shown the need to expand the teaching of professional ethics in all the 18 faculties of the university, that is why a new specialty "business communication" was included in the FSES of HE (The Federal State Educational Standards of Higher Education) and two editions of the federal textbook were released (Sidorov et al. 2004, 2010). In addition, ethical blocks in a series of 10 specialized books and guides were enhanced. The NSMU experience allowed justifying the need to expand the teaching of medical ethics in all clinical departments and students training in the ethics in business communication.

Today, *students of medical faculties* study biomedical ethics in the amount of 72 hours (2 units) with the task of mastering the *general cultural competencies* (GCC-8): "the ability and willingness to carry out their activities in view of socially accepted moral and legal norms, comply with the rules of medical ethics, laws and regulations on handling confidential information, maintain the patient confidentiality."

The same amount of hours is devoted to the master's degree in "Public Health," where the general cultural competence (GCC-8) is extended to "the ability and willingness to organizing of productive interaction with representatives of various segments of the population, including risk groups." In exactly the same, but the European master's program in the Arkhangelsk International School of Public Health (since 2007, certificates of the Russian Federation and Tromso University, Norway), bioethics has 2.5 times more time (180 hours / five units) with a fixation on verbal and behavioral patterns of business communication. If for professional arrangements of basic general cultural potential of these hours as part of a humanitarian cycle may be enough, then the immersion into the moral diagnosis and propedeutics requires a systematic and comprehensive participation of all departments.

The long-term educational and methodical, preventive and corrective, therapeutic rehabilitation activity showed that in medical institutions of the country in order to improve the efficiency of moral diagnosis and propedeutics, moral education of students and provide adaptive professiogenesis of medical and social, psychological and pedagogical community, the development and implementation of *"Innovative integrated block -module program of clinical medical ethics"* is required; and for non-medical universities - the ethics in business communication.

Program Global Platform - "The Universal Declaration of Bioethics and Human Rights," UNESCO (2005), the principles of which 191 states have agreed.

Program Matrix – "The Basic Training Program on Bioethics of UNESCO"

Program Objective – organization of a focused and systematic training of medical ethics in the process of continuous education and medical practice for the application of ethical principles of the "Universal Declaration of ethics and human rights."

Major objective – block-modular principle of the program to account for the specifics of stages of medical education and professional development of the target group peculiarities.

Program Blocks are defined on the basis of the definition of the target groups for medical students, nurses, graduate students, interns, residents, physicians (including participating in clinical trials of new medical products), members of ethics committees and others.

Modules are part of the blocks, and their number is determined depending on the purpose and content, as well as the target group.

The proposed program has all the hallmarks of *innovation*:

1) the existence of the invariant module - education is created, and training is organized in the framework of the enshrined in the UNESCO Declaration of Principles of Bioethics, which do not cause controversy;

2) the presence of the variable part of the program, consisting of modules, where the education and ethics in business communication can be built around specific medical problem that is solved in different ways in different countries;

3) the availability of additional modules of moral diagnosis and propaedeutics, correction and rehabilitation, the contents of which significantly expands the scope of bioethics, bringing a clinical paradigm;

4) the presence of a synergistic biopsychosociospiritual methodology of systematic monitoring of educational and working environment, social and mental health, assessing the effectiveness of the program (Starodubov, Sidorov, Vasilieva 2013).

The NSMU educational management has developed several versions of the program. So, for the FSES of HE (The Federal State Educational Standards of Higher Education) 060101.65 “Medical care” it is offered in all 954 hours / 26.5 units, incl.:

1) humanitarian, social and economic cycle (20% of labor intensity), in all

225 hours / 6.25 units:

A) basic section:

- Philosophy - 36 hours.
- Bioethics - 72 hours.
- History of Medicine - 23 hours.
- Psychology and Pedagogy - 22 hours.

B) variative section:

- Business Communication 72 hours.

2) Mathematics, Natural Sciences course (5% of the labor input), a total of 45 hours / 1.25 units:

A) basic section:

- Hominal Physiology - 12 hours.
- Pharmacology -12 hours.
- Pathoanatomy - 15 hours.

B) variative section:

- Human Ecology - 6 hours.

3) professional cycle (10% of labor input), total 684 hours / 19 units for all clinical disciplines:

A) basic section - 620 hours
B) variative section - 64 hours

For the FSES of HE (The Federal State Educational Standards of Higher Education) 060500.62 "Nursing care" it is offered in all 639 hours / 17.75 units, incl.:

1) humanitarian, social and economic cycle (20% of labour intensity), in all

144 hours / 4 units:

A) basic section:

- Philosophy - 22 hours
- Psychology - 36 hours.

B) variative section:

- History of Medicine and Nursing - 14 hours
- Medical Bioethics - 72 hours.

2) Mathematics, Natural Sciences course (5% of the labor input), a total of 45 hours / 1.25 units:

A) basic section:

- Hominal physiology - 8 hours
- Pharmacology - 6 hours
- General pathology - 8 hours

3) professional cycle (10% of labor input), total 450 hours / 12,5 units for all clinical disciplines:

- Healthy human and his environment
- Psychology in professional activity
- Pedagogy with teaching methodology
- Nursing care

A) basic section - 324 hours
B) variative section - 126 hours

The new clinical paradigm of biomedical ethics, of course, requires a broad multidisciplinary discussion, but the latest challenges and threats to public and professional conscience as surely require the mobilization of new spiritual and moral formation of resources and strengthening of the nation's mental immunity.

Only program and systematic approach can allow medical ethics, forming the ethical modality of the mentality of a doctor, an ethical diagnosis and propaedeutic of the condition of the patient, to become the new paradigm for the development of clinical practice, medical research and education.

28.4. Moral and Axiological Basics of Happiness

Studying the level of happiness of people with different moral orientation, I. V. Nekhorosheva (2013) interviewed 407 respondents, of which only 18% had *positive moral orientation*, and only 4% had high moral qualities. People with *negative moral orientation* were twice more - 36%. The remaining respondents were assigned to a group with *unexpressed moral orientation*, although half of them (45%) were formed one or two negative moral convictions - the admissibility to assign things of someone else and to take bribes (!). The reference of theft and corruption to the unexpressed moral orientation is a testament to the catastrophic moral degradation of Russian society. A proof of this is the fact that people with negative moral orientation are happier and with positive - less, especially people with high moral character. The society of happy, but immoral people have no future. That is why the spiritual and moral education and personality development become an important national priority today.

The moral psychodiagnosis effectively uses a method of forming an advanced life strategy, based on the method of value orientations of M. Rokeach and which allows direct rankings of the terminal and instrumental values of the client.

In the process of teaching of psychology and ethics in business communication, the NSMU students in the training mode master the art of "personal happiness strengthening."

1. *Harmonious distribution of time and effort,* trying to give equal time to work and our health, communication and self-development, increases resistance to stress.
2. *Creating and maintaining a good mood*, that depends only on us, and it needs to be cultivated (small daily gifts for ourselves, favorite music in the morning, funny photos on the desktop, etc.)
3. *Ability to enjoy the current situation.* As the ancient proverb: "The past is no longer, and the future might not be. Live the present." It is important to enjoy the pleasure of every, even routine moment of life.
4. *Moderation in responsibility*, which is objective and subjective. It is always important to define the boundary of that things, which in life really depend on you and to worry about the rest is meaningless.
5. *Proper planning* is required to set goals, achievement of which really depends on the person and the concrete steps to achieve them. Inflated and unattainable goals lead to a sense of failure.

6. *Communication with relatives.* Ask for help if you need it, and tell them what they mean to you.

For working in the mental preventology, we designed a multimodal "formula for happiness" and multivariate path of destiny, integrating the moral sense and a healthy lifestyle with the acronym SUNAPCE (as synapse), where S - is save and U - use N - need, A - activate, P - pay attention to, C - create. After all, synapses provide development and design of stages of mirror neurons of the cerebral cortex that are possible receptor matrices of mental representations, of which the trajectory of human destiny is created.

Save: • optimism and constructiveness • openness to novelty • criticality to the world • practicability to yourself • flexibility and plasticity • principles and beliefs • honesty and wisdom • self-esteem and self-determination • realistic expectations • faith in God, family and yourself	Use: • system strategy • resource planning • concentration on priorities • training and coaching • auxiliary materials • commitment and responsibility • persistence and consistency • caution and circumspection • judgment and prudence • goals tree as the tree of life
Need: • the joy of life • the purpose and objectives of growth • meanings and images of the future • reasons to smile and humor • methods of stress "sewage" • opportunities and new resources • time for yourself and your family • irony of stories and jokes of fate	Activate: • reserves and resources • the vision of life perspectives • perception of new challenges • love and self-respect • adaptability and tolerance • search for positive alternatives • forecasting and prediction • competence and relevance • experience for new discoveries
Pay attention to: • life is a moment - everything passes • winning is not always necessary • friendship is more important than money • envy is nonsense • self-criticism is dullness • do not advertise good things • you can not borrow time • happiness is in sensations • self-esteem is more important than the fact • your origins, parents and friends	Create: • a team of friends and supporters • yourself and your family • success without illusions • profession as a vocation • identity and mentality • spiritual immunity • on the moral foundation • positive reality • the road to the Temple under the general personal plan • trajectory of Fate according to the compass of Soul

Psychologists believe that you can become happier if you use the method of "randomized good deeds." It says every day to make a little good deed, for which nobody precisely gives praise or reward. Only then you can have a chance to feel a good hand of fate on your own shoulder...

Finally, the pursuit of happiness is possible only when you find the meaning of life and its active lifetime. Not by chance in the existential analysis of V. Frankl (1990), the principle of pleasure and hedonistic motivation are not relevant to the normative goal-setting of human aspirations. They are only the result of a side effect of achieving the goals, structuring the meaning of life:..". if there is a reason for happiness, happiness derives from it automatically and spontaneously" (p. 56). The hedonistic mental trap is in this fact, that when making happiness as the object of own desires and aspirations, a human inevitably loses sight of the reasons to create it and happiness escapes...

The most capacious and concise is a formula of self-actualization in the path of human destiny, formulated by Karl Jaspers (1991), who said: "A man becomes what he is, because of an affair, which he does as his own."

Chapter 29

Religious Resources of Mental Medicine

The systemic crisis of psychiatry updated the search for new and the redefining of the traditional conceptual and methodological approaches to improve the effectiveness of therapy. One of these areas is the spiritual and integrated care, based on the potential of both formal religious confessions and "faith without intermediaries," becoming the resource of mental medicine.

Mental medicine, which has the synergetic biopsychosociospiritual methodology, allows expanding the prenosological field and improves the implementation of religious life for the strengthening of the mental health in preventive-rehabilitative programs and treatment-rehabilitation technologies of clinical psychiatry. This methodology allows measuring the resources of the human body as a mentality biogenetic matrix; faith as a universal psychogenetic person matrix, stabilizing its structure and prioritizing lifestyle; religion as animogenetic matrix, filled with the image of God with moral and philosophical and value-ideological senses; the Church as sociogenetic component of infrastructure of society and the state.

The urgent task today is to systematize the remaining zones of tension between religion and psychiatry, as well as opportunities to overcome them in the methodology of mental medicine; review of historical and contemporary forms of religious participation in strengthening mental health and treatment of mental illnesses; the evaluation of the effectiveness of spiritually-integrated, preventive rehabilitative and treatment rehabilitation programs of mental medicine; allocation of mechanisms for the implementation of religious resource; substantiation of promising areas for further synergistic research.

29.1. Mental Health as a Canonical Religious Priority

Mental health has the important component - the spiritual and moral. Every world religion contains in its canons the compulsory care of moral and mental health, the prevention of stress and dependencies. Only a truly healthy and free person can fully develop its spirituality and humanity.

Conceptual and methodological, operational and technological resources of the world's religions were developed and perfected over the centuries. At the maximum level of generalization and regarding mental medicine, *the mission of any denomination is in the adaptive control of public conscience.* Mechanisms for implementation of the mission depend on the chosen by person perception model of reality: Orthodox or Catholic, Muslim or Jewish, etc. It is essential to note that any of these models allows a person to strive and approach the high Image and deeper Meaning of his God.

Long-term parallel attempts of the science to insert the human in the framework of certain social and ideological trends have come a long way from the model of a "social animal" to "psychosocial human" and "synergistic person," i. e. biopsychosociospiritual (Sidorov 2006, 2013). It is clear that no model or scheme can approach the diversity of human nature; it only fixes the methodological resources of time. Today, four-dimensional synergistic approach to adaptive control of public conscience can be attributed to the last approximation. It is instructive to recall that Einstein's theory of relativity was created precisely for the four-dimensional space. It is no coincidence that we have developed the *sanogenetic therapy* (Sidorov 1988) as adaptive biopsychosociospiritual control of patient's or client's conscience and it is a scientific and technological embodiment of the base multi-faith mission. Sanogenetic therapy has become the synergistic tool for mental medicine, designed to not only treat mental illnesses and strengthen the mental health but also to ensure the adaptive protection of social conscience, that is, to implement the mental paradigm of national security.

Without immersing in a huge amount of interesting studies, which reveal parallels and relationship of theology with psychology and psychotherapy, philosophy, sociology, medicine and preventative care, neurolinguistics and psychophysiology et al., we will focus only on the religious potential of tetracyclic mental medicine: somatogenesis and psychogenesis, animogeneze and sociogenesis.

Religious resource of somatogenesis is represented by multivariate *nutritional therapy*. It is Christian fasting and Muslim Ramadan, vegetarianism of Kundalini Yoga, Brahmanism and Buddhism moving. *Neuro-physiotherapy* implies tempo-rhythmological and intonation-emotional subconscious resonance tuning of social conscience arrival. Mono- and binaural psychophysiological effects of church music and choral singing, church bells and trumpets, gongs and drums harmonize the bioelectric activity of the brain.

Religious resource of psychogenesis is represented by Christian and Buddhist, Muslim and Jewish, and other *psychologies and psychotherapies* (hundreds of types and methods). Huge multi-faith prayer and meditation experience, practices of inspired sermon facilitate and purify the confession soul. Variety of appeals to God launches the interactive mechanisms of the internal dialogue.

Religious resource of animogenesis is represented by moral and value understanding of Christian duty in the spirit of the Holy Gospel, the Muslim duty in the spirit of the Quran, the Jewish duty in the spirit of the Talmud, etc.; multivariate and multi-confessional ethics of interpersonal communication; the unity of the humanitarian and compassionate mission of religion and medicine; and etc.

Religious resource of sociogenesis is presented in various forms and methods of social service, obedience, and counseling; behavioral and social models of confessional (or theological in the understanding of the church) socially-public, socially-private and public-private partnerships, providing the construction of the church and spiritual creation; various forms of religious child and adolescent, youth and women's associations, sisterhoods of mercy and volunteer movements, Sunday schools, religious communities of doctors and teachers, social workers and teachers, patrons and benefactors, and others.

As an example, several illustrations can be cited from a huge variety of confessional forms of religious, social allegiance.

Thus, the basic principles of the Orthodox counseling, which are quite compiled on all forms and methods of spiritual and integrated therapy, are the provisions, established in the Pastoral Center in the name of St. John of Kronstadt:

1. Confession of the Orthodox faith and the addition of its spiritual truth and purity in medical, psychological and psychotherapeutic activities.
2. Basing of the pastoral practice on the religious-philosophical and psychological-paternal and patristic heritage.
3. Rejection of the occult and mystical techniques.
4. Pastoral care:
    - pastoral conversations and sermons;
    - group lessons for the Holy Scriptures study;
    - inclusion in the life of the Church: the Holy Sacraments of Baptism, Confession, Communion, Anointing of the Sick;
    - Liturgical life, prayer service, pilgrimages to holy places (Berestov et al. 2002).

In the history of the Russian Orthodox Church of the early twentieth century, there are spectacular *sociogenetic models* of social alcoholism epidemic confrontation. The constraining of this social malaise increase could be achieved only by multilevel macro- (state) and meso- (province, city, town), milli - (family) and micro- (person) social mobilization and intergovernmental synchronization of the activities of government, public and spiritual church institutions, enhancing the moral potential of the nation. Short periods of the effective opposition to drunkenness arose only when the *state* legislation regulated the production and sale of alcohol. The *church* strengthened public morality and spiritual immunity, which was the only "multivalent vaccine" against all social ills. The *police* prevented but not covered the manufacture violation and alcohol sale, as well as consistently reacted to the abuse of alcohol in society and on the country's roads. The *school* systematically inculcated anti-alcohol education and training. The *medicine* performed professional tasks of patients' detoxification and depsychotization. *Public organizations* created societies of "public health protection" by organizing a broad front of resistance to social evil. Such experience in Russia and the Russian Orthodox Church already exists, but today it is implemented in the compartmentalized format: in the activities of "All-Russian Society of Orthodox Doctors," "Association of the ROC Sisterhoods" without echelon multiple-level and multi-institutional systematicity.

Another historical example of the effective religious anti-drug campaign was the activity of the American Jewish Community half a century ago. For example, during the epidemiological study, it was found that about 20% of treated drug users in San Francisco were the Jews, and the rate of increase in the prevalence of drug addiction among Jewish children became closer to traditionally vulnerable ethnic groups (Cekiera 1994). The Jewish community has experienced what could be called a shock, after finding a high tolerance of the Jewish religion to the psycho-active substances (PAS) and defenseless in front of the growing scale of addiction. At some point in the community, the panic started, because parents literally "lost their heads from the problems», inducing the surge of publications in the media about the new suicidal genocide of the Jewish nation.

In response to the international level, involving the Government of Israel, it developed a comprehensive program, which systematically mobilized resources of state-private and public-state partnerships, based on a chain of religious congregations and the main focus of efforts on primary prevention of drug addiction in the family. The synagogues organized the centers for drug addicted Jews. The special Committee on Families and Children at the Federation of Jewish Philanthropy was organized in New York. Even then it became clear that the *prevention of destructive addictions - is the strengthening of the adaptive dependence on the religious and spiritual traditions, moral and value potential of the family and the capitalization of the future of the nation in the upbringing and education of children.* The Orthodox document "Halakhis" was revised, it strictly forbid the Jews to use drugs, especially marijuana. As in Judaism, the source of motivational and orientational interpretation of the interpersonal communication ethics is the Torah, the recommendations for warning the faithful from the use of PAS were systematized. It is crucial to note that the "spiritual vaccination" was not made in rigid way "against PAS," but the mental and behavioral patterns of the trajectory of fate were formed, focused on success and health, wealth and well-being, etc. depending on personal and family, moral and resource Jewish typology.

Positive results were obtained for ten years and are summarized in the first Jewish monograph on the struggle against drug addiction (Landman 1973), where the religious and ethnic, ethical and psychological, sociological and medical aspects of drug addiction were described in the multidisciplinary mode. The book of L. Landman (1973) became the first sign of the future synergetic methodology in drug preventology (Sidorov 2005) and was recommended especially to parents, whose children might be vulnerable in the case of PAS.

It is noteworthy that from the conceptual and methodological basis of the preventology as a new interdisciplinary specialty till the creation of Russia's first preventology department (Head. Prof. L. S. Shpilenya) at the Institute of Special Pedagogy and Psychology n. a. Raoul Wallenberg (St. Petersburg) almost a decade has passed.

The psychoprophylactic program effect was provided with a complexity and systematicity, as well as the delicate and harmonious setting of mental and behavioral patterns, which take into account the multilevel matrix projection of Jewish religious traditions ↔ public political and social design ↔ family habits ↔ personal priorities. Only with such echelon approach, "the act as an implicit judgment" (by Rubinstein S. L.) is a consequence of "spiritual anti-drug immunization."

The effectiveness of the religious resources use in preventive and correctional, remedial rehabilitative, spiritually-integrated protocols and programs of psychiatry and mental medicine is not studied enough, and at present, there are too little scientific and longitudinal follow-up data.

29.2. "Faith without Religion" as a New Mental Paradigm

In the United States during the General Social Survey in 2012, it was found that almost 15% of the population is among the "believers without religion": people did not associate themselves with any denomination, and they did not need temples and priests. Several global studies of the world's religiosity confirmed the extent of a new phenomenon "faith without intermediaries." The world is faced with a new reality, which was predicted by Viktor Frankl (1990), in the interview for US magazine "Time," where he said that ..". there is a tendency to move away not from religion, but from those beliefs, which are engaged only in poaching of believers from each other. We are moving not towards a universal, but personal, profoundly personalized religiosity, by which everyone can communicate with God in his own, personal, intimate language" (p. 337).

At the international conference, organized by one of the largest centers of sociology in the world in 2012, (Gallup, Pew Research Center) "The new irreligious" received a special name - "nones" or "people no," "none." It has been shown (Table 29.1), they make up a significant portion of the world's population (over 1 billion). They save their own religious views: 30% "none" French and 68% of such Americans believe in God, 44% "none" Chinese people make worship at the graves of their ancestors. However, they do not consider themselves as traditional believers. In a survey, "no people" 9 out of 10 said they were not looking for a religion, which suited them. They do not look for something; they have found their "no," which means the communication and reunion with God without intermediaries.

Gallup members try to explain this phenomenon as a new attitude of people to the labels and avoiding stigmatization. Other researchers pay attention to the growth of "no people" only in the category of respondents with liberal views, while the conservatives are loyal to the old religions, perceiving it as a symbolic protest against religious "right-wing."

Table 29.1. Top ranking countries of "believers without religion"

Country	Number of believers (thousand people)
China	700680
Japan	72120
USA	50980
Vietnam	26040
Russia	23180
South Korea	22350
Germany	20350
France	17580
North Korea	17350
Brazil	15410

All researchers note that "nones" refer mainly to the same generation, born between 1966 and 1975, although their predecessors and descendants show much greater clerical certainty and traditionalism.

The refusal of religious labels has not led to greater cooperation and openness among people yet. According to the Pew Research Center (2012) the "nones" differ with total disunity, they tend to say "no" not only to religion but also to other people.

The Chairman of the Synodal Department for Church Charity and Social Service of the Russian Orthodox Church, the Chairman of the All-Russian Society of Orthodox Doctors the Bishop Panteleimon refers "none" to "poor faith," reflecting the global trend of deethization and demoralization of conscience, reducing the level of culture and education.

In the expansion of "nones" subpopulation the modern tendencies of individualism and separatism can be seen, but the extent of the phenomenon requires careful attention to possible tomorrow "crystallization" of the new religious paradigm in the same virtual space because the "no" is the first screening sign of creativity.

The famous Russian religious philosopher Nikolai Berdyaev (2002) wrote: "The official church people, professionals of religion, tell us that the matter of personal salvation is the only necessary thing, that creative work for this purpose is unnecessary and even harmful... A simple woman, they say, can be saved more successfully than a philosopher, and it is not necessary to have knowledge and culture for saving her. However, one may doubt that God needs only simple Women, and that exhausts the plan of God for the world." The person is taken to the church for that he did NOT do: did not kill, did not commit adultery, did not steal, etc. And all things, which he did: created, wrote, discovered, invented, that is actually the multiplication of talents, received from the Creator - the church does not ask about it, it is outside its interests. But we are directly responsible to God for these things, and this is a key to the understanding of the "poor faith."

In 2012, the non-profit sociological service "Environment" conducted a large study in the framework of the project "Atlas of religions and nationalities in Russia," interviewing 57,000 people in almost all regions of the country. According to these data, 41% of the population identify themselves as Russian Orthodox, but not 80% as previously thought. In second place - 25% - were people, who just believe in God and do not confess any particular religion. 4% ecumenists, i.e., Christians, who do not identify themselves to any denomination, can be added to them. Such "poor believers" rather than "totalitarian sects" are now the main rival of the traditional religions in Russia. The "Poor Faith" to a significant extent is an achievement of educated people: the share of "non-confessionalists" among students is the highest - 46%. Preeminently, these people can make a tomorrow breakthrough in the development of civil society, requiring a new quality of mental health (Epstein 2014) and the evolution from non-conformism to constructivism. This is confirmed by the fact that about a quarter of the representatives of different religions in Russia, as well as "believers without religion," hopes to get closer to God than they are now (Table 29.2).

In essence, that is an indirect marker of realized and unrealized resources of religiosity and spirituality, increasing the epidemic threshold of mental and social epidemics.

H. M. van Praag (2013) noted the progressive loss of prestige of the Church and ecclesiastical institutions against the background of religiosity growth, considered as a normative component of human personality. The author is inclined to regard it as a biologically fixed and genetically determined, that is evidenced by a recorded change of the neural activity in the brain, depending on the intensity and depth of religious experience (Inzlicht et al. 2009; Perroud 2009). However, neurobiological processes only mediate religious, psychological nature of which is filled with multi-function image of God as:

1) symbol of unlimited creative potential and absolute morality;
2) idealized form of paternal and maternal qualities, accumulated in God formation;
3) symbol of unification with a person's conscience, purification from sin and vice;
4) finding of meaning and purpose.

Table 29.2. Would you like to believe in God more than you believe now?

Religion group	% gave a positive response in different religion groups
I do not believe in God	4
I believe in God (higher power), but do not profess a particular religion	26
I profess Christianity but do not consider myself neither Orthodox nor Catholic nor Protestant	23
I profess Orthodox Christianity and belong to the Russian Orthodox Church	21
I profess Orthodoxy; I am an Old Believer	34
I profess Orthodoxy, but do not belong to the Russian Orthodox Church, and I am not an Old Believer	26
I profess Catholicism	31
I profess Protestantism	28
I profess Sunni Islam	23
I profess Shiite Islam	21
I profess Islam, but I am neither Sunni nor Shiite	14
I profess Judaism	0

The image of God is a key tool for personal support, which do not always require the church incarnation. Religiosity is the characteristic of the human mind. Religion is its product, institutionalized in the church (Norenzayan, Sharif 2008; Verhagen, Cox 2010).

If the construction of the traditional spiritual and rehabilitation program involves the tandem of priest and psychiatrist, the new realities require from psychological and psychiatric professional community more profound spiritual and moral and religious-culture training. Undoubtedly, the psychiatrist in circumstances of sense, style and mandate will never become a confessor. The total stigmatization will prevent it, but within the biopsychosociospiritual methodology of mental medicine, the religious resource becomes a mandatory integral element of spiritual therapy.

29.3. Animogenesis as a Pattern of Mentally and Spiritually Integrated Psychotherapy

Anima, animus (Lat. anima - soul and animus - spirit) - are the concepts expressed in the ancient Greek culture as a phenomena of spiritual. They are the evolution stages of spirituality understanding: if the anima (soul) is inseparable from their physical carrier, the animus (spirit) has the status of autonomy.

Animogenesis - is ontogenetic spiritual and moral development of the individual, structuring the mental health. It is a central part of the tetracyclic biopsychosociospiritual model of mental medicine, which allows assessing and predicting the fractal trajectory of conditions and diseases of the "synergistic person." It systematically builds a multidisciplinary preventive and corrective (mental preventology) and the medical treatment and rehabilitation (clinical psychiatry) care protocol.

In the Orthodox ascetics the understanding of "mental illness" is much broader than in psychiatry. Ascetics means not only intensed psychopathology, accentuation of character, borderline states, various forms of personality disorders, but also the "immoral state of mind and the human heart, a strong-willed failure to state in the good" (Eumenes 1999).

According to Metropolitan Anthony of Sourozh (2002), it is important to distinguish *spiritual and heartful.*

"When the question is about the spirituality and warm-heartedness, these areas are often confused. If you ask people about their spiritual life, very often in response, they describe their state of mind, as if the spiritual life can be expressed in physical and psychological manifestations. However, if we turn to the Holy Scriptures, we see that from the very beginning of human history, it is quite clearly to define two areas: the spirit and the flesh. And between them there is a field of the human mentality, the human soul, is very reminiscent of the twilight between darkness and light.

Warm-heartedness - is an area of imagination, fantasies, false interpretations; it needs to be cleansed, enlightened and filled with God. Our task is to open the access to Him by way of own sobriety, the relentless struggle with imagination. Nevertheless, we can know neither God or grace nor many relations except on this level."

In the Old Testament (Sirach 40, 1-15), there is a commandment concerning the treatment to the doctor: "Honour a doctor with the honor when you need Him, as the Lord created him, and the healing is from the Highest... God created ... a doctor and a wise man will not neglect him. My son! In your disease do not be careless, but pray to the Lord and He will heal you. Leave sinful life, and mend your hands, and from all sin cleanse the heart... So give a place to the doctor, for the Lord created him: and let him not go from you: as he is needed... Who sins in front of his Creator, falls into the hands of a doctor!"

As the psychologist T. A. Florenskaya noted (1994): "the history of Russian science suggests that *spiritless psychology is soulless too - "the science without a soul."* Becoming a discipline of natural science, psychology "divides the soul into pieces" slaying it. So the soul dies, divorced from the spirit; spiritless psychology loses itself, its original vocation. Psychology begins to develop rapidly the heritage (global and domestic) of religious philosophy, the spiritual experience of faith of confessors, ascetics of the spirit, to expand the experience with the subjective world of a human, his mind, and most importantly - to build a new outlook, a new vision of human reality in its subjective view. The appearance of the second pole of psychological objectivity - spirituality - opens up the prospect of becoming a true leader in the psychology, and in many respects the legislator in the human sciences."

The importance of spiritually-integrated approaches is suggested by the classics of different directions of psychotherapeutic schools. Prominent Austrian psychotherapist, author of Logotherapy, Viktor Frankl (2000) says: "The medical service is not intended to be a replacement of the treatment of souls, what is practiced by a priest. What is the interrelation between psychotherapy and religion? In my opinion, the answer is very simple: the goal of psychotherapy - is to treat the soul, make it healthy; the purpose of religion - is something substantially different - to save the soul. But the wonderful side effect of religion - is psychohygienic. Religion gives a person the spiritual anchor with a sense of confidence, which he cannot find anywhere else. ... It is impossible to take religion to a neurosis or "collective unconscious." *The spiritual dimension can not be ignored, it specifically makes us the people."*

V. Frankl (2000) reminded psychologists and psychotherapists that the final resolution of human problems was impossible without an understanding of his relationship with God: "A religious person is different, apparently, from the secular by the experience of its existence as not just as a task, but as a mission. This means that he apperceives as the Person of the One, who poses this problem, he knows the Source of his mission. For thousands of years, this source is called God."

The president of the Association for Humanistic Psychology, Professor of Seiber University, James Bugental (2001) has the same opinion. In "The Art of the Psychotherapist" he wrote about the opportunities, opened with the process of self-discovery and inner workings of clearing the way to the spiritual plan of human existence: "We are all looking for God, all." Atheists and agnostics do it not less than the prayers. We can abandon this quest of not more than to stop the flow of our conscience. Our thoughts throw together what we have with what we want, and soon we have to present ourselves as we might be, and consequently, join the path of seeking God. I believe that the *search for God coincides with the deepest aspirations of the human being to his own."*

Prominent psychologist and psychotherapist Rollo May (1994), a classic of existential-humanistic psychology, believed that before starting work with the person, psychotherapist should make a portrait of the person for himself, consisting of four components: freedom, individuality, social integration and depth of religiosity. "Personal spirituality is a sign of great opportunities. This is the occasion for celebration because the spark of God disturbed the darkness inside our earthly shell... Portrait of a person will be incomplete if we ignore its inner spiritual tensions. Systems of psychotherapy, coming from purely naturalistic principles, doomed to failure. We can conclude that a healthy person should adapt creatively to the understanding of the boundedness and that the *key to health is a conscious sense of spirituality.* The task of the consultant - is to teach the client to accept adequately and make sustainable that spiritual tension, which is inherent in human nature."

Robert Dilts (2000), one of the leading specialists in the field of neuro-linguistic programming (NLP), thinks that *"to respond to questions, concerning the mission (of a person in this world) is quite impossible without affecting the subject of God."* The psychotherapists of this direction in its work with the problems of patients use logic levels table, work on which leads persons to a deeper understanding of themselves and their place in the world.

Psychotherapists, who use NLP as a general procedure, assume that to solve the psychological problems of getting rid of the painful symptoms, the person eventually has to come to the question of awareness of his own place in this world, the meaning of his mission in life, his relationship with God. Therefore, we can say that the statement that psychology, psychotherapy, and even more so, the mental medicine, can be an atheist - is a myth, refuted by time and by the experts.

Speaking of spirituality, we should remember the responsibility for ourselves and our lives. The spirituality - is high, significant category for people, having the responsible attitude to life. *Personality in Christian anthropology is regarded in the unity of spiritual, mental and physical symptoms.* So this unity is achieved only upon condition of the prevailing influence of the spirit sphere. According to St. Theophan the Recluse (2007), the spiritual sphere in person is awe and life in the fear of God, the conscience and the search for God. "The spirit is, first of all, a person's ability to distinguish the highest values: good and evil, truth and falsehood, beauty and ugliness. If the choice is made in this regard, the spirit seeks to subordinate its decision the body and soul. The human communicates with God through his spirit. Without communion with God, the spirit of a human is not able to find the true criterion for determining the highest values, as only God, who Himself is an absolute good, trouth and beauty can specify the right solution to man" (Orthodox Catechism 2000).

29.4. From Spiritually Integrated Psychiatry to Biopsychosociospiritual Mental Medicine

The theme of interaction between religion and psychiatry has a long history, full of vivid examples of complementarity and unity in the social service and merciful mission. In his book, "Spirit, soul and body" (1997) St. Luke (Voyno-Yasenetsky) quotes his famous contemporaries.

One of the founders of Russian psychiatry, a professor at the St. Petersburg Medical-Surgical Academy I. P. Merzheyevskiy wrote: "The ideal concept of happiness ... is expressed in the faith, that it is possible in another life, in the afterlife. It is the only hope of all the suffering and offended in life; this is a shelter, specified by the religion, especially of the Christian, for all the suffering and grief, for which there is no medicine." Another founder of Russian psychiatry the professor P. I. Kovalevsky, Rector of the University of Warsaw, alone among prominent psychiatrists the graduate of the seminary, the author of the resonant "Psychiatric studies of history," wrote: "Knowledge and Faith will find a decent Union and give the person comfort and reconciliation."

Leading European psychiatrists have virtually the same point. One of the founders of sexology the professor Richard von Krafft-Ebing states: "Happy is who finds in religion the right anchor against the storms of life." The French psychiatrist Laurent in his book "Soul Medicine" adds: "Joining the Holy Mysteries - is a great remedy for body and soul. It is a great relief for the afflicted and bereaved; it uplifts the spirit and fills the heart with joy and hope." The professor of psychiatry L. A. Koch writes: "Nothing is achieved without religion, i.e., without a personal relationship with God. The best forces are in religion ... for the prevention of many nervous diseases».

The illustration of the principle of subsidiarity, formulated by Niels Bohr in 1927, can become a quote from the book "The Psychology of the soul" of the famous French psychiatrist Professor Fleury: "religion and science, each has their method and field. They may perfectly exist side by side and both serve its purpose."

A formula of the integral mission of religion and psychiatry is the message to Simferopol eparchy priests of the Aarchbishop of Luke: "Are there many among you, priests who are similar to serious doctors? Do you know how much effort and attention are devoted to the serious patients by good and experienced doctors? ... However, the task of the doctor is only healing of disease, and our task is immeasurably more important. After all, we are put by God for the great work of human souls healing, deliverance from everlasting suffering." He finished his book, "Science and Religion" St. Luke (2001) with the words of N. I. Pirogov: "When we believe that the main ideal of the teachings of Christ is in its inaccessibility, we will remain forever and will ever affect the souls, seeking peace through inner connection with the God. We cannot doubt for a moment that this doctrine is destined to be an unquenchable lighthouse on the twisting path of our progress." Ended a quarter-century ago, the ordeal for the Orthodox faith in Russia left terrible wounds and deep scars in the public conscience and the mental health of the nation, but clearly demonstrated that the light of God's lighthouse is enduring.

Tension and mistrust between psychiatry and religion in the twentieth century were often dependent on the idea of the incompatibility of the worldview, based on science and faith (Barbour 1974). A substantially lower level of religiosity of psychiatrists as compared with the population in general (Shafranske 2000); underestimation by the professional psychiatric community of the role of religion in the treatment and rehabilitation of patients (Pergament, Lomax 2013); lack of medical, psychological and social education for the mobilization of religious resources of the mental health and treatment of mental illnesses (Larson et al. 1997; Sidorov 2005) – all this contributed to the misunderstanding.

The situation changed at the turn of the twenty-first century, reflecting the growth of research in the field of spiritual and integrated treatment and rehabilitation, preventive and rehabilitative programs. Numerous studies have confirmed the mission of religion as the first and most accessible resource, which is accessed by patients and clients. According to the generalized estimates, from 50% to 90% of patients reported the relief of symptoms in the process of appeal to religion. Pain, reduced anxiety and stress reduction of anosognosia and early treatment, improving of coping strategies and compliance, self-control and social adaptation, finding the meaning of life and peace of mind, self-esteem and self-confidence, acceptance and compassion, hope and love (Tepper et al. 2001; Rammohan et al. 2002; Jangarber-Hicks 2004; Prado et al. 2004; Canada et al. 2006; Fridman et al. 2006; Mohr et al. 2006; Greeuberg 2013). It is confident to say that *religion is the oldest and most versatile protective and compensatory civilizational resource,* allowing the satisfying a wide variety of human needs, structuring his mentality and identity.

The effectiveness of spiritually-integrated treatment was convincingly shown in different groups of patients and clients: anxiety disorders and depression (Azhar et al. 1995); schizophrenia (D`Souza et al. 2002); eating disorders (Richars et al. 2006); subclinical anxiety and alarm (Rosmarin et al. 2010); related disorders (Avants et al. 2005; Sidorov 2005); PTSD in combatants (Harris et al. 2011) and women who have been sexually abused (Murray-Swan, Pargamen 2005) and etc.

Religious resource of mental health in psychological and psychotherapeutic, psychiatric and addictologic practice serves several functions:

1) adaptation to the problem or illness;
2) source of meaning and catharsis;
3) achieving of emotional comfort and reducing of anxiety;
4) means of self-regulation and self-development;
5) improving the quality and style of life;
6) adaptive and social professiogenesis (Huguelet, Mandhouj 2013).

Assessment of the spirituality degree of the patient or client and his religious beliefs are not just important but required spiritual, moral, social and psychological blocks in the diagnosis and treatment of mental medicine.

Only mental medicine enables to unfold maximally widely and effectively the biopsychosociospiritual mechanisms, mobilizing resources for the mentally- and spiritually-integrated treatment. These mechanisms are the adaptation and compensation, protection and coping, releasing and training, immunomodulation and restitution, restoration and regeneration, remission and chronicity, implemented in different fractals of conditions and diseases. All of these mechanisms are accumulated in the *sanogenetic therapy* - adaptive biopsychosociospiritual mind control, which results in destabilization of stable pathological state, activation of personal resources and reserves of the body, as well as a renewal of structural and functional life support systems.

A significant contribution to the explanation of the complex relationship between religion and mental illness was the creation of the WPA section on "Religion, Spirituality and Psychiatry" (www.religionandpsychiatry.com), publication of WPA manual "Psychiatry and Religion: beyond the borders" (2010) and the management of "Religion and Health" (2012), edition of the newsletter "Psyche and Spirit."

In this area in 2000, in the Northern State Medical University (NSMU) the *Mental Health Service* (MHS) as a synergetic biopsychosociospiritual φ-cluster, providing protection for mental health and treatment -rehabilitation assistance in mental illnesses was established. The activity of MHS is coordinated by the *Institute of Mental Health*, created in 2009. In 2011, in the NSMU together with Arkhangelsk Archdiocese, organized by the *Community Mental Health Department*, has five branches: the spiritual and moral education, the Orthodox medicine, population policy, the protection of public health and confrontation to social ills, Orthodox psychology and psychotherapy. The faculty is in control of Scientific Methods and the Board of Trustees. The Department appeared after ten years of work on the NSMU basis of the initial Orthodox educational courses and training of the Sisters of Charity, the creation of the Arkhangelsk branch of the Russian Society of Orthodox Doctors, annual conferences of Ioannovsky Voyno-Yasenetsky readings, many scientific and practical forums. The working efficiency was rated by the *system monitoring of mental health.*

The *promising areas for further research* on the relationship of religion, psychiatry and mental medicine can identify:

1) the need to expand multicultural research field;
2) inclusion in the diagnostic and therapeutic tools of the ways to identify the religious problems and religious resources;
3) the importance of longitude studies of the complex interactions of psychopathology and religion;
4) adaptive forms of religious life for persons with mental illness;
5) etiopathogenetic differences of religious and non-religious psychopathological disorders;
6) the development and implementation of new training programs, taking into account the religious and cultural components of the spiritually-oriented methodology for psychiatrists and clinical psychologists, social workers and experts in bioethics;
7) spiritual and integrated research in all fields of psychiatry and mental medicine;
8) study of the impact of religious involvement on health;

9) differential assessment of dramatic spiritual experience and mental disorders;
10) epidemiology of the relationship between religion and health;
11) instrumentalization and operationalization of the definition of spirituality;
12) measurement of religiosity in the context of the multi-confessional;
13) trans- and cross-cultural investigations of features of religious manifestations;
14) resilience of religiosity and spirituality on the prenosological nosological fractals of psychopathological process;
15) the role of religion in the formation of individual and social, ethnic and professional identity;
16) the volume and quality of the religious component in the spiritual and spiritually-integrated treatment and rehabilitation programs (Sidorov 2005; Baetz 2013; Blass 2007; Koenig 2011; Moriera-Almeida 2013; Puchalski et al. 2001).

The Nobel Laureate in Physics, Albert Einstein wrote: "To know that there are things in the world that are not directly accessible to us but which really exist. The things that are learned by us and hide a supreme wisdom and supreme beauty; to know and feel it - is the source of true religion. In this sense, I belong to religious people." The same idea was formulated more vividly and concisely by another Nobel Laureate in Physics, Werner Heisenberg: "The first sip from the cup of natural science begets atheism, but at the bottom of the pot God is always waiting for us."

As a part of a universal logic model S. G. Handsdak, R. Paulraj (2013) noted that psychiatry and religion were wrong enemies yesterday, but today remain old friends. *It is possible to add that tomorrow they will be partners in the synergetic methodology of mental medicine and open the door to a new paradigm of spiritual medicine.*

Section VII. Synergetic Technological Platform of Mental Health Service

Chapter 30

Synergetic Integrativity and Health-Oriented Optimisticity of Mental Medicine

30.1. From Mythologization of Psychiatry to the Development of Mental Health Services

Modern descriptive psychiatry is currently suffering from the lack of trust of both doctors and patients. It is because pharmaceutical companies' marketing resources distribute extensively psychiatric diagnoses convincing doctors that everyday life problems are in fact mental disorders caused by a chemical imbalance which can be easily treated by a high-priced pill (Francis 2013). Therefore, in the last 20 years, the prevalence of attention deficit hyperactivity disorder (ADHD) has tripled; bipolar disorder has doubled, the child diagnosis cases have increased fortyfold; autism spectrum cases are diagnosed 20 times more often (Batstra et al. 2012). In the USA the mental disorders prevalence totals up to 20-25%, the lifetime prevalence is about 50% (Kessler et al. 2005), the amount followed up by Europe (Graaf et al. 2012). The American perspective juvenile study has showed that the overall frequency of mental disorders will amount to 83% by 2021 (Copeland et al. 2011).

In the meantime, only 5% of the population has a severe mental disorder and 15-20% of the psychotropic drugs consumers go through "common everyday life experiences." They are the ones who contribute the most to the income of the USA pharmaceutical industry: $18 billion a year accounts for antidepressants, and $8 billion is spent on ADHD medications. Moreover, 80% of psychotropic drugs are prescribed by doctors of the primary medical network (Mark et al. 2009). It is no coincidence that the number of overdoses and fatal cases as a result of the psychotropic drug usage prescribed by doctors exceed the number of those done by narcotic drugs. Only one-third of the USA patients suffering from severe depression are under actual medical treatment (Francis 2013). This means that the social epidemic of induced deformation of the qualified conscience of medical community triggered by the pharmaceutical industry is at least mercenarily biologically destroying the public conscience of the valid part of the modern civilization.

The intensity of the controversy about the pharmacotherapy effectiveness in treating mental disorders forced Mario Maj, President of WPA (2013) to declare that "we shouldn't saw off the bough, on which we are all sitting, realizing that each of us may or may not like the rest of the exit branches." However, the problem is far more complex here and deals, metaphorically speaking, not with branches and leaves, but with roots and the tree of psychiatry itself, which demands new conceptual-methodological approach, one of which is the biopsycosociospiritual methodology of mental medicine.

According to European Brain Council, one-third of all modern civilization pathologies are brain disorders, which by 2030 will outnumber cardiovascular diseases and oncology. In Russia, the population of which had gone through the severe post-Soviet psychosocial stress (Kara-Murza S., 2013), the number of mentally sick accounts to 27 million people. Also, there are about 10 million victims of natural and industrial disasters, wars, local armed conflicts, terrorist attacks, criminal assaults, rape, abduction, kidnapping etc. Most of these people show signs of PTSD, reactive state, neurosis, depression (Muhamednev, Hollander 2011). Almost a third of the country's population is in need of medical care from psychiatrists, who are only 11117 persons left in Russian healthcare system (2011). Together with psychotherapists, sexologists and forensic experts, they hold 21577 vacancies in office. There are 37-38 thousand real and potential patients per one psychiatrist (Gurovich 2012). In the frames of the long-lasting campaign of psychiatric care development, there is a reduction not only in the number of psychiatrists but also in the asylums' bed stock without an adequate replacement with the specialized ambulatory care (Andreev, Nazarova 2013).

In Russia, the relative share of stationary section of psychiatric service is almost 90% while of the healthcare is 67.9%. The best possible share in the context of structural effectiveness, according to the Ministry of Healthcare of the Russian Federation, was considered to be of about 40-45% (Vyalkov 2003). Subject to compliance with the Russian Federation government decree (№2599-p 28.12.12) this indicator, showing the effectiveness of healthcare, was slightly adjusted and fixed in the workflow chart at a level of 60.3% in 2013 and 50.3% by 2018.

It is noteworthy that throughout the decades despite all the reforms on optimization of bed stock this figure in psychiatry stays unchanged and confirms the "low structural effectiveness of the service" (Schevchenko et al. 2013). If truth be told, the longer the waiting of the industry to reform itself is, the more dangerous the galloping increase of destructive social epidemics from alcohol and drug addiction to extremism and terrorism is to the national security.

The joint burden of mental disorders per the number of the USA population equaled $817.2 billion or 7.2% GPD in 2005 (Yastrebov et al. 2012). The components of the cost burden are medical and economic costs, living standards degradation and indirect expenses.

The evaluation of mental disorders burden in Russia turned out to be 2-4 times lower than that in the USA, which can be accounted for the differences in the structure of the expenses of mental health care services and the lack of a correct statistics (Gurovich, 2010; Kulikov, Dedyurina 2011).

Unfortunately, in the last 20 years, psychiatry has been under steady paradigmatic mythologization (Anthony et al. 1994) which slows down the development of the multidisciplinary approach to rehabilitation and innovative technologies in the environment of mental health. These are the following psychiatric myths:

1) Most of the patients who have mental disorders recover successfully.
2) The increase in the patient's motivation to drug-assisted treatment improves the recovery results.
3) Traditional treatment methods used at hospitals such as psychotherapy, group and medication therapy contribute to the better recovery.
4) New methods of hospital treatment such as environmental therapy, encouragement therapy ("coupon economics") and attitude therapy positively contribute to the recovery results.
5) Occupational therapy in psychiatric facilities positively contributes to work skills of patients.
6) Outpatient care treatment at a place of residence achieves a better rehabilitation effect than a hospital one.
7) Ambulatory care clinics at a place of residence are more popular among mentally deranged people than hospitals.
8) It is more important where to treat a patient, rather how to treat.
9) The rehabilitation effect is highly correlated to the symptom profile of mental disorders.
10) Nosological diagnosis says a lot about the prognosis of rehabilitation actions.
11) Skills of a patient largely depend on the medical signs of a disease.
12) The patient's ability to function in one environment (for example, hospital) helps to foresee how he will function in a different environment (for example, work).
13) The result of rehabilitation can be precisely predicted by an expert.
14) The result of rehabilitation of a specific patient depends on qualifications of the working expert of the mental health environment.
15) The prognosis of rehabilitation is in a direct correlation with the cost of the intervention.

Myth, according to C. Jung, is a cognitive scheme which struggles to present itself as a system of facts. It concerns both myths, which are specific to a society as a "social order" and expectations from psychiatry, and the delusions of the psychiatrists themselves. It is a system of their, to a large extent, irrational thinking concerning their practice and its theoretical basis, the occurrence of which in some integration systems in psychotherapy is very questionable. The defining characteristics of such thinking are the following:

- the misperceptions are fairly generalized;
- they are based solely on "belief" without sufficient argumentation and deny facts which are in contradiction to those beliefs;
- they are not critical and tolerate the internal conflicts of thinking; they mix up cause and effects;
- they are hardly subject to self-reflection;
- they are hard to be constantly maintained (Vinokur, Novikova 2015).

To avoid misperception in a profession entirely is impossible, but through understanding its influence on a working process one is capable of making the psychiatrist's professional activities more constructive.

Among the main factors which determine the mythologization of psychiatry the following are pointed out (Skorik et al. 2014):

1) The unreliability of information.
2) Violation of social ethics by the mentally deranged.
3) Mythopoetic thinking.
4) Protective function.
5) The universality of the social myths existence.

Inertial preservation of psychiatric myth creation is, at a very least, the evidence of a sufficient underdevelopment of psychiatry comparing to other sciences in a singular modern era when the rate of development of scientific and technical revolution is exponentially rising.

According to the same authors (Anthony et al. 1994), the necessity in the development of multidisciplinary rehabilitation services in the USA was particularly acute when the number of psychiatric beds in 1960-1970s has diminished by two-thirds. This reduction resulted in a large increase of people who found themselves in the suburbs or even in the main streets of cities instead of a hospital ward. The following intensive establishment of psychosocial rehabilitation centers in the USA (from 18 in 1976 to 148 in 1981) gave a rise to the development of multidisciplinary rehabilitation practices as well as the multiple-path structure of mental health services. Russia went through this process in the tough early 90s when all former psychiatric hospital's patients without exception were left homeless on the streets and this subpopulation equifinally died out (Kazakovcev 2009), because of the lack of the necessary money and resources.

One has to agree with D. Bolton (2013) that XXI century will bring not so much the establishment of psychiatry as a medical profession, bringing up the same century-old problems. The new time will make psychiatry a union of genetic and neurobiological, psychological and social health determinants that will together create a new consultative profession which deals with mental health issues. This will allow improving the quality of care provided to patients and clients, optimizing the costs and finding a solution to the problem of selecting experts.

Professor B. Pivan (2014) was even more critical when stating that "so far nothing new has come into existence in clinical psychiatry except for new terminology." We can add the perception of the necessity of a new methodology, the example of which is the synergetic biopsychosociospiritual methodology of mental health care. The global crisis has added new economic factors to the growing multidisciplinary teamwise care in psychiatry as a result of which the cost of psychiatrist services is 50% more expensive than ones of a clinical psychologist and two times more expensive than a help from a social worker (Motov 2003; Piven 2010).

The creation of mental ecology and mental epidemiology, mental health care and mental preventology, which are almost brought to life in a new synergetic methodology of mental health care service, and systematic monitoring of mental health – all this are the specific steps taken as a part of an existing professional and civilization trend.

30.2. Mental Medicine as a Psychiatric Paradigm of Integrative Medicine

Descriptive psychiatry in two centuries of its existence has evolved into phenomenological (illusory-compensatory euphemism), having saved the adherence to subjective conclusions being a deficit in objective markers.

The first crisis of trust for descriptive psychiatry happened early in the 1970s. It was evoked by the publication of research showing the inaccuracy of psychiatric diagnosis and ambiguity of treatment. Therefore, (Kendell et al. 1971) have shown that British and American psychiatrists came to different diagnostic conclusions after watching a videotape of the same patient. In the other research done by D. L. Rosenban (1973), students had continued to reside in a psychiatric ward over the claim that they hear voices despite the fact that their behavior was normal from the very first day of hospital admission. This evoked a vast discussion of the reliability of diagnosis and specificity of psychiatric treatment which in turn led to a sufficient renewal of DSM and ICD.

The second crisis is happening now due to the release of DSM-5, which has broadened the diagnostic boundaries of a number of mental disorders ("diagnostic inflation"). The biggest problems have become the removal of a bereavement factor for major depression, the addition of a very vague "somatic symptoms disorder," the threshold reduction for childhood ADHD and PTSD, the introduction of a 'behavioral dependency' term, the addition of "mild neurocognitive disorder" and "binge eating disorder." Elastic borders of psychiatry have substantially broadened, because of the absence of a clear dividing line between a healthy anxiety and mild mental disorder. During the preparation of DSM-5 classification a petition concerning the independent scientific analysis using evidence-based medicine supported by 50 associations of mental health environment was ignored (Francis 2013)

The irony is that any attempts to change the paradigm, trying to replace or extend descriptive psychiatry by a different approach to the etiopathogenesis of mental disorders are not yet perceived. Again and again, the necessity of a forced usage of the descriptive psychiatry alone to conclude a right and sustainable diagnosis, to order an effective and safe treatment is declared. Meanwhile, the prospects for the future development are focused on finishing up the ICD-11 preparation and new hopes for reevaluating of psychiatric diagnosis. This reminds more of walking in circles instead of the classical spiral development of scientific methodology.

One cannot disagree with V. Engelgardt (1970) who said that reductionism, not going further from the descriptive analyses of human individuality, had become a terrible phenomenon for human sciences. Reductionism means that regularities of one level of individuality apply to the regularities of another, identify with them and, therefore, lose their specific essence (Merlin 1964). Per se, reductionism "from below" and "from above" methodically provides "diagnostic inflation" confirming the additive strategy of a client's individuality research and clinical characteristics of a patient's decease.

Reductionism appears in psychiatry as a tendency for reification and objectification leading to an existential vacuum. V. Frankl (1990) pointed out the bygone nihilism as an existential vacuum and visual nihilism which identifies in reductionism: "This is referring to the feeling of the inner emptiness, the feeling of the deepest loss of meaning which we, psychiatrists, encounter at every turn" (p. 47). Unfortunately, today we can only state with sadness that the warnings about the underestimating of the devastating effect of reductionist doctrines on psychiatry have been left unheard.

The counterbalance to reductionism is *integratism as a systematic model of perception which allows uniting the parts into one whole providing the formation of a new quality* (Belous 2009). That is exactly why multidisciplinary and integrative synergetic biopsychosociospiritual methodology of mental health care is perceived as a productive vast alternative to a narrow descriptive reductionism of phenomenological psychiatry. The mental healthcare itself continues the number of earlier created integrative human sciences: a human study by B. Ananyev (1977), humanology by V. Merlin (1986), integrative anthropology by B. Nikityuk (1995), integrative psychotherapy A. Katkov (2013), etc.

V. Bekhterev (1917) conducted pioneer research in psyconeurology integratism principles; he wrote in his main research paper "General Principles of Human Reflexology": "The world is built in a form of closed system which features special individualities. Each individuality can be different in complexity, but it always represents a specific harmony of its parts and posesses its form and relative system stability." V. Bekhterov's close relation between conceptually-methodological and theoretical-practical world outlook showed itself as a whole holistic attitude concerning diagnosis and mental disorders treatment.

From S. Rubinstein's point of view (1959) the whole individuality had been filled up with characteristics of different levels, which is an integration of biological and social. The interdisciplinary approach of B. Ananyev (1977) to the wholeness of human development included integral characteristics of a human being as species, individual, personality, and mankind. V. Merlin (1986) relying on systematic numbering approach (a mathematical term which underlies in the distinction of "horizontal," one-one and "vertical" multidigit dependency) outlined in integrative individuality theory the sub-systems in the "human society" macro-system which nowadays are one of the subjects of mental ecology:

1) The sub-system of an organism: biochemical, somatic and neurodynamic patterns.
2) The sub-system of an individual: psychodynamic characteristics and their interrelation.
3) The sub-system of a personality characteristics and their interrelation.
4) The sub-system of sociopsychological characteristics and their interrelation.
5) The sub-system of sociocultural community and their interrelations.

The total of the listed sub-systems forms the individuality defined by the unity of liner and non-linear dependence. Every hierarchical level has its specific functional invariants (FI) linear as well as non-linear, its own characteristics package, which allows it to defend self-sufficiency and relative independence. The numbering principle not only prevents the reducibility of the patterns of one sub-system to another but also allows defining the levels earlier unknown. This principle takes a new special meaning for clinical psychotherapy helping to withstand "diagnostical inflation." In short, V. Merlin came close to fractal dynamics of dissipative structures (sub-systems, systems, macro-systems) development in synergetic FI model.

In the research of psychodynamic and personal levels of integrative individuality, V. Belous, I. Boyazitova (2013), in a synergetic parlance, have discovered fractal characteristics of FI, explained apodictic (necessarily true) connections between behavioral models, pointed out the non-linear invariant, described the multidimensionality of dissipative self-control and self-organized personality system. The authors showed the infinity of occasional changes of separate variables with a finiteness of relations of such variables and suggested over-typed structure of individuality. It can be said that the functional invariant as a fractal has already come into basic terms usage in differential psychology, *becoming a matrix of symptom formation in a psychological diagnosis of mental medicine.*

Reductionism and holism (integratism) obviously shouldn't be mechanically contradistinguished. The truth always lies in between the opposing points of view. Yu. Odum (1986) wrote: "Both holistic and reductionist approaches have to be used equally without setting them against… Ecology aims for synthesis, not division." Poetizing this point of view, G. Rosenberg (2014) underlines that the two-ways road to the temple of truth (reductionism plus holism) is hard and thorny, but by fearlessly continuing the journey, we don't risk to find ourselves on the sideways of science.

30.3. Resource-integrated and Person-Centered Synergetic Technological Platform of Mental Medicine

Personified (individualized, personalized) medicine – is a resource-integrated and patient-centered healthcare which main concern is a potential and adaptational self-actualization of a human body and an increase of its active lifetime based on the consideration of genetic, external environmental and local factors (Jain 2009).

I. Ushakov, A. Bogomolov (2014) point out eight basic biomedical concepts of drug-free preventive treatment, monitoring, and increase in adaptive abilities of human beings.

1) *The concept of occupational health* based on the characteristics of the genetically determined process of normal biological aging in a particular socio-economic environment.
2) *The concept of multistage preventive changes* based on the realization of dose risk-metrical approach to the effects of health risk factors and individualized course of its maintenance from medical and occupational selection to recovery and rehabilitation.
3) *The concept of syndrome-like conditions* based on confirmation of syndrome-like complexes of changes at molecular-cellular and tissue levels. Meanwhile, the more acute the noci-influence on the body is, the more acute its response will be.
4) *The concept of biological age* allows one to compare age change of physiological systems of a specific organism to average population changes.
5) *The concept of living standard* is an integrated characteristic of physical and emotional, psychological and social functioning of a human being.
6) *The concept of mathematical support* of health risk-measurement providing a differential evaluation and prediction of human's state of health.
7) *The informative telecommunicational concept* which provides a technological monitoring of a psychophysiological state of health in a non-contact mode.
8) *The informative concept of passportization of health* providing an uninterrupted monitoring of personified occupation health control programs based on the national standard of medical informatics.

Prognostic preventive-intervention personified healthcare will be much more effective than a population one. That is exactly why *the technological platform of the mental medicine pilot project developed by us* is able to become the actual form of realization of public-private partnership and a tool to shape the innovative policy of mental health advocacy of the nation as the most important modernization resource and the basis of national security.

The overriding priority of the technological platform "Mental Healthcare" is the development of breakthrough technologies of adaptive mental health protection and opposition to mental epidemics based on national defense multidisciplinary synergetic methodology. Mental medicine can be one of the approaches of the federal technological platform "Medicine of the future." It will create a medico-biological segment of an advanced development based on a summation of innovative technologies. In turn, this will define the possibility of entry of new high-technology production and services markets and also the rapid distribution of cutting-edge technologies in medical and pharmacological sectors (Ogorodova 2011; Gustap 2014).

Technological platform as an institute of innovation-driven growth stimulation can enable the solution to topical problems as a part of cooperation between businessmen, producers, researchers and government.

Personalized medicine is based on the ideology of the new interdisciplinary model of health care organization. According to forecast estimates, up to 50% of current research of pharmaceutical companies account for personalized medicine. In 2016, the proportion of personalized remedies will amount to one-third of all drugs in the total world production (Paltsev 2015).

Personalized medicine is based on the principles of the four P: predictivity and prevention, personalization and participativity.

Predictivity is based on a probabilistic forecast of health.

Preventivity is the prevention of the development of disease and its complications.

Personalization of treatment consists of detecting individual biomarkers that determine the development of the disease.

Participativity appears in a motivated and active participation of the person in the prevention and treatment of diseases.

As stated by the Minister of Health of the Russian Federation, V. I. Skvortsova (2015): "Russia is on the way of formation of preventive medicine as the most efficient and profitable, the most personalized medicine." In this context, mental medicine, based on the synergetic biopsychosociospiritual methodology, is a practical implementation of the principles of the personalized medicine. The mission of the mental medicine, consisting in adaptive engineering and management of mind and health, is implemented in a multidisciplinary block-module design and realization of programs and protocols of the brigade care. It allows prenosological screening and predicting the development trajectory of conditions and diseases, expanding effective personalized early intervention. In fact, on the particular model of mental medicine, we have developed and tested a synergetic methodology of integrative medicine, reinforcing its reform potential as a global trend of innovative development of the contemporary medicine.

Chapter 31

Mental Health Service as an Interface of Public Conscience

31.1. System Monitoring of Mental Health

Socioeconomic situation existing in Russia over the last years objectively caused mental health deterioration among the population and worsening of mental health in patient's cohort at the same time.

The actual prevalence rate of mental and behavioral disorders considerably exceeds the one given in official statistics. Thus, a mental disorders prevalence rate of a non-psychotic level is 27.3% of an adult population (according to official data this number is 1,4%) (Churkin, Tvorogova 2006). According to V. S. Yastrebov et al. (2009) nearly 14% of Russian population (which corresponds to 21 million people) needs psychiatric care. This number is described by the author as "the real number of people experiencing mental disorders." At the same time, the number of mental disorder episodes occurring in undiagnosed patients can reach 27 million people. Moreover, nearly 7.5 million people suffer from episodic disorders of mental activity while approximately 10 million is the number constituting the patient cohort.

Over the last years, some suggestions about Russian mental health service reorganization have been made. And these suggestions are characterized by multiple approaches. The major emphasis here is made on a long-term improvement of existing psychiatric care system by means of efficient use of existing resources, interdepartmental interaction, and psychiatric care delivery in general medical settings.

Mental disorders are listed among the most socially important diseases in the concept of a federal "Prevention and control of socially important diseases (2007-2011)" target-oriented program implemented by the Russian Federation Government. The main objective of the "Mental disorders" subprogram was the development of the system of complex preventive measures, diagnosing, treatment and rehabilitation in cases of mental disorders. At the same time, effective implementation of these measures is impossible without objective statistical data concerning mental pathology prevalence rate.

Thus, the necessity in mental health system monitoring is explained by the acuteness of society's up-to-date problems connected with mental and behavioral disorders. Mental illnesses not only deteriorate population wellbeing and public health but also undermine Russian economics in general.

In a broad sense, the term "monitoring" (from the Latin word "Monitor" meaning "admonitory") denotes specially organized systematic observation over the state of the objects or processes for the purpose of their estimation, control, and prognosis. Monitoring systems are the basic examination mechanism of how the environment influences the population health.

The objectives of any monitoring organization are as follows: the choice of the monitoring object and collecting data about it; estimation of possible unfavorable environment influence on the population health on the basis of collected data; decision making about the way to eliminate or reduce this unfavorable influence.

Currently, dozens of monitoring systems are carried out in Russia. They are: atmospheric air, natural waters and soils monitoring (Ministry of Natural Resources 1972); government ecological monitoring (1993, Ministry of Natural Resources); socio-hygienic monitoring (Russian Federation Ministry of Public Health 1994); rational environmental monitoring (Ministry of Natural Resources 1995); bad habits monitoring among children and teenagers (RF Ministry of Public Health 1997); tuberculosis monitoring (RF Ministry of Public Health 1997); congenital defects monitoring (RF Ministry of Public Health 1998); all-Russian monitoring and prognosis of natural and anthropogenic character emergency situation by EMERCOM, Russia (Ministry of Civil Defence of the Russian Federation 1999); critically important objects monitoring (Roscosmos, EMERCOM, MIA, FSS 2005).

System ecological monitoring is a complex contrastive monitoring engaging cosmic, geophysical, meteorological, hydrological, social and medical components. This monitoring is aimed at cause-effect relation finding between outer impacts, people's health, and life quality, and at unfavorable phenomena and processes prognosis. It is considered to be the most important priority of national security and the country's sustainable development (Sidorov 2006).

Socio-hygienic monitoring in the Russian Federation is a government observation system over the population health state and environment, their analysis, estimation, and prognosis, as well as a system of cause-effect relation finding between the population health state and environmental factors influence. It is one of the most effective mechanisms of sanitary-and-epidemiologic population well-being provision, as it was based on creation and analysis of health and environmental factors databases, and on cause-effect relation finding between sickness rate indicators within specific areas and influence of harmful environmental factors on population.

Contemporary tendencies in research of mental health pathology prevalence rate are characterized by emphases shift towards more universal ones, based on the understanding of mental health as a combination of mental, social, psychological well-being and balance between an individual and environment. Thus, N. K. Dyomcheva (2006; 2015) suggests viewing life quality and social functioning as a criterion for population's mental health.

System monitoring concept and monitoring objects are represented in Figures 31.1 and 31.2.

Structurally functional model of mental health system monitoring (MHSM) includes the following (Figure 31.3): objective, measurement process, organization, forms, means, methods, ways, estimation process and monitoring results identification.

At the maximum generalized level, *MHSM* is a complex multidisciplinary monitoring based on synergetic methodology and aimed at cause-effect relation finding in the "Environment – Society – Person" system with the purpose of the high level provision of adaptive professiogenesis, mental health and population's quality of life.

MHSM requires informational support and telecommunication systems large-scale adoption, the absence of which makes such processes as regulation, processing, and analysis of semantic data masses provided by associated automated informational systems, impossible. "Informational system of automated diagnosing" (ISAD) program product created by L. N. Blagov and A. A. Loschinin (2013), based on the model of clinical and practical activity in psychiatry and addictology, hastens MHSM adoption.

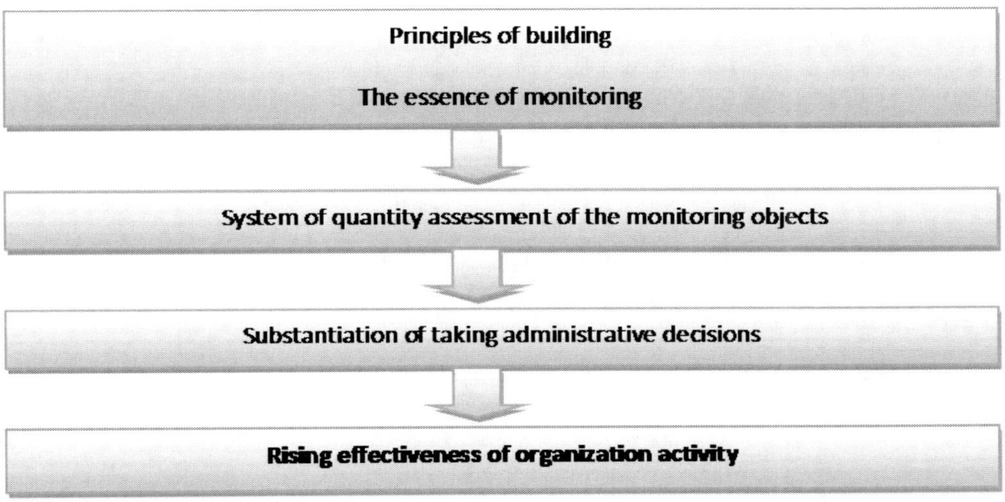

Figure 31.1. Concept of system monitoring.

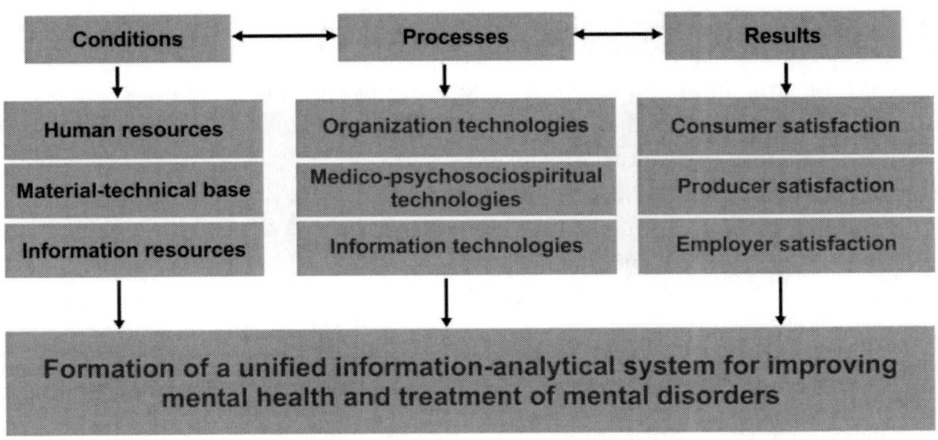

Figure 31.2. Objects of system monitoring.

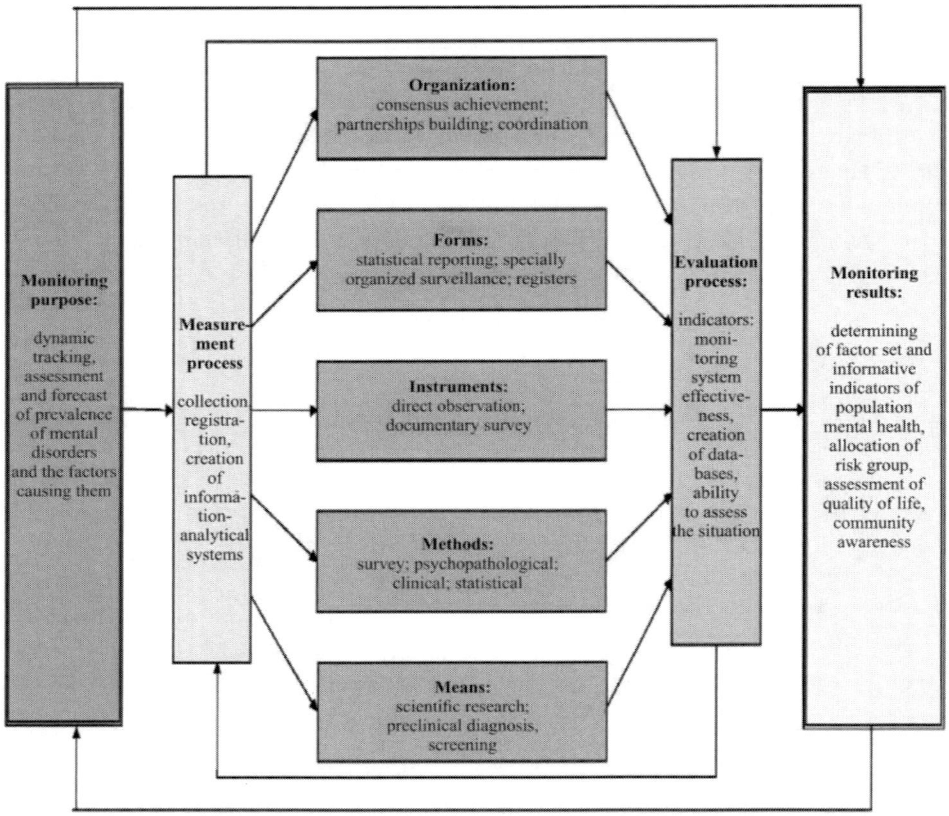

Figure 31.3. Structural and functional model of the mental health system monitoring.

Conceptual model of mental health system monitoring consists in monitoring methodology and organization development; carrying out mental disorders monitoring; forming of integral information base; results estimation and prognosis; forming of risks management strategies; development of multi-level prevention programs.

System monitoring requires solving the following strategic tasks: getting real rates of mental health quality and mental illnesses prevalence rate; creation of a common database and registers of mental disorders; development of multi-level multidisciplinary prevention programs; economic effectiveness increase.

Currently, the interface becomes a very popular and widely-spread interdisciplinary term in scientific and practical discourse. It serves to explain and project the systems and mechanisms of selective nondestructive relationships among wildlife and inanimate nature objects. In a broad sense, an interface is a specified by standards boundary between independent interacting objects. Interface sets interactional parameters, procedures and characteristics. MHSM can be defined as interface of individual and public conscience.

The main features of human conscience defining it as an interface between the subject and the world of physical reality include:

1) *Conscience selectivity* towards all the forms of stimulation: physical and social, spiritual and psychological.
2) *Conscience flexibility* providing creation, manifestation and restriction of freedom degrees within the framework of human personality and body integrity.
3) *Conscience universality* preserving functionality features by changing the content in different corporeal forms.
4) *Conscience individuality* which is defined by perceptive systems mechanisms, forming subjective reality.
5) *Conscience clear transparency,* when the subject does not distinguish constructs created in the brain from constructs, emerging in conscience under the influence of physical reality stimuli on perceptive systems (Sergeev 2014; Sidorov 2014).

Interface features of conscience and perceptive systems of a person should be taken into consideration when planning and adopting MHSM.

A necessity for further development and adoption of government and corporate, social and government, public and private models of MHS and mental health system monitoring is dictated by question solution of early effective mental disorders prevention. Medical, mental, social and spiritual care in cases of mental disorders, which was developed on the basis of synergetic methodology, includes medical and psychological, social, moral and spiritual units, and also *presupposes* multidisciplinary teams' involvement in prevention, correction, treatment, and rehabilitation.

Without the creation of MHS and mental health system monitoring of nation, it will be merely impossible to withstand modern challenges of globalizing system aggression and mental terrorism, which are chronizated in lifestyle through stresses and permanent crises. This problem is particularly urgent nowadays when global web triggered *schism* of modern world public conscience into real and virtual while social *autism* of gamers and Internet addicts' subpopulations started the mechanisms of various users' selection and destructive degradation of their conscience (mental terrorism).

If previously all screening functions of candidates selection and classification for work in special services were carried out by employment agencies and training centers, neo-cults and network marketing (from business corporations to youth movements), nowadays even personalized recruiting becomes a history, because individual and public conscience control with the help of Internet is more effective. Thus, the NSA (whose illegal activity was disclosed by Edward Snowden) not only has been controlling electronic communications all over the world for a long time but also purposefully and tenaciously tracks even personal Internet playing areas. According to expert estimations, behavioral analysis of military games players makes it possible to detect a certain level of technical skills, the inclination to venturesome and romantic adventures, risk and resistance to stress among these persons. For this purpose, American special services created their personal virtual characters and communicated like this with real gamers in order to detect the most interesting persons for recruiting. It is possible to judge the scale of this testing network according to the fact that only World of Warcraft (game controlled by them) engaged nearly 8 million people by the end of 2013 (Andreev, Nazarova 2014).

Another version of using online games in the NSA activity is conditioned by the fact that under the guise of virtual characters activity, it is possible to undertake mental manipulations in order to activate text and voice channels of intergame communications for coordination of real activity and hacker's acts by terrorists and subversives, as well as for data collection and pictures exchange.

It is for a reason that the Internet is still an American private company property. The USA fights against international control establishment on behalf of the UNO in every possible way. Such control concerns the Internet content and protection provision from any unauthorized interference. The country is also against forming of international control principles over recourses and regimes of the Worldwide Web functioning.

31.2. Principles of Organization and Functions of the Mental Health Service

Mental health service is a synergetic bio-, psycho-, socio- and spiritual Ψ-cluster of both society and government, providing preventive and correctional protection of mental health as well as treatment and rehabilitation assistance in cases of mental illnesses.

The first pilot model of MHS was developed and adopted at the premises of NSMU in 2000, demonstrating a fundamentally new quality of mental health and adaptive professiogenesis provision for a team by means of multidisciplinary synergetic methodology.

It is possible to single out the main *organization principles* for mental health service:

1) *Individual approach* to every patient and client with a gradual transition to group forms of work.
2) *Taking socio-psychological, moral and spiritual peculiarities* of a patient and his family *into consideration*, the realization of family-centered strategies.
3) *Complex and systemic* medical, mental, social and spiritual approach to the planning of preventive, correction, treatment and rehabilitation programs.
4) *Screening of* a person and organism's *prenosological resources*, prognosis of states and diseases trajectory development.
5) *The quality of life estimation* for the objectification of technologies effectiveness in mental preventology and medicine.
6) *Multivariance and multidimensionality* of multidisciplinary resources mobilization in planning and realization of personalized programs and schedules.
7) *Broadening of traditional resource* and instrumentally technological healthcare approaches.
8) *Synergetic effects attainment* within the framework of economically inexpensive and resource saving technologies.
9) *Integration* of psychiatric care into general practice.
10) *Destigmatization of the technological field* and multidisciplinary specialists' team.
11) *Holistic approaches and partnership relations* inside the professional and therapeutic community.
12) *Health-oriented priorities* in the unity of healthy lifestyle and moral life sense.
13) *Interactive info-communicative provision* of adequate health level in patients, clients, establishments and organizations.
14) *Humanistic position* and the presumption of mental individuality of clients and patients.

15) *Brigade and team forms* of polyprofessional activity organization.
16) *System monitoring of mental health* and mental illnesses, resources allocation and usage, services effectiveness estimation.
17) *Mobilization of resource-constructive strategies* of adaptive professiogenesis and adequate quality of life provision.
18) *The inclusive direction* in correction process together with specialized care delivery character.
19) *Continuity* of correction, preventive, treatment and rehabilitation work on every age steps, taking patients and clients' mental peculiarities specifics into consideration.
20) *The key role* of patient's interests while choosing instrumental and technological approaches.
21) *Planning and realization of religiously integrated* programs and schedules.

The following *MHS functions* can be distinguished within the framework of developed four-dimensional bio-, psycho-, socio- and synergetic spiritual methodology of mental medicine.

A. *Medical-oriented MHS functions (psychiatric, addiction, psychosomatic, etc.):*

- psycho-pharmacotherapy organization;
- screening and medical diagnostics carrying out for patients and clients, members of their families, staff;
- organization and delivery of medical care;
- informing the patients and clients or their guardians about their health state, diagnosis, and prognosis;
- home nursing for patients and their families;
- informing the patient about his or her rights to receive medical care and procedure of its delivery;
- sanitary, hygienic and psychoeducation.

B. *Socially-oriented MHS functions:*

- screening and social diagnostics carrying out for patients and clients, members of their families, staff;
- development and carrying out individual programs and schedules of social correction, therapy, and rehabilitation for a patient or client;
- organization and carrying out of measures for social defense and support, employment and living settlement, continued studying and professional education;
- representation of patients and/or clients interests needing social care in government agencies;
- assistance and prevention of socially dangerous acts;
- creation of rehabilitation social infrastructure;
- informing the patients about benefits and other types of social defense;
- assistance in solving social, living and accommodation problems, pensions and benefits payments;

- training on social skills and family resistance or flexibility, communicative family styles;
- interaction with the Mass Media and population in the sphere of forming a resource-constructive attitude towards socio-medical problems.

C. *Mentally-psychotherapeutic oriented MHS functions:*

- screening and psychological diagnostics carrying out for patients and clients, members of their families, staff;
- development and carrying out of individual programs and schedules in psychotherapeutic care and psychological correction;
- mobilization of coping mechanisms of diagnostic distress control;
- risk factors detection and assistance in stress situations;
- family questions consulting, family psycho-correction and psychotherapy;
- education in the sphere of communication techniques with "troubled patients";
- staff education in the sphere of self-regulation and self-help methods;
- organization and delivery of training on communication, self-assertion, decision making, etc.;
- delivery of Balint groups, support groups, T-groups, therapy by creative self-expression, coaching, etc.;
- individual and group hypnotherapy;
- rational and positive psychotherapy;
- play and music therapy;
- interaction with the Mass Media and population in the sphere of adaptive extension of public conscience.

D. *Morally and spiritually oriented MHS functions:*

- screening and moral diagnostics carrying out for patients and clients, members of their families, staff;
- development and carrying out of individual programs and schedules of moral and spiritual care and rehabilitation in cases of syndromes of destructive professiogenesis and demoralization, existential hopelessness, etc.;
- organization and carrying out of religiously integrated preventive, correction, treatment and rehabilitation programs with official confessions involvement;
- delivery of moral and spiritual propedeutics, sense-oriented and psychosocial psychotherapy;
- organization of training in business communication ethics and personal happiness growth;
- monitoring of moral climate, prognosis and conflict situations solving (mediation);
- mandate widening and increasing activity effectiveness of ethical committees in health care organizations;
- early correction of disturbances in forming and development of moral and spiritual feelings, image and position, behavioral and communication ethics.

E. *Integrative-synergetic MHS functions:*

- integration of diagnostic, analytical, organizational and coordination resources;
- the government, public and private partnership provision in assistance delivery for patients and clients, staff and employees families;
- mental health system monitoring implementation for patients/clients and their families, staff, and population including modern computerized interactive forms;
- organization of multidisciplinary preventive, correction, treatment and rehabilitation programs;
- synergetic therapy delivery;
- adoption of team forms of assistance delivery within the framework of individual schedules and interdisciplinary protocols;
- provision of synchronism and harmony in efforts on micro-, milli-, meso- and macro-social levels, provision of multichannel program financing and multidisciplinarity of staff support, polymodality and resonance of synergetic efforts;
- socio-medical expertise and rehabilitation implementation;
- legal consultancy in medical, mental, social and spiritual spheres;
- organization of volunteer movement and therapeutic communities in self- and mutual help among patients and clients, their families and staff.

MHS principles and functions listed above resulted from the last pilot project of its organization on the basis of departments of leucosis and children surgery of NSMU in Arkhangelsk regional children's clinical hospital in 2013-2014. Many specialists were involved in the working process including oncologists, psychiatrists, psychotherapists, clinical psychologists, social workers, teachers, educators, nurses, patients' parents, hospital clowns and volunteering students of NSMU. The project of MHS regulations was offered to the ministry of public health in Arkhangelsk region administration after receiving the study results.

Implementation of functions mentioned above makes it possible to form synergetic functional diagnosis consisting of clinical, psychological, social and ethical diagnosis as well as comorbide and associated disorders. Individual preventive, correction, treatment and rehabilitation schedule for a patient or client is based on this functional diagnosis. Mission and scale of efforts made by each specialist are given in full in multi-professional team protocol.

The key element of MHS is a team permitting to trigger resonant and cumulative socio-genetical, animogenetical, psychotherapeutic and biogenetical mechanisms accumulated in sanogenetic therapy by means of multichannel and polymodal efforts.

31.3. Adaptive Professiogenesis as a Priority of Corporate Mental Health Service

Organizationally-functional provision of adaptive professiogenesis becomes a priority of *mental health corporate services,* enterprises or organizations. Their infrastructure exists, but only in an uncoordinated and rudimentary form. Synergetic effect can be provided by medical, psychological, social and ethical integration and realization of a *staff's mental health system monitoring* aimed at finding cause-effect relation in the "working environment – person" system. Within the framework of unified synergetic methodology MHSM unites profile information bases, giving a real picture and dynamics of significant socioeconomic trends.

Areas of mental health service work are represented in Figure 31.4. While medical (EMERCOM, trade union committees), psychological (psychological service) and social (departments of labor protection, social work, veterans administrations) areas were established long ago, ethical area requires radical mandate editing, existing in every medical establishment of ethical committees.

Strategies and targeted factors of mental health services activity are represented in Figure 31.5.

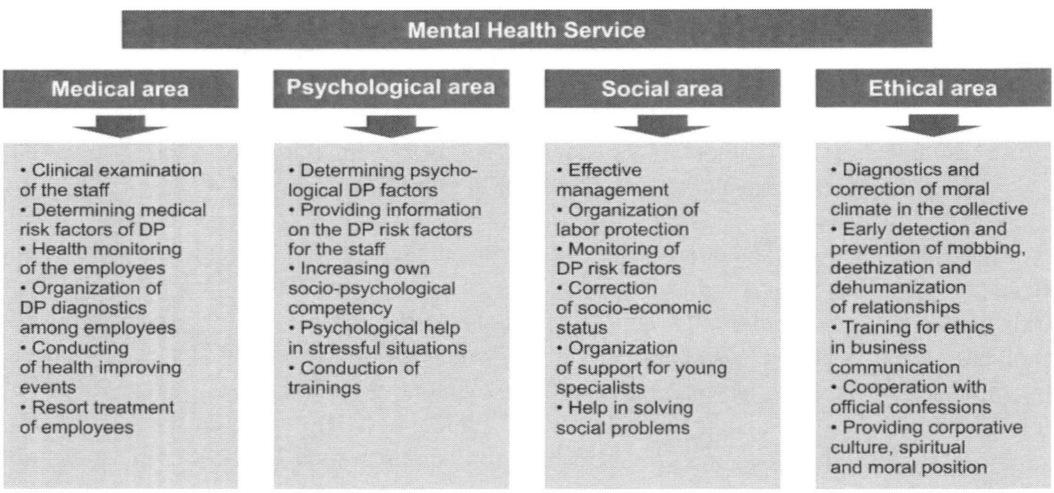

Figure 31.4. Provision of adaptive professiogenesis.

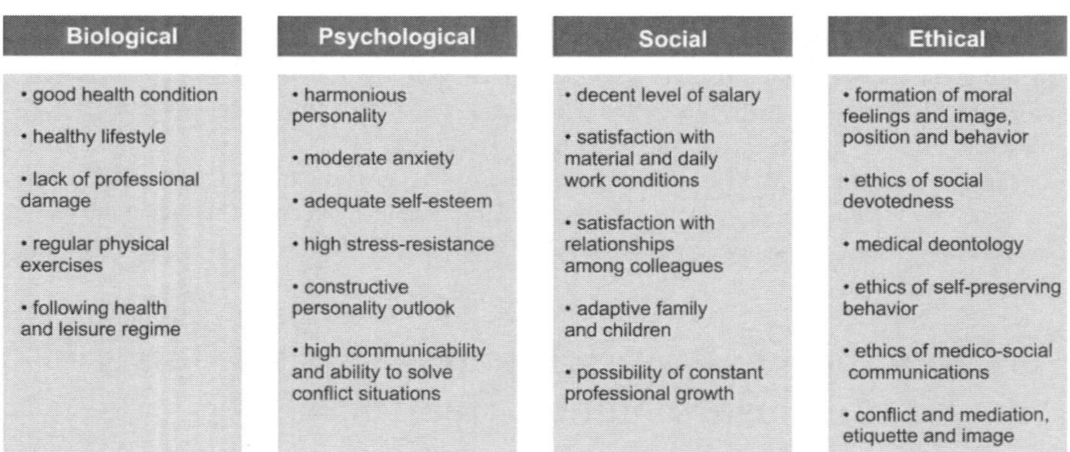
Biological
Psychological
Social
Ethical
• good health condition
• healthy lifestyle
• lack of professional damage
• regular physical exercises
• following health and leisure regime
• harmonious personality
• moderate anxiety
• adequate self-esteem
• high stress-resistance
• constructive personality outlook
• high communicability and ability to solve conflict situations
• decent level of salary
• satisfaction with material and daily work conditions
• satisfaction with relationships among colleagues
• adaptive family and children
• possibility of constant professional growth
• formation of moral feelings and image, position and behavior
• ethics of social devotedness
• medical deontology
• ethics of self-preserving behavior
• ethics of medico-social communications
• conflict and mediation, etiquette and image

Figure 31.5. Strategies and target orientation of the mental health service.

In the Northern State Medical University, *mental health service* (MHS) was established as a pilot version in 2000. It includes the following elements: clinics for educators and students, psychotherapeutic and addiction clinics, psychological and sociological services, ethical committee, departments of labor protection, educational and social work, centers of trainings and business technologies, consulting and recruitment, volunteer student communities, clubs (of international friendship, literature, movie discussion), student and veterans councils. Assistance for students, employees and members of their families is provided for free.

MHS activity is controlled by the *Mental medicine institute* which was established in 2009 and comprises departments of psychiatry, addictology and clinical psychology, neurology and neuropsychology, pedagogy and psychology, as well as the faculty of clinical psychology and social work, the students of which carry out their volunteer practice by means of assistance delivery (including assistance for veterans of the higher-education establishment).

The *Public faculty of mental health* was established in NSMU in 2011. It includes five departments: the Departments of spiritual education, orthodox medicine, demographical politics, public health protection and social illnesses withstanding, orthodox psychology and psychotherapy. The faculty accumulated multidisciplinary approaches towards moral and spiritual education within the framework of government, private and public partnership with Arkhangelsk and Holmogorsk metropolitan towns and business community.

Fully valid mental health service can implement the program of medical, psychological, social and spiritual prevention measures against destructive professiogenesis. Essentially this program is a *multidisciplinary protocol of teamwork*, revealing synergetic effect by means of combined efforts.

However, corporate level of preventive measures is not sufficient. The systemic and multilevel approach is required (Figure 31.6).

Countrywide measures are implemented on a *macrosocial* level. There are data about t he fact that employees' salaries increase favors reduction of BS development rate. Thus, BS symptoms occur in medical employees of private clinics less frequently (Yuryeva L. N., 2005).

Measures on a *mesosocial* level (work personnel) include improvement of socially-psychological climate and work activity conditions. Psychologist or psychotherapist from mental health service should control and provide prevention measures against destructive professiogenesis on the level of work personnel.

Employee's family as an object of preventive measures occurs on a *millisocial* level. A psychologist can provide family relationship correction and family psychotherapy if needed. Also, psychologist should provide preventive measures against destructive professiogenesis on a *personal micro-social* level. Therefore, it is necessary for a medical establishment to employ a psychologist or psychotherapist as a staff member, who can deliver assistance not only for patients but also for establishment employees.

The following basic areas are included into psycho-psychotherapeutic work in DP prevention by mental health service: lectures on informing about DP and its prevention principles; DP diagnostics and risk factors detection; employees education in the sphere of self-regulation methods; education on self-help methods; psychological assistance in stress situations; assistance in conflict situations solving; trainings carrying out (communicative, self-assertion, decision making); professional communicative skills correction; psychological correction of personal attitudes; education in the sphere of communication techniques with troubled patients; therapy by means of creative self-expression; delivery of Balint groups, support groups, T-groups; using techniques aimed at personal happiness growth.

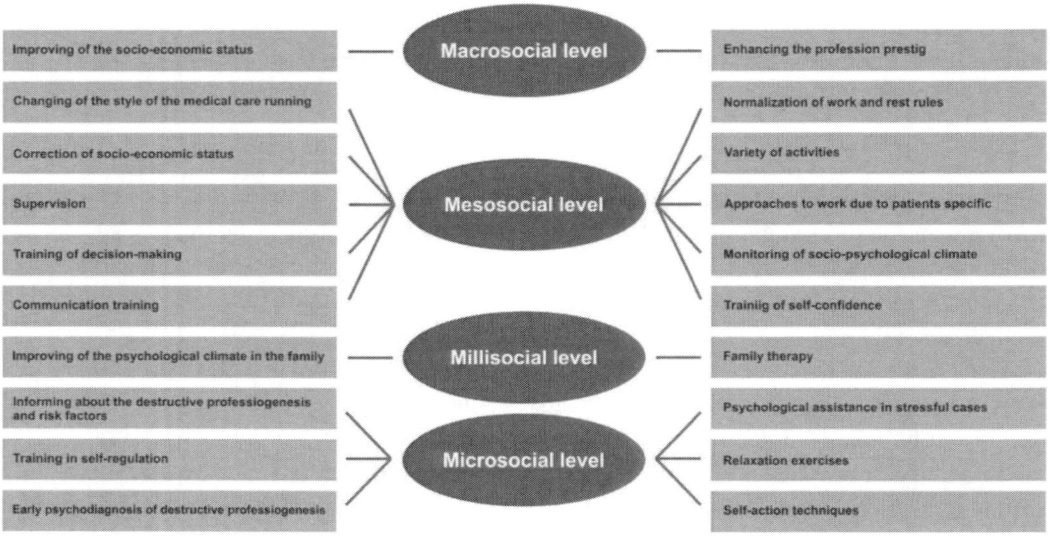

Figure 31.6. Algorithm of multilevel prevention of destructive professiogenesis among health care workers.

MHS differs from existing mental health services by moral and spiritual unit involvement and synergetic methodology of mental medicine.

Thus synergetic methodology of mental medicine makes it possible to organize preventive measures even on the prenosological level and realize individual treatment and rehabilitation schedules on the basis of corporate mental health services. The suggested multilevel multidisciplinary system of adaptive professiogenesis provision should become a priority in socio-medical protection of any professional community. Current provoking of country reforming requires radical changes in the modality of public and professional conscience of work personnel, i.e., replacement of pessimistic and catastrophic paradigm of world perception by resource creative life strategy, predetermining adaptive professiogenesis and sustainable development.

Chapter 32

Mental Engineering of Public Conscience

One of the major means of mental engineering is the cinema art which has an immense influence on young viewers. There have been empirical researches of the influence of existential-themed movies and TV-shows on the self-actualization of the viewers. The results of the researches show that such movies and TV-shows can be classified as means of adaptive (or disadaptive) mind control. For example, V. S. Gryazeva-Dobshinskaya (2013) figured out that general artistic effect of the modernism and post-modernism production can be summarized by saying that the audience develops discomfort states of instability and ambiguity which intensity varies from "incomplete harmonization" to "open catastrophe" as the uttermost unstable, ambivalent condition. Contrastingly, classic and neo-classic production lead to a harmonizing effect of catharsis. Every artist has his own specific semantic influences on viewer's personality. These influences are personological effects manifesting themselves in resonating or confrontation of Self-identities with The Different, mirrored by themselves and created by connatural or extraneous director's meanings. A method of detection of such influences has been suggested. It is substantiated that symbolic cinema art can be classified as cultural means of influence on a person, and its specific character allows understanding their evolutionary meaning in modern culture as the implement of meaning-making and specify the vectors of the most probable personal and semantic transformations of the subjects and subpopulations.

In the modern society the television has turned into a major socializing institution (Zhuravleva 2013), and in this capacity has substantially supplanted the influence of books, family, and school teachers. Any kind of asocial behavioral role models, as well as obscene language, occur on a daily basis in everlasting TV series overfilled with strong sexual content, murders, maniacs, homosexuals, prostitutes, strippers, gangsters and detectives. All of this intensifies the accumulation of "existential vacuum," destroying traditional standards and values, socially and culturally fixed in viewers' mind. A. P. Nazaretyan (2010) draws attention to the fact that TV-industry often uses "evil charm of violence and fear" (same book, page 432) and regularly uses such concepts as "a corpse livens up the scene" (page 428). It turns any scene into "necrophilous feast" thus, creating an image of modern society as a totally violent and criminalized community in the mass conscience. According to E. U.

Strizhenov (2011), about 85% of the youth regard fraudulence as completely acceptable means of earning a living. Virtually every hero of youth subculture originates from the television subculture.

In this context, the popular English TV series "Sherlock" is a typical example of modern manipulative mythogenesis. The authors created an exotic image of an ingenious detective, full of modern, up-to-date traits that have nothing in common with the original prototype but perform the very same historic mission - the mythologization of the public conscience which needs regular confirmation of inevitable victory of The Good over The Evil. While watching, the viewer is plunged into the intrigue of the plot, enjoying the process of psycho-aesthetic consuming of the artistic product, thus being unable to notice that he becomes a target of hidden manipulation.

Regardless all its illusiveness, any myth implements a very important socializing function of reproduction and substantial structuring of public conscience. The characters of Holmes and Watson are more than 100 years old. They are close and loved personages for many generations of readers all over the world. Their original patriarchal classics were brilliantly personified by Vasiliy Livanov and Vitaliy Solomin in the Soviet period. However, the ethics in business and person-to-person communication of the characters corresponded with the traditions and moral values of that era. The modern age has demanded drastic personality reform as well as the ethic and aesthetic modernization.

It appears relevant to analyse mental engineering of virtual images and the plot meanings of the "Sherlock" series in the frame of the synergetic biopsychosociospiritual methodology of mental medicine. The description of phenomenology and mechanisms of realisation of pathoplastic factors of Anglo-Saxon mentality accumulates major characteristics of public conscience and self-identity. The substantiation of necessity of systematic monitoring of mental health has the purpose of upgrading the efficiency of adaptive control of the public conscience.

32.1. Mental Designing of a Virtual Image and Real Meaning

A. L. Zhuravlev et al. (2013) suggested a two-component model of "psychosocial man" and the ground rules of its designing. We developed the quad-core and four-dimensional model of biopsychosociospiritual "synergetic man" (Sidorov 2013) built basically on the same ground rules of mental engineering.

1) Semantic system integrity-presence of correlations among attitudes, relations and mechanisms.
2) Positive "Self-concept" as a core of the semantic system.
3) The dynamic balance of actions and meanings.
4) Formation of behavior by means of social learning.
5) Harmony of the semantic sphere and symbolic systems, particularly ethics in business communication.
6) Ontogenetic development, accumulating peculiarities of individual biopsycho-sociospiritual resources.

7) Fractal multidimensional dynamics of life journey and multivariant trajectory if the fate, changing its vector at bifurcation points.
8) The tendency to understand the outside world and reflection.

Any model of a human is undoubtedly a simplification and schematization, which can be justified only because of the necessity of fixation of the level of conceptual immersion predetermined by chosen methodology. The synergetic biopsychosociospiritual methodology of mental medicine is equally applicable to the assessment of mental health as well as mental diseases. Despite its conditional and artificial character, the clinical analysis of a movie character appears important for detection of personifications of new time challenges.

Psychogenesis of the main character is designed like a mosaic collection of various personality disorders, deep-rooted action and intellection patterns characterized by reflection and counter reactions manifesting themselves with a vengeance. Synonyms of such personality disorders are psychopathy, deviant personality, sociopathy. Essentially, personality is the aggregate of stable and lasting characteristics of individuality. Sherlock, performed by Benedict Cumberbatch displays many clinical pieces ofevidence:

- -flat affectivity and emotional strangeness (autism) accompanied by very choosy hypersensitiveness and vulnerability;
- deficiency and disorder of interpersonal relationships in relative social isolation;
- devaluation of respect for social convention and decorum, social rules of conduct;
- eccentric and impulsive behavior, scandalousness and persistence, self-absorption and narcissism;
- avoidance of intimate contacts and distrust, lack of responsibility and empathy;
- alluring and attractive, but disrespectful and unpopular among others behavior pattern;
- almost pathological frankness and self-actualisation (obviously in accordance with scenario demands for the sake of better audience perception).
- The highlighted characteristics formally relate to schizotypal and paranoid, narcissistic and hysterical, asocial and emotionally labile types of personal disorders. This fact might only show the authors' desire for designing of a simulacrum of total marginality which literally blows up and widens the limits of public conscience.

With the same purpose, there is a pronounced cyclothymia of the hero, when periods of hypomanic agitation (particularly in anticipation of another investigation or murder) give place to subdepressiveness accompanied by excessive smoking and narcotization (in the original – cocaine and morphine, which at those times had not been put on the drug schedule). In the "Prolog" (1 episode of 1 season) Sherlock detects high tolerance of the murderer (a taxi-driver) to a drug attack thus, revealing his own personal disorders.

Holmes' dependence disorders are represented or annotated nearly by all possible clinical versions:

- chemical one: smoking or “3 nicotine patches problem,” narcotization;
- non chemical one: extreme, aggressive and self-destructive detective activity, risk of possible gambling reflected by distinctive cry: “The game is on !”- with almost ecstatic agitation;
- vicarious one, filling moral and psychological emptiness: workaholism, mental terrorism;
- latent sexual perversions which have become one of the nearly normative traits of multiculturalism.

No wonder that the image of a modern European hero has demanded from its creators broad hints and ambiguities about Sherlock's latent homosexuality manifesting itself particularly in reckless boldness and sadistic verbal activity as well as inability and unwillingness to predict the outcome of his eccentric actions. From the beginning of the very first episode of the first season, a viewer is intrigued by tedious waiting: when and how Holmes will manage to fulfill himself sexually. Categorical asexuality, excessively declared by Sherlock (“I am married to my job”) is mimically perceived by Watson as the opposite.

Sociogenesis of Sherlock's image is conditioned by relative social deprivation in his childhood, disharmony of relationship in his parents' family that later on manifested themselves in defective forming of adaptive behavior and response patterns as well as in estrangement and dissociation from collective actions. Thus, being “white crow” in one's young days, the one becomes almost an outcast in his middle age and tends to “leadership notwithstanding the current situation” by virtue of intellectual uniqueness, but outside the formal career field. That's why he obtains an exotic status of a consulting detective. He is busy with his favorite job and focused solely on the process of investigation, being completely indifferent towards the result and its capitalizing. That is why he doesn't care for his routine honorarium (Perelman-like novel), as opposed to the doctor Watson who appears half-contused by Afghan reality.

Social behavior patterns of Sherlock are somehow ambivalent and ambitendent. Thus, illusive-compensatory relationships with Watson become constructive and reality-based only occasionally, when the moment is crucial. Being an autonomous introvert, Holmes uses Watson in an unpretentiously one-sided way. Watson though naively flatters himself with an idea of business-based partnership. A conversation taken by Watson as a dialogue is nothing but a monolog for Holmes. He sees, feels and listens only to himself. Against such a background, Sherlock's rare touching human enlightenments almost make viewers weep. No wonder that in his interview with a Psychologist magazine (January of 2015, page 20) Benedict Cumberbatch himself calls “Holmes a rare stinker.”

Holmes' favorite methods of management and manipulating people are scandalous behavior and provocation, deception and verbal aggression borrowed from an arsenal of a mobbing-terrorist. It is only the genre's canons that prevent Sherlock from outraging all decency and save pro-social anchors.

Holmes' milieu are almost identically problematic and sociopathic as Holmes himself: Watson is a grave neurotic with the post-traumatic syndrome, his wife Mary is a killer, missis

Hudson is a former mama-san, his assistants are drug-addicts and swindlers, his elder brother Mycroft Holmes is a boss of high-ranked functionaries mob, etc. With such an abundant past and impressive present, this model of society will undoubtedly manage the task of destroying the modern world from within, against a background of the global crisis. Whether is it this idea that the producers want to embed in viewers' minds or maybe following series are to be amended, but the impression is that the measured semantic inoculations or enemas are given to public conscience as a part of global dehumanizing mental trend.

Animogenesis of the Holmes' image starts with difficulties and problems of upbringing in his parents' family. It is no coincidence that Sherlock literally despises his parents who were unable or didn't want to introduce harmonious shaping of basic spiritual and moral senses, attitudes, and behavior at early stages of his moral socialization and civil maturing. It manifested itself in many factors, such as his unpreparedness to harmonious self-responsible behavior; undevelopment of moral self-conscience of the personality; deformation of his patience, tolerance, mercifulness, humanism and ability to be friendly and affectionate; non-critical estimation of his own motives, attitudes, intentions and thoughts; incomprehension of unconditional value of the family and its moral basis; giving up professional and career development; deficit of personal responsibility; and substantial devaluation of legal awareness. The entire mentioned above are characteristics of a demoralization syndrome which originates addiction and personal disorders.

Somatogenesis of the main character is not detailed. So, basing on random fragments, we can only conjecture his periodic psychosomatic decompensation, conditioned by somatization of multiple unreacted stresses and troubles, conflicts, and complexes as well as comorbid and associate disorders.

These are main biopsychosociospiritual qualities of the virtual construct named "Sherlock" in the frame of the multidisciplinary methodology of mental medicine.

32.2. Mentality and Identity of Virtual Characters and Real Adherents

On the16 of March of 2004, in London, some personal documents of Sir Arthur Conan Doyle were discovered. More than 3000 pages were found in an office of a law firm. Among them, there were diaries and manuscripts of his unpublished works which allowed extending significantly our understanding of the personality of the writer himself and his characters literary destiny.

Psychologic and patographic bibliography of Arthur Conan Doyle and his characters is very extensive. The personal traits and qualities that the author inserted in the original Sherlock's image and its evolution in multiple screens and theatrical versions are traced back a long time ago. It is important, though, to focus on mechanisms and matrices of the modern era challenges' projection on changing mentality and identity of the heroes themselves and their fans. The duality of mentality and identity consists in the fact that mentality, figuratively speaking is a way of seeing the outside world, and identity is a look inside, in other words – personal identity. The objects of mental medicine are the quality of mental health and risk of mental diseases development. These factors are in direct relation to how well the images and meanings of exo- and endo-reality are balanced and harmonious.

There are pathoplastic factors of the modern world's mental ecology, which substantially predetermined features of scenario designing and the actor's embodiment of the last Sherlock. They are:

- extended and uncontrollable reproduction of all the forms of destructive social epidemics varying from alcoholism and narcotization to fanaticism and terrorism, that no longer can be restrained by traditional medical, social and law enforcement authorities, which leads to globalization of violence and aggression creating the situation of "war without rules" (e.g., Ukrainian Revolution in Kiev, in February of 2014) and Sherlock's "mental terrorism";
- galloping compaction of infosphere; supplanting of traditional interpersonal and cultural interaction by technogenic, virtual form of communication; formalization and stereotypization of communications, manifesting themselves in Sherlock's behavior by emotional and social deficit;
- the increase of estrangement and marginalization, incompetence (Lestrade, constables, etc.) and psychological illiteracy, legal regulation efficiency impairing, which Sherlock displays by deformation of his civil responsibility, empathy and syntonia;
- line mass cult production and moral disorientation, increase of de-ethisation and dehumanization of public conscience, revealing themselves in Sherlock's demoralization syndrome development.

Formal logic has a classic check of assertion validity- its exaggeration. In this context, Sherlock's transfer to the present is an obvious exaggeration, and one has to admit it's quite a successful one in the frame of adaptive manipulating of public conscience. It manifests itself in another reloading of national, social, group and individual identity, as well as in strengthening of the unity and cohesiveness of all generations. The thing is that Holmes has already become a core brand, which culturally structures English mentality. Metaphorically speaking, the identity is a major lens in the telescope of our mentality as a way of viewing the world. It is the mental medicine that has techniques and methods of adaptive adjustment of one's life- and self-perception, mobilizing resources of the organism and personality, strengthening mental health and preventing mental diseases.

An integral quality of mental health is public conscience which in many respects predetermines personal and social identity. Personal identity means physical, intellectual and moral self-determination of a person. Social identity means social, group (confessional, professional, elite, etc.) self-determination. Seren Kierkegor said: "A human is a social animal and can be happy only within a herd. No matter if it is absolute nonsense or a horrible villainy. As soon as it is the herd law and he can be a part of the herd, the human will feel easy and calm" (Sas 2007). That is why the identity is the most important moral value and socio-psychological construct within social engineering. It appears as the major marker in the frame of systemic monitoring of mental health (SMMH) which was designed and introduced by us at the premises of SSMU. In the modern global world, SMMH is becoming an important instrument of national security which makes it possible to predict and prevent any destructive social epidemics.

32.3. Adaptive Widening of the Public Conscience as Mental Evolution

Hopefully, that the reincarnated Sherlock appeals to young viewers not only because of his sociopathic characters but because of his deeply hidden, mutilated but still preserved humanitarian, merciful nucleus of his personality, which preserved him from turning into an outright monster. He impresses and charms with broad range of traits of his multidimensional personality that widen within borderline areas virtually to a fault. Holmes is busy with widening his conscience and actualises searching for new personal resources, almost artificially putting himself in deadlocks, but always miraculously gets out, thanks to creative efforts of script writers. This is, of course, self-destructive and almost sadomasochist lifestyle which is presented to viewers as normative manifestation of multiculturalism.

The main target of the “serial mirror-world” is undoubtedly a viewer, whose soul the authors try to get hold of and make resonate, offering, even more, exotics and originality, varying modalities and registers of the main hero's personality. They know perfectly well the zero-risk rules of their “digital roulette”: if the direct induction of bright, startling characters does not work, then the backward one definitely will. Although none of the viewers would ever say that he or she would like to become a bit Watson or Holmes or that he has visited unpretentious missus Hudson's brother or has worked retroactively for some local Magnuson, etc. Anyway, the immensity of the hero's personality and his ability to widen the viewers' conscience is the essential condition of viewers' affection based on conscious or (which is more frequent) subconscious self-identity. And in such a case, there are no holds barred.

Such an approach represents the global trend of widening conscience, manifesting itself with new facets and fresh paint of new interpretations of classic characters, loaded with modern neurolinguistics and aesthetics. We can try to ask some rhetorical questions- are there any limits of such a widening of conscience? What speed should the process have? How does this process correlate with resources of a personality? How and with what strings the expanding universe resonate with the expanding conscience? Moreover, finally, what is to collapse earlier and when is it going to happen?

Psychotechnics of figurative space-time widening of conscience, which creates a sense of immersion by means of trance and altered state of conscience is achieved by transferring classic story in the present; filling the classic plot with modern agenda; childhood's reminiscences; fantasies; dreams. The “Sherlock” has almost all of these traits, aimed at another editing and correction of our problem identity and borderline mentality which are easier to rule and manipulate in such a condition. In the frame of mental medicine, for therapeutic purposes, we designed a technique of sanogenetic therapy which is the adaptive biopsychosociospiritual management of conscience for the purpose of mobilization of the personality resources and the organism reserves (Sidorov 1988, 2008).

32.4. TV Series as a Mental Matrix of Life and Death Image and Meaning

Adaptive TV-accompaniment of the public conscience safety is traditionally based on code of journalistic ethics, besides it has various forms of presentation of facts as well as aesthetic and graphic arrangements of the presentation. During last decades, there are more and more various TV series within television broadcast which aimed to certain mental subpopulations and their topical problems. TV series, in fact, perform a mission of parapsychotherapeutic substitute-TV-marathons (additional interactivity of cable TV drastically increases psychotechnological effectiveness), promoting actualization of moral values potential of the audience. This clear mechanism can be marked as "forestalling reflection," full of images, stimuli, and meanings that contain urgent challenges of forecast tomorrow and provide adaptive development of public conscience. Only if today's reflection is forestalled then it becomes possible to achieve an effective moral and psychological immunization, thus shaping a desirable form of future spiritual immunity. Virtually all the talk-shows and TV-discussions familiarly kick about the issues that have already taken place. Mental medicine and mental ecology, with the help of the synergetic methodology, make it possible to predict and calculate space-time trajectories of events and conditions, social epidemics and diseases in the frame of quantum fractal dynamics, meanwhile consistently calculating preventive, correctional and rahabilitation resources.

Modern domestic cops-and-robbers series, including classic Holmes-Poirot-Marple films, persistently suggest to the viewers an idea that criminal pandemic is next door to us. It is clear that society is in an extreme need of professional and effective law enforcement institution. TV series though are the only imitation of the reality which destroys even an illusion of safety. Moreover, the excessiveness of the police theme and the viewers' surfeit provoke the opposite effect, and the Ukrainian February revolution is an evidence of the statement. There is still time to think things over and get an idea on how to change approaches.

A sophisticated viewer of the "Sherlock" series will easily find lots of reasons to heap reproaches on the producers about fragmentariness and mosaicism of the characters, sketchiness and artificiality of the plot lines; rigidity of the Holmes' image who substitutes intellectuality and creativity with trite impulsiveness and adventurousness; noisy excessiveness of actions accompanied by deficit of real meaning and furthermore-heaps of exuberantly bombastic and folk stupidity (gunshot-operation, family soporifics, Chinese arbalest etc.).

Meanwhile, those of viewers who got interested in the movie will note a good rhythm and the plot dynamics, vivacity and currency of the dialogues, minimalism of the necessity and sufficiency of resonant modulations which revive the mask on a nearly wax-made figure of the main hero.

It is not a secret that modern world is not just undemanding about creativity and extraordinariness but hardly tolerates these two qualities which threaten the traditions of the past, the consumption of the present and expected prosperity of the future. This statement can be proven by the abundance and diversity of artificial movie- and TV-heroes, long-playing show-business superstars who are only supposed to fill existential and spiritual emptiness. Endless resuscitations and reincarnation of new either Sherlocks or Holmeses are phenomena of the same field. It is much more urgent to create tomorrow's hero of the present because any hero of our time already accomplished all his heroic deeds (the real ones as well as the mythical ones) in the past and now the hero is simply getting his fair rent.

In the character of Sherlock, there is a clearly visible effect of polarization and dramatization of psychotic personal diversity in the periods of another civilizational cycle. Modern Holmes chooses a role of creative ranger, defending sacred meanings and foundations of the System with sometimes not entirely legal methods. He realizes very well that crimes and criminals are procreated by the very System that he serves, being de facto an elite prostitute who inevitably manifests in increase of the burden of demoralization syndrome and various self-destructions.

It is not by mere chance that both Holmes and Moriarty are narcissistic mirror reflections ("I am you"), frenetically exhausting themselves in the hysterical marathon of self-destructive life for the sake of ecstatic inspirational death. Such a literal suicidal message to the young generation of viewers looks more like an outspoken curse on the growing at an exponential rate army of unemployed or partially unemployed young people. At least, this is manipulation of the conscience which is supposed to impart an easier perception of the life and the death. Besides, again and again, everything happens according to classic Shakespeare formula "all the world is a stage, and all the men and women are merely players": enjoy the process; there are others who care for the results. This very much reminds anti-psychiatric formula of Lord Robert Webb-Johnston: "Neurotics build cloud-castles, schizophrenics live in them, psychopaths destroy them and alcoholics guzzle away the ruins. Everybody enjoys the process, but it is only the psychiatrists who collect the rent money."

In the frame of the public life, the mission of conventional psychiatrists (the ones who make diagnoses based on intraprofessional convention) is performed by politicians creating social diagnoses of self-made global or colourful crises. It goes along with multi-billion "treatment and rehabilitation programs and routes" in the direction of another exceptionally bright future, illusive for the "patients" and very concrete for the "doctors."

Such features as universal computer code (season 2, episode 3), an actor-clone, and four (why not thirteen!) international killers, etc. look like background spam. The fact that Moriarti works for the elder brother Mycroft's organized criminal group looks more realistic. Besides, Mycroft was so kind to inform Moriarty about juicy biographic details of nearly uncontrollable Sherlock, who is potentially able to threaten unmasking to both the spiders and their spiders' net. Only because of that the consulting detective should be guided and loaded with work on a regular basis, as this would create an illusion of self-fulfilment for him. This is an easy task for a dependent and unsound personality of Sherlock.

Whatever "dances of the little swans" the members of villainous chorus perform – it is just an execution of the "Elder Brother" will, on whose behalf Mycroft articulates something, but nobody will ever witness true puppeteers. This is the principle of life, according to either the codes of the underworld or decorative standards which are independent of ethnocultural national platform, acting language and the genre of another world première, padding noospheric spiritual vacuum. As for the impressed viewers, the meaning of the performance is an imitation of real life accompanied by obtrusion of illusive, compensatory roles and patterns being integrated into the social and personal identity and more importantly, leading away from constructive activity. Indeed, people who are capable of such activity do not watch TV series but produce them.

Producers have already gladdened viewers with Moriarty's comeback in the 4th season, although one, even disregarding this fact, could have guessed that the elder brother Mycroft as a leader of "Westminster gang," showing concern about his young brother, would recruit a new generation of the Moriarty-like clones. At the end of the day, why to slash jobs of the huge army of professionals on both sides of the moral-legal barricade made from a historical junkyard and chaotic conglomeration of the Criminal Code articles. One may state that Sherlock is an agent of influence 001, working for English royalty, whose civilizational anchors demand even more strengthening nowadays to prevent the islands from washing away from human history and culture, in a literal and figurative sense. The whole paradoxically-borderline image of the main hero is nothing but a convulsive grimace, being washed away and blown up by the multiculturalism of English identity and mentality. It is so tempting to say, using Holmes' words "elementary, my dear Watson!," i.e., there is going to be a complete elemental disintegration of the modern degradating and unhumanized system of limitless consumption, which is destroying itself and the whole world. It is hoped, that this a bit sorrowful trajectory can somehow be changed, at least during the inter-season period between soap operas...

As can be seen from the above, the TV in the modern world is still the main issuer of social, moral and cultural values, practically supplanted such traditional institutions of socialization as school, family, public organizations. It models in mass conscience a given image of reality and behavioral stereotypes of the heroes of modern time. That is why it is essential to conceptually-methodologically and instrumentally-technologically secure adaptive development of public conscience and strengthening of mental health that becoming an important priority of mental medicine performing a mission of interiorization of identity and forming spiritual immunity to destructive social phenomena.

32.5. Mental Health Service as a System of Adaptive Defense of Public Conscience

At the highest level of generalization, the **mission of mental medicine** is the interactive guaranteeing of civilizational trends and the instrumentarium of the coverage of the operative field (adaptive management and engineering of public and individual conscience and health). It can be collected in the process of consistent monitoring of mental health which is supposed to forecast and prevent threats to the public conscience of the nation, monitoring the whole path of human life, from parental development to active senility. SMMH is a multi-disciplined, complex monitoring aimed to reveal cause-and-effect links within the "environment-society-individual" system. It clusters core databases within a framework of integrated synergetic methodology, providing objective sight and dynamics of socially-important mental and behavioral trends. In the absence of the instrument, any programs of development and modernization will be very vulnerable. System monitoring of mental health (SMMH) is a part of system monitoring of public health as an anthropogenic block of *Global monitoring* which is supposed to provide interactive maintenance of the evolution of civilizational trends and global safety.

Mental health service (MHS) is a new synergetic productive cluster which is being formed nowadays in Russia. This service carries out mental medicine tasks in a system, programmatic and target-oriented mode, mobilizing federal, regional, corporative and private resources of the state-private and society-state partnerships. MHS is a synergetic biopsychosociospiritual Ψ-cluster of the society and the state. It provides the mentally-ill with preventive and correctional defense of the mental health along with medical and rehabilitation care (Sidorov 2013).

Health-centered priority of mental medicine is strengthening of mental health, which is in line with the strategy of mentality alteration suggested by A. L. Zhuravlev et al. (2013) *changing mentality strategy*. In the words of A. S. Pushkin, “the best and the firmest changes are those which happen due to folkways improvement, without forcible distress.”

Assignment of such a strategy requires an answer to a question about guidelines of the society development and evolution of mentality. The most cogent answer was given in 2010 by the French Committee on the effectiveness of economics and social progress under auspices of Nobel Prize Winners – J. Stiglitz and A. Sen along with J.-P. Fitoussi. They noted that economic indexes are important not as an end in itself, but inasmuch as they make people happy and the society stable. “*It is time to shift an emphasis from measuring economic production to measuring people's well-being* and...maintenance at least the current level of well-being for the future generations” (page 18). In the committee's report there are subjective estimations of well-being analysed, as well as its anticipated objective correlates, e.g., general health, education, leisure activities, political liberties, etc. However, there is no analysis of their correlation and the nature of the very phenomenon of well-being and its dependence on moral values systems of a human. It is important to note that well-being is the main characteristic of mental health which is measured with various multiple questionnaires of quality of life.

Alteration of strategic socio-economic modalities of well-being is a mission of a state policy, but the tactical alteration of its subjective perception has already become a routine practice of psychological and psychotherapeutic functioning. Moreover, conceptualization of strategic and tactical priorities are progressively inverted while synergetic trajectories of conditions and situations development may dramatically change at points of bifurcation due to even superweak influences. It’s for a reason that MHS, integrating resources of psychiatrics and clinical psychology, social work and ethic consulting, basically becomes an *institution of adaptive management of the patient or client's mentality* due to alteration of the motivational and attitudinal mechanism and moral-values priorities along with correction of social and personal identity.

In this context, A. F. Bondarenko (2006) describes the western psychotherapy as an obtrusion of ideology and mentality that suits ruling class: *“The genuine goal of psychotherapy is the maintenance of conventionalism, befitting “decent style” of the social standard”* (same book, page 73). He thinks that positive strategy for Russian psychotherapy is the strengthening of historical and genetic bases of Russian mentality and “is not to destroy naturally-historical tissue of native culture with artificial cultivation of foreign culture stereotypes, values and myths. But, on the contrary, undertaking deliberate and very delicate steps aimed at strengthening of dignity, self-conscience, and self-identity of a Russian man who found himself without up-to-date conscience and spiritual guardianship on the universal draughts of globalization. The strategy should assist a man in obtaining that peace of mind and spiritual greatness which could help us to regain an ability to conduct dialogue with the rest of the world on equal ground; to have an ability to create and stand up for not unfamiliar for us world of the Russian life” (same book, page 75).

According to A. L. Zhuravlev et al. (2013), the choice of the optimal vector of mentality development supposes a concrete analysis of the most important goals for the society. The authors-psychologists suggest a "model of optimal mentality" for every situation, which will assist a person in the goals realization in the frame of his institutional role, using all his energy and eagerness. Given a huge variety of possible situations and types of personal typology, the approach is going to be exceptionally extravagant. *The mental preventology strategy aims at maintaining the necessary and sufficient quality of mental health* (measured by "Personal mental ecology index") for adaptive reaction to every possible situations and challenges looks much more effective. Upon that, available resource- and personality-dependent mental models of behavior and reaction internalize from educational programs and training of mental representation styles, ethics in business communication and mediation.

Such goal-setting enables to classify legitimately mental medicine as a *strategic science* with the following criteria: 1) influence on country's power and competitive ability along with destiny and health of a large social stratum. 2) conceptually-methodological instrumentarium enables to obtain practically significant and useful results. Both these criteria are convincingly represented in mental medicine which has the multi-disciplined synergetic methodology that enables to mobilize effectively the resources of a person and society which makes it an innovative paradigm of not merely the whole clinical medicine but of the national security as well. Moreover, mental medicine with its biopsychosociospiritual instrumentarium accumulates the whole *technological complex of the strategic breakthrough*: nano-, bio-, informational, cognitive and social sciences (Kovalchuk 2011).

Undoubtedly, conceptually-methodological, instrumental and technological apparatus of mental medicine is acquiring strategic significance for the society and the state only upon condition of organizational and functional institutionalization in the frame of mental health service. MHS will enable to combine harmoniously on synergetic basis various mutually supportive forms of psychiatric, psychologic, addictologic, psychotherapeutic, social, spiritual and moral care, supplementing inertial post-Soviet standard medical examination with systematic monitoring of mental health. It is crucially important in this crisis situation when the mental health, in particular, turns into especially significant civilizational priority. It happens because satisfaction of material needs and guaranteeing of decent living standards of the population is about to reach a certain level. So "*it is a sensation that becomes the main condition of welfare rather than material goods*" (Florida 2002) and public conscience increasingly fixates on security and safety.

That is why the strategic health-centered goal of mental medicine is optimization and harmonization of public conscience as an integral quality of nation's mental health and fundamental priority of stable development. One would think it is enough, just to choose and adopt one or another socio-economic model which has already shown its effectiveness, along with a package of proper institutions. However, it is impossible to borrow the mentality that launches those models and institutions (Zhyravlev 2014). Essentially, it is MHS, based on new synergetic methodology of mental medicine that is supposed to realize interactive task of designing and introduction of mechanisms and technologies of forming the mentality and mental health that would be adequate to modern time challenges. One could fulfill this task only relying upon our model of biopsychosociospiritual "synergetic man," allowing forecasting and realizing multi-dimensional and multi-optional trajectories of development of a person and society. MHS prioritizes on maintenance of adaptive professiogenesis, sociogenesis, psychogenesis, somatogenesis, and animogenesis. All the tasks are perfectly executable, which has been convincingly demonstrated since 2000 in the frame of a pilot model of MHS based on Northern State Medical University (Sidorov 2014).

Here would be instructive to recall the speech of Russian President V. V. Putin that took place on general meeting of RAS in 2008, when he sorrowfully told to the academics that western technologies, procured by KGB, turned out to be uncalled in the Soviet Union. The cadre of science and technology sector of dying USSR with their mentality and infrastructure simply was not ready to innovations. One can imagine what would have happened in modern Russia if the modernization that loomed on the horizon of the noughties had been launched at those times. In a best-case scenario, the country would have got the early Gorby "syndrome of acceleration of the armoured train" from the sidetrack of civilization.

Without fulfilling the task of *forming innovative mentality* of the critical mass of such subpopulations as the entrepreneurship, state employees, science and education, it is impossible to take even a step closer to full-scale reforms. Solely in the present, and as usual, in the years of imminent peril, it is possible to achieve a new quality of understanding innovative tasks and cohesion of the nation.

Chapter 33

Mental Preventology as a System of Integration of Healthy Way and Moral Meaning of Life

33.1. From Psychoprophylaxis to Mental Preventology

The recent decade in the history of the Russian society is characterized by rapid changes from almost full neglect of personal health to its comprehension as a leading value. The paradigm of the entire medicine is changing from disease-oriented to health-oriented. At the same time, the preventive orientation of the health care is not efficient as it exists in the current medical practice. It is approved by the result of the public health evaluation – in recent decades, the level of health is progressively declining.

As early as in 2002, the Board of the Ministry of Healthcare of the Russian Federation adopted the Concept of Preventative Health care. It marked the development of a new activity area – the transition from the system oriented to disease treatment, to the system of the public health care, based on the priority of healthy lifestyle and the disease prevention. The key problem in this concept is the formation of the health culture, promotion of the prestige value of health and responsibility for the preservation of personal health. It started the practical implementation of new approaches to the promotion of preventive health care and became the background for creation of a methodological and ideological base of preventology.

General preventology is a field of knowledge about the ways of formation and support of optimal health level, its strengthening and disease prevention by any available means and with the involvement of a wide circle of specialists.

The necessity of training for preventologists having as the leading motivation for their activities the task of health loss prevention is currently being realized with increasing urgency.

The area of the preventologist's professional activities is the evaluation of individual and public health resources, of influence of environmental factors (natural, social, industrial) on human health, organization and implementation of preventive programs and events, learning of technologies and skills for health formation and strengthening, prevention of special diseases, individual consulting on the issues of health strengthening, teaching preventology in educational institutions of all forms and levels, conducting the field-specific scientific and marketing researches etc.

Professional field of preventology includes medical centers, consulting rooms and hospital departments of medical prevention, rehabilitation and health improvement centers, health resorts and rest houses, medical and social centers, educational institutions, schools of special diseases prevention (school "Diabetes," asthma-school etc.), communities and associations of patients and their relatives, physical training and sports facilities, etc.

The existence of a doctor called preventionist, specializing in preventive medicine and qualified for work in this area is a common phenomenon in Europe and the USA. Thus, in Great Britain, it is a doctor, completed an internship of Public Health Faculty, in the USA it is a doctor received the Certificate of the Preventive Medicine Counsel (Frank 1991).

Mental preventology is a special section of multidisciplinary preventology, dealing with prevention of mental disorders and preservation of mental well-being of a person, which allows realizing personal potential.

The object of *mental preventology* is factors and conditions of a mental pathology development; screening and prediction of mental disorders; preventive programs of various purpose; upbringing and formation of self-preserving behavior in family, at school, in higher educational institution, and at work; preventive resources of all the authorities concerned; strategies and mechanisms of overcoming a mental pathology etc. The main characteristic of mental preventology is its wide cross-disciplinary approach, which became possible due to the change of the disease-oriented paradigm to the health-oriented one.

Traditionally the problems of mental health preservation were the issue of psychoprophylaxis. The main provisions of mental preventology are originated from psychoprophylaxis; thus, we will further consider the main stages of psychoprophylaxis.

Table 33.1 shows the types of psychoprophylaxis and various fractals of disease epidemic development. Mental medicine provides full interpenetration of prevention and treatment. This is the medicine of mental health strengthening and treatment of mental disorders.

Table 33.1. Psychoprophylaxis in different fractals of diseases

Fractals	Predisposition: disharmonious family	Latent: diathesis	Initial: functional disorder	Full-scale clinical picture of the disease	Chronization: forms and types of the disease	Outcome: somatic-neurologic complications
Types of psychoprophylaxis	Primary			Secondary		Tertiary
Condition	Health			Disease onset and exacerbation		Disease outcome:
Epidemicity	Public Health Public Conscience			Mental epidemic	Destructive mental epidemic	Pandemic

Psychoprophylaxis is a section of general prophylaxis, including the complex of measures, providing mental health together with the prevention of personal and professional crises, prevention of neuropsychic diseases and their distribution.

The main difference between mental preventology and psychoprophylaxis is in the fact, that mental preventology is based on synergetic methodology, and it is multidisciplinary.

In Russia, the international classification of psychoprophylactic stages is accepted. Psychoprophylaxis is divided into primary, secondary and tertiary.

Primary prophylaxis is a complex of events, aimed at prevention of adverse influence on the human psyche. At this stage, the psychoprophylactic system consists of the investigation of mental resistance to harmful factors of environment and possible ways of increasing this resistance, as well as of prevention of psychogenic diseases. Actually, it is a preventive medical examination of healthy people accompanied by a wide range of psychohygienic events. Because both negative social and psychological human conditions (information overloads, mental traumatization and micro-social conflicts, poor upbringing in childhood, etc.) and biological factors (somatic diseases, brain traumas) can give rise to neuropsychic disorders. The psychoprophylaxis system at this stage should also be focused on studying the psycho-traumatic factors, mental resistance to harmful factors of environment and possible ways of increasing this resistance. It is reasonable to include in this stage the value and holistic upbringing of an infant, as well as the psycho-hygiene of a family and pregnant women; timely application of methods of clinical, pedagogical and psychological diagnostics and correction.

Primary psychoprophylaxis means the system of general government measures on health promotion. The role of psychology here is in the development of the bases of promotion and integration of a healthy lifestyle, in overcoming carelessness towards personal health, in the promotion of the health culture.

Previously the limit of mental health protection was the state of pre-existing disease. It was considered that for contraction of a disease it was necessary to have a certain correlation between the reason, causing the disease and the conditions, making possible the development of its mechanisms and symptoms. In the states of pre-existing disease both, the reason and a part of the conditions necessary for starting the disease process are formed, but initial manifestations still have not become clinical, and the disease vicious circle has not been generated, in which some symptoms complicate the manifestation of the others and vice versa. Thus, even if the possibility of a disease development is very high, it is possible to prevent it by timely psycho-prophylactic and psycho-corrective intervention.

Mental preventology made more progress in the prenosological field, separating the fractals not only of a pre-existing disease but also of diatheses and family predisposition. It allows predicting threats to normative biopsychosociospiritual ontogenetic development as early as possible, by conducting early interventions and preventive-correctional programs.

Secondary psychoprophylaxis is the earliest detection of initial phases of neuropsychic diseases and their timely (early) active treatment. Secondary psychoprophylaxis consists in the control overexaggeration or prevention of negative consequences of the starting mental disease or psychological crisis. Secondary psychoprophylaxis requires broadly defined psychotherapy. It includes the work with higher risk groups of neuropsychic disease incidence.

Tertiary psychoprophylaxis is the prevention of exacerbations of neuropsychic diseases and recovery of an ability to work with a person, who went through the disease. Tertiary psychoprophylaxis is focused on prevention of the disablement of a person suffering from a neuropsychic disease. The activities of a psychologist and psychotherapist at this stage include consulting, recovering and rehabilitation care. Professional rehabilitation (search of new resources to professional activities, the opportunities for professional advancement), social adaptation (creation of the most favorable conditions for a patient at his/her return to his/her habitual family environment) and search of the ways of self-actualization (conscience of personal resources of growth and development) play a special role in the supportive therapy.

One of the main aspects of tertiary psychoprophylactic work is connected with disabled people whose disability is the result of congenital or evoked severe somatic or mental diseases. The main problem is in the necessity to provide the involvement of these people into the active public life, in the development of their sense of self-sufficiency and realistic perspectives of their further existence in the world, the ability to live with their peculiarities, building an adequate relationship with the surrounding people.

33.2. Mental Resilience

Modern diagnostic, preventive, clinical and rehabilitation measures, as well as personal inner resources, help a person to preserve his/her mental health. The results of research works on mental resilience, which means an active use of personal inner resources in order to cope with various negative situations, are being published in foreign periodicals for over 40 years.

The history of recovery study started when the first results of a research were published, touching upon the epidemiologic aspect in order to reveal both harmful and protective factors, contributing to the formation of "resilience" (Garmezy, Streitman 1974). Emmy Werner was one of the first researchers, using term "resilience" in 1970 (Werner 1982). She studied children, growing in dysfunctional families (alcohol-dependent parents; parents with mental disorders; underprivileged families, etc.). According to the results of the research, 2/3 of the studied children demonstrated destructive behavior in later life (chronic unemployment, illegitimate births, addictions), while 1/3 of the youth did not reveal such forms. Later the researcher called this group "flexible" (Masten, Best, Garmezy 1990).

In 1980s children of schizophrenic mothers were studied in order to reveal mental resilience (Masten 1989). According to the results of this study, it was stated that the children of schizophrenic mothers got less emotional warmth and caring in comparison with the children of healthy mothers. This fact influenced the development of a majority of children, but some children of schizophrenic mothers developed sufficiently, were socially competent and had good adequate achievements, which required conduction of new studies to explain this phenomenon (Cicchett, Rogosch 1997).

It is not acceptable to consider resilience as only an individual characteristic (Routter 2008). It allows coping with the current situation and it is a factor contributing to the tolerance towards the same situations in future, as well as to the psychological well-being of an individual (Masten 2009; Zautra et al. 2010). In the opinion of foreign researchers, the strategies of coping as well as good families and schools, communities and social politics also contribute to the development of recovery (Leadbeater et al. 2005). In resilience as a process, there are two compounds: risk (situation of misery, stressor) and positive adaptation to it (Ungar 2004).

Thus, *resilience may be considered as a phenomenon of recovery after long-lasting and suddenly emerged traumatic situation* (Davidson 2000; Gleser et al. 1981). Also, resilience means the ability of an individual or community to find a way to psychological, social, cultural, and physical resources, which provide a well-being (Suarez-Orozco et al. 2009). This is a dynamic process, concluded in a positive behavioral adaptation (Luthar et al. 2000); and this is a positive outcome in the situation of increased risk (Masten et al. 1990).

The concept "resilience" has the following synonyms: resistance, learned optimism by M. Seligman; Rosenbaum's learned resourcefulness; resourcefulness, individual self-healing by G. Friedman, etc. (Anthony 1987). The human ability to prosper and realize personal potential despite various negative influences is the definition of resilience in humanistic psychology. Thus, people having sufficient level of recovery, are more prone to consider their problems as opportunities for their growth and development; while people with low level of resilience likely perceive stressful situations negatively and dejectedly.

The relationship, providing caring and support, love and confidence, is the main protective factor; supplementary aspects are the ability to make realistic plans, self-reliance, developed communicative skills, ability to control strong feelings and impulses (Werner 1995).

D. Cicchetti et al. (1993) separate three groups of resilience factors, where absence or their opposite qualitative transformation can lead to absence or abruptly decrease the ability to resilience:

1) Sociability and positive self-image.
2) A family where there is a close relationship with at least one member or an emotionally stable parent.
3) The community as a source of support.

There are the following individual characteristics of people, being "flexible" in severe conditions (Marunyak 2012):

4) The ability to "bounce back," recover from something.
5) The tendency of perceiving problems as opportunities for growth and development.
6) The ability to see even small positive aspects of a situation and to use them to the full extent.
7) A healthy and solid network of social support.
8) The firm belief in the system of purposes.
9) Skills and abilities to cope with a number of various situations.
10) A wide comfort zone.

Resilience is not a blissful givenness - one should learn and train it. The training may be spontaneous or systematical and purposeful. Resilience can be learned through preventive programs, which allow minimizing psychological harm and significantly saving the energy, required for work with the people without sufficient ability to recover after their exposure to traumatic factors. Development and growth of mental resilience are illustrated with the formula (Figure 33.1.)

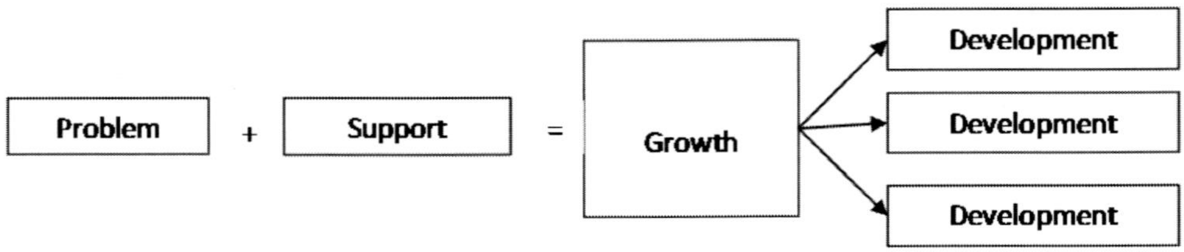

Figure 33.1. Mental resilience growth and development formula.

According to it, the problem of any size and intensity can be the source of growth and development for an individual only in case of quantitive and qualitative support correlating with the problem. In case there is an absolute lack of support or it is not enough, the problem can reveal itself as a serious harm to a human health.

The core of mental resilience is authenticity – individual nature and biopsychosociospiritual uniqueness of a person, unifying all his personal characteristics and the fractals of the faith track.

Authenticity as a resource of personal self-organization can be manifested in situational aspect through its uniqueness and wholeness, contributing to specific (not always adequate from the eye of a passive onlooker) interaction with the environment. On the other hand, trying to achieve social adaptation against personal authenticity, a person pays the price equal to mental and somatic problems (Umanskiy 2014).

The American Psychological Association offers ten ways of resilience development (10 WRD), which should be applied complexly because they are not an efficient instrument for development of psychological resilience, when applied independently (*http://www.wilderdom.com*):

1) To maintain good relationship with close family members, friends, etc.
2) To avoid viewing crises and stressful events as an insolvable problem.
3) To accept the circumstances that can't be changed.
4) To develop and achieve realistic goals.
5) To undertake decisive actions in negative situations.
6) To look for the opportunity of self-revealing after a struggle with loss.
7) To develop self-reliance.
8) To have a long-term perspective; to consider stressful events in a wider context.
9) To have a support of an encouraging perspective, positive expectations, visualization of desirable things.
10) To care of soma and cognitions, to have regular training, to pay attention to personal needs and feelings, to have a rest for pleasure.

The results of the research approved the connection between resilience and the peculiarities of individual emotional manifestations (Tugade et al. 2004). Thus, widows with a high level of resilience feel more positive and more negative emotions than widows with a low level of resilience. The first group shows high emotional complexity, which is an ability to support differentiation of positive and negative emotional states. The authors suppose, that adaptive consequence of resilience is the function of emotional complexity increasing (differentiation of emotions) (Ong et al. 2006). People with a high level of resilience have a low level of depression and low propensity for addictions (e.g., smoking); while people with a low level of resilience are characterized by difficulties in control over negative feelings, sensitivity to everyday stressors (Bonanno et al. 2007).

In the literature positive influence of religion and ability to resilience are underlined. Thus, young people, who join in with church, show improvement of academic achievements, apparently caused not by belief, but by social life of the church, which in its turn contribute to better emotional, social and partially physical health of the people, considering the factors of resilience (Johnson 2002).

The history of resilience study is 40 years old, as it is seen from the represented data. The ability to actively involve inner resources of a person into the operation allows him/her to cope with a traumatic situation and to teach proper application of personal resources in future. This skill will give the opportunity to increase psychological, social, moral, and physical well-being both of the person and of a certain community. The concept of "resilience" represents a qualitatively new aspect of recovery of personal mental health.

In the opinion of S. V. Marunyak (2012), the most appropriate is to consider the peculiarities of mental resilience synergetically, founding on the theory of disasters by V. I. Arnold. A. Chulichkov (2009) describes a number of variants when a scientific thought discovered many examples of precipitous changes of system under small influences. It was realized that any system when developing, comes through the stages of sharp change, with rebuilding of balance on them. These stages are characterized by the temporary prevalence of one of the forces, which leads to chaos, destructing previous structures. Further there will be harmonization, recovery of balance, but in another, qualitatively new state. One of the mathematical theories, describing such abrupt transitions is the theory of disasters. An important advantage of this theory is the fact, that it can define the situations not "quantitively," but "qualitatively."

A simple explanation of the theory of disasters belongs to English mathematician K. Zeeman, contained in a popular book by V. Arnold "Theory of Disasters." The author describes creative process of scientist and characterizes his/her achievements depending on the involvement and acquisition of the research technique and skills. If the involvement is low, the achievements increase slowly and monotonously with the growth of professional skills. However, if the involvement is high then qualitatively new phenomena take place: with the growth of professionalism, the achievements can increase abruptly. The area of high achievements, in this case, is called "geniuses." But if the growth of involvement is not supported by the corresponding growth of professionalism, then a disaster takes place: the achievements decrease abruptly, and this results in "maniacs." According to the theory of the disasters by V. Arnold, a genius and a maniac having equal involvement, differ from each other only by the level of achievement.

In certain situations - at the points of disasters and bifurcations – even insignificant movements can influence the process. One may find indirect indicators of the fact that studied system is situated near the point of disaster – set so-called "flags of disasters," i.e., the peculiarities of the system behavior, which are the gage of the approaching critical point:

- several various (stable) conditions;
- existence of unstable conditions, from which the system is taken out by weak "pushes";

- the ability to change the system quickly under little changes of external circumstances;
- inconvertibility of the system (inability to return to previous conditions);
- hysteresis.

Today on the level of mathematical theory it is stated, that any system which is complicated enough, interacting with its environment, comes through certain stages in its development. Firstly, "new forms" - a number of structures is being built from random parts of a system and begins to grow at a great rate. Due to opposite, "destructive" tendency, the speed of its growth gradually slows down; some forms vanish, the other become stable. This tendency sooner or later wins, putting everything into the initial chaos, and a crisis takes place, originating the structures of the following stage. Thus, mathematical model develops according to the scenario: a destruction of harmony – conflict necessary for development, – puts the system into the vivifying chaos, giving birth to new life.

Chaos is an inevitable, obligatory attribute of life of any system which is complicated enough. The stage of crisis is characterized by an extreme inconsistency: a little movement away from the track can make the system change the scenario of its development. It can go to "the second circle" of its evolution, slightly different from the first one, but can also move over to another, new circle. For studying the dynamics of systems, it is necessary to know the principle of the "offset." Synergetics gives the answers to such questions (Chulichkov 2009).

The mathematical apparatus of the theory of disasters, appropriate for the description of many self-organizational processes was developed by a Russian mathematician V. I. Arnold and by a French mathematician René Thom.

The common feature for all the evolving systems is nonequilibrium, spontaneous formation of new microscopic (local) structures, changes at macroscopic (system) level, origination of new peculiarities of a system, stages of self-organization and fixation of new qualities of the system. At the transition from a chaotic state to the state of order, all the developing systems behave the same way. Developing systems are always open and exchange energy and substance with the environment, which results in the processes of local order and self-organization. In the states of strong nonequilibrium, systems begin to perceive the factors of external influence, which would not be perceived by them in a more equilibrium state. In nonequilibrium conditions relative independence of the system elements gives place to corporate behavior of the elements: near the equilibrium, the element interacts only with the neighbor, far from equilibrium it "sees" the whole system and the coherence of the elements behavior increases. Under the conditions which are far from equilibrium, bifurcation mechanisms come into force – short-term points of bifurcation of transition to one or another relatively long-term system mode called attractor. It is impossible to predict, which attractor will be occupied by the system. The fundamental principle of self-organization is the emergence of new order and complication of the systems through fluctuations (random deviations) of the states of their elements and sub-systems. Such fluctuations are suppressed in every dynamically stable and adaptive system, but in more complicated open systems, due to the external energy supply and increase of nonequilibrium, the deviations grow with the time, accumulate and lead to "loosening" of the previous order and through relatively short-term chaotic state of the system, lead either to the destruction of the previous structure, or to new order. The fluctuations are accidental; that is why the state of the system after bifurcation is caused by the influence of a number of accidental factors.

Thus, in accordance with the evolutionally-synergetic paradigm, development is understood as the consequence of long-term periods, corresponding to stable states of a system, which are interrupted by short-term periods of chaotic behavior ("bifurcations"). After this a transition to the next stable condition takes place, which can be determined, as a rule, by fluctuations in the point of bifurcation.

Generalizing all said above, we can say that mental resilience is a main biopsychosociospiritual resource of mental preventology, accumulated in quality and style of life, its healthy way and spiritual purpose. Factors and instruments of mental resilience are: neuroplasticity and the force of personality, musical and vocal therapy, dance therapy and physical activities, somnology, sexual management, etc.

33.2.1. Neuroplasticity

In the 1990s it was found, that new neurons are constantly generating in the brain of adults. This phenomenon was called *neuroplasticity* – the abilities of the brain to change under the influence of experience. Actually, it became the biological basis for mental resilience and allowed accomplishing the revolutionary breakthrough in the development of new unique methods of neurorehabilitation.

A new technology of central nervous function recovery was the methodic "BrainPort" developed in the 1960s by Paul Bach-y-Rita (2005) and today it is used in clinical practice. By mobilizing the mechanisms of neuroplasticity, the methodic allows recovering central nervous functions. Thus, *BrainPort balance device* (registered in Russia, UE, Canada and Brazil) is used to help patients, who went through strokes, brain injuries, hereditary cerebellar ataxia, meningoencephalitis, etc. The device helps to recover vestibular function. Even after 20 minutes of the therapeutic session, a person can stand up and walk without assistance. This effect lasts from 4 to 24 hours and several weeks for some patients.

The second one is *BrainPort vision device*, which helps the blind to see through their tongue. The source of information, translated into the tongue is a digital camera, fixed on the head of a patient. After 2-10 hours of training, the patients learn to "see" contrast objects and distinguish faces, correctly estimate the direction and the speed of the moving objects.

The advanced technologies influencing the control neuron connections help not only to recover lost functions but also to overcome severe pain. Thus, an American professor Hunter G. Hoffman (2013), Laboratory Chief of Virtual Reality of the Washington University of Seattle, has developed the system of *immersive virtual reality*, which immerses a patient into the virtual world, significantly soothing painful procedures and senses. Application of this methodic allows decreasing painful feelings of a patient by 30-50%, which can be comparable to the effect of strong anesthetics but has no side effects.

For the patients with severe burns the variant of this methodic called "Snow world" was developed, imitating snowy landscapes and reducing the body temperature and the edge of the painful senses of the patients.

Mental resilience predetermines not only style and quality of life but also its longevity. Thus, analysis of 68 thousand anamneses of people at the age over 35 (Watson et al. 2012), showed that those exposed to stresses and prone to negative feelings die before the normal age. The risk of untimely death is directly proportional to the level and length of psychological, social, moral and emotional feelings.

Melatonin, the hormone regulating emotional profile and anxiety level, caused by stress, plays the role of biological mediator of mental resilience. Besides, melatonin participates in the regulation of body biological rhythms, stimulating the immune system, having an antioxidant effect, protecting the cells from destruction by free radicals and providing antineoplastic activity.

If to take the production of melatonin in 10 years as 100%, then in 25 years it is equal to 50%, in 45 – 10%, and in 75– 1-3%. The decrease of melatonin level leads to weakening of protective body functions, decreased libido and display of external aging symptoms. This is precisely why it is recommended to supply melatonin by courses beginning from 25-30. It is principal that such biological therapy should work well together with suitable physical load, intellectual and moral training (Macrae 2012). As a Russian poet said: "A soul must work hard."

33.2.2. Musical and Vocal Therapy

Therapeutic effects of music are known from the earliest times. It was firstly mentioned in the Old Testament. There is a parable in the Bible, where David cured Saul, the king of Israel, of melancholia by playing the harp. The Aesculapians of ancient Egypt advised the people suffering from insomnia to listen to choristry. There were also historic cases when music helped to stop social epidemics. Thus, in the 14th century, the chorea epidemic (also known as "saint Vitus dance") broke out in the Western Europe. The crowds of possessed people moving bizarrely were walking along the streets of the cities and villages; they cried out something inarticulate and convulsed with foam at the mouth. The epidemic was abruptly stopped only where the authorities were able to call the musicians, playing slow, calm, and melodic music as soon as possible.

According to folk tales, it was considered that each musical note has a special effect on a certain part of the body. Thus, "do" predominantly influences the stomach and pancreas functions; "re" - gall bladder and liver; "mi" – visual and hearing organs; "fa" - urogenital system; "sol" – heart functions; "la" – lungs and kidneys; "si" - energy and heat exchange of the body. Low sounds resonate with lower part of the body while high sounds resonate with the upper one.

One out of four patients with depression is healed thanks to musical composition or execution while anti-depressant therapy helps to heal only every 7-16 patients. Music pieces allow reducing anxiety and relieving stress even of people with severe depression (Erkkila et al. 2011).

In the course of the experiments in mice, the Japanese researchers (Uchiyama et al. 2012) succeeded to show that music reduces the incidence of heart transplants rejection, influencing the immune system in a good way. Classical music significantly extended the time of operating of a transplanted organ and prevented its rejection, while contemporary music did not have such effect. Classical music significantly reduced the concentration of interleukin-2 and gamma interferon in the mice blood, while the concentration of anti-inflammatory interleukins increased. The concentration of DM4^{+} and DM25^{+} cells, regulating peripheral immune responses increased as well. All these changes slowed down the processes of transplanted tissue rejection or suppressed them entirely.

Music reduces the anxiety of the patients during surgeries while vocal therapy cures stammering and neurotic disorders (Holmes 2012). Moreover, the vocal therapy can be the instrument of neurorehabilitation. Thus, a member of Congress of the USA Gabrielle Giffords got a gunshot wound to the head with a severe damage to the left brain hemisphere. The trauma had deprived her of the ability to speak, but she began to sing with the help of her music therapist. She began with small song parts and developed a serious repertoire. Then she learned to sing separate colloquial phrases and finally learned to speak them out (The Lancet 2012, No. 6).

Vocal therapy is an effective technology of poststroke patient's neurorehabilitation. A majority of the connections between brain sectors, responsible for movements and speech, are located in the left hemisphere. The American researchers showed: when the patients learn to sing, the active connections begin to form in the right hemisphere as well (Levitin 2006), leading to growth and change of the axon structure (Swinnen 2008). Professor (Schlaug et al. 2003) showed that children, who had been studying music during 15 months not less than two and a half an hour per week, had the corpus callosum volume – the structure responsible for the information exchange between the hemispheres – increased by 25% at average. Apparently, this is the biological resonance resources of music neuroplasticity.

L. S. Vygotskiy (1998), when quoting the music description in "The Kreutzer Sonata" by L. N. Tolstoy, agreed that: "Music makes me forget my real situation. It transports me into a state, which is not my own. Under the influence of music, I seem to feel what I do not feel, to understand what I do not understand, to have powers which I cannot have …». Moreover, further developing the idea: «…music does not draw us upon something certain, it just creates an undefined need for some actions, it opens the way and clears up the road to our deepest powers; it acts like an earthquake, revealing new layers of our living…." As Anna Akhmatova said: "Leave us alone with music and we will agree soon."

33.2.3. Dance Therapy

A synthetic variant of the biopsychosociospiritual therapy is *dance therapy*, where movements and music ensure the development of social and spiritual, as well as psychological and physical life of a person. Dance therapy helps people to solve emotional problems and addictions, severe chronic diseases and intellectual deterioration.

The founder of this type of therapy is an American dancer Marian Chace, who in the 1940s paid attention to the fact, that some students were interested not in the technique of a dance, but in feelings and emotions, which could be expressed through movements, having improved their mental health. Chace separated remedial and releasing elements of dance and became the first dance therapist, who worked in public service. Among her patients were alcoholics and narcomaniacs, schizophrenes and people with post-traumatic stress disorder.

Development of dance therapy together with Jungian analysis and Cognitive behavioral therapy (CBT) led to a modern practice of "authentic movement," when patients dance their inner images and feelings out, getting rid of fears and anxieties, stresses and emotional tension. Dance allows expressing emotions, even if the person is not able to verbalize them. New comprehension of opportunities of body and relaxation, empathy and creative self-expression are harmonically represented in dance therapy. It allows overcoming inner barriers and seeing new perspectives of personal development.

Dance therapy is an effective form of therapy for psychosomatic diseases (coronary heart disease, diabetes mellitus, and rheumatoid arthritis). Application of short-term dance therapy allowed expanding the motional space and communicative abilities of the patients, reducing the activity of asthenia and anxiety (Oganesyan, Ilyina 2010).

An impressive clinical achievement of dance therapy is a three-month experiment of the English National Ballet and the employees of the Roehampton University in London (Houston, Mc Gill, Jokes et al. 2011) in teaching the ballet parts of "Romeo and Juliette" to 24 *wheelchair invalids with Parkinson disease*. The people suffering from a degenerative brain disease were able to get on feet and dance, got rid of depressions and complexes, acquired sense of confidence and the vision of life perspective.

33.2.4. Physical Activity

According to the World Health Organization, the life expectancy of human life and the condition of health are by 60% determined by the lifestyle and firstly – by *adequate physical load* as the main biological resource of mental resilience.

Multicentre and transcultural epidemiologic study found that lack of physical activities increases the risk of cardiac failure by 6 %, breast cancer – by 7%, bowel cancer – by10%. Health-detrimental behavior annually becomes the reason of 9% of untimely deaths. At the same time, even small increase in the level of physical activities can decrease the morbidity level by 10-25%. The elimination of hypodynamia increases average life expectancy of the Earth population by 0,68 years. Maximal level of physical activity is preserved in the south-eastern Asia, minimal – in the Mediterranean countries (Lee et al. 2012).

Generalizing a great amount of researches of lifestyle and risk of disease development it may be said, that people, spending more than ten years at sedentary work are twice as more exposed to tumorigenesis in the distal large intestine, have by 44% higher risk of rectal cancer and by 30% higher risk of prostate cancer.

Numerous researches showed that *regular physical exercises* have mainly the same effect as anti-depressants. Thus, the researchers from Georgetown University (Murray et al. 2010) showed that after a several-week course of physical exercises, there is an increase in the level of galanin in brain – the peptide, regulating the exchange of serotonin and noradrenaline, while the imbalance in this process leads to depression. The scientists supposed that human brain is programmed evolutionally and genetically to a certain level of physical activities, and its reduction leads to system mental decompensation.

In order to prevent depression, the researchers recommend performing 30-minutes exercises not less than five times a week, including tramps or intensive 30-minutes aerobics three times a week.

There are obvious advantages of physical training for overcoming depression: 1) no negative consequences and complications comparing with the medications; 2) training without assistance does not require money; 3) physical load increases mood and tonus immediately and fast.

The study of the scientists from University of Aberdeen (Grey et al. 2012) showed that there is no need in exhausting oneself in long and severe training. It was found that those, who had 30-minute walks every day, decreased the level of fat in their blood by 11% comparing with those, who did not do any exercises. However, those, who practiced short intensive exercises (30 seconds of cycling machine, 4 minutes of rest – 4 sets), decreased their level of fat by 33% as if they were running for 90 minutes! Though, they ate fat foods, including mayonnaise and cheese for breakfast and dinner.

The Taiwanese researchers took things a step further (Wen et al. 2011, 2012). Having analyzed the anamneses of 400000 people, they proved that 15-minute moderately intensive physical exercises on a daily basis reduce the mortality risk by 14%, sustaining life by three years.

Almost all the researchers agree that the optimal recipe for preventing the senile psychosis is a "*golden duet*" – the combination of intellectual activities and sport. The quality of brain training, i.e., its mental resilience should correlate with the level of physical activities, providing a harmonious biopsychosociospiritual balance.

The irony of the mankind history and any personal faith is in the fact, that only perfect physical shape in the years of youth can be the pledge of well-being and mental health in old age. Thus, the scientists from University of Gothenburg (Aberg et al. 2012) found that regardless of the muscle power, the poor functional state of heart-vascular system in 18 years predetermines the twofold increase in the risk of depression with the age, and this correlation maintains even in 30-40 years. This information was obtained in the research of 1 million people, approving the necessity of holistic approach to the study of neuroplasticity (the ability of brain cells to change), balancing at non-linear and multidimensional somatic-mental, psycho-somatic, social-psychological and spiritual and moral correlations. It may be said, that today the most adequate method of studying the factors and resources of mental resilience is the biopsychosociospiritual synergetic methodology of mental medicine.

33.2.5. Somnology

The World Health Organization designated a healthy sleeping to one of the leading conditions of healthy lifestyle. Every third person, applying for medical assistance, suffers from sleep disturbance.

Human biological rhythms are the leading characteristic of biogenesis, predetermining the quality of mental health. In the singular modern world basic biological rhythms are constantly disturbed, which leads to chronic stress and psycho-emotional tension, development of psycho-somatic and somatic-mental disorders.

Main natural biological rhythms are alternation of day and night, tidal motion, alternation of seasons, the sun and moon phases change, time zones etc. The most frequent indicator of natural biorhythms disturbance is insomnia, effecting 10-20% population of Europe.

The researchers from University of Chicago (Leproult, Van Canter 2011) found, that young men, sleeping less than 5 hours per day, have the reduction of testosterone level by 10-15%. It is displayed in the decrease in muscle mass and bone density, decreased libido, powers, and energy.

The people suffering from insomnia have 6 times higher risk of diabetes and heart diseases (Walley et al. 2009). This mechanism appeared to be connected with a genetic defect of an everyday launch of biological clock: very rare gene-mutations of MT2 melatonin receptor were found, influencing the risk of diabetes.

The researchers from the English University of Surrey (Möller-Levet et al. 2013) found that even 1 week of sleep deprivation is able to provoke incorrect functioning of 700 genes, increasing the risk of psychosomatic diseases, a decrease in immunity and increase inflammations.

Study of gender peculiarities of sleep deprivation indicated (Alexander 2012) greater vulnerability of women in the progress of heart diseases and type 2 diabetes.

The fault of biological clock can lead not only to somatic but also to mental disorders. The researchers from University of Oxford (Geddes et al. 2012) developed a hypothesis that schizophrenia is connected with the fault of body circadian rhythm, resulting in the fault of the "central clock," located in the brain and "peripheral clock," locating in the other organs. A majority of patients with schizophrenia suffer from sleep disturbance. In an experiment in mice with SNAP25 (synaptosomal-associated protein of 25kDa) gene defect (also connected with human schizophrenia), the researchers were able to describe the defects of circadian rhythms and mental disorders of the animals.

Somnology as a study of sleep has a great importance for developing the strategies of mental health provision and mental disorders prevention.

33.2.6. Sexual Management

The concept of sexual health accepted by the World Health Organization in 1975 is based on three main elements:

1. human ability to have pleasure and control sexual and reproductive behavior according to social and personal ethics;
2. freedom from fear and shame, feeling of guilt and false beliefs, suppressing sexual reactions and worsening sexual intercourse;
3. absence of organic disorders, diseases and defects, damaging sexual and reproductive functions.

Sexual health is a normative biopsychosociospiritual complex of social and reproductive human behavior, enriching the personality and increasing communicative abilities, based on the right to have the information in the sphere of sexuality and sexual education, and the right to have pleasure as well. These rights should be realized in harmony and balance with the responsibility, without which mutual love is impossible.

Sexual management is an effective achievement of sexual and reproductive goals of a person by means of planning, organization, leadership and control over circumstances. Fractal dynamics of sexual management ontogenetic development is represented by self-understanding and self-education, self-improvement and self-organization, self-regulation and self-control, personal identity and personal management, oriented to the achievement of certain goals.

Sexual management is represented in biogenesis (biorhythms, genetic programs) and psychogenesis (psychology of infatuation and desires), sociogenesis (ontogenetic development of gender roles and relationship) and animogenesis (ethics of interpersonal interaction).

Sexual management is characterized by poor signal management and orientation to unexpected things. It is not limited by internal processes but includes perspectives of the environment and development, consideration of the partner's peculiarity and changing circumstances.

Slightly rephrasing the definition of a human by J. Sartre, we can say that "Sexual management is a result of the implementation of your own project." Sexual management creates not closed and introvert, but open and extravert personality. Entering the sphere of sexual relationship, a person does not revolve around him/herself. Only orienting to his/her partners the person is able to understand and comprehend him / her, organizing and implementing his/her life project with the same projects of the reference environment.

Sexual management is the access to new resource levels of control over the intimate interpersonal relationship, where the most important personal problems are solved on the basis of a selected way of organization. It should not be perceived only as a simple set of some rules, all the more defined in folklore and jokes. It is an individual technology of a unique self-organization, integrating biopsychosociospiritual individuality of a human life and faith.

Built on pluralistic value systems, sexual management is closely connected with the religious way of life organization and considers unique coverage of world religions as well as various religious denominations. In the search of new opportunities and launch of the mechanisms of self-development, sexual management allows strengthening spiritual and moral sphere, mortifying inadequate desires and enriching self-esteem.

Sexual management allows a person to include all the biopsychosociospiritual resources of personal mental health reasonably and deliberately, not falling within the power of circumstances or psycho-social sexual manipulation. That is exactly why sexual management is a creative process and improvisation, an unconventional approach to problems and situations. As it is always multivariant and multidimensional, polymodal and interdisciplinary and that is exactly why the synergetic biopsychosociospiritual methodology of mental medicine is the only effective way of its studying.

Sexual management is the experience, which is sometimes enough traumatic. It is connected with revelation, apprehension of mistakes and vices. It is a creative laboratory, search of trouth and personal overcoming, when "my drawbacks" are often rated higher than "your virtues."

Sexual management is not just a fashion or solace for modern people. It is filled and enriched with the knowledge of the intimate human relationship, being faced to the widest circles of population, striving for self-development and harmonious relationship with surrounding people and their families.

There are the following main goals of sexual management and self-management:

- personal development as the basis for success;
- rational organization of sexual lifestyle;
- development of personal sexual abilities;
- learning the lessons and analysis of the mistakes, prediction of dangers and losses in sexual activities;
- the design of an important sphere and overcoming the difficulties, strengthening sexual health and self-assertion.

Sexual management is one of the universal biopsychosociospiritual resources of mental resilience. Thus, the researchers from Princeton University (Lenner et al. 2010) found that sex stimulates growth of neurons in hippocampus responsible for memory and learning. The experiment was conducted on two mice groups: one group males had access to females while the other group didn't. In the course of the research the mice glucocorticoid (stress hormone) level was measured. It was found that the hippocampus neurons of the mice from sexually active group grew, directly proportional to the increase in sexual contacts. Their level of anxiety was lower than those, who were less sexually active. In the opinion of the researchers, the experiment showed negative influence of stress on brain and positive role of sex.

It was confirmed by the researches (Greco et al. 2013) that the process of neuron regeneration (neuroplasticity) is much more intensive for those, who are in love in the process of sex. Besides, sexual activities increase the level of immunoglobulin, boosting body resistance by 30%. Especially important is hormonal splash during sex, boosting the level of oxytocin fivefold, thus contributing to improvement of mood and relaxation, regulating sleep and general state.

Analgetic effect of sex is connected with the rush of endorphins in the moment of orgasm. B. C. Evans, R. Couch (2001) showed that 61% of women, having sex during a headache noted the decrease in its intensity and 20% of them felt total relieve from a headache. However, it is worth noting that the headache itself may be the indicator of sexual disharmony or abstinence.

It is known that women, involved in social fashion epidemic, are too fastidious and demanding and sometimes illusionary-compensative about their underwear and clothes, shoes and bags, hats and gloves, perfume and cosmetics and other attributes of "sexual battle suit."

Unfortunately, often clothes are not only the way of attracting people, but also the way of acquiring various problems: discomfort and tension, stresses and depressions. British Osteopathic Association (Jones 2012) conducted a survey and found that more than 50% of women suffered from pain senses caused by uncomfortable underwear, squeezing headwear, control belts, heavy bags, high-heeled shoes and even slippers. Unsuitable bras appeared to be the main reasons of back pains for six out of ten women. Large bags caused the same pains for four out of ten respondents. Every fifth women suffered from skin inflammation caused by thongs and deformation of toes because of flips.

According to the research of American traumatologists, 40% of patients applied to doctors with the complaints about arthritic pains, had worn uncomfortable shoes, mostly high-heeled (Rome et al. 2011).

It is seemingly the simplest truth that clothes and shoes should be not only pretty, but comfortable as well, but the women involved in the world *fashion pandemic*, keep increasing the number of their problems and diseases through the experiments with their wardrobes. The researchers among osteopaths and arthrologists, dermatologists and general practitioners stop at this level of generalization and studying the problem. They do not want to and cannot note that clothes and shoes is a "litmus test" of a much more serious problematics, connected with conscious or unconscious complexes and syndromes of loveless, abandoned, cast-off and unhappy women. Because the lower self-esteem is, the higher are the heels…

One thing is doubtless: sexual management is always the art of discovery of yourself in the world and the discovery of the world in yourself, which means that it is always a secret, and its revelation is an endlessly engrossing process, good for mental health and self-improvement.

Thus, a huge variety of registers of mental resilience behaviorally embodies mental resources of the *mental immunity* - of the biopsychosociospiritual system of spiritual defense of the individual and society. It is the mental immunity that provides a high level of psychophysiological resistance and stress tolerance, awareness of values and meanings of life, enshrined in the patterns of individual and social identity, implemented in effective behavioral strategies and adaptive professiogenesis.

33.3. Main Directions of Mental Preventology

There are the following directions of mental preventology:

1) *Pedagogical.* At developing primary prophylaxis, it is important to develop positive inner moral and mental potential of a person, which can be achieved by promotion and advertising healthy lifestyle. Formation of the value of health in the family and at school plays here an important role. It is necessary to integrate health-reserving approaches in educational institutions.
2) *Medical.* It is concluded in preventive aspects of the healthcare system activities. General medical practice and the institutions of general medical network play a significant role in prevention. A family doctor, knowing the family living conditions and the relationship between its members, can be the main figure of conducting preventive measures in the family. Besides ordinary medical work, focused on revealing some health problems of patients, early intervention is a rather new method of mental preventology. Among the tasks of a family doctor, there are revealing the high-risk groups of mental and psychosomatic disorders during the examination; their directing for further examination to a psychiatrist, psychotherapist, medical psychologist; control of treatment; active participation in preventive programs.
3) *Social.* In the formation of mental disorders, the process of social labor decompensation can develop, when family and work relationship are broken, which can result in the loss of family or work. Developing social maladaptation of patients requires conducting rehabilitation and recovery of the patient's social status. That is why the goal of social work is in mental preventology, which is recovery of a disturbed social network of patient and social support for him/her.
4) *Psychological.* A criterion of mental disorders is an absence of adaptation to everyday life, which is connected with the culture, where the quality of living is the main value. By psychological help in mental preventology it is meant the supply of emotional, rational and existential support of a person or a group in severe situations, arising in the process of their personal or social existence. One of the tasks of prevention is destigmatization of patients and their relatives from the side of society in order to increase the quality of treatment.
5) *Infocommunicative***.** The world information space, exponentially expanding, requires unification of information and communication technologies, provision of balanced development of information service market. Synergetic medico-psychosociospiritual methodology of mental medicine allows estimating and predicting, preventing and correcting clinically and behaviorally significant effects of virtual "mental virology"

across the spectrum. It is possible to stop the dangers of destructive social epidemics development in proper time in early prenosological fractals, only by early "mental immunization," forming quite measurable Spiritual immunity to any social diseases and mental toxic agents. Moreover, the methodology of mental medicine is significantly grown out of the synergetics of controlled chaos of information-psychological wars. Not by accident treatment and rehabilitation technologies of mental medicine are the conversion versions of mental weapon of modern terroristic wars (e.g., system of immersive virtual reality etc.).

6) *Culture-based.* Ethnical differences, as well as individual behavior, also contribute to the development of mental and psychosomatic pathology, because they provide a special attitude towards material (food, clothes), and social (organization and structure of society) phenomena. They have differences in formation of nonpsychotic mental pathology in various ethnical populations. Building the preventive politics is undoubtedly based on the knowledge of history, culture and ethnic-ecological peculiarities, which gives an opportunity to consider personal psychological peculiarities and the peculiarities of behavior of people, living in this region, to the full extent.
7) *Administrative-legal.* The main principle of legal regulation politics in the sphere of healthcare should be social priorities, contributing to increasing of duration and quality of living.
8) *Spiritual and moral.* Spiritual and moral education and personal development is the most important condition of effective mental health formation, predetermining successful self-realization and adaptive professiogenesis, the ability to overcome stresses and taking an active part in the development of society. Modern forms of social and governmental partnership allow having a productive cooperation with religious organizations. Any world religion contains in its canons obligatory care of moral and physical health. Spiritual methods are alternative ways of help. Though, it is an important and serious aspect of rehabilitation, and spiritual rehabilitation is aimed at recovery of the highest human values – singularity of life and love, faith and patience. Healthcare institutions and organizations have a unique opportunity to use the infrastructure of ethical committees for spiritual and moral supply of mental health, with their expanded power instruments, which allow not only predicting and preventing conflict situations and conducting mediation, but sanitizing moral climate of a working staff in the context of system monitoring of mental health.

The Russian society is currently in a spiritual and ethical crisis. The existing situation is the reflection of changes, happened in the social conscience and national policy. Spiritual and moral educational and upbringing functions of the current educational system appeared to be minimized. It resulted in the fact that complex of value mindsets characterizing mass conscience (including conscience of the youth) is mostly destructive from the perspective of the development of personality, family and state. *The biggest danger for our society today is not in the economic collapse or change of political system but in the destruction of personality.* The young generation has lost the main factor of the development, which is rising out of spirit. Material values dominate over spiritual that is why the concepts of kindness, benevolence, nobility, justice, civil conscience and patriotism are falsified. High level of criminality is caused by general increase in aggressiveness and cruelty in the society.

Destruction of the institution of the family is going on: extraconjugal, anti-parental and antifamily mindsets are being formed. The forms of collective activities are gradually diminishing. A strong system of spiritual and moral upbringing in schools and higher educational institutions, which was effective in the Soviet time, is now almost destructed.

The system of higher education changes its orientation to the labor market. The leading tendency in reformation of the modern higher education is professional orientation, but the content of education cannot be limited just to professional training.

To a large extent these risks are becoming more and more real at this precise point of time. For recent decades, there is a tendency towards an increase in a number of the university students with a lower level of common moral and behavioral culture. In the process of living, a person acquires three spheres: spiritual, social and natural world. The content of the modern university education regulated by federal standards includes only learning of social and natural spheres. Unfortunately, human spiritual content is slightly reflected in the educational standards.

Professional training should be obligatory supplemented with spiritual and moral upbringing as the instrument of acquiring human purpose of living.

In the Russian universities during the recent 15 years, there has been a search of the creation of new ways of spiritual and moral upbringing system for the youth based on the values of Christian Orthodox culture. It should be exactly the system, but not separate attempts. In the universities of Kursk, Ryazan, Belgorod, Smolensk, Kemerovo, Yaroslavl, Lipetsk, Voronezh, Stavropol and others the work under spiritual and moral upbringing of students is represented by various forms of educational and extracurricular activities. The students of the universities study such disciplines as “Basics and Values of Orthodox Christianity,” “Christian Orthodox Pedagogics,” “Christian Orthodox Culture,” “Rhetoric,” “Christian Orthodox Psychology,” “Orthodox Christianity and Russian Literature” and others, the university churches are being established. Regular seminars, round tables, meetings and conferences on the problems of formation of the spiritual and moral basis of the future specialists contribute to the scientific and methodological supply of the work under spiritual and moral upbringing of the students. The festivals of the Slavic culture and literature, art exhibitions, scientific and pedagogical readings: “Znamenskie,” “Pokrovskie,” “Rozhdestvenskie,” “Glinskie” and others, spiritually-oriented scientific forums and scientific and theological conference have become traditional.

Spiritual and moral raising and development of students is supported by the diversity of forms and content of the extracurricular activities. Curatorial hours on the spiritual and moral subject are held. Such holidays as “Christmas ball,” “Day of Saint Tatyana,” “Day of Christian Orthodox Youth,” “Students’ Eastern,” the memorial day of a saint patronizing university church. An integral part of the spiritual and moral upbringing of students is excursions to saint places, cathedrals, monasteries. Pontifical meetings become regular in a number of universities.

The experience of the universities of the central Russian regions gives the evidence of the revival of the Christian Orthodox traditions in the higher education. Specifically spiritual and moral upbringing of students based on the values of Orthodox Christianity creates positive background for formation of highly qualified specialists.

An example is Northern State Medical University, which has a wide experience in the Christian Orthodox education at the preliminary Christian Orthodox theological courses (since 2000), “Visiting nurse” courses (since 2002); the Society of Christian Orthodox

Doctors is established (since 2003); the conferences with the representatives of the Christian Orthodox Church are held. NSMU long-term constructive experience of cooperation with Arkhangelsk metropolitanate has shown the necessity of transition of the existing relationship into more official functional organization like the Public Faculty of Mental Health (2011), which is able to occupy a unique niche on the modern stage of the Russian education development and formed in the USSR by “faculties of social professions.”

Modernization of the country is impossible without high quality of mental health, provided by new forms of social and governmental partnership as well. Polymodal resources and technologies of mental preventology in defense of mental health allow providing integration of healthy lifestyle and spiritual purpose of living, forming and strengthening mental immunity of the nation.

Chapter 34

Mental Immunity as the Matrix of Identity and the Basis of Security

Epidemic growing diversity of threats and challenges of the singular world has ensured the wide relevance and expansion of the semantic field of the classical medical term of immunity. Today, the concepts of psychological and social, moral and spiritual immunity become common in virtually. However, the entirety and systematicity of approaches to security issues require the synergetic reading of the concept of *mental immunity (MI) as a biopsychosociospiritual protection of the identity and security basis of the individual and society.*

The relevant task is a conceptual and methodological grounding of the synergetic approach to the mental immunity and mental security (MS), a description of their structural and functional features on the clinical model of the acquired mental immunodeficiency syndrome, accentuation of strategies of new resources provision to ensure national security in today's crisis-ridden reality.

34.1. Functions of Mental Immunity

Mental immunity is an integral protective and compensatory buffer of singularly growing globalization pressure. Numerous attempts to mentally design the socio-political and socio-economic activities in these conditions were not reducible to the classical models of co-evolutionary, harmonious and sustainable human existence. On the personal and society level, the globalization pressure is equilibrated with the balance of "globalization from below," which is provided by the *natural mental immunity* of adaptive extension of conscience, and "globalization from above" with *artificial mental immunity* of "transplantation of conscience" and unobvious prospects of integration. Natural mental immunity appears in ontogenetically harmonious expansion of vision of picture and meanings of the human world, development of its moral and cultural values and ideas, understanding of the variety of levels and lifestyles. Artificial mental immunity is an imposed from outside, manageable and stereotyped technique of universalization of achievements and values of the world, global on a scale, but hybrid in the matter.

In the conceptual MI frameworks, the most dramatic and ontogenetically last defensive reaction is death as a result of conscious or unconscious inability or impossibility of the terrestrial life. Numerous evidence in the writings of the church on prior notice of the death of the outstanding ascetics of Orthodoxy the examples, in contemporary language, of the interface of the Spirit over the passions of the Body and the World. In the brilliant philosophical essay of the Professor I. L. Andreev (2015), ethnopsychological mechanisms and multicultural diversity of mental matrices of "life after life" are revealed.

Not coincidentally, the Noosphere doctrine of V. I. Vernadsky, as a planetary shell of the human mind or global conscience, to a large extent was supplemented by Marie-Pierre Teilhard de Chardin with notions of spiritual evolution of the Universe, the formation and development of the "homo sapiens" and the prospect of his integration with the Creator (Rezhabek 2008). Mechanisms for interactive work of "noosphere mirror" as a global accumulator of civilizational resilience (Sidorov 2015a), reviewed by us on a number of models, allow approaching the hypothetical understanding of the effectiveness both of a heartfelt prayer and of an inspiring creative dream in the fate ecology.

It is possible to single out the following basic functions of the mental immunity.

1) Regulatory, providing control of all protective resources.
2) Integrative, uniting all kinds of immunity.
3) Coherent, creating the harmonious integrity and dynamic succession of layered protection.
4) Interface, provided by the system and polymodal focus of all kinds of immunity.
5) Adaptive, manifesting in adaptation to constantly changing external and internal conditions and protection resources.
6) Resonant, with the complementary setting for the protection systems under tempo-rhythmic dynamics of challenges.
7) Interactive correction of the protection front with respect to the dynamics of its gradual results.
8) Mirror, accumulating the meanings and characters from the past, the present, and the future in the bifurcation correction of the fate trajectory.
9) Symmetrical, providing the compliance of polymodal protection resources to the variety of challenges.
10) Cumulative, being to perform the gradual accumulation and instantaneous ("explosive") mobilization of protecting resources in the critical periods.
11) Prognostic, outperforming the challenge dynamics by updating and mobilization of new levels of security (the acceptor of action by P. K. Anokhin).
12) Interiorization, forming the internal patterns of protection through the assimilation of external algorithms.

The synergetic MI concept has evolved from the earlier ideas about the reactions and mechanisms of adaptation and accommodation, resilience and coping resources, protection and compensation, and others. It allows to measure and to predict the resources of the body and the individual, group and collective, society and the state in tetranuclear and four-block-modular mode.

Persistent conceptual and terminological discrepancies in the current resource estimate of somatogenesis and psychogenesis, sociogenesis, and animogenesis, certainly require the further integration efforts within the synergetic methodology. However, already today many available methods of psycho-semantics allow receiving mathematically and graphically the categorical structure (Vorona et al. 2015) or mental matrix (Sidorov 2015a) of conscience, which is essentially the MI screening. The variety of both existing and potential constructed polymodal protective resources screening batteries makes the task of quantitative and qualitative MI typing promptly carrying.

As an example, it is possible to mention a working version of qualitative MI criteria among preschoolers, consisting of skills, available to psycho-sociometric quantifiable:

- explanation of events causes, behaviors, and reactions to it;
- analysis and explanation of their emotions and reactions;
- reconstruction of the situation;
- setting goals and finding a constructive way out of the situation (the constructive goal-setting);
- explaining and defending their choice of the decision;
- evaluation and the quality of the act and the result, themselves and the situation (reflection of the situation, the results and themselves);
- awareness and verbalization of the situation (Burkova 2013).

Minimally overdrawing, we can say that the age of onset of the MI formation is determined by the date of verbalization of the intention to conceive a future citizen; and the efforts of his independent strengthening are directly reflected in the trajectory of human destiny.

34.2. Mental Immunodeficiency Epidemic

The radical dismantling of the Soviet mental matrices and systems, life attitudes and behavior models, values, and meanings, having occurred a quarter of a century ago, is phenomenologically described in the picture of the *population posttraumatic stress disorder* (PPTSD) (Sidorov 2015b).

Russia's sticking to the early stages of PPTSD development or *transformation society* appears in deformation and loss of the old collective identity, but not finding a new one. This is evident in the numerous examples of renaming without content, work without result, promises without achievement, abundance of words without real cases, repairs for repairs, investment for kickbacks, etc.

Applying to the modern Russian society the *sociocultural trauma theory* of P. Sztompka (2001), it is proposed to define six stages (fractals) of PPTSD or the *traumatic public disorder* (Zhapuev 2013):

1) pre-reform crisis state – changeover time;
2) destructive changes in the permanent crises of transformation (1991, 1993, 1998, 2008-2009, 2014-2015), appearing more often and risking to go into the equifinality development;

3) reinterpretation of the historical experience with the release of a single history textbook (Russia today);
4) structural modernization of the country;
5) overcoming the consequences of population mental trauma and access to a new level of development;
6) stabilization of public life and sustainable development.

Unfortunately, it seems that the singular nonlinearity of the modern world significantly reduces the possibility of long-term forecasting and futurology.

In the situation of globalization pressure and systemic crisis, when the MI is diminished or deformed, the *identity crisis* develops, the most common initial symptom of which is the appearance of the *mass human* as a carrier of *mass conscience* (Dubrovsky 2013). Such psycho-type is self-centered and narcissistic, ambitious and demanding, cynical and cruel. This "image of success" replicated in the media squeezes virtually all the traditional positive personal qualities from kindness and humility to the warm-heartedness and justice. The core of the mass human personality becomes the thirst for consumption, reaching the consumer ecstasy with various forms of dependence disorders (shopping addiction, etc.). The subject loses the need for critical and autonomous thinking, is quite satisfied with reactive tips, perceiving them as a transfer of responsibility for himself. Reflection is no longer needed, since all you need in order to maintain the illusion of personal solvency is available off the shelf. That is how a predictable and obedient, conformal and controlled mass human arises (Moscovichy 1998; Kormochy 2015). However, the question about the true plans of the producers of the population psycho-surgery remains unsolved.

The leading weapon of this war is globalization, which dilutes and evaporates the traditional socio-economic and civil-political differences between people and societies and more recently, the states themselves – at a rate of a chain reaction of "noosphere atomic explosion." In this situation, the last safety boundary for the personality is a protective cage of *identity*, interiorized from culture representations and norms, patterns and behaviors.

In the methodology of mental medicine the *identity crisis syndrome* (ICS) is described in the *animogenesis* by a symptom complex of demoralization, in the *psychogenesis* by depressive and asthenic-apathetic, dependent and perverse disorders, in the *sociogenesis* by reactions of care and downshifting, in the *biogenesis* by a wide range of psychosomatic disorders. When the ICS occurs, the MI resources help to save from the deformation and transformation of the public conscience, to reduce emotional stress and existential despair, to reduce the "sharpness of discomfort" (Erikson 1996), and destructive behavior, to prevent the collapse of individual and collective relations, to preserve important values and moral priorities (Stepin 2013).

Increasing the level of generalization, we can say that sweeping the whole world pandemic of demoralization and dehumanization is a population manifestation of the *acquired mental immunodeficiency syndrome (AMIS),* distinguished by us on the clinical models of combatants and migrants, alcoholism and drug abuse (Sidorov 2005).

Numerous social psychological studies reveal the terrible scope of *mental immunodeficiency epidemic* in modern Russia. For example, the Institute of Sociology of the Russian Academy of Sciences (Gorshkov 2014) studied the changes of people over the past 15-20 years: 78% reported the increase of aggression and ¾ the reduction of respect for elders, 70% - the increase of malignity and insincerity, the growth of selfishness and lack of altruism, 67% - lack of respect for the woman and the disappearance of cordiality, 68% - marked the growth of cynicism, 70% - a decline of integrity and 47% - a decline of partnership, 37% - the weakening of responsibility to the family. Such critical and self-critical assessment indicates the erosion of social identity, but still persisting mental immunity, allowing, at least, to notice and with the urgency to accept the collapse of moral values.

The deformable reality inevitably leads to various pathologies of conscience. Thus, there is a return to the *existential despair syndrome* of 90-ies of the last century: with anxiety and depressed mood, decreased performance, loss of zest for life, distraction, and confusion (Zobov et al. 2014; Sidorov 2014). The authors see the reasons for the growth of psychopathological phenomena of social and individual conscience in massive pressure of values and norms, which are not compatible with the traditional archetypes.

Evidence of serious deformation of the law enforcement system, as the basis of national security, is a complete lack of protection of the victims of criminal attacks and their formal defenders: 90% of victims and witnesses said that in the face of threat to their life or health, they would be forced to refuse to testify or would give false testimony; 95% of judges and law enforcement officials confirmed the change of indications and only 0.2% of them recognized the effectiveness of their security (Revyagin et al. 2014). Such evidence of accumulation of total legal and social, psychological and moral insecurity are still amortized by the mental resilience, but the deepening of social and economic crisis will inevitably lead to a cumulative explosion of public conscience. Not coincidentally Russia is ranked the first place in Europe for citizens' distrust of the police (Dubnyakova 2013).

The drama of the situation is that the MI is the last frontier of national security, just as the rise in the melee in the digital field of the hybrid war. After all, the social conscience of the country-target is cumulatively blown within it, and the economically motivated race of traditional armament is only way of "budget suicide" and the illusory-imitated trance for aboriginals, doomed at the best case for dreary survival (no wonder, that People's Republic of China in September 2015 launched a program to reduce the army for 300 thousand). However, the survival as a way of adaptation with minimal resource costs and amorphous value priorities, stoical fanaticism and reductionism, paternalism and infantilism repeatedly saved the Slavs at all times (Andreev 2007). We can only recall the classics – never say never.

The AMIS epidemic is phenomenologically described by the following blocks of symptom complexes:

a) *destructive biogenesis:*
   - deterioration in the quality and reducing the level of public health;
   - depopulation trends in demographics;
   - the growth of mental (depression, etc.) epidemics;

b) *destructive sociogenesis:*
   - growing social deformation and catastrophic social stratification of society;
   - reduction of social mobility and the growth of migration activity (up to 50% of the population would like to leave the country (Gorshkov 2011);
   - strengthening of deprivation and isolation trends;
   - expansion of simulation-imitational pseudo-public institutions;
   - loss of labor productivity, destructive professiogenesis;

- the increase in the gap between the people and the authorities;
- lack of social trust in society;
- the growth of social (alcoholism, drug addiction, etc.) and antisocial (extremism, terrorism, etc.) epidemics;

c) *destructive psychogenesis:*
- the crisis of individual and collective identity;
- deformation of national and civil conscience;
- depersonalization of business and functional relationships;
- infocommunication transparency and vulnerability of individual and social conscience;

d) *destructive animogenesis:*
- growing cultural deformation;
- the decline of the value of the human personality and life;
- violations of moral socialization;
- deformation of the family institution, the growth of family violence and aggression, severity and homelessness;
- degradation of education and training systems;
- lack of moral values and meanings in the mode and style, quality, and standard of living;
- marginalization and unification of social life, the rise of mass culture;
- devaluation and the loss of spirituality traditions.

Unfortunately, present-day Russia is almost literally "split society," which is characterized by "*conflict of fundamental values of justice*" (Konstantinova, Konstantinov 2012). A critical thing here is the avalanche of increasing dynamics of social inequality and polarization, destruction and annihilation of the integrity of spiritual and cultural space of still united country... According to M. K. Gorshkov (2014): "Two cultures – "ruble" and "Rublevsky," two morals – collectivist and individualist..." – all these are faults and cracks in the mental matrix of the Russian social identity, which requires prompt and effective correction.

That is why the style of passive-inertial contemplation and expectations on the side of the society may become a suicidal catalyst for the collapse of the state. *The imperative of modernization of the country requires the mobilization of new mechanisms and tools for engineering and management of public conscience and public health, accumulated in the synergetic technological platform of mental medicine.*

34.3. Target Levels of Mental Security

Safety Of Living (SOL) is the science of the human safe interaction with the environment. As an independent specialty, it first started in Russia in 1991 with a profile council for doctoral and master's theses organized by us in Arkhangelsk State Medical Institute.

The new direction of SOL is the *mental safety* (MS) – the science of safe engineering and management of individual and social conscience. This issue was actualized by us ten years ago with the release of psychical (mental) terrorism as a non-lethal weapon of mass destruction (Sidorov 2005). Essentially, this is a new method in the synergetic methodology of mental medicine for the old problems of occupational safety of intellectual work and psycho-technological inversion, information, and hybrid wars, etc. MS accumulates and focuses the MI resources and registers of mental resilience (MR), which in specific clinical cases and epidemic situations are measured and predicted, modeled and managed by the various *mental health services* (MHS) (Table 34.1).

MR is flexibility and plasticity of individual and public conscience and the MHS is synergistic biopsychosociospiritual Ψ-cluster of society and state, providing the MS.

Table 34.1. Matrix of mental immunity and security levels

Ontogenesis vectors	Types of immunity	Target levels of mental security
Biogenesis	Biological	Protection of the body and the population against infections and invasions, and own altered cells providing the adaptive level of physical health
Psychogenesis	Psychic Psychological	Protection of the individual and society from the psycho-traumatic factors of external and internal environment, which provides the adaptive level of psychic (psychological) health
Sociogenesis	Social	Protection of the individual and society from the destroying sociogenic factors of external and internal environment, which provides the adaptive level of social health
Animogenesis	Spiritual and moral	Protection of the individual and society from destructive animogenetic factors of external and internal environment, which provides the adaptive level of spiritual and moral health

The basic integral MS indicators, as protection of individual and social conscience from the external and internal threats, are:

- prevalence of psychic and behavioral disorders, mental and social epidemics;
- levels of crime and violence in society;
- levels of poverty and unemployment, social stratification, and justice;
- the degree of social vulnerability of sick and disabled people;
- prevalence and severity of anomie and permissiveness;
- synchrony and symmetry, glassiness and interactivity in dynamics and rhythmic of fate trajectory and ecology;
- harmonious balance in the interface of individual and social conscience of resources and opportunities, rights, and duties, freedom and responsibility, competence and ambition, aspirations and self-esteem, etc.;
- the integrity of perception of the individual and society in all ethnocultural and socio-psychological, spiritual-moral and biomedical diversity;
- the balance of mechanisms of self-development and self-actualization, triggering the mental and social epidemic processes;

- confidence in the future and a sense of security, realization and satisfaction;
- stress resistance and reliability of psychoemotional stress canalization;
- the effectiveness of screening and prediction, correction, and automediation in critical periods of the ontogenetic development;
- polymodal unity of style and quality, healthy mode and moral meaning of life;
- the balance of all-human and national spiritual-moral values and priorities;
- the quality of resonant and coherent interaction between the individual and society;
- positive and constructive perception of the world and our place in it;
- professiogenesis adaptability and education continuity, the effectiveness of education and self-management;
- maturity and stability, activity and realization of moral feelings and image, position and behavior;
- equal starting opportunities and non-discrimination in the fate ecology;
- the level of public consolidation and trust to state institutions;
- the degree of society polymodal polarization;
- nature and extent of social mobility and migration;
- the quality of public health and public conscience;
- dynamics of demographic development (a type of reproduction, indexes of fertility and mortality, marriage and divorce, etc.);
- the level of patriotism, civic and political activity.

At the maximum level of generalization, MI is the interface of polymodal and multilevel MS of the individual and society. Biopsychosociospiritual resources of MI are behaviorally translated into registers of MR, making the functional and dynamic MS basis, enshrined in the mental matrix of individual and social identity. MS as the protection system of the inner world of the man is the most important prerequisite for effective business cooperation and adaptive professiogenesis. Without its ensuring there can not be neither constructive, creative activity of the person, nor real modernization of society and the state.

Prediction and prevention of MS threats provide the *system monitoring of mental health* (SMMH), which is one of the MHS tools.

The integral sense-forming marker of MI is identity. If *personal identity* is understood as the self-determination of the individual in terms of its biological and physical, psychological and spiritual-moral traits, then *social identity* is as self-determination within the framework of social groups and social roles. In the context of MS consideration, the level of generalization increases to collective and ethnic, social and political, civil and state identity.

Herewith the civic identity is understood not only as loyalty to the state and a marker of the power legitimization but also as their identification with the citizens (Drobizheva 2014). This is an extremely polymorphic and multimodal concept, which is changing under the influence of actual challenges of the past and the crisis present, the socio-political and socio-economic situation both for each individual and collective identity. Operational categories of MI and MS allow instrumental and technological filling and measuring, predicting and simulating the multi-dimensional functionality of the formation and nonlinear development of *state-civil identity as an actual priority of the national security*.

Not by chance, even the WHO definition (2001) of *mental health* (MH) is completed with civil and political focus. It is not just the absence of psychic disorders and mental well-being of the person, which allows realizing own potential, helps to resist stress, to work productively and to *contribute to the development of society*. All MH specifications are biopsychosociospiritually multidimensional. Moreover, it can be said that MH is a *polymodal welfare*. It is important to emphasize the fundamental importance for the identity of the moral component of the "well-being" and "self-realization," "stress resistance" and "performance," which are impossible without the ethics in business communication. That is why, for all the social service professions, involved in the MS ensuring – doctors and teachers, psychologists and social workers, law enforcement officers and clergy – there should be a single *Set of ethical codes*.

34.4. Integrated Strategies of Mental Security

At the maximum level of generalization it is possible to define the following basic strategies for mental security.

Self-development strategy (individual, society, etc.) is presented as updated and deepen with the spiritual and moral and biopsychosocial potential, which is accumulated in the MI, providing the successful integration into the public conscience and functioning of multilevel society. All MI resources are systematically and harmoniously integrated into MR registers. Thus, adaptive animogenesis allows effective and timely ensuring the coherence of global and universal humanistic priorities with the patriotic and civic national interests. Adaptive sociogenesis synchronizes and symmetrizes the multilevel pyramid of social roles and relationships. Adaptive psychogenesis provides the response effectiveness to the stress of singular-crisis reality. Adaptive biogenesis is responsible for resistance to traditional infectious and emerging viral and other agents.

Forms and types, techniques and tools of implementation of this strategy are exclusively multivariate: from polymodal formulation of canonical revelation of the Apostle Paul: "Do not conform to the pattern of this world, but be transformed by the renewing of your mind," - to the modern secular classics of education and training through, but not for the whole life. This MS strategy allows, in particular, confronting the generalization mechanism of mental and social epidemics.

The *strategy of adaptive conscience expansion* is traditionally realized by the media, TV and the Internet in relation to the actual event-driven "anchors" from everyday disasterization of the picture of the world to gender mainstream. Among many undoubtedly successful recent TV projects, it is important to note the expanding representation of frankly illusory-compensatory mental matrices of the archival genre of a hystero-demonic renaissance, which always and quickly comes to life in all crises and marks them with marginal magical and shamanistic rites. If the professional psychologist annually treat not more than 10% of Russians, then the extrasensory perception experts and magicians – about 25%. That's more than the number of taking part in the sacraments. Only the third of respondents denies the phenomenological reality of occultism, the other, in varying degrees, were involved in the occult atmosphere. So the occultism, but not religion, displaces the Soviet atheism. About 300 thousand of different magicians, healers and extrasensory perception experts are officially registered in the country. The actual numbers are much bigger, and the dynamics of growth leaves no doubt that tomorrow it will be the main "psycho-technological subpopulation," manipulating the public conscience. Moreover, the progressively decreasing subpopulation of professional scientists is already less than 400 thousand (Yurevich 2015).

History has repeatedly demonstrated the lameness and suicidal nature of artificial prosthesis or blurring of reality, displacing the creative forms of personal and public business activity. Even with the fairly common hyper-indulgent assessment of domestic TV- sewage production, sometimes it seems that mainly the task of the destruction of the nation social conscience is executed.

The mission of MI strengthening and MS ensuring becomes feasible only when maintaining consistency and continuity of transmitted constructive moral position in the sense-figured design of created virtual reality. The work genre and technique of contemporary stupid artists of digital shop become a secondary task. They equally may be the socialists or the surrealists, modernists or primitivists – in any case, the mental variety of potential audience is guaranteed to provide the force imposed consumer demand for "mental allowance" of even surrogate information. It is essential only to preserve the diversity of the palette of colors and meanings. It is much noticed in the reborn vogue, again as in all times of crisis, on the talk show of "everything and nothing": in spite of tactical actuality of present-day issues, the strategic items often fall out of focus or are illusory disguised.

It is not by chance that peculiarities of mental ecology of simultaneous expansion of Russian culture and public conscience, reflections of diverse and vast natural spaces in the national character are historically reflected in all projects of Eurasian integration. So, N. A. Berdyaev (1990) wrote: "The immensity of the Russian land, the absence of borders and the limits are expressed in the structure of the Russian soul. The portrait of the Russian soul corresponds to the Russian landscape with the same boundlessness and shapelessness, urgeness into infinity and the breadth." Namely, the MI interface provides the assessment and selection of challenges and threats in the public conscience on the vast field of problems and resources, as well as the launching of directly related induction of new and alternative ways of development.

Permanent self-identification strategy (or identities drift by V. A. Tishkov (2013), which allows in all ontogenesis fractals to maintain the current perception of one's personal identity in case of change of the social one. Just as the lack of calcium in the body can lead to osteoporosis and fracture of the skeleton, so the internal moral and evaluative framework of personality is formed with sense-figures of mentality and skeletonizes the identity.

It allows to save critical and balanced assessments of changing kaleidoscopic picture of reality: with the habitual-normative anomie and permissiveness; gallopingly growing demoralization and dehumanization of the world, immersed in a system civilization crisis; with irreversibly destroyed national-patriarchal grids of ethic customs and traditions as a mental matrix of civilizational diversity, which are replaced by ritual performance and gamization, simulation and simulacrum, centaurisms and antinomies. The soaking of this "crazy charm" of crisis reality under the pretentious administrative ecstasies of self-destructive import substitution is only allowed by reliable identificational MI skeleton, woven from traditional humanistic ideas and values, tools and techniques of system biopsychosociospiritual evaluation of norm and pathology.

Just as love lasts forever or at least for a long time, but every day, every day starting from the beginning, so the MI of personality is preserved only in the constant renewal of identity during the real creative work. After all, even the correct vaccinations of good, not to mention the divine commandments, are impossible to be made in the childhood and for the rest of the life...

Not coincidentally, namely this strategy to a large extent is manifested in the steadily growing subpopulation of "believers without religion," who disclaim any intermediaries in their communion with God and show the high MI level. This trend was predicted even by Viktor Frankl (1990) in an interview with the US magazine Time, where he said that "We are moving not to the universal, but to personal, profoundly personalized religiosity, by which everyone can communicate with God in his own, personal and intimate language." However, the degree and depth of the personal ethical self-determination and autonomation are in danger of turning into another mental pit-trap in a situation of gallopingly growing Internet globalization, which virtually facilitates the instant and efficient access to the conscience of users.

That is why the "noosphere resilience," accumulating the potential of civilizational MI, should be provided with adaptive engineering and management of the network and, ideally, transparent services of mental health, which until recently operated worldwide exclusively within national security systems.

The separated strategy allows to substantially neutralize or, at least, to counterbalance the mechanisms of anonymity and identity destruction in the development of anti-social and mental epidemics.

Asymmetric coherence strategy consists of systemacity and integrity of the perception of values and meanings, space and time of real and virtual world with the unconditional priority of the real one. The name of this strategy is associated with one of the basic principles of cosmology – baryon asymmetry of the universe, consisting in the observed prevalence in its visible part of matter over antimatter (Sidorov 2015).

Today, in usual everyday situation of engineering and management of global (noosphere) conscience by virtual instruments and techniques, humanity imperceptibly is drawing into a giant black hole or a mental trap of reality inversion. In fact, the TV and the Internet have almost convinced the world that really thing is only what we are said and shown to us, and without which we simply can not live tomorrow.

The scale and pace of growth of the computer and the Internet addiction become a factor, which threatens the MS and requires the protection of public conscience by strengthening the MI.

Polymodal (cross-, trans-, interactive, etc.) resonance strategy is actualized by singularly-crisis situation of the tectonic civilizational shift, which has exhausted the traditional resources of the world order. This strategy is in tempo-rhythmological focusing and MI self-adjustment to operational forecasting and non-linear response to the challenges and threats, mobilizing in proportion the resources and protection registers. Passive watching and waiting with the naive hope of surviving being an innocent observant, or even in a highly protected palace, as in the mental mousetrap with very ecstatic oil and gas illusions, - all this dooms beyond retrieve to repeat the Russian Empire disaster. Like now at those times everybody with the ability to think understood and spoke about the inevitability of the collapse, but, generally speaking, did not do anything. It is highly naïve to enjoy yourself watching a fly splashing in sanctions milk, hoping to turn it into the import substitution butter. The uniting and inspiring, creative and technologically mobilizing national defense programs and programs of strategic development are necessary.

Multidimensional conscience glassiness strategy lies in metered and selective passage through the mental lens of conscience of images and meanings of surround and the inner human world. MI can be compared to a protective layer of such optics, creating the mirror effect. Herewith the illusion thoughts and forms of the unconscious are as important for the individual conscience, as the challenges of the outside world. Mirror neurons of the brain, providing the mental representation can be designated as mental immunocompetence cells. Mental immunomodulation lies in regulation and setting of glassy multidimensional optics of conscience interface. Instrumental and methodological issues have been described by us in a synergetic technological platform of mental medicine, which mission is the engineering and management of conscience and health (Sidorov 2015a).

The proposed approach is equally implemented on both clinical models of individual conscience and the epidemic models of public conscience, reflected in the "noosphere mirror" (Sidorov 2015a).

In this regard, the recent (August 2015) confrontation on the Korean peninsula is representative, when towards the "loud-speaking" mental attacks of southerners in the XXI century, the northerners asymmetrically responded with artillery salvos from the XX century. The producers of the most longlasting deprivation-sanctions experiment demonstrated again to the world that the protection is in principle possible without development, but the victory – never. This is especially important for the Russian Federation, for which many opponents predict the North Korean path of destiny, with full reproduction of self-destructive scenarios of not still forgotten life behind the Soviet Iron Curtain.

That is why, the *mobilization strategy for modern Russia becomes uncontested*, requiring for MS updating of MI resources and MR registers. This is especially true because hybrid wars have practically ceased to be visible in the cruelest way of competitive fighting for the same resources of the hybrid world. It is significant that comprehensively suicidal Ukrainian Front became a world event largely as a generalization of the experience of "successful" Korean mirrored population experiment. At the same time the party, which is doomed to a life in civilizational illusion, was announced long before. Just do not break the "noosphere mirror" as crystallized (by C. G. Jung) in the World Wide Web global conscience. And tomorrow to say with certainty who and at whom is looking, where the reflection is, and most importantly – on which side the reality is – will not be easy.

After all, a hybrid war has neither fighting nor labor fronts – all the resources and tools of life-support have become the weapon. Therefore, the continuation of waiting that moment, when Motherland calls, is naive carelessness. In the planetary cataclysms of singular epoch only completely accidental survivors with severe post apocalyptic syndrome may silly suspect themselves as winners...

These integral strategies for MS provision and MI development are just a small illustration of still unclaimed resources of synergetic technological platform of mental medicine and ecology, mental epidemiology and preventology, practically embodied in the work of many, but not co-ordinated services of mental health: medical and psychological, sociological and pedagogical, legal and corporate. *The breakthrough in the new system and supradepartmental performance becomes vitally necessary.*

Moreover, the civilizational singularly-globalization trends are made of extremely categorical branchy tree of internationalization and informatization, stereotyping and unification, integration and differentiation, trans-gendering (feminization of men and women masculinity) and migration pandemic, generalization of mental and asocial epidemics, etc. *All this requires new tools and resources, supradepartmental organizational-functional structure and synergetic methodology of the work to ensure the mental safety of the world.*

Conclusion

Development Strategies for Mental Epidemiology and Medicine

Problems of ethical and social, mental and physical relations are among the most complex and unresolved, despite the ongoing interest from many generations of researchers from various fields to this side of a human nature. It is the first time when synergetic biopsychosociospiritual methodology of mental epidemiology allowed measuring and predicting the focus and the way of epidemic process development applying instrumental and technological methods.

Mental medicine and epidemiology based on the synergetic methodology enables us to solve a number of burning issues in today's health care:

- develop and implement the technologies of *mental health system monitoring*, supporting and transforming traditional health survey that allows to evaluate the quality of life and social functioning providing an adaptive professiogenesis and avoiding anachronistic psychiatric stigma;
- develop organizational forms of *mental health services* to assist both people with difficulties in adaptation and patients with psychosomatic and mental disorders, comorbid disorders of somatic and mental health, falling back upon governmental help and resources of public and state, state and private as well as public and private partnership;
- develop common approaches to *screening and prediction*, early detection, and diagnosis of psychiatric and psychosomatic disorders, preventive and correctional, medical and rehabilitative tactics;
- provide primary prevention of diseases in early prenosological fractals based on *synergistic functional diagnostics*;
- put into practice a *synergetic personalized model of biopsychosociospiritual care provided by a multidisciplinary team*, including general practitioners, psychiatrists and psychotherapists, clinical psychologists and teachers, specialists in social work and bioethics and others;

- professionalize *mental preventology and recreation therapy* establishing specialization like "preventologist" and "recreation therapist" which are already provided with specialists in social work;
- develop new *biopsychosociospiritual technologies* in combination with somatic and psycho pharmacotherapy, spiritual and moral rehabilitation, social and psychotherapy, that help to start sanogenetic mechanisms;
- *fill medical ethics with clinical content*, expanding functional diagnostics with moral syndromology;
- integrate *health promotion and moral purpose of life* technologically as a part of the biopsychosociospiritual methodology of mental preventology;
- justify and measure the weight characteristics of *mentality as a factor of public health;*
- introduce a new approach to the *evaluation of the quality of life as the endemic mental representation* (20%);
- justify *the classification and mechanisms of mental, social and anti-social epidemics,* beginning with alcoholism and drug addiction ending with extremism and terrorism;
- describe *terrorism as a polymodal asthenic disorder and prioritize mental ecology of national security;*
- point out the *mental immunity* as a matrix of identity and basis of personal and public safety;
- justify the new direction of *mental safety* as a priority of national security in the epoch of hybrid wars;
- justify the methodology of construction and introduce *spiritual and religious-integrated treatment and rehabilitation programs* into clinical practice;
- develop *mental preventology as a social institution* for adaptive protection and *engineering of social conscience;*
- organize forms and methods, approaches and resources of *mental resilience;*
- expand the use of *sanogenetic therapy for patients in somatic departments;*
- strengthen the basic training of *general practitioners in mental health.*

Borderline personality disorders now are responsible for about a half of all mental disorders. Clinical psychopathology pathomorphosis is shown in the growth rate of somatoforms. This emphasizes the relevance of a strong interdisciplinary cooperation of various specialists in providing care to patients with mental disorders.

One of the primary tasks is a timely diagnosis and adequate treatment of borderline personality disorders associated with physical disorders. Primarily the patient should receive treatment in the outpatient departments. Taking into consideration this fact, a synergistic approach in the treatment should be a fundamental one. From one-third to a half of therapeutic patients are in need of specialized and psychopharmacological or psychotherapeutic assistance. To provide the population with access to psychological, psychotherapeutic and psychiatric care, the interaction of the certain forms with a system of general medical network and the initial integration in territorial clinics is required.

The interdisciplinary character of mental epidemiology is to bring to the study and form a human personality, prevent from mental health problems of the whole society, teachers and psychologists, doctors and social workers, etc.

In recent years biopsychosociospiritual paradigm is actively promoted in personalized medicine, which takes into consideration all the components of patients' treatment and rehabilitation. However, little attention is still paid to the primary prevention measures of mental and physical disorders. Principles of diagnosis and rehabilitation of disorders at the so-called prenosological level are not developed.

There are the following development strategies of mental epidemiology and medicine:

1) *Program and target-oriented strategy* are to change the approach to solving problems from departmental and administrative one to system and software based one. The benefits of the supra-departamental program based method are defining issues, the possibility of targeting risk groups, compliance with the principles of consistency and continuity in the work of various specialists.
2) *The extranosological strategy* is a specific methodological requirement for mental epidemiology, which is noticeable for polyetiology and interdisciplinary, dynamic and changeable, unstable and reversible characteristics. Causes and consequences of mental disorders affect different spheres of life and at the same time are different in the monotony of etiological factors and conditions of development. The extranosological approach provides the most appropriate prevention measures and correction of mental disorders by different specialists - doctors, psychologists, social workers, teachers, etc.

Mental epidemiology is an applied science and it is based on care provided by specialists' brigade led by the reference specialist, a professional in the field of social programs and social management, preventive and corrective or therapeutic and rehabilitation activities.

3) *Humanistic strategy* includes the realization of individuality as the desire to agree on self-ideal and self - real mainly through internal mechanisms and ethics in business communication. This idea opens great prospects for participation not only secular but also religious institutions in providing preventive measures.

Humanistic strategy combined with all the dimensions of the individual - mental, social, spiritual and moral, biological - which has a strong potential for the development of mental epidemiology. Development of social skills and roles, formation of moral values and identity, providing mental immunity and resistance to various forms of addiction is a strategic objective of strengthening public health and public awareness, national security and sustainable development.

4) *Pedagogic-educational strategy* is the primary mental preventology aimed at healthy lifestyle filled with moral sense. Healthy lifestyle is only a means to reach the goal, which is self-actualization and self-development of personality. There are two main approaches to the formation of centric and morally valuable mentality in this strategy: people's skills and organization and reorganization of the environment so that it may contribute to the development of the individual and does not contain sources of chronic stress (mobbing prevention and destructive professiogenesis etc.). Educational strategies can be implemented in several ways. One of the most famous

is education on mental health. The purpose is to assist in gaining knowledge about the factors that form a healthy way of life and moral sense. We seek to strengthen mental stability and well-being of people through the popularization of knowledge about physical and spiritual health, bringing all the media. The second way is the direct training of skills, for example ethics of communication, solutions of difficult problems and social skills training. One of the types of work in this area is public support group: professional and paraprofessional. Cooperation of many social groups, aimed at minimizing the threat of social pathology is required. This is an impact on psychological and moral climate of the family and school, workplaces and neighborhood, which could be called engineering and management of the public conscience.

5) *The forward-looking strategy* is needed for the prediction of the reliability and efficiency of adaptive response with the clearest focus on the choice of specific preventive programs. The prevalence of mental, social and anti-social epidemics has an endemic nature and poses a real threat to public health and national security. Therefore, the earliest assessment of mental immunity and health factors and resources, identification and correction of initial symptoms of possible mental disorders are the most important aspects.
6) *The environmental strategy* should include biological, social, psychological and ecologically dependent aspects of preventive measures. The primary emergence of this strategy is due to the appearance of factors accumulation of biogeochemical destruction of biological structures in a closed production cycles as well as due to changes in weight of various routes responsible for input of extraneous substances into the body. In the context of mental ecology, this strategy requires taking into account the spiritual, moral and social reason complexes (in particular demoralization, mobbing syndromes, etc.) to develop preventive programs.

In the year of environmental culture and environmental protection (2013) in Moscow, Novosibirsk, Volgograd, Samara, and Ufa a national interdisciplinary project called “Ecology of the brain,” organized by the Association of interdisciplinary medicine under the international program “Brain Age” was launched. The purpose of the project is training of people to preserve mental health in a rapidly changing world, prevention and treatment of brain diseases. The project involves a broad interdisciplinary cooperation of representatives of a wide variety of specialties in the treatment and prevention of psycho-neurological diseases and behavioral disorders.

7) *The integrated strategy* involves a complex interaction of mental epidemiology with related fields of social work and clinical psychology, pedagogy, and bioethics. It means establishing integral links between social policy as a whole and its individual parts, among all the preventive and correctional facilities as well as treatment and rehabilitation process. A single synergetic methodological and technological approach to strengthen the mental health and treatment of mental disorders excludes artificial opposition of “health medicine” and “ disease medicine.” Moreover, the centric component of mental preventology will in future prevail over noso -centric component of clinical psychiatry, providing harmonious redistribution of power and

resources within a single integrated mental medicine, focused on the synergistic functional diagnosis.

The integral synergetic methodology of mental medicine made it possible to overcome the inertial descriptive reductionism of clinical psychiatry, providing it with new resources and technologies. Integratism of individual clinical practice in mental medicine is supplemented with integralism of the epidemiological phenomenology of public health and public awareness fully represented in a new concept of the mental and social epidemic.

The concept of "integralism" was introduced by the greatest macrosociologist of the twentieth century, Pitirim Sorokin. He published the scientific basis of his study in the work called "Social and Cultural Dynamics" - a sort of a "Bible" of integralism while the work called "The main trends of our time" serves as "The New Testament."

Mental medicine is a psychiatric paradigm of the integrative medicine global trend of integrative and personalized medicine.

8) *Economic strategy* of mental medicine demands full inclusion of market sticks confronting to mental epidemics. The modern concept of prevention focuses people on the perception of medicine as a socioeconomic category. This means that health care including prevention should become a real economic entity in the overall economy. Socially oriented market of mental health is unprecedented in the scale and capital coverage. It requires a new legal quality of public-state and state-private partnership to guarantee mental health and the protection of the public conscience of the nation by means of psycho-technological methods. This will create the conditions to minimize the shadow market of pathogenic agents and techniques of rapid resource support (drugs, sects, and others) and essentially to minimize mental terrorism within the framework of permanent hybrid wars of the modern world.

We have established the synergetic methodology for the development of mental epidemiology and mental medicine. Thus today we have some practical pilot models to manage the system monitoring and mental health services. Economic cost-effectiveness and resource availability make them functional, adaptive and anti-crisis instruments of the state and society.

9) *The regulatory strategy* reflects the quality of legislative support for mental epidemiology. An urgent task is to develop and improve legal policy to protect public conscience. The development and adoption of the "Psychotherapy" law draft can radically enhance the legal support for psychotherapists and clinical psychologists, increasing guarantees for the protection of the mental health of the nation.

In the XXI century not only the formation of psychiatry as a medical specialty raising 100-year-old problems again should be expected, but association of genetic and neurobiological, psychological and social determinants of health in a new profession, engaged in mental health (Bolton 2013). This will improve the quality of medical treatment, costs and solve the problem of specialists training.

Establishment of mental ecology and epidemiology, mental medicine and preventology embodied in the new methodology of mental health services and mental health system monitoring is a step in existing professional and civilizational trend, accumulating multidisciplinary resources and providing healthcare personalization. This allowed *mental medicine to realize the mission of adaptive engineering and management of conscience and health,* reflecting new conceptually methodological and instrumentally-technological stage of development of personalized medicine in Russia.

In conclusion we would like to note that the above-mentioned development strategies of mental medicine and epidemiology are polydisciplinary and multivariant ones. They should take into account the characteristics of professional and social, age and gender, ethnic and religious, economic and cultural target groups.

The research of mental medicine and epidemiology was a strategic response to medical science to the current challenges of global crisis and a need to modernize our society. All this requires a radical change in the technological basis of strengthening of mental health, as well as in the modalities of public and professional awareness: to change pessimistic and catastrophic paradigm of perception of the world into the resource and mobilization life strategy that predetermines adaptive professiogenesis and sustainable development.

References

"Nones" on the Rise: One-in-Five Adults Have No Religious Affiliation. Pew Research Center. 2012. 80 p.

Ababkov V.A., Karvasarskij B.D. *Psihoterapija* [Psychotherapy]. SPb. Piter, 2012. 672 p.

Aberg M. et al. Cardiovascular fitness in males at age 19 and risk of serious depression in adulthood: Swedish prospective population-based study. US National Library of Medicine National institutes of Health. 2012. N. 201(5). P. 352-359.

Akulenko L.V., Ugarov I.V. *Medicinskaja genetika* [Medical Genetics]. Ed. O.O. Janushevicha, S.D. Arutjunova M.: GEOTAR-Media, 2011. 208 p.

Aleksander F. *Psihosomaticheskaja medicina. Principy i primenenie* [Psychosomatic medicine: Its Principles and Applications]. Transl. from English A.M. Bokovikova, V.V. Starovojtova. M.: Institut obshhegumanitarnyh issledovanij, 2009. 319 p.

Aleksandrov A.A. *Integrativnaja psihoterapija* [Integrative psychotherapy]. SPb.: Piter, 2009. 352 p.

Alexander S. Women wake up grumpier than men because they need more sleep. *The Telegraph*. 12.03. 2012.

Allen L.A., Woolfolk R.L. Cognitive Behavioral Therapy for Somatoform Disorders. *Psychiatric Clinics of North America*. 2010. Vol.33. P. 579-593.

Alleyne R. If you dream of weight loss, try having a good sleep. *The Telegraph*. 29.03.2011.

Alleyne R. Viewing art gives same pleasure as being love. *The Telegraph*. 09.04.2013.

Ametov A.S. *Izbrannye lekcii po endokrinologii* [Selected lectures on endocrinilogy]. M.: Medicinskoe informacionnoe agentstvo, 2009. 496 p.

Ananyev V.A. *Konceptual'nye osnovy psihologii zdorovya* [Conceptual basics of health psychology]. SPb.: Rech, 2006. 384 p.

Andreev I.L. Mikrobiologicheskie aspekty psihiatrii [Microbiological aspects of psychiatry]. *Psihicheskoe zdorovye* [Mental health], 2015. №1. P. 72-81.

Andreev I.L., Nazarova L.N. Gorkij sahar diabeta [Bitter Sugar of Diabetes]. *Vestnik RAN* [RAS Bulletin], 2014. V. 84. № 2. P. 78-83.

Andreev I.L., Nazarova L.N. Igrajushhij mozg. Kto igraet v azartnye igry: gejmer, ego mozg ili oba? [Playing brain. Who gambles: a gamer, his brain or both?] *Psihicheskoe zdorovye* [Mental health], 2014. № 4. P. 87-96.

Andreev I.L., Nazarova L.N. Psihicheskoe zdorovye naselenija Rossii: chto den' grjadushhij nam gotovit [Mental health of the Russian population: what will it be like in the future]. *Psihicheskoe zdorovye* [Mental health], 2013. № 9. P. 75-83.

Ansari S. et al. Report. XXII World Congress on Psychosomatic Medicine. 2013. 12-14 Sept. Lisbon (Portugal).

Antropov Ju.F. *Osnovy diagnostiki psihicheskih rasstrojstv. Rukovodstvo dlja vrachej* [Basics of diagnostics of mental disorders. Handbook for general practitioners]. Ju.F. Antropov. M.: GEOTAR-Media, 2010. 384 p.

Appleton A.A., Buka S.L., Loucks E.B. et al. A prospective study of positive early-life psychosocial factors and favorable cardiovascular risk in adulthood. Circulation. 2013. Vol. 127, N 8. P. 905–912.

Apriansyah M. et al. Report. XXII World Congress on Psychosomatic Medicine, Lisbon, 12-14 Sept. 2013.

Argajl M. *Psihologija schastyja* [Psychology of Happiness]. M., 2003.

Arnold V.I. *Teorija katastrof* [Theory of catastrophes]. 4th ed. M.: Editorial URSS, 2004. 128 p.

Atak Dzh. Kusochek chistogo neba. Habbard. Dianetika i Sajentologija bez prikras [A Piece of Blue Sky. Habbard. Dianetics and Scientology Unmasked]. M., 1990.

Atlas religij i nacional'nostej. Nekommercheskaja sociologicheskaja sluzhba [Atlas of religions and nationalities. Nonprofit sociological service]. «Sreda," 2012.

Baetz M. Religion and psychiatry: from conflict to consensus. *World psychiatry*. 2013. V.12. № 1. P.35-36.

Baile W., Constantini A. Differences of the traditional approach to communication in medicine and models of communication focused on interrelationships. *Psycho-oncology*. London. 2013.

Bakhtin M. Towards a Philosophy of the Act. Austin: University of Texas Press, 1993.

Balabolkin M.I., Klebanova E.M., V.M. Kreminskaja. *Differencialnaja diagnostika i lechenie endokrinnyh zabolevanij* [Differential diagnosis and treatment of endocrine diseases]. M.: *Medicinskoe informacionnoe agentstvo* [Medical Information Agency], 2008. 752 p.

Batstra L. et al. Child emotional and behavioral problems. *Dev. Med. Child Neurol*. 2012. № 54. P. 492-494.

Bauer A.M., Fielke K., Brayley J. et al. Tackling the Global Mental Health Challenge: A Psychosomatic Medicine. Consultation–Liaison Psychiatry. *Psychosomatics*. 2010. Vol. 51. P. 185-193.

Bauman Z., Donskis L. Moral Blindness. The Loss of Sensitivity in Liquid modernity. Cambridge: Polity Press, 2013.

Beck U. Twenty Observations on a World in Turmoil. Cambridge: Polity Press, 2012.

Behrend C., Prasarn M., Coyne E. et al. Smoking cessation related to improved patient-reported pain scores following spinal care. *Journal of Bone and Joint Surgery*. December. 05.2012.

Bejtson G. *Ekologija razuma* [Mind ecology]. M.: Smysl, 2000. 476 p.

Bekke-Hansen S., Pedersen C.G., Thygesen K. et al. Faith and use of complementary and alternative medicine among heart attack patients in a secular society. *Complement Ther. Med*. 2012. Vol. 20, №5. P. 306–315.

Belenkov Ju.N. *Kardiologija. Nacionalnoe rukovodstvo* [Cardiology. National Handbook]. Ju.N. Belenkov, R.G. Oganov – M.: GEOTAR-Medicina, 2010. 1232 p.

Belous V.V., Bojazitova I.V. Integratizm – sistemnaja model poznanija psihologii individualnosti [Integratism - system model of perception of personality psychology]. *Psihologicheskij zhurnal* [Journal of Psychology], 2013. V.34. № 6. P. 112-117.

Bernini O. et al. Report. XXII World Congress on Psychosomatic Medicine, Lisbon, 12-14 Sept. 2013.

Bilder L. Cancer - a family event: the patient's illness - a look through the eyes of family. *Psycho-oncology*. London. 2013.

Biondi M., Pasquini M. Psychopharmacotherapy in oncology. *Psycho-oncology*. London. 2013.

Bjudzhental D. *Iskusstvo psihoterapevta* [The art of psychotherapist]. SPb. Piter, 2001. 304 p.

Bojko O.E. et al. Vlijanie psihologicheskih osobennostej bolnyh bronhialnoj astmoj na ih socialnuju adaptaciju [Effect of the psychological characteristics of patients with bronchial asthma on their social adaptation]. *Uchenye zapiski Sankt-Peterburgskogo gosudarstvennogo universiteta im. akad. I.P. Pavlova* [Scientific notes of the St. Petersburg State University named after Acad. I.P. Pavlov], 2010. V.XVII, №2. P. 46-47.

Boldueva S.A. et al. Vzaimosvjaz narushenij psihiki s sostojaniem vegetativnoj reguljacii serdechnogo ritma i vnezapnoj smertju bolnyh, perenesshih infarkt miokarda [The relationship of mental disorders to the state of the autonomic regulation of the heart rhythm and sudden death in patients after myocardial infarction]. *Rossijskij kardiologicheskij zhurnal* [Russian Journal of Cardiology], 2008. №1. P. 26-31.

Bolton D. Should mental disorders be regarded as brain disorders? 21st century mental health sciences and implications for research and training. *World Psychiatry*. 2013. № 2. P. 21-22.

Bondarenko A.F. Psihoterapija: tip socialnosti i setevoj marketing [Psychotherapy: type of sociality and network marketing]. *Psihologija. Zhurnal Vysshej shkoly ekonomiki* [Psychology. Journal of Higher School of Economics], 2006. V. 3, № 1. P. 68–76.

Bondyreva S.K., Bezjuleva G.V., Sochivko D.V. Rossijskaja molodezh v riskogennom prostranstve sovremennoj dejstvitelnosti [Russian youth risk-taking in the space of contemporary reality]. *Psihologija nravstvennosti* [Psychology of morality]. Ed. A.L. Zhuravleva, A.V. Jurevicha. M.: Institut *psihologii RAN* [RAS Institute of Psychology], 2010. P. 261–300.

Bouthoul G. Histoire de la socialogie. Paris: PUF, 1958.

Bowman G.L. et al. Nutrient biomarker patterns, cognitive function, and MRI measures of brain aging. Neurology. Published online before print 28. 12. 2011.

Briko N. I. et al. *Epidemiologija* [Epidemiology]. V. 2. M.: MIA, 2013. 832 p.

Brojtigam V. et al. *Psihosomaticheskaja medicina* [Psychosomatic medicine]. Transl. from German. M.: GEOTAR- Medicina, 1999. 376 p.

Brown S., Kim M., Mitchell C. et al. Twenty-five year mortality of a community cohort with schizophrenia. *Br J Psychiatry*. 2010. N. 196. P. 116-21.

Buhanovskij A.O., Buhanovskaja O.A., Shostakovich B.V. *Psihicheskie rasstrojstva u serijnyh seksualnyh prestupnikov* [Mental disorders in serial sex offenders]. Rostov-na-Donu: Feniks, 2003.72 p.

Burikova I.S. Formirovanie chelovecheskogo kapitala kak osnova dejatelnosti vlasti v epohu globalizacii [The formation of human capital as the basis for the activities of government in the age of globalization]. *Psihoterapija* [Psychotherapy], 2015, № 1, P. 75-77.

Burikova I.S. Televidenie v socialnoj psihoterapii: perehod ot usilivajushhej obratnoj svjazi k uravnoveshivajushhej [Television in social psychotherapy: the transition from reinforcing feedback to counterbalancing one]. *Psihoterapija* [Psychotherapy], 2014. № 12. P. 62-63.

Burno M. E. *Terapija tvorcheskim samovyrazheniem* [Therapy of creative self-expression]. M., 2010.

Burton-Chase A., Gritz E., Peterson S. Peculiarities of genetic counseling and revealing predisposition to hereditary cancer. *Psycho-oncology*. London. 2013.

Canada A.L., Parker P.A., deMoor J.S. et al. Active coping mediates the association between religion/spirituality and quality of life in ovarian cancer. *GynecolOncol*. 2006. №101. P. 305-317.

Chitlova V.V. Trevozhnye i affektivnye rasstrojstva v obshhej medicine: obzor materialov 26-go Kongressa Evropejskoj kollegii nejropsihofarmakologii 5-9 oktjabrja 2013g., Barselona, Ispanija [Anxiety and mood disorders in general medicine: a review of the materials of the 26th Congress of the European College of Neuropsychopharmacology, October 5-9, 2013, Barcelona, Spain]. *Psihicheskie rasstrojstva v obshhej medicine* [Mental disorders in general medicine]. 2013. № 4. P. 46-48.

Chochikov H.M. et al. Psychosomatic Medicine and Integrated Care. *The Journal of Lifelong Learning in Psychiatry*. 2013. 11(4): I. 210-216.

Constantini A., Levenson J., Bersani E. Psychological and Psychopathological Reaction to the Disease Psychological and Psychopathological Reaction to the Disease. *Psycho-oncology*. London. 2013.

Copeland W. et al. Cumulative prevalence of psychiatric disorders by young adulthood. *J.Am.Acad.Child Adolesc. Psychiatry*. 2011. № 50. P. 252-261.

Cross-Disorder Group of the Psychiatric Genonics Consortium. Identification of risk loci with shared on five major psychiatric disorders: a genome-wide analysis. *Lancet*. 2013. 381 (9875). P. 1371-9.

Daniljuk A.Ja., Kondakov A.M., Tishkov V.A. Koncepcija duhovno-nravstvennogo razvitija i vospitanija lichnosti grazhdanina Rossii [Concept of spiritual and moral development and education of a citizen of Russia]. M.: Prosveshhenie, 2009. 17 p.

Dawkins R. The Selfish Gene. Oxford University Press. 1976.

Dawkins R. Viruses of the Mind. Dennet and His Critics: Demystifying Mind, ed. Bo Dalhbom. Cambridge, Mass.: Blackwell, 1991.

Debor G. Obshhestvo spektaklja [Society of the Spectacle]. M.: Logos, 2000. 184 p.

Dedov I.I. Patogenez saharnogo diabeta [The pathogenesis of diabetes]. I.I. Dedov, M.I. Balabolkin. *Medicinskij akademicheskij zhurnal* [Medical academic journal], 2006. V.6. №3. P. 3-15.

Dedov I.I., Shestakova M.V. Algoritmy specializirovannoj medicinskoj pomoshhi bolnym saharnym diabetom [Algorithms of specialized medical care to patients with diabetes mellitus]. I.I. Dedov, M.V. Shestakova. Saharnyj diabet [Diabetes mellitus], 2011. №3, app. 72 p.

Demcheva N.K. Rasprostranennost psihicheskih rasstrojstv v RF v 1991-2012 gg. [The prevalence of mental disorders in the Russian Federation in 1991-2012 years]. *Vestnik nevrologii, psihiatrii i nejrohirurgii* [Journal of Neurology, Neurosurgery and Psychiatry], 2014. № 5. P. 3-12.

Diagnostika i lechenie arterial'noj gipertonii [Diagnosis and treatment of hypertension]. Rekomendacii Rossijskogo medicinskogo obshhestva po arterialnoj gipertonii i Vserossijskogo nauchnogo obshhestva kardiologov [Recommendations of the Russian Medical Society of hypertension and the All-Russian Scientific Society of Cardiology].

Kardiovaskuljarnaja terapija i profilaktika [Cardiovascular therapy and prevention], 2010. № 7(6), app. 2.

Dilts R. *Izmenenie ubezhdenij s pomoshhyu NLP* [Changing beliefs with NLP]. M.: Klass, 2000. 192 p.

Dimsdale J., Sharma N., Sharpe M. What Do Physicians Think of Somatoform Disorders? *Psychosomatics*. 2011. Vol. 52. P. 154-159.

Dirton E.S. et al. Herpervirus latency confers symbiotic protection bacterial infection. Nature. May 2007. V.447/17. P. 326.

Dmitrieva T.B. *Etnokulturalnaja psihiatrija* [Ethnocultural psychiatry]. T.B. Dmitrieva, B.S. Polozhij. M.: Medicina, 2003. 448 p.

Doklad Komissii po izmereniju jeffektivnosti jekonomiki i social'nogo progressa [Report of the Commission on the Measurement of Economic Performance and Social Progress]. M.: Research Institute of the Account Chamber, 2010.

Domorackij V.A. Psihoterapija psihosomaticheskih rasstrojstv [Psychotherapy of psychosomatic disorders]. *Psihoterapija* [Psychotherapy], 2014. № 10. P. 18-23.

Drozhdina E.N. et al. Rol psihotravmirujushhih faktorov v dezadaptacii deteĭ i podrostkov, stradajushhih juvenilnym artritom [The role of stressful factors of maladjustment in children and adolescents with juvenile arthritis]. *Socialnaja i klinicheskaja psihiatrija* [Social and clinical psychiatry], 2012; (1): 44–50.

Dube S.R., Fairweather D.L., Pearson W.S. et al. Cumulative childhood stress and autoimmune diseases in adults. *Psychosom Med*. 2009; 71(2): 243–50.

Dzhekobson Dzh.L., Dzhekobson A.M. *Sekrety psihiatrii* [Secrets of Psychiatry]. Ed. acad. P.I. Sidorov. M.: Medpress-inform, 2005. 576 p.

Dzhidaryan I.A. Psihologija schastya i optimizma [The psychology of happiness and optimism]. M.: Institut psihologii RAN [RAS Institute of Psychology], 2013.

Eidemiller E.G., Klinicheskaja psihologija i psihoterapija semyi i detstva: tradicii i sovremennost [Clinical Psychology and Psychotherapy of the family and childhood: traditions and modernity]. *Psihicheskoe zdorove* [Mental Health]. 2015. № 2. P. 45-50.

Einsle F., Kraft D., Köllner V. Post-traumatic stress disorder (PTSD) in cardiology and oncology – which diagnostic tools should be used? *Journal of Psychosomatic Research*. 2012. Vol. 72. P. 434-438.

Elsukov A.N. Stigmatizacija kak sredstvo omassovlenija informacii [Stigma as a massification of information]. *Sociologicheskie issledovanija* [Sociological researches], 2014. № 2. P. 3-10.

Engel G.L. Biopsychosocial model and medical education: who are to be the teacher? *N. Eng. J. Med*. 1982. V. 306. P. 802-805.

Engel G.L. The need for a new medical model: a challenge for biomedicine. *Science*. 1977. Vol. 196, N 8. P. 129-136.

Engelgardt V.A. Integratizm - put ot prostogo k slozhnomu v poznanii javlenij zhizni [Integratism - the way from simple to complex in the understanding the phenomena of life]. *Voprosy filosofii* [Problems of Philosophy]. 1970. № 11. P. 115.

Epidemiologicheskij slovar [Epidemiological dictionary]. Ed. John M. Last. M., 2009. 316 p.

Epshtein M.N. *Religija posle ateizma. Novye vozmozhnosti teologii* [Religion after atheism. New features of theology]. M.: AST-Press, 2014. 416 p.

Erikson E. *Identichnost: junost i krizis* [Identity: Youth and Crisis]. M.: Progress, 1996. 197 p.

Erkkila J., Punkanen M., Fachner J. et al. Individual music therapy for depression: randomized controlled trial. *British Journal of psychiatry*. (2011) 199. P. 132–139.

Escobar J.I., Cook B., Chen C.N. et al. Whether medically unexplained or not, Heree or more concurrent somatic symptoms predict psychopathology and service use in community populatioms. *J. Psychosom. Res*. 2010. V. 69. N. 1. P. 1-8.

ESH/ESC Guidelines for the management of arterial hypertension: the Task Force for the management of arterial hypertension of the European Society of Hypertension (ESH) and of the European Society of Cardiology (ESC). *J. Hypertens*. 2013. Vol. 31, N 7. P. 1281–1357.

Estruch R., Ros E., Salas-Salvadó J. et al. Primary prevention of cardiovascular disease with a Mediterranean Diet. *The New England Journal of Medicine*. 370 (9): 886. 25.02.2013.

Faustov Je. Religioznost studentov i narkomanija [Religious students and addiction]. *Vysshee obrazovanie v Rossii* [Higher education in Russia]. 2011. № 1. P. 95-99.

Feldman J.M., Siddique M.I., Thompson N.S., Lehrer P.M. The role of panic-fear in comorbid asthma and panic disorder. *Journal of Anxiety Disorders*. 2009. Vol. 23, Issue 2. P.178-184.

Fisun A.Ja., Shamrej V.K., Goncharenko A.Ju. et al. Psihologija i psihopatologija informacionnyh vojn [Psychology and psychopathology of information warfare]. *Voenno-medicinskij zhurnal* [Military Medical Journal]. 2014. № 6. P. 4-12.

Florida R. The rise of the creative class and how it's transforming work, leisure and everyday life. New York : Perseus Book Group, 2002.

Frankl V. *Chelovek v poiskah smysla* [Man's search for meaning]. M.: Progress, 1990. 368 p.

Frankl V. *Osnovy logoterapii. Psihoterapija i religija* [Fundamentals of logotherapy. Psychotherapy and religion]. SPb. Rech, 2000. 286 p.

Frensis A. Proshloe, nastojashhee i budushhee diagnoza v psihiatrii [Past, present and future of the diagnosis in psychiatry]. *Psihiatrija i psihofarmakologija* [Psychiatry and psychopharmacology]. 2013. V. 15. № 5. P. 64-66.

Freud S. *Psihologija bessoznatelnogo* [Psychology of the unconscious]. M.: Prosveshhenie, 1990. 448 p.

Freudenberger H. Burnout: The high Cost of higt achievement. 1974.

Friedman L.C., Kalkidas M., Elledge R. et al. Medical and psychosocial predictors of delay in seeking medical consultation for breast symptoms in women in a public secotr setting. *J. Behav Med*. 2006. № 19. P. 327-334.

Fromm E. *Anatomija chelovecheskoj destruktivnosti* [The Anatomy of human destructiveness]. M.: AST-LTD, 1998. 147 p.

Fuko M. *Istorija bezumija v klassicheskuju epohu* [History of madness in the classical age]. SPb. Universitetskaja kniga [University Book], 1997. 213 p.

Fulford K. Looking with both eyes open fact and value in psychiatric diagnosis? *World Psychiatry*. 2005. Vol. 4. №2. P.78-86.

Fuller Torrey E. *Shizofrenija* [Schizophrenia]. SPb: Piter Press, 1996. 446 p.

Gabbasova Je.R. et al. Osobennosti orientacij u bolnyh, perenesshih infarkt miokarda [Features of orientation in patients with myocardial infarction]. *Uchenye zapiski Sankt-Peterburgskogo gosudarstvennogo medicinskogo universiteta im. akad. I.P. Pavlova* [Scientific notes of the St. Petersburg State University named after Acad. I.P. Pavlov], 2010. V.XVII, №2 (app.). P.56-57.

Gasperin D. et al. Effect of psychological stress on blood pressure increase: a meta-analysis of cohort studies. *Cad. Saúde Pública*. 2009. Vol. 25, N 4. P. 715–726.

Geddes L. Disrupted body clock may prime you for schizophrenia. *New Scientist*. 19.01.2012.

Ghaemi N. The rise and fall of the biopsychosocial model. *J. Psychiatry*. 2009. № 195. P. 3-4.

Gilinskij Ja. I. *Sovremennyj terrorizm: kto «vinovat» i chto delat?* [Modern terrorism: "who to blame" and what to do?]. Psihologija i psihopatologija terrorizma. Gumanitarnye strategii antiterrora [Psychology and Psychopathology of Terrorism. Humanitarian anti-terror strategies]. Coll., ed. M. M. Reshetnikov. SPb. 2004. P. 20.

Goff D. C. Future perspectives on the treatment of cognitive deficits and negative symptoms in schizophrenia. *World Psychiatry*. 2013. V. 12. № 2. P. 95-102.

Gois C. et al. Report. XXII World Congress on Psychosomatic Medicine, Lisbon, 12-14 Sept. 2013.

Goodman M. et al. Parental viewpoints of trajectories to borderline personality disorder in femaile offspring. *J Pers. Disord*. 2010. P. 2004-2016.

Goodwin R.D., Pagura J., Cox B., Sareen J. Asthma and mental disorders in Canada: Impact on functional impairment and mental health service use. *Journal of Psychosomatic Research*. 2010. Vol. 68, Issue 2. P. 165-173.

Gostoli G. et al. Report. XXII World Congress on Psychosomatic Medicine, Lisbon, 12-14 Sept. 2013.

Graaf R. De et al. Prevalence of mental disorders and trends from 1996 to 2009. *Soc. Psychiatry Psychiatr. Epidimiol*. 2012. № 47. P. 252-261.

Greco R., Tassorelli C., Mangione S. et al. Effect of sex and estrogens on neuronal actiovation in an animal model of migraine. US National library of medicine National Institutes of Health; IRCCS National Neurological Institute C.; Mondino Foundation and University of Pavia. 02.2013.

Greed F., Guthrie E., Fink P. et al. Is there a better term than "medically unexplained symptoms"? J. Psychosom. Res. 2010. V. 68. N. 1. P. 5-8.

Greenberg D. Religion and mental health: a double-edged sword or a life-giving medicine? 2013. V.12. № 1. P.37-38.Sept. Lisbon (Portugal).

Grigoryev A.I. et al. Sposob interaktivnogo lechenija zavisimogo povedenija [Interactive method of treatment of addictive behavior]. Invention patent № 2252038, 2005. 15 p.

Guo X., Zhang X., Guo L. et al. Association between pre-hypertension and cardiovascular outcomes: a systematic review and meta-analysis of prospective studies. Curr. Hypertens. Rep. 2013. Vol. 15, N 6. P. 703–716.

Guovanini E. et al. Framework to measure the progress of societies, OECD Working Paper, 2009.

Gurovich I.Ja. et al. Bremja depressivnyh rasstrojstv v otechestvennyh psihiatricheskih sluzhbah [The burden of depressive disorders in the local mental health services]. *Zhurnal nevrologii i psihiatrii* [Journal of Neurology and Psychiatry], 2010. №2. P. 4-13.

Gurovich I.Ja. Sostojanie psihiatricheskoj sluzhby v Rossii [State of mental health services in Russia]. *Socialnaja i klinicheskaja psihiatrija* [Social and clinical psychiatry], 2012. № 4. P.5.

Gustap N.N. Tehnologicheskaja platforma «Medicina budushhego» kak instrument obespechenija ekonomicheskogo rosta [The technological platform "Medicine of the Future" as a tool for economic growth]. *Fundamentalnye issledovanija* [Basic Research], 2014. № 11, p. 1599-1603.

Haken H. *Sinergetika. Ierarhija neustojchivostej v samoorganizujuschihsja sistemah i ustrojstvah* [Synergetics. The hierarchy of instabilities in self-organizing systems and devices]. M.: Mir, 1985. 419 p.

Hamer M., Batty G. D., Stamatakis E., Kivimaki M. Hypertension Awareness and Psychological Distress. Hypertension. 2010. N 56. P. 547–550.

Handsdak S.G., Paulraj R. Are we doing harm by omission? Addressing religiosity of the mentally ill. *World Psychiatry*. 2013. V.12. № 1. P.36-37.

Hansel A., von Kanel R. Psychosomatic medicine and arterial hypertension - love it or leave it? Ther Umsch. 2012. Vol. 69, N 5. P. 315–323.

Harris J.I., Erbes C.R., Engdahl B.E. et al. The effectiveness of trauma focused spirituality integrated intervention for veterans exposed to trauma. J.I. Harris, C.R. Erbes, B.E. Engdahl et al. *J. ClinPsychol*. 2011. № 67. P. 1-14.

Hillman B. G. et al. Behavioral analysis of NR2C Knockout mouse reveals deficit in acquisition of conditioned fear and working memory. *Neurobiol Learn. Mem.* 2011. N. 95. P. 404-14.

Holdevici I. The use of Ericksonian hypnosis in somatic disorders. I. Holdevici, B. Crăciun. *Procedia – Social and Behavioral Sciences*. 2012. Vol.33. P. 75-79.

Holmes D. Music therapy's breakthrough act. D. Holmes. *The Lancet*. Vol. 11. Issue 6. P. 486-487. 06.2012.

Holzner B., Grisinger J., Efficace F. On the modern computerized options for assessing the quality of life of cancer patients. *Psycho-oncology*. London. 2013.

Houston S. et al Dancing ballet 'can relieve Parkinson's symptoms'. *The Telegraph*. 04.06.2011.

Huang Y., Cai X., Li Y. et al. Prehypertension and the risk of stroke: a meta-analysis. *Neurology*. 2014. Vol. 82, N 13. P. 1153–1161.

Huguelet P., Mandhouj O. Spiritual assessment as part of routine psychiatric evaluation: problems and implications. *World Psychiatry*. 2013. V.12. № 1. P. 32-33.

Iain B. McInnes, Georg Schett. The Pathogenesis of Rheumatoid Arthritis. *N Engl J Med*. 2011; (365): 2205-19.

Ikeda A., Iso H., Kawachi I. et al. Social support and stroke and coronary heart disease: the JPHC study cohorts II. Stroke. 2008. Vol. 39, N 3. P. 768–775.

Ilic N. P01-377. Psychosomatic diseases and depression with general practice physicists. *European Psychiatry*. 2011. Vol. 26, Suppl. 1, P.380.

Inzlicht M. et al. Neural markers of religious conviston. *Psychol. Sci*. 2009. № 20. P. 385-392.

Isachenkova O. Report. XXII World Congress on Psychosomatic Medicine, Lissabon, 12-14 Sept. 2013.

Isaeva E., Ivanova G. Report. XXII World Congress on Psychosomatic Medicine, Lissabon, 12-14 Sept. 2013.

Islamskih radikalov budut lechit [Islamic radicals will be treated]. *Argumenty nedeli* [Arguments of the week]. 2013. № 21 (363). URL: argumenti.ru/talks/n391/259380 (accessed date: 17.01.2014).

Isurina G.L. Integrativnyj podhod v psihoterapii [Integrative approach in psychotherapy]. *Rossijskij psihoterapevticheskij zhurnal* [Russian Journal of Psychotherapy], 2012. № 1-2, p. 9-20.

Ivashkin V.T. *Gastroenterologija: Klinicheskie rekomendacii* [Gastroenterology: Clinical recommendations]. M.: GEOTAR-Medicina, 2009. 208 p.

Jakushev I. *Mentalnaja medicina postkrizisnogo mira. Mentalnaja medicina i sovremennaja paradigma* [Mental Medicine of the Post-Crisis World. Mental Medicine and the Modern Paradigm]. I. Jakushev, P. Sidorov. LAP Lambert Academic Publishing, 2011. 196 p.

James R. Rundell Factors Associated with Depression Treatment-Response in an Outpatient Psychosomatic Medicine Practice: An Exploratory Retrospective Study. *Psychosomatics*. 2012. Vol. 53, Issue 4. P. 387-391.

Jastrebov V.S. et al. Psihicheskoe zdorovye naselenija mira: socialno-ekonomicheskij aspect [Mental health of the world population: the socio-economic aspect]. *Zhurnal nevrologii i psihiatrii* [Journal of Neurology and Psychiatry]. 2012. № 3. P.4-13.

Join K.K. Textbook of Personalized Medicine. Springer, New York. 2009. 419 p.

Jones T. We are the nation of fashion vicitims, and too tight bras and surprized bags are causing the biggest damage. *The Dailymail*. 24.01.2012.

Jung C.G. O psihogeneze shizofrenii [On the psychogenesis of schizophrenia]. *Psihologija Dementia praecox* [Psychology of Dementia praecox]. Minsk: Harvest, 2003. 400 p.

Jung C.G. *Ob otnoshenii analiticheskoj psihologii k pojetiko-hudozhestvennomu tvorchestvu. Fenomen duha v iskusstve i nauke* [On the relation of analytical psychology to poetic and artistic creativity. The phenomenon of the spirit in the arts and sciences]: Transl. from German. Coll. in 19v. - V. 15. M.: Renessans, 1992.

Jung C.G. Otnoshenija mezhdu Ja i Bessoznatelnym [The relationship between I and the unconscious]. C.G. Jung. Collected Works. Psychology of the Unconscious. M.: Kanon, 1994. P. 251.

Jung C.G. Problema dushi sovremennogo cheloveka [The problem of the soul of modern man]. C.G. Jung. *Problemy dushi nashego vremenini* [The problems of the soul of our time]. M.: Publishing Group Progress-Univers, 1994. P. 314.

Jung C.G. *Psihologicheskie tipy* [Psychological Types]. SPb. Juventa; M.: Publishing Group Progress-Univers, 1995. 716 p.

Jung C.G., Neumann E. *Psihoanaliz i iskusstvo* [Psychoanalysis and Art]. M., 1996.

Jung C.G. Psihologija perenosa [Psychology of transfer]. C.G. Jung. Psychology of transfer. Articles. M.: Refl-book.; Kiev. Vakler, 1997. P. 187.

Jung C.G. Sovremennyj mif o «nebesnyh znamenijah» [The contemporary myth of the "heavenly signs"]. C.G. Jung contemporary myths. M.: Praktika, 1994. P. 55, 171, 173.

Jung C.G. *Sovremennyj vzgljad na shizofreniju* [The modern view of schizophrenia]. Psihologija Dementia praecox [Psychology of Dementia praecox]. C.G. Jung. Minsk: Harvest, 2003. 400 p.

Jurevich A.V., Ushakov D.V. Nravstvennoe sostojanie sovremennogo rossijskogo obshhestva [Moral state of the modern Russian society]. *Psihologija nravstvennosti* [Psychology of morality]. Ed. A.L. Zhuravlev, A.V. Jurevich. M.: *Institut psihologii RAN* [RAS Institute of Psychology], 2010. P. 177–208.

Juryev A.I. Posleslovie recenzenta [Afterword of a reviewer]. Reshetnikov M.M. Psihologicheskie faktory razvitija i stagnacii demokraticheskih reform [Psychological factors of development and stagnation of democratic reforms]. SPb. 2013. P. 241–259.

Kampinskij A. *Psihologija shizofrenii* [Psychology of schizophrenia]. SPb. 1998.

Kara-Murza S.G. *Anomija v Rossii: prichiny i projavlenija* [Anomie in Russia: causes and manifestations]. M.: Nauchnyj ekspert [Scientific Expert], 2013. 264 p.

Karateev D.E. Novoe napravlenie v patogeneticheskoj terapii revmatoidnogo artrita: pervyj ingibitor Janus-kinaz tofacitinib [A new direction in pathogenetic therapy of rheumatoid arthritis: the first inhibitor of Janus-kinase tofacitinib]. *Sovremennaja revmatologija* [Modern Rheumatology], 2014; (1): 39-44.

Karpov Ju.A. Novye rekomendacii po arterialnoj gipertenzii [New recommendations on arterial hypertension]. *RMOAG/VNOK* [RMSAH/SCRF] 2010. Voprosy kombinirovannoj terapii [Issues of combination therapy]. *Russkij medicinskij zhurnal* [Russian Medical Journal], 2010. №22. P.1290.

Katkov A.L. *Integrativnaja psihoterapija* [Integrative Psychotherapy]. SPb. Publ. Mezhdunarodnyj institut socialnoj psihoterapii [Publishing House of the International Institute of Social psychotherapy], 2013. 300 p.

Katkov A.L. Normy I etika v professionalnoj psihoterapii [Standards and ethics in professional psychotherapy]. *Psihoterapija* [Psychotherapy], 2014. № 6. P. 2-12.

Kazakovcev B.A., Demcheva N.K., Jazdovskaja A.V. Obespechennost psihiatricheskih sluzhb specialistami s nemedicinskim obrazovaniem [The provision of mental health services with experts with non-medical education]. *Psihicheskoe zdorovye* [Mental Health], 2015. № 23, p. 11-19.

Kekow J., Moots R., Khandker R. et al. Improvements in patient- reported outcomes, symptoms of depression and anxiety, and their association with clinical remission among patients with moderate-to-severe active early rheumatoid arthritis. *Rheumatology*. 2011; (50): 401–9.

Kenny P.J., Johnson P.M. Shows Compulsive Eating Shares Same Addictive Biochemical Mechanism with Cocaine, Heroin Abuse. The Scrips Research Institute (SRI); News Release Scropps Research Study. 23.03.2010.

Kissane D., Doolittle M. Depression and demoralization. *Psycho-oncology*. London. 2013.

Kocjubinskij A.P. et al. Holisticheskij diagnosticheskij podhod v psihiatrii [Holistic diagnostic approach in psychiatry]. *Socialnaja i klinicheskaja psihiatrija* [Social and clinical psychiatry], 2014. V. 24. № 1. P. 65-69.

Koenig H.G. Schizophrenia and other psychotic disorders. In: Peteet J.R., Lu F.G., Narrow W.E. (eds). Religious and spiritual issues in psychiatric diagnosis: a research agenda for DSM-V. Arlington: American Psychiatric Association. 2011. P. 31-51.

Komaki I. et al. Report. XXII World Congress on Psychosomatic Medicine, Lisbon, 12-14.09.2013.

Körber S., Frieser D., Steinbrecher N., Hiller W. Classification characteristics of the Patient Health Questionnaire-15 for screening somatoform disorders in a primary care setting. *Journal of Psychosomatic Research*. 2011. Vol. 71, Issue 3. P. 142-147.

Kovalchuk M.V. Konvergencija nauk i tehnologij – proryv v budushhee [Convergence of Science and Technology - a breakthrough in the future]. *Rossijskie nanotehnologii* [Russian Nanotechnologies], 2011. № 12. P. 13–23.

Krasnov V.N. Napravlenija razvitija nauchnoj i prakticheskoj psihiatrii: rashozhdenija i vzaimosvjazi [Fields of science and practice of psychiatry: differences and relationships]. V.N. Krasnov. *Socialnaja i klinicheskaja psihiatrija* [Social and clinical psychiatry], 2008. № 1. P. 5-7.

Kravchenko S. A. «Normalnaja anomija»: kontury koncepcii ["Normal anomie": the contours of the concept]. *Sociologicheskie issledovanija* [Sociological researches], 2014. № 8. P. 3-10.

Kretschmer E. Geniale menschen. Berlin-Gottingen: Heidelberg Springer, 1958.

Kross E., Berman M.G., Mischel W. et al. Social rejection shares somatosensory representations with physical pain. Proceedings of the National Academy of Sciences. 22.02.2011.

Kuprejchenko A.B., Vorobyeva A.E. Psihologicheskie tipy nravstvennogo samoopredelenija rossijskoj molodezhi [Psychological types of moral self-determination of the Russian youth]. *Psihologija nravstvennosti* [Psychology of Morality]. Ed. A.L. Zhuravleva, A.V. Jurevich. M.: *Institut psihologii RAN* [RAS Institute of Psychology], 2010. P. 237–260.

Kurpatov V.I. Integrativnaja psihoterapija v psihosomaticheskoj medicine [Integrative Psychotherapy in psychosomatic medicine]. V.I. Kurpatov, A.N. Erichev, G.A. Ivanova et al. *Psihosomaticheskaja medicina – 2008: Sbornik materialov. III Mezhdunarodnyj congress* [Psychosomatic Medicine - 2008: Proceedings. III International Congress]. SPb. Chelovek. P. 14-17.

Lauks G., Mjoller H. Ju. *Psihiatrija i psihoterapija: Spravochnik* [Psychiatry and Psychotherapy: Handbook]. Transl. from German. Ed. Acad. P.I. Sidorov. M.: MEDpress-inform, 2010. 510 p.

Lee I-M., Shiroma E.J., Lobelo F. et al. Effect of physical inactivity on major non-communicable diseases worldwide: an analysis of burden of disease and life expectancy. *The Lancet*. 2012. Vol. 380. Issue 9838. P. 219-229.

Leentjens A.F.G. Reprint of: Psychosomatic medicine and consultation-liaison psychiatry: Scope of practice, processes, and competencies for psychiatrists working in the field of CL psychiatry or psychosomatics. A consensus statement of the European Association of Consultation-Liaison Psychiatry and Psychosomatics (EACLPP) and the Academy of Psychosomatic Medicine (APM). A.F.G. Leentjens, J.R. Rundell, D.L. Wolcott et al. *Journal of Psychosomatic Research*. 2011. Vol. 70, Issue 5. P. 486-491.

Leonov V. *Osnovy pravoslavnoj antropologii* [Fundamentals of Orthodox anthropology]. M.: Publishing House of the Russian Orthodox Church of the Moscow Patriarchate, 2013. 456 p.

Leproult R. Effect of 1 week of sleep restriction on testosterone levels in young healthy men. R. Leproult, V.E. Canter. *The Journal of the American Medical Association*. 2011. V. 305(21): 2173.

Leuner B. Sexual experience promotes adult neurogenesis in the hippocampus despite an initial elevation n stress hormones. B. Leuner, E.R. Glasper, E. Gould. PLoSONE. 14.07.2010.

Levin T. Psychooncology—the state of its development in 2006. Detailed abstract. T. Levin, W.D. Kissane. *Mental Disorders in General Medicine*. 2007. Vol.3. P. 59-65.

Levy-Bruhl L. Les fonctious mentales daus les societes inferieures. 1910.

Lichnostnye i psihicheskie rasstrojstva u patsientov s arterialnoj gipertenziej (obzor literatury) [Personality and psychiatric disorders in patients with hypertension (review)]. B.A. Volel, E.S. Ternovaja, A.A. Ermusheva, E.A. Syrkina. *Psihicheskie rasstrojstva v obschej medicine* [Mental disorders in general medicine], 2013. № 4. P. 23-29.

Lifintsev D.V., Seryh A.B., Lifintseva A.A. Socialnaja podderzhka kak psihologicheskij fenomen [Social support as a psychological phenomenon]. *Voprosy psihologii* [Questions of Psychology], 2014. № 5. P. 105-117.

Linde N.D. *Sutra o shizofrenii. Psihoterapija* [Sutra about schizophrenia. Psychotherapy], 2014. (6): 82-89.

Linden M. et al. Report. XXII World Congress on Psychosomatic Medicine, Lisbon, 12-14 Sept. 2013.

Lisitsyn Ju.P., Sidorov P.I. *Alkogolizm. Mediko-socialnye aspekty* [Alcoholism. Medical and social aspects]. M.: Medicina, 1990. P. 453.

Lisitsyna T.A., Veltishhev D.Ju., Nasonov E.L. *Stressovye faktory i depressivnye rasstrojstva pri revmaticheskih zabolevanijah. Nauchno-prakticheskaja revmatologija* [Stress factors and depressive disorders in rheumatic diseases. Scientific-practical rheumatology], 2013; (2): 98–103.

Ljejard R. *Schastye: uroki novoj nauki* [Happiness: Lessons from a new science]. M.: Publishing House of Gaidar Institute, 2011.

Ljuban-Plocca B. *Psihosomaticheskie rasstrojstva v obschej medicinskoj praktike* [Psychosomatic disorders in general practice]. B. Ljuban-Plocca, V. Peldinger, F. Kreger. SPb. Psychoneurological Institute. named after V.M. Bekhterev, 2000. 288 p.

Macrae F. Taking your brain for a walk. *The New York Times*. 07.02.2011.

Mahovskaja O.I., Marchenko F.O. Formirovanie u doshkolnikov solidarnyh ustanovok sredstvami televidenija [Formation in preschoolers of solidarity by means of TV]. *Psihologija nravstvennosti* [Psychology of Morality]. Ed. A.L. Zhuravleva, A.V. Jurevich. M.: Institut psihologii RAN [RAS Institute of Psychology], 2010. P. 439–459.

Maj M. (October 2008). «The WPA Action. Plan 2008-2011." M. Maj . *Word Psychiatry*. № 7 (3). P. 129.

Maj M. Adherence to psychiatric treatments and the public image of psychiatry. *World Psychiatry*. 2013. Vol. 12. N 3. P. 177-178.

Makarov V.V. *Ekspedicii dushi: psihoterapija, duhovnost* [Expeditions of the soul: psychotherapy and spirituality]. V.V. Makarov, G.A. Makarov. M.: Academic Project, 2012. 305 p.

Makarova G.A. Sindrom emocionalnogo sgoranija [Syndrome of emotional burnout]. *Psihoterapija* [Psychotherapy], 2003. №11. P. 18-20.

Makolkin V.I. *Vnutrennie bolezni* [Internal diseases]. V.I. Makolkin, S.I. Ovcharenko, V.A. Sulimov. M.: GEOTAR-Media, 2011. 768 p.

Malfertheiner P. European Helicobacter Study, Group. Management of Helicobacter pylori infection - the Maastricht IV. P. Malfertheiner, F. Megraud, C.A. O'Morain et al. Florence Consensus Report. 2012. Gut 61 (5). – P. 646-664.

Mann S. J. Psychosomatic research in hypertension: the lack of impact of decades of research and new directions to consider. *J. Clin. Hypertens*. 2012. Vol. 10, N 4. P. 657–664.

Margaretten M., Julian L., Katz P., Yelin E. Depression in patients with rheumatoid arthritis: description, causes and mechanisms. *Int J Clin Rheumtol*. 2011; 6 (6): 617–23.

Marilov V.V. *Psihosomatozy: Psihosomaticheskie zabolevanija zheludochno-kishechnogo trakta: Monografija* [Psychosomatoses: Psychosomatic diseases of the gastrointestinal tract: Monograph]. M.: Miklosh, 2010. 154 p.

Mark T.L. et al. Data points: psychotropic drug prescriptions by medical specialty. Psychiatr. Serv. 2009. 1167 p.

Martens U. Motivation for Psychotherapy in Patients with Functional Gastrointestinal Disorders. U. Martens, P. Enck, A. Matheis et al. *Psychosomatics*. 2010. Vol. 51, Issue 3. P. 225-229.

Medvedev V.A. Terror kak osnovanie kommunikativnoj kultury XXI veka: ot ponimanija k interpretacii [Terror as the basis of communicative culture of the XXI century: from understanding to interpreting]. *Psihologija i psihopatologija terrorizma. Gumanitarnye strategii antiterrora* [Psychology and Psychopathology of Terrorism. Humanitarian anti-terror strategies]. Coll. ed. M. M. Reshetnikov. SPb. 2004. P. 102–130.

Medvedev V.Je. Lichnost patsienta kak faktor zabolevaemosti ishemicheskoj boleznyu serdtsa [The personality of the patient as a factor in the incidence of ischemic heart disease]. *Kardiologija i serdechno-sosudistaja hirurgija* [Cardiology and Cardiovascular Surgery], 2010. V.3. №5. P. 18-23.

Mendelevich V.D. *Psihiatricheskaja propedevtika. 5-e izd* [Psychiatric propaedeutics. 5th ed]. M.: GEOTAR-Media, 2014. 570 p.

Merlin V.S. *Ocherk integralnogo issledovanija individualnosti* [Outline of the integrated research of individuality]. M.: Pedagogika, 1986.

Merton R. Socialnaja teorija i socialnaja struktura [Social Theory and Social Structure]. *Sociologicheskie issledovanija* [Sociological researches], 1992. № 2. P. 10-18.

Miller G. Music Builds Bridges in the Brain. *Journal Science NOW*. 16.04.2008

Mironenko I.A. Problema nravstvennosti v sovremennoj rossijskoj psihologii [The problem of morality in contemporary Russian psychology]. *Psihologija nravstvennosti* [Psychology of Morality]. Ed. A.L. Zhuravlev, A.V. Jurevich. M.: *Institut psihologii RAN* [RAS Institute of Psychology], 2010. P. 15–28.

Mjasnikova L.K. Recenzija na knigu «Psihoonkologija» [Review of the book "Psycho-oncology"]. *Psihicheskie rasstrojstva v obshhej medicine* [Mental disorders in general medicine], 2013. № 3. P. 68-72.

Mjej R. *Iskusstvo psihologicheskogo konsultirovanija* [The art of psychological counseling]. M.: Klass, 1994. 144 p.

Mohr D.C., Lovers J., Brown T. et al. A randomized trial of stress management for the prevention of new brain lesions in MS. *Neurology*. 11.07.2012.

Möller-Levet C.S., Archer S.N, Bucca G. et al. Effects of insufficient sleep on circadian rhythmicity and expression amplitude of the human blood transcriptome. Proceedings of the National Academy of Sciences. 23.01.13.

Moreno C., Nuevo R., Chatterji S. et al. Psihoticheskie simptomy imejut polozhitelnuju svjaz s somaticheskimi zabolevanijami nezavisimo ot nalichija diagnoza psihoticheskogo rasstrojstva: rezultaty issledovanija VOZ World Health Survey (Vsemirnoe issledovanie zdorovya) [Psychotic symptoms have a positive relationship with somatic diseases regardless of a diagnosis of a psychotic disorder: results of the WHO World Health Survey]. *Vsemirnaja psihiatrija* [World Psychiatry], 2013. № 12. P. 251-257.

Moriera-Almeida A. Religion and health: the more we know the more we need to know. World Psychiatry. 2013. V.12. № 1. P. 34-35.

Moshhelkov E.N. et al. Sovremennyj terrorizm: prichiny, suschnost, principy postroenija gumanitarnyh modelej protivodejstvija [Modern terrorism: the causes, nature, principles of human models to counter]. *Sovremennyj terrorizm i borba s nim: socialno-gumanitarnye izmerenija* [Modern terrorism and the fight against it: social and humanitarian dimensions]. S.A. Afonin et al. Ed. V.V. Jashhenko. M.: MCCME, 2007. P. 19–26.

Murray P.S. Locus coeruleus galanin expression is enhanced after exercise in rats selectively bred for high capacity for aerobic activity. P.S. Murray, J.L. Groves, B.J. Pettett et al. *Peptides*. 2010. V. 31. N. 12. P.2264-2268.

Nanni M. et al. Report. XXII World Congress on Psychosomatic Medicine, Lisbon, 12-14 Sept. 2013.

Nasonov E.L., Karateev D.E., Chichasova N.V. Novye rekomendacii po lecheniju revmatoidnogo artrita (EULAR, 2013): mesto metotreksata [New recommendations for the treatment of rheumatoid arthritis]. *Nauchno-prakticheskaja revmatologija* [Scientific and practical rheumatology], 2014; (1): 8-26.

Nazaretjan A.P. *Civilizacionnye krizisy v kontekste Universalnoj istorii*. 2-e izd [Civilization crises in the context of universal history. 2nd ed]. M.: Mir, 2004. 367 p.

Nazaretjan A.P. Psihologicheskie issledovanija duhovno-nravstvennyh problem [Psychological studies of spiritual and moral issues]. Ed. A.L. Zhuravlev, A.V. Jurevich. M.: Publishing House of the "Academy of Sciences Institute of Psychology," 2011. P. 428, 432.

Nazlojan G.M. *Maskoterapija* [Mask therapy]. Simferopol: Di Aj Pi, 2005. 341 p.

Nehorosheva I.V. Uroven schastya ljudej s razlichnoj nravstvennoj napravlennostyu [The level of happiness of people with different moral orientation]. *Voprosy psihologii* [Questions of psychology], 2013. № 3. P. 22-31.

Nikolaev Ju.A. Distantsionnye informatsionnye vzaimodejstvija u bakterij [Remote informational interactions in bacteria]. *Biohimija* [Biochemistry], 2000. № 5.

Novák M. Psychosomatic medicine and consultation-liaison psychiatry in Hungary. M. Novák, G. Gazdag, F. Túry. *Journal of Psychosomatic Research*. 2009. Vol. 66, Issue 2. P.187-188.

Nuevo R., Chatterji S., Verdes E. et al. The continuum of psychotic symptoms in the general population: a cross-national study. *Schizophr Bull*. 2012. N 38. P. 475-85.

Nuller Ju. L. Smena paradigm v psihiatrii? [Paradigm shift in psychiatry?]. *Psihiatrija i psihofarmakoterapija* [Psychiatry and psychopharmacotherapy], 2008. V. 9, №5. P. 4-7.

Oganesjan N.Ju. Tancevalnaja psihoterapija bolnyh psihosomaticheskimi zabolevanijami [Dance therapy of patients with psychosomatic diseases]. N.Ju. Oganesjan, D.V. Ilyina. *Uchenye zapiski Sankt-Peterburgskogo gosudarstvennogo medicinskogo universiteta im. akad. I.P. Pavlova* [Scientific notes of the St. Petersburg State Medical University. named after Acad. I.P. Pavlov], 2010. V.XVII, №2 (app.). P. 101-102.

Oganov R.G., Maslennikova G.Ja. Profilaktika serdechno-sosudistyh zabolevanij - realnyj put uluchshenija demograficheskoj situacii v Rossii [Prevention of cardiovascular disease - the real way to improve the demographic situation in Russia]. *Kardiologija* [Cardiology], 2007. №1. P. 4-7.

Onkologija. Nacionalnoe rukovodstvo [Oncology. National Handbook]. Ed. Chissov V.I., Davydov M.I. M.: GEOTAR-Media, 2014. 576 p.

Orlova E.V., Denisov L.N., Arsenyev A.O., Karateev D.E. Otsenka priverzhennosti bolnyh revmatoidnym artritom farmakologicheskim i nemedikamentoznym metodam lechenija i ee dinamika pod vlijaniem obrazovatelnoĭ programmy [Evaluation of patients with rheumatoid arthritis in commitment to pharmacological and non-drug therapies and its dynamics under the influence of the educational program]. *Nauchno-prakticheskaja revmatologija* [Scientific-practical rheumatology]. 2012; (3): 68-74.

Ortega-i-Gasset H. *Vokrug Galileja (shema krizisov)* [Around Galileo (Crises scheme)]. H. Ortega-i-Gasset. Selected works. M., 1997. 322 p.

Ovchinnikov B.V. et al. *Psihicheskaja predpatologija* [Psychic pre-pathology]. SPb.: ELBI-SPb, 2010. 368 p.

Ozhirenie i izbytochnyj ves [Obesity and overweight]. Informacionnyj bjulleten VOZ [WHO Information Bulletin], 2014. №311. 22 p.

Parsons T. *O socialnyh sistemah* [About social systems]. M.: Academic Project, 2002. 832 p.

Pedak A.A. *Psihicheskie i psihosomaticheskie rasstrojstva v klinike vracha obshhej praktiki – semejnoj mediciny* [Mental and psychosomatic disorders in the clinic of a general practitioner - family medicine]. M.: MedBooks, 2011. 696 p.

Perez A., Fleury J., Shearer N. Salud de Corazon: Cultural Resources for Cardiovascular Health among Older Hispanic Women. *Hisp Health Care Int*. 2012. Vol. 10. №2. P.93–100.

Pergament K.I., Lomax J.W. Understanding and addressing religion among people with mental illness. K.I. Pergament, J.W. Lomax. *World Psychiatry*. 2013. V.12. № 1. P.23-29.

Perinatalnaja psihologija i psihiatrija: V 2 t [Perinatal Psychology and Psychiatry: In 2 v.]. Ed. N.N. Volodin, P.I. Sidorov. M.: Akademija, 2009. V.1. 300 P.; V.2. 251 p.

Perroud N. Religion/spirituality and neuropsychiatry. Perroud N.; In: Huguelet P., Koenig H.G. (eds). Religion and spirituality in psychiatry. Cambridge: Cambridge University Press, 2009. P.48-64.

Pilevina Ju.V. *Psihosomaticheskie osobennosti i komplaentnost u pacientov hronicheskoj serdechnoj nedostatochnostju: avtoreferat* [Psychosomatic features and compliance in patients with chronic heart failure: the author's thesis]. SPb., 2012. 22 p.

Pitceathly C., Watson M., Cawthorn A. Counseling and specific psychological treatment. *Psycho-oncology*. London. 2013.

Piven B.N. Novaja sut ili tolko novye nazvanija? [New meaning or just new names?]. *Zhurnal nevrologii i psihiatrii* [Journal of Neurology and Psychiatry], 2014. № 5. P. 104-107.

Plahov V.D. *Norma i otklonenie v obshhestve. Filosofsko-teoreticheskoe vvedenie v socialnuju etologiju* [Norm and deviation in society. Philosophical and theoretical introduction to the social ethology]. SPb. Publishing House of the Institute of Law, 2011. P. 52.

Popov L.M., Maksumova A.O. Tipologija ljudej v eticheskoj psihologii lichnosti [Typology of people in an ethical personality psychology]. *Psihologija nravstvennosti* [Psychology of Morality]. Ed. A.L. Zhuravlev, A. V. Jurevich. M.: *Institut psihologii RAN* [RAS Institute of Psychology], 2010. P. 95–115.

Popova S.M., Shahraj S.M., Janin A.A. *Izmerenija progressa* [Measuring progress]. M.: *Nauka* [Science], 2010.

Poppito S., Tait G. The organization of training for oncologists and palliative care physicians. *Psycho-oncology*. London. 2013.

Porter R. *Kratkaja istorija bezumija* [Brief History of Madness]. M.: AST-Astrel, 2008. 224 p.

Powell-Wiley T.M., Banks-Richard K., Williams-King E. et al. Churches as targets for cardiovascular disease prevention: comparison of genes, nutrition, exercise, wellness and spiritual growth (GoodNEWS) and Dallas County populations. *J. Public. Health* (Oxf). 2013. Vol.35. №1. P. 99–106.

Psychooncology. Editors: Wise T. et al. London, 2013.

Pushkina M.A. Vlijanie SMI na formirovanie patologij massovogo soznanija [Influence of media on the formation of pathologies of mass conscience]. *Psihoterapija* [Psychotherapy], 2014. № 12. P. 63.

Rafanelli C. Psychological correlates in patients with different levels of hypertension. C. Rafanelli, E. Offidani, S. Gostoli, R. Roncuzzi. *Psychiatry Research*. 2012. Vol. 198, Issue 1. P. 154-160.

Rajh O.I. *Tip lichnosti D u bolnyh s aterosklerozom razlichnoj lokalizacii: rasprostranennost, vlijanie na kachestvo zhizni: avtoreferat* [Type D personality in patients with atherosclerosis of various localization: prevalence, impact on quality of life: the author's thesis]. Kemerovo, 2012. 24 p.

Rakitjanskij N.M. Kategorija mentaliteta v prostranstve psihologii very [Category of mentality in faith psychology space]. *Vestnik SPbGU* [SPbGU Bulletin], 2009. Ser. 12. № 4. P. 205–210.

Reshetnikov M.M. *Psihologicheskie faktory razvitija i stagnacii demograficheskih reform* [Psychological factors of development and stagnation of democratic reforms]. SPb. 2013. 260 p.

Reshetnikov M.M. Vozmozhen li kontrol mentalnoj evoljucii cheloveka, chtoby sdelat ego ustojchivym protiv psihozov zhestokosti i razrushenija? Perepiska Z. Frejda s A. Einshtejnom [Is it possible to control the mental evolution of man, to make him resistant against the psychoses of violence and destruction? Correspondence of Z. Freud to A. Einstein]. *Psihoterapija* [Psychotherapy], 2014. № 7. P. 2-8.

Ribeiro A. et al. Report. XXII World Congress on Psychosomatic Medicine, Lisbon, 12-14 Sept. 2013.

Rome K., Frecklington M., Mcnair P. et al. Footwear characteristics and factors influencing footwear choice in patients with gout. *Arthritis Care & Research*. 2011. Vol. 63. Issue 11. P. 1599-1604.

Rosari A. et al. Report. XXII World Congress on Psychosomatic Medicine, Lisbon, 12-14 Sept. 2013.

Rosmarin D.H., Pargament K., Piroutinsky S. et al. A randomized controlled evaluation of spirituality integrated treatment for subclinical anxiety in the Jewish community, delivered via the Internetn. D.H. Rosmarin, K. Pargament, S. Piroutinsky et al. *J Anxiety Disord*. 2010. № 24. P. 799-808.

Rozenberg G.S. *Holizm + redukcionizm: dve dorogi k hramu* [Holism + reductionism: two roads to the temple]. Vestnik RAN [RAS Bulletin]. 2014. V. 84. № 9. P. 830-833.

Saharnyj diabet: ostrye i hronicheskie oslozhnenija [Diabetes: acute and chronic complications]. Ed. I.I. Dedov, M.V. Shestakova. M.: MIA, 2011. 380 p.

Sanina A.G. Genezis idei identichnosti v sociologii i smezhnyh naukah [Genesis of the idea of identity in sociology and related sciences]. *Sociologicheskie issledovanija* [Sociological researches]. 2014. № 12. P. 3-.

Sartorius N., Schulze H. Reducing the stigma of mental illness. Cambridge University press. 2005. 238 p.

Schneider A. Joachim Szecsenyi Depression and panic disorder as predictors of health outcomes for patients with asthma in primary care. A. Schneider, B. Löwe, F. Joachim Meyer et al. *Respiratory Medicine*. 2008. Vol.102, Issue 3. P. 359-366.

Schneider K. Clinical psychopathology. New York: Grune and Stratton. 1959.

Schröder A., Fink P. Functional Somatic Syndromes and Somatoform Disorders in Special Psychosomatic Units: Organizational Aspects and Evidence-Based Treatment. A. Schröder, P. Fink. Psychiatric Clinics of North America. 2011. Vol. 34, Issue 3. P. 673-687.

Schröder H. et al. Kompetenzals Zielgrössefür Persönlichkeitsstructer und Verhaltensmodofocation. M. Vorwerg (Hrsg.) Probleme der Persoulichkeitsforschung. Leipzig, 1978.

Schulte I.E., Petermann F. Somatoform disorders: 30 years of debate about criteria: What about children and adolescents? I.E.,Schulte, F. Petermann. *Journal of Psychosomatic Research*. 2011. Vol.70. Issue 3. P. 218-228.

Scott D., Wolfe F., Huizinga T. Rheumatoid arthritis. *Lancet*. 2010; 376(9746):1094-1108.

Seligman M. *Put k procvetaniju: novoe ponimanie schastya i blagopoluchija* [Path to Prosperity: a new understanding of happiness and well-being]. M.: Mann, Ivanov i Ferber, 2013.

Semenov V.E. Budushhee Rossii v kontekste rossijskoj polimentalnosti [Russia's future in the context of Russian polymentality]. *Vestnik SPbGU* [SPbGU Bulletin]. 2009. Ser. 12. № 3, part. 1. P. 153–165.

Semenov V.E. Duhovno-nravstvennye cennosti i vospitanie kak vazhnejshie uslovija razvitija Rossii [Spiritual and moral values and education as the most important conditions for the development of Russia]. *Psihologicheskie issledovanija duhovno-nravstvennyh problem* [Psychological studies of spiritual and moral issues]. Ed. A.L. Zhuravlev, A.V. Jurevich. M.: *Institut psihologii RAN* [RAS Institute of Psychology], 2011. P. 60–70.

Sergeev S.F. Psihologicheskie aspekty problemy interfejsa v tehnogennom mire [Psychological aspects of the interface in technogenic world]. *Psihologicheskij zhurnal* [Psychological Journal], 2014. V. 35. № 5. P. 88-98.

Sharpe L. Psychological Treatment for Rheumatoid Arthritis Works: Now We Need to Know What Elements Are Most Effective and for Whom. *J Rheumatol*. 2013; 40(11):1788-90.

Shenoi S.D. Role of cultural factors in the biopsychosocial model of psychosomatic skin diseases: an Indian perspective. S.D. Shenoi, S. Prabhu. *Clinics in Dermatology*. 2013. Vol. 31, Issue 1. P. 62-65.

Shhigolev I.I. *Psihicheskie epidemii v Rossii* [Mental epidemics in Russia]. Brjansk. BSU Publ., 2001. P. 3-13.

Sidorov P. I. Sistemnyj sintez mentalnoj mediciny [System synthesis of mental medicine]. *Ekologija cheloveka* [Human ecology]. 2013. № 10. P. 37–48.

Sidorov P., Novikova I. Strategy for occupational burnout prevetion among physicians. *Occupational Health and Safety*. 2011. Vol. 14, N 3. P. 72–75.

Sidorov P.I. Destruktivnyj professiogenez v onkologii [Destructive professiogenesis in oncology]. P.I. Sidorov, A.V. Krasilnikov, I.A. Novikova, A.A. Kuznecova. *Ekologija cheloveka* [Human ecology]. 2009. №5. P. 16-24.

Sidorov P.I. Duhovno-nravstvennye resursy psihiatrii i mentalnoj mediciny [Spiritual and moral resources of psychiatry and mental medicine]. *Psihicheskoe zdorovye* [Mental health]. 2014. № 6. P. 22-39.

Sidorov P.I. Ekologija mentalnyh epidemij [Ecology of mental epidemics]. *Ekologija cheloveka* [Human ecology]. 2015. № 6. P. 36-50.

Sidorov P.I. From bullying to pandemy of terrorism: synergetic biopsychosociospiritual methodology of mental health protection. Handbook on Bullying: Prevalence, Psychological impacts and intervention Strategies. NY: NOVA Science Publishers, 2014. P. 177-214.

Sidorov P.I. From mental epidemics to terrorism pandemic: synergetic biopsychosociospiritual methodology of public conscience protection. Handbook «Focus on Terrorism." NY: NOVA Science Publishers, 2015. P. 182-221.

Sidorov P.I. Mehanizmy socialnyh epidemij i sinergetika effektivnogo otveta [Mechanisms of social epidemics and synergetics of effective response]. *Psihicheskoe zdorovye* [Mental Health]. 2014. № 5. P. 32-44.

Sidorov P.I. Mental terrorism of Hibrid Wars and Defense Synergetics. Handbook Surveillance Systems and National Security of the 21s Century: New Developments. NY: NOVA Science Pablishers, 2015. P. 200-237.

Sidorov P.I. *Mentalnaja medicina: metodologija i praktika* [Mental Medicine: methodology and practice]. P.I. Sidorov, I.A. Novikova. LAP Lambert Academic Publishing, 2012. 692 p.

Sidorov P.I. *Mentalnaja medicina: Rukovodstvo* [Mental Health: Handbook]. P.I.Sidorov, I.A. Novikova. M.: GEOTAR-Media. 2014. 728 p.

Sidorov P.I. *Narkologicheskaja preventologija. 2-e izd* [Narcological preventology. 2nd ed.]. M.: MEDpress-inform, 2006. 820 .

Sidorov P.I. Pandemija terrorizma i sinergetika zashhity [Pandemic of terrorism and defense synergetics]. *Psihicheskoe zdorovye* [Mental Health]. 2014. № 2. P. 31-40.

Sidorov P.I. Psihicheskij terrorizm – neletalnoe oruzhie massovogo porazhenija [Psychic terrorism - non-lethal weapons of mass destruction]. *Rossijskij psihiatricheskij zhurnal* [Russian Journal of Psychiatry]. 2005. № 3. P. 28–34.

Sidorov P.I. *Psihologija katastrof* [Disaster Psychology]. P.I. Sidorov, I.G. Mosjagin, S.V. Marunjak. Aspekt-Press, 2008. 415 p.

Sidorov P.I. *Psihosomaticheskaja medicina: Rukovodstvo dlja vrachej* [Psychosomatic medicine: Handbook for general practitioners]. P.I. Sidorov, A.G. Solovyev, I.A. Novikova. Ed. acad. P.I. Sidorov. M.: MEDpress-inform, 2006. 568 p.

Sidorov P.I. Resursy i napravlenija mentalnoj preventologii [Resources and direction of mental preventology]. *Ekologija cheloveka* [Human ecology]. 2014. № 10. P. 31-43.

Sidorov P.I. Sanogeneticheskaja terapija zavisimogo povedenija [Sanogenetic dependent behavior therapy]. P.I. Sidorov, T.V. Cyganok, K.V. Shelygin, V.V. Sinickij. *Narkologija* [Narcology]. 2008. № 1. P.13-21.

Sidorov P.I. *Seksualnyj menedzhment* [Sexual management]. P.I. Sidorov, G.B. Derjagin, I.A.Konopleva. Arhangelsk: Publ. NSMU, 2009. 488 p.

Sidorov P.I. Sinergeticheskaja koncepcija zavisimogo povedenija [Synergetic concept of addictive behavior]. *Ekologija cheloveka* [Human ecology]. 2005. №10. P. 27–32.

Sidorov P.I. Sinergeticheskaja paradigma shizofrenii [Synergetic paradigm of schizophrenia]. *Psihicheskoe zdorovye* [Mental health]. 2014. № 8. P. 19-34.

Sidorov P.I. Sinergetika sluzhby mentalnogo zdorovya [Synergetics of mental health service]. *Psihicheskoe zdorovye* [Mental health]. 2015. № 1. S. 14-27.

Sidorov P.I. Sposob ocenki mentalnoj ekologii lichnosti [Method for evaluating mental ecology of the person]. P.I. Sidorov, I.A. Novikova. Patent for invention №2347528 reg. 27.02.2009.

Sidorov P.I. Sposob skriningovoj ocenki faktorov zdorovya [A method of screening evaluation of health factors]. P.I. Sidorov, I.A. Novikova. *Gigiena i sanitarija* [Hygiene and sanitation]. 2010. №2. P. 85-89.

Sidorov P.I., Novikova I.A. Professionalnyj stress i ego posledstvija u medicinskih rabotnikov [Occupational stress and its impact on health care workers]. *Professionalnaja patologija* [Professional pathology]. M.: GEOTAR-Media, 2011. P. 603–614.

Sidorov P.I., Parnjakov A.V. *Klinicheskaja psihologija. 4-e izd* [Clinical Psychology - 4th ed]. M.: GEOTAR-Media, 2010. 880 p.

Sidorov P.I., Putin M.E., Konopleva I.A. *Delovoe obshhenie* [Business communication]. M.: GEOTAR-Media, 2004. 848 p.

Sidorov P.I., Rezvyj G.G., Andersen T. «Otkrytyj dialog» kak novyj etap v evoljucii psihiatricheskoj terapevticheskoj sredy ["Open dialogue" as a new stage in the evolution of psychiatric therapeutic environment]. *Nezavisimyj psihiatricheskij zhurnal* [Independent psychiatric journal]. 2000. № 2.

Sidorov P.I., Sovershaeva E.P. Sinergeticheskaja biopsihosocioduhovnaja koncepcija revmatoidnogo artrita [Synergetic biopsychosociospiritual concept of rheumathoid arthritis]. *Ekologija cheloveka* [Human ecology]. 2014. № 12. P. 34-44.

Sidorov P.I., Sovershaeva E.P. Sinergeticheskaja biopsihosocioduhovnaja koncepcija arterialnoj gipertonii [Synergetic biopsychosociospiritual concept of arterial hypertension]. *Ekologija cheloveka* [Human ecology]. 2015. № 1. P. 49-60.

Sidorov P.I., Sovershaeva E.P. Sinergeticheskaja biopsihosocioduhovnaja koncepcija socialnoj epidemii bronhialnoj astmy [Synergetic biopsychosociospiritual concept of bronchial asthma social epidemic]. *Ekologija cheloveka* [Human ecology]. 2015. № 2. P. 42-50.

Sidorov P.I., Sovershaeva E.P. Sinergeticheskaja biopsihosocioduhovnaja koncepcija socialnoj epidemii jazvennoj bolezni [Synergetic biopsychosociospiritual concept of peptic ulcer social epidemic]. *Ekologija cheloveka* [Human ecology]. 2015. № 3. P. 43-51.

Sidorov P.I., Sovershaeva E.P. Sinergeticheskaja biopsihosocioduhovnaja koncepcija socialnoj epidemii onkologicheskih zabolevanij [Synergetic biopsychosociospiritual concept of oncological diseases social epidemic]. *Ekologija cheloveka* [Human ecology]. 2015. № 4. P. 41-50.

Sidorov P.I., Sovershaeva E.P. Sinergeticheskaja biopsihosocioduhovnaja koncepcija socialnoj epidemii ozhirenija [Synergetic biopsychosociospiritual concept of obesity social epidemic]. *Ekologija cheloveka* [Human ecology]. 2015. № 5. P. 40-51.

Sidorov P.I., Sovershaeva E.P. Sinergeticheskaja biopsihosocioduhovnaja koncepcija mentalnoj epidemii saharnogo diabeta [Synergetic biopsychosociospiritual concept of diabetes mellitus social epidemic]. *Ekologija cheloveka* [Human ecology]. 2015. № 8. P. 38-51.

Sidorov P.I., Sovershaeva E.P. Sinergeticheskaja biopsihosocioduhovnaja koncepcija mentalnoj epidemii ishemicheskoj bolezni serdca [Synergetic biopsychosociospiritual concept of coronary heart disease social epidemic]. *Ekologija cheloveka* [Human ecology]. 2015. № 9. P. 39-48.

Sidorov P.I., Sovershaeva E.P. Sinergeticheskaja biopsihosocioduhovnaja koncepcija mentalnoj epidemii psihosomaticheskih rasstrojstv [Synergetic biopsychosociospiritual concept of psychosomatic disorders social epidemic]. *Ekologija cheloveka* [Human ecology]. 2015. № 10. P. 31-45.

Sidorov P.I., Sovershaeva E.P. Sinergeticheskaja biopsihosocioduhovnaja koncepcija mentalnoj epidemii somatoformnyh rasstrojstv [Synergetic biopsychosociospiritual concept of somatoform disorders social epidemic]. *Ekologija cheloveka* [Human ecology]. 2015. № 11. P. 34-48.

Sidorova T.A. Metodologicheskie voprosy issledovanija normy i normativnosti v biojetike [Methodological issues of rules and regulations research in bioethics]. *Bioetika* [Bioethics]. 2014. № 2. P. 9-12.

Silverman M. et al. The course of anxiety disorders other than PTSD in patients with borderline personality disorder and axis II comparison subjects: a 10-year foiiow-up study. *J Pers Disord*. 2012. P. 804-816.

Skorik A.I. et al. Psihiatricheskaja mifologija i problema sotrudnichestva [Psychiatric mythology and the problem of cooperation]. *Socialnaja i klinicheskaja psihiatrija* [Social and clinical psychiatry]. 2014. № 3. P.31-36.

Smolen J.S., Landewe R., Breedveld F.C. et al. EULAR recommendations for the management of rheumatoid arthritis with synthetic and biological disease-modifying antirheumatic drugs: 2013 update. *Ann Rheum Dis*. 2013; 1-18.

Smulevich A.B. *Psihicheskie rasstrojstva v klinicheskoj praktike* [Mental disorders in clinical practice]. M.: Medpress-inform, 2011. 720 p.

Sosin V.A. *Psihologija sovremennogo terrorizma* [Psychology of modern terrorism]. M.: Forum, 2012. 160 p.

Spitzer C., Wegert S., Wollenhaupt J. et al. Gender-specific association between childhood trauma and rheumatoid arthritis: a case-control study. *J Psychosom Res*. 2013; 74(4): 296-300.

St. Luke [Svjatitel Luka Vojno-Jaseneckij]. *Duh, dusha i telo* [Spirit, soul and body]. M.: Orthodox St. Tikhon Theological Institute, 1997. 54 p.

St. Luke [Svjatitel Luka Vojno-Jaseneckij]. *Nauka i religija* [Science and religion]. Feniks. Orthodox Library "Trinity word," 2001. 320 p.

Starodubov V.I., Sidorov P.I. Konopleva I.A. *Upravlenie personalom organizacii* [Personnel management]. V.I. Starodubov, P.I. Sidorov, I.A. Konopleva. M.: GEOTAR-Media, 2006. 1104 p.

Starodubov V.I., Sidorov P.I. Vasilyeva E. Ju. *Ocenka kachestva obrazovatelnoj sredy* [Assessment of the quality of the educational environment]. M.: GEOTAR-Media, 2013. 464 p.

Starodubov V.I., Sidorov P.I. Vasilyeva E. Ju. *Sistemnyj monitoring obrazovatelnoj sredy* [System monitoring of the educational environment]. M.: GEOTAR-Media, 2013. 304 p.

Starostina E.G., et al. Epidemiologija naibolee chastyh psihicheskih rasstrojstv u bolnyh saharnym diabetom [Epidemiology of the most common mental disorders in diabetic patients]. *Almanah klinicheskoj mediciny* [Almanac of the clinical medicine]. 2014. № 32. P. 17-23.

Steinbrecher N. The prevalence of medically in explained symptoms in primary care. N. Steinbrecher, S. Koerber, D. Frieser et al. *Psychosomatics*. 2011. V. 52. N. 3. P. 263-271.

Stiefel F., Krenz S. Psychological support of dying patients. *Psycho-oncology*. London. 2013.

Stojanovich L. Stress and autoimmunity. *Autoimmunity*. 2010; 9(5): 271–76.

Straub R.H., Kalden J.R. Stress of different types increases the proinflammatory load in rheumatoid arthritis. *Arthritis Research & Therapy*. 2009; 11(3): 114-15.

Strayer D. et al. A walk outdoors away from gadgets can boost brain power by half. *The Dailymail*. 13.12.2012.

Strizhov E.Ju. Psihodiagnostika nravstvennyh determinant moshennichestva [Psychodiagnostics of swindle moral determinants]. *Psihologicheskie issledovanija duhovno-nravstvennyh problem* [Psychological studies of spiritual and moral issues]. Ed. A.L. Zhuravlev, A.V. Jurevich. M.: *Institut psihologii RAN* [RAS Institute of Psychology], 2011. P. 336–354.

Suharev A.V. Etnofunkcionalnyj podhod k profilaktike socialno-nravstvennyh otklonenij [Ethnofunctional approach to the prevention of social and moral deviations]. *Psihologija nravstvennosti* [Psychology of morality]. Ed. A.L. Zhuravlev, A.V. Jurevich. M.: *Institut psihologii RAN* [RAS Institute of Psychology], 2010. P. 401–417.

Szasz T. *Fabrika bezumija* [Manufacture of Madness]. Ekaterinburg: Ultra. Kultura, 2008. 516 p.

Thomec S. et al. Information portal Paininfo.ru. 10.02.2015.

Toshhenko Zh.T. Antinomija – novaja harakteristika obshhestvennogo soznanija v Rossii [Antinomy - a new feature of public conscience in Russia]. *Novye idei v sociologii* [New ideas in sociology]. M.: UNITI-DANA, 2013. P. 339-358.

Troshin V.D., Pogodina T.G. *Terrorizm i nervno-psihicheskie rasstrojstva: diagnostika, lechenie, profilaktika* [Terrorism and neuro-psychiatric disorders: diagnosis, treatment, prevention]. N. Novgorod, 2007. 314 p.

Trunova M.S., Orlov A.B. Metod biologicheskoj obratnoj svjazi: psihoterapevticheskaja perspektiva [Biofeedback: psychotherapeutic perspective]. *Voprosy psihologii* [Questions of psychology]. 2014. № 6. P. 33-43.

Tully P. Report. XXII World Congress on Psychosomatic Medicine, Lisbon, 12-14 Sept. 2013.

Uchiyama M., Jin X., Zhang Q. et al. Auditory stimulation of opera music induced prolongation of murine cardiac allograft survival and maintained generation of regulatory $CD4^+$ $CD25^+$ cells. *Journal of Cardiothoracic Surgery*. 23.03.2012.

Umanskij S.V. Proschenja lozh il iskrennosti mest [Forgiveness of lies or revenge of sicerity]. *Psihoterapija* [Psychotherapy]. 2014. № 3 (135). P. 40-45.

Ushakov I.B., Bogomolov A.V. Informatizacija programm personificirovannoj adaptacionnoj mediciny [Computerization of programs of personalized adaptive medicine]. *Vestnik RAMN* [RAMS Bulletin]. 2014, № 5-6, p. 124-128.

Van der Boom K.J., Van den Hout M.A., Huntjens R.J.C. Psychoform and somatoform dissociation, traumatic experiences, and fantasy proneness in somatoform disorders. *Personality and Individual Differences.* Vol. 48, Issue 4, March 2010, P. 447-451.

Van Praag H.M. *Religiosity*, a personality trait to be reckoned within psychiatry. H.M. Van Praag. *World Psychiatry*. 2013. V.12. № 1. P. 30-31.

Vasserman L.I., Trifonova E.A., Shhelkova O.Ju. *Psihologicheskaja diagnostika i korrekcija v somaticheskoj klinike* [Psychological diagnostics and correction in somatic clinic]. SPb.: Rech, 2011. 271 p.

Vejn A.M., Voznesenskaja T.G., Vorobyeva O.V. *Vegetativnye rasstrojstva: klinika, lechenie, diagnostika. Rukovodstvo dlja vrachej* [Autonomic dysfunctions: clinical features, treatment, diagnosis. Handbook for general practitioners]. M.: *Medicinskoe informacionnoe agentstvo* [Medical Information Agency]. 2010. 640 p.

Verhagen P.J., Cox J.L. Multicultural education and training in religion and spirituality. In: *Religion and Psychiatry. Beyond boundaries*. New York: Wiley, 2010. P.587-613.

Vescovelli F. Report. XXII World Congress on Psychosomatic Medicine, Lisbon, 12-14 Sept. 2013.

Vinokur V.A., Novikova I.A. Sistemnyj analiz processa integracii v psihoterapii [System analysis of the integration process in psychotherapy]. *Ekologija cheloveka* [*Human Ecology*], 2015. № 4, p. 58-64.

Vodopyanova N.E. *Profilaktika i korrekcija sindroma vygoranija: metodologija, teorija, praktika* [Prevention and correction of a burnout syndrome: methodology, theory, practice]. SPb.: SPbGU Publ., 2011. 160 p.

Voigt K. Towards positive diagnostic criteria: a systematic review of somatoform disorder diagnoses and suggestions for future classification. K. Voigt, A. Nagel, B. Meyer et al. *J. Psychosom*. Res. 2010. V. 68. N. 5. P. 403-414.

Volkov V.S., Poseljugina O.B. Essencialnaja arterialnaja gipertonija i arterialnaja gipertonija pri metabolicheskom syndrome [Essential hypertension and hypertension in metabolic syndrome]. *Klinicheskaja medicina* [Clinical Medicine], 2011. №2. P. 64-65.

Volovikova M.I. Duhovno-nravstvennaja reguljacija socialnogo povedenija lichnosti [Spiritual and moral regulation of social behavior of the person]. *Psihologija nravstvennosti* [Morality Psychology]. Ed. A. L. Zhuravleva, A. V. Jurevicha. M.: *Institut psihologii RAN* [RAS Institute of Psychology], 2010. P. 15–28.

Volovikova M.I. K probleme psihologicheskogo issledovanija sovesti [On the problem of psychological research of conscience]. Psihologicheskie issledovanija duhovno-nravstvennyh problem [Psychological studies of spiritual and moral issues]. Ed. A. L. Zhuravlev, A. V. Jurevich. M.: *Institut psihologii RAN* [RAS Institute of Psychology], 2011. P. 71–86.

Voronkov B.V. Razmyshlenija o sushchestve i obshhestvennoj znichimosti konformnosti i konformizma [Reflections on the being and the social significance of conformity and conformism]. *Nezavisimyj psihiatricheskij zhurnal* [Independent Journal of Psychiatry], 2014. № 4. P. 58-61.

Vorontsova L.V., Frolov D.B. *Istorija i sovremennost informacionnogo protivoborstva* [History and modernity of information warfare]. M.: *Gorjachaja linija – Telekom* [Hotline - Telekom], 2006. 192 p.

Voznesenkaja T.G. Rasstrojstva pishhevogo povedenija pri ozhirenii i ih korrekcija [Eating disorders in obesity and its correction]. Farmateka, 2009. №12. – P. 91-94.

War or Health. Foreword by the UN General Secretary Kofi Annan. Comp. I. Tajpale; ed. acad. P.I. Sidorov. Arhangelsk, 2004. 688 p.

Watson L. Even low levels of stress put you more at risk of dying from a heart attack or a stroke. *The Dailymail*. 01.08.2012.

Wen C.P., Man Wai J.P., Tsai M.K. et al. Cardioholic Improve your heart health with 2.5 minutes of intense exercise. *Lancet*. 2012. V. 23. 20.11.2012.

Widlin B. Differences in the impact of the frequency and enjoyment of joint family activities on adolescent substance use and violence. B. Widlin, E. Kuntshe. *J Health Psychol*. 2012, May. Vol. 17. N 4. P. 509-519.

Wiles N., Thomas L., Abel A. et al. Cognitive behavioral therapy as an adjunct to pharmacotherapy for primary care based patients with treatment resistant depression: results of the CoBalT randomized controlled trial. *The Lancet*. P. 375-384. 02.02.2013.

Williams AC., Eccleston C., Morley S. Psychological therapies for the management of chronic pain (excluding headache) in adults. Cochrane Database Syst Rev. 2012: 1-26.

Williams D.T., Harding K.J. Somatoform Disorders. D.T. Williams, K.J. Harding. *Encyclopedia of Movement Disorders*, 2010, P.121-127.

Xu W.L., Atti A.R., Gatz M. et al. Midlife overweight and obesity increase late-life dementia risk. *Neurology*. 03.05.2011. Vol. 76, no. 18. P. 1568-1574.

Yoon S. S., Gu Q., Nwankwo T. et al. Trends in Blood Pressure Among Adults With Hypertension: United States, 2003 to 2012. *Hypertension*. 2014. [Epub ahead of print].

Zahoor A.S., R-c. Li, Ahmad A.S. et al. How dark chocolate may guard against brain injury from stroke. Johns Hopkins Medicine release. 05.05.2010.

Zajchik A.Sh. *Patohimija (endokrinno-metabolicheskie narushenija)* [Patho-chemistry (endocrine and metabolic disorders)]. A.Sh. Zajchik, L.P. Churilov. SPb. Jelbi, 2007. 768 p.

Zhang Y. et al. Inhibition of NMDARs in the nucleus reticucaris of the thalamus produces delta frejuency bursting Front Neural circuits. 2009. N. 3. P. 20.

Zhuravlev A.L., Jurevich A.V. Kollektivnye smysly kak predposylka lichnogo schastja [Collective senses as a prerequisite for happiness]. *Psihologicheskij zhurnal* [Psychological Journal], 2014. V. 35. № 1. P. 5-15.

Zhuravlev A.L., Jurevich A.V. Psihologija nravstvennosti kak oblast psihologicheskogo issledovanija [Psychology of morality as an area of psychological research]. *Psihologicheskij zhurnal* [Psychological Journal], 2013. V. 34, № 3. P. 5–14.

Zhuravlev A.L., Kuprejchenko A.B. Nravstvennaja elita v sovremennom rossijskom obshhestve: socialno-psihologicheskij aspekt [Moral elite in the contemporary Russian society: socio-psychological aspect of morality]. Psihologija nravstvennosti [Psychology of Morality]. Ed. A.L. Zhuravleva, A.V. Jurevich. M.: *Institut psihologii RAN* [RAS Institute of Psychology], 2010. P. 209–236.

Zhuravlev A.L., Ushakov D.V., Jurevich A.V. Perspektiva psihologii v reshenii zadach rossijskogo obshhestva [Prospect of psychology in solving the problems of Russian society]. Parts I–III. Psihologicheskij zhurnal [Psychological Journal], 2013. V. 34, № 1. P. 3–14; № 2. P. 70–86; № 6. P. 5–25.

Zhuravleva N.A. Dinamika orientacij molodezhi na moralno-eticheskie cennosti – aktualnaja problema sovremennogo rossijskogo obshhestva [Dynamics of orientations of young people in the moral and ethical values actual problems of modern Russian society]. *Psihologicheskij zhurnal* [Psychological Journal], 2013. V. 34, № 5. P. 46-57.

Zinchenko Ju.P., Shilko R.S. Vyjavlenie grupp riska, predstavljajushhih resursy razvitija terrorizma, i obosnovanie principov antiterroristicheskoj dejatelnosti na etom napravlenii [Identifying risk groups, representing the resources of terrorism and the study of the principles of anti-terrorist activities in this area]. *Sovremennyj terrorizm i borba s nim: socialno-gumanitarnye izmerenija* [Modern terrorism and the fight against it: social and humanitarian dimensions]. S.A. Afonin et al. Ed. V.V. Jashhenko. M.: MCCME, 2007. P. 36–37.

Zoccola P., Figueroa W., Rabideau E. et al. Dwelling on Stressful events can increase inflammation in the body, study funds. Ohio University. 13.03.2013.

Index

A

a full-scale, 59, 81, 88, 89, 90, 91, 99, 102, 104, 106, 115, 116, 117, 125, 127, 129, 130, 132, 138, 140, 142, 143, 150, 151, 154, 167, 171, 172, 173, 175, 176, 177, 186, 190, 217, 320, 322
accentuation, 42, 211, 294, 378, 441
Acceptable limits, 28
acquired mental immunodeficiency syndrome, 441, 444
activity, 9, 14, 16, 25, 28, 40, 45, 52, 54, 55, 76, 84, 87, 91, 101, 106, 107, 108, 119, 124, 125, 137, 138, 143, 146, 155, 157, 160, 161, 164, 165, 167, 176, 178, 185, 190, 191, 192, 207, 208, 209, 211, 212, 221, 226, 227, 238, 250, 256, 257, 262, 267, 275, 276, 277, 278, 279, 280, 281, 290, 291, 297, 299, 300, 309, 312, 319, 320, 321, 322, 323, 326, 328, 329, 330, 331, 332, 334, 338, 339, 343, 349, 361, 364, 366, 372, 373, 376, 382, 395, 397, 399, 401, 402, 404, 405, 410, 415, 421, 430, 432, 445, 448, 450, 474
adaptation, 6, 10, 19, 24, 33, 42, 54, 72, 75, 76, 80, 84, 92, 99, 105, 113, 115, 118, 127, 131, 138, 144, 145, 146, 148, 149, 153, 157, 162, 166, 167, 168, 171, 177, 178, 185, 188, 190, 216, 226, 239, 250, 254, 256, 272, 288, 290, 293, 294, 298, 301, 306, 310, 319, 323, 325, 328, 335, 345, 348, 350, 351, 353, 381, 382, 423, 424, 425, 426, 437, 442, 445, 455, 463
adaptive management, 146, 416, 417
adaptive professiogenesis, 24, 82, 91, 158, 179, 207, 231, 241, 262, 263, 313, 364, 397, 400, 401, 403, 404, 406, 418, 437, 438, 448, 455, 460
adaptive protection, 35, 41, 82, 372, 456
adaptive psychosocial and, 229
addiction, 8, 44, 46, 48, 57, 64, 90, 161, 199, 206, 208, 209, 215, 221, 222, 223, 224, 225, 226, 227, 229, 231, 238, 246, 248, 262, 279, 320, 321, 322, 323, 324, 325, 326, 328, 351, 352, 353, 358, 360, 374, 388, 401, 405, 411, 444, 446, 451, 456, 457, 466
addictive behavior, 45, 137, 221, 222, 224, 225, 228, 229, 231, 310, 321, 323, 326, 328, 352, 467, 479
addictive disorders, 90, 228, 230, 332
addictogenic diatheses, 228, 230, 272, 282
addictogenic family, 228, 229, 230, 272, 282
adequate physical, 432
adipogenic diathesis, 162, 163, 166
adipogenic family, 162, 163, 166, 167
Aim(s), 19, 24, 25, 91, 145, 176, 227, 294, 302, 312, 323, 326, 332, 344, 345, 352, 393, 418
air blast, 267
Alcoholism, 5, 42, 44, 46, 48, 57, 199, 203, 222, 223, 224, 225, 229, 246, 260, 262, 278, 351, 354, 358, 360, 373, 412, 444, 446, 456, 472
alexithymia, 81, 98, 115, 128, 140, 165
Algorithm of multilevel prevention, 406
alimentary-addictive, 332
and destroy, 64, 212, 229
anhedonic diathesis, 307, 308, 310
Anhedonic family, 306, 307, 308, 310, 311, 313
Anima, 30, 38, 39, 40, 41, 42, 44, 211, 262, 303, 377, 447, 450, 470, 471
Anima, animus, 30, 303, 377
animogenesis, 8, 9, 22, 30, 31, 33, 37, 43, 46, 51, 53, 55, 59, 67, 74, 81, 86, 89, 94, 95, 100, 104, 114, 116, 126, 130, 139, 141, 143, 151, 152, 163, 165, 172, 175, 178, 186, 187, 199, 210, 211, 226, 228, 229, 239, 253, 255, 272, 274, 279, 290, 291, 293, 294, 296, 307, 308, 309, 311, 320, 324, 326, 358, 372, 377, 378, 411, 418, 434, 442, 444, 446, 447, 449
Animogenesis of ME, 43
Anomia, 249, 258, 262, 263, 267, 268

anomie, 38, 39, 40, 41, 42, 44, 211, 262, 447, 450, 470, 471
anonymous weapon, 266
Antidepressants, 93, 107, 132, 154, 155, 176, 189, 202, 311, 332, 333, 334, 387
anti-psychiatric, 14, 15, 16, 18, 19, 20, 61, 271, 278, 415
Anti-psychiatry, 14, 15, 16, 18, 19, 20, 61
antithesis, 16, 18, 19, 20, 271
approach, 13, 15, 17, 20, 27, 29, 31, 47, 48, 54, 55, 68, 71, 72, 73, 79, 82, 84, 85, 99, 107, 111, 121, 124, 132, 145, 154, 155, 156, 158, 184, 191, 192, 196, 197, 209, 222, 229, 238, 245, 251, 266, 279, 337, 338, 341, 343, 345, 348, 349, 354, 359, 367,372, 374, 388, 391, 392, 393, 400, 405, 413, 418, 422, 433, 435, 441, 452, 456, 457, 458, 462, 469, 470, 481
arctic hysteria, 46, 191, 193, 194, 196, 203
Arterial hypertension, 46, 71, 78, 83, 86, 89, 92, 98, 101, 102, 159, 164, 306, 332, 466, 468, 470, 479
arthritic diathesis, 171, 172, 175, 177
arthritic family, 171, 172, 176, 177, 179
artificial mental immunity, 441
Asocial epidemics, 48, 247, 452
associated disorders, 59, 130, 142, 158, 175, 179, 186, 223, 254, 273, 279, 294, 403
asthmogenic diathesis, 125, 127, 130, 131
asthmogenic family, 125, 126, 130, 131
Asymmetric coherence strategy, 451
attribute, 47, 125, 127, 141, 199, 200, 258, 269, 277, 288, 428
autism, 47, 61, 73, 142, 294, 296, 297, 303, 357, 387, 399, 409
autogenous training, 46, 108

B

basis for moral conduct and ethics may devalue, 212
behavior ethics and communication, 56
Behavioral strategies for avoiding mobbing, 240
Behavioral Training in Extremal Situations, 344
believers without religion, 270, 273, 375, 376, 451
bifurcation points., 226, 409
biogenesis, 30, 32, 33, 44, 199, 296, 303, 320, 326, 433, 434, 444, 445, 447, 449
Biogenesis of ME, 44
biological theories of schizophrenia, 286
biopsychosocial triad, 6
biopsychosociospiritual methodology, 225, 260, 262, 278, 279, 359, 365, 377, 408, 456
biopsychosociospiritual model of ontogenesis, 30, 32, 94
biopsychosociospiritual technologies, 456
bloodless color revolution, 248
Borderline personality disorder, 257, 456, 467, 480
bossing, 82, 143, 158, 178, 233, 237, 238, 313
Bossing as a compensation for personal complexes, 238
Bossing as a lifestyle, 237
brainwashing, 252
Bronchial asthma, 46, 71, 78, 123, 124, 126, 463, 480
brotherhood duel, 280
bullying diathesis, 253, 256, 257
bursts of anger, 234

C

cancerous family, 149
Capacity for work, 339
cardiogenic diathesis, 99, 100, 101, 104, 105
cardiogenic family, 99, 104, 105
cardioneurosis, 77, 101, 102
causative complexes, 350
certain perception of both, 67
chaka, 194, 195, 197, 198
change conductors, 348
changing mentality strategy, 417
chronization, 37, 59, 73, 74, 76, 80, 81, 86, 87, 90, 91, 92, 99, 100, 104, 105, 113, 114, 117, 118, 125, 126, 130, 131, 139, 142, 143, 144, 152, 153, 163, 166, 171, 172, 175, 176, 177, 185, 186, 187, 188, 189, 210, 216, 227, 228, 230, 254, 255, 256, 258, 259, 273, 274, 275, 277, 278, 282, 288, 290, 296, 298, 301, 307, 309, 310, 320, 322, 323, 324, 325, 326, 422
Circumstances of idea's genesis, 28
civilization degradation, 256, 275
civilizational suicide, 261, 268, 269
civilizational war, 265, 266, 268, 281
classification and mechanisms of mental, social and anti-social, 456
Classification of risk factors, 11
clinical diagnostics, 34
clinical medical ethics, 364
clinical picture, 24, 31, 37, 59, 71, 73, 74, 80, 81, 86, 87, 88, 89, 90, 91, 92, 99, 100, 101, 102, 104, 105, 106, 113, 114, 115, 116, 117, 118, 125, 126, 127, 128, 129, 130, 131, 132, 138, 139, 140, 141, 142, 143, 144, 149, 150, 151, 152, 153, 154, 162, 163, 164, 166, 167, 171, 172, 175, 176, 177, 185, 186, 187, 188, 189, 203, 206, 210, 216, 217, 228, 230, 290, 293, 294, 295, 305, 307, 308, 309, 310, 311, 320, 322, 324, 325, 326, 347, 422
Clinical Psychiatry, 23, 24, 25, 41, 59, 246, 262, 271, 371, 378, 390, 458, 459, 465, 468, 470, 471, 480

Community Mental Health Department, 382
comorbid pathologies, 223
compensation, 108, 146, 226, 238, 251, 288, 290, 291, 294, 309, 318, 319, 350, 354, 382, 442
competence, 6, 67, 109, 145, 184, 234, 295, 339, 363, 364, 368, 447
Concept, 4, 5, 6, 7, 10, 11, 13, 14, 19, 23, 24, 25, 28, 29, 30, 31, 34, 40, 49, 52, 62, 66, 71, 73, 79, 90, 104, 111, 117, 124, 138, 140, 143, 146, 147, 151, 157, 159, 164, 167, 169, 179, 185, 191, 205, 206, 208, 215, 224, 225, 231, 233, 239, 244, 247, 253, 262, 268, 272, 276, 279, 286, 287, 293, 297, 299, 303, 323, 328, 338, 348, 349, 351, 354, 358, 359, 362, 380, 393, 395, 396, 397, 408, 421, 425, 427, 434, 441, 442, 448, 459, 464, 471, 479, 480
concerned, 15, 184, 280, 287, 292, 341, 422
conflict of fundamental values of justice, 446
conformal subculture, 42
conscience, 3, 4, 8, 14, 31, 35, 37, 38, 41, 42, 43, 44, 45, 46, 47, 48, 49, 50, 53, 55, 56, 63, 64, 67, 71, 82, 90, 104, 116, 130, 142, 146, 161, 175, 179, 201, 202, 206, 212, 226, 229, 243, 244, 245, 247, 248, 250, 253, 254, 255, 256, 259, 261, 262, 263, 265, 266, 267, 268, 269, 270, 271, 272, 273, 274, 275, 276, 277, 278, 279, 280, 281, 290, 320, 339, 341, 342, 348, 356, 357, 358, 359, 360, 361, 362, 367, 372, 376, 377, 379, 380, 381, 387, 395, 398, 399, 402, 406, 407, 408, 409, 411, 412, 413, 414, 415, 416, 417, 418, 422, 424, 438, 441, 442, 443, 444, 445, 446, 447, 448, 449, 450, 451, 452, 456, 458, 459, 460, 476, 478, 481, 483
constant discussion, 234
contemporary hybrid epoch, 279
Contemporary terrorism, 250
content, 4, 7, 18, 25, 28, 36, 39, 49, 52, 62, 117, 159, 160, 193, 229, 249, 276, 279, 280, 290, 291, 295, 297, 301, 331, 347, 350, 365, 399, 400, 407, 439, 443, 456
Coronary heart disease, 46, 48, 71, 78, 88, 97, 98, 99, 100, 105, 106, 159, 164, 432, 468, 480
Counseling on Mind Transformation, 341
counterterrorism, 243, 244, 263
Crime, 48, 64, 223, 246, 351, 359, 361, 447
crisis, 4, 7, 18, 21, 22, 23, 38, 39, 41, 47, 54, 67, 82, 97, 98, 99, 236, 237, 247, 256, 271, 275, 276, 278, 294, 312, 345, 347, 351, 357, 371, 390, 391, 411, 418, 423, 428, 438, 441, 443, 444, 445, 446, 448, 449, 450, 451, 459, 460, 466, 469
Crisis of Psychiatry, 22
critical period, 267, 442, 448
crowding terrorism, 256, 257
culture, 3, 4, 10, 17, 18, 22, 30, 36, 39, 43, 45, 50, 52, 55, 60, 63, 64, 94, 97, 179, 191, 192, 195, 196, 199, 203, 212, 237, 240, 245, 247, 249, 260, 270, 271, 328, 338, 342, 351, 352, 359, 361, 376, 377, 407, 416, 417, 421, 423, 437, 438, 439, 444,446, 450, 458, 473
cumulative charges, 267

D

dance therapy, 429, 431, 432, 475
death from workaholism, 205
decarceration, 17
decivilizational rating, 266
decoherent, 287, 288, 289, 295
decrease in, 37, 78, 111, 117, 141, 145, 165, 209, 211, 239, 263, 323, 327, 329, 330, 433, 434, 436
dehumanization and de-ethization of professional, 212
demonology occurred, 197
demoralization syndrome, 55, 56, 58, 59, 81, 82, 90, 104, 106, 117, 130, 143, 154, 158, 175, 179, 186, 203, 206, 228, 245, 246, 253, 256, 273, 294, 296, 308, 309, 313, 360, 411, 412, 415
dependence on drugs, 222
dependent behavior, 221, 224, 226, 227, 228, 229, 230, 231, 255, 256, 259, 263, 277, 278, 282, 479
Depressive disorder, 106, 107, 154, 164, 170, 171, 176, 184, 214, 305, 306, 307, 309, 310, 311, 312, 467, 472
destruction of a moral position, 212
destructive professiogenesis, 43, 46, 81, 82, 90, 143, 154, 158, 175, 178, 179, 186, 203, 206, 207, 209, 210, 212, 215, 216, 217, 235, 236, 238, 239, 277, 296, 308, 311, 313, 357, 402, 405, 406, 445, 457, 478
destructive social epidemic, 47, 48, 243, 245, 247, 249, 251, 254, 256, 258, 261, 262, 267, 268, 269, 279, 280, 388, 412, 438
development mechanisms of mental epidemics, 44
Deviant behavior, 59, 210, 211
Dextrocerebral thinking, 28, 29
Diabetes, 46, 47, 48, 78, 98, 102, 135, 136, 137, 138, 139, 140, 141, 142, 143, 144, 145, 146, 159, 161, 164, 296, 306, 330, 332, 354, 422, 432, 433, 434, 461, 464, 477, 480
diabetogenic diathesis, 138, 139, 141, 144
diabetogenic family, 138, 143
dialectics of casualty and necessity, 352
diathesis, 31, 73, 74, 76, 77, 80, 85, 86, 87, 90, 92, 99, 100, 101, 104, 105, 113, 114, 115, 116, 118, 125, 126, 127, 130, 131, 138, 139, 141, 144, 149, 152, 153, 162, 163, 164, 166, 171, 172, 175, 177, 185, 187, 188, 216, 253, 255, 256, 257, 274, 275, 290, 293, 294, 307, 308, 310, 320, 326, 422

Direction, 7, 21, 25, 28, 30, 58, 63, 64, 93, 128, 132, 138, 156, 160, 189, 262, 293, 294, 296, 298, 299, 301, 341, 348, 349, 379, 401, 415, 429, 446, 456, 470, 479
directions of mental preventology, 437
disadaptation, 74, 86, 89, 100, 114, 126, 129, 139, 141, 151, 152, 163, 170, 171, 172, 187, 205, 206, 210, 211, 212, 226, 228, 231, 255, 256, 274, 275, 307, 324, 351
disease of homeostasis, 137
diseases, 3, 5, 6, 8, 10, 11, 12, 13, 22, 30, 31, 33, 34, 35, 36, 44, 46, 47, 50, 57, 58, 59, 61, 62, 71, 72, 73, 76, 78, 79, 81, 85, 97, 99, 112, 113, 119, 124, 125, 126, 127, 131, 132, 135, 136, 146, 147, 148, 149, 151, 153, 158, 160, 161, 162, 164, 170, 171, 185, 190, 195, 196, 197, 198, 199, 202, 206, 211, 212, 213, 222, 223, 227, 228, 229, 230, 238, 247, 266, 271, 278, 282, 292, 305, 306, 320, 323, 324, 329, 332, 334, 348, 350, 351, 352, 353, 354, 356, 358, 378, 380, 382, 388, 394, 395, 400, 409, 411, 412, 414, 422, 423, 424, 431, 432, 433, 434, 436, 438, 455, 458, 462, 465, 468, 471, 472, 473, 474, 475, 478, 480
diseases of homeostasis, 99
disharmonious and deformed moral character, 212
disharmonious family, 89, 129, 209, 210, 238, 422
displacement of the workplace, 234
distortion of psychosomatic development, 77
dramatization of the situation, 234, 250
Drug addiction, 44, 46, 48, 57, 64, 206, 223, 224, 225, 229, 246, 248, 351, 358, 360, 373, 374, 388, 446, 456
Dynamics, 12, 19, 22, 24, 28, 30, 31, 32, 34, 37, 40, 47, 50, 53, 67, 73, 76, 86, 99, 100, 107, 108, 113, 114, 125, 126, 139, 152, 163, 172, 185, 187, 205, 209, 210, 224, 225, 228, 239, 252, 255, 260, 265, 267, 272, 274, 287, 289, 290, 293, 307, 324, 348, 349, 392, 404, 409, 414, 416, 428, 434, 442, 446, 447, 448, 449, 459, 475, 484

E

Ecology of Global Security., 281
Economic strategy, 459
ecopolicy of happiness, 65
engineering of social conscience, 456
environmental strategy, 458
Epidemic of mental terrorism, 269, 276
Epidemic stigmas, 42
epidemic suicidal behavior, 245
epidemics, 30, 35, 36, 37, 38, 42, 44, 45, 46, 47, 48, 50, 54, 69, 71, 72, 82, 181, 191, 192, 197, 198, 219, 231, 247, 248, 249, 259, 261, 263, 278, 283, 360, 445, 446, 452, 456, 478
epidemiology, 1, 35, 41, 42, 50, 51, 54, 67, 123, 266, 290, 356, 383, 455, 457, 459, 460, 463, 481
Epidemiology of noncommunicable diseases, 35
equivalence paradox, 340
ethical codes., 449
Ethics, 6, 19, 24, 33, 41, 43, 44, 50, 52, 54, 56, 59, 60, 81, 82, 90, 91, 106, 156, 158, 178, 179, 203, 206, 212, 229, 248, 250, 260, 287, 291, 296, 299, 301, 303, 313, 339, 357, 358, 363, 364, 365, 367, 372, 374, 390, 402, 408, 414, 418, 434, 449, 456, 457,458, 470
European Federation of psychoanalytic psychotherapy, 363
evaluation of the quality of life as the endemic, 456
evil and immoral behavior, 59
evolution, 6, 10, 11, 18, 27, 30, 33, 50, 54, 72, 206, 224, 227, 259, 260, 261, 268, 278, 293, 294, 297, 299, 349, 359, 376, 377, 411, 413, 416, 417, 428, 442, 476, 479
existence of the meaning of life, 67
existential despair syndrome, 445
existential vacuum, 54, 360, 391, 407
External outline of actions, 28
extranosological strategy, 457

F

faith without, 371, 375
family variant of the terrorist demoralization, 245
fashion pandemic, 436
fatalistic, 303, 361
Focus, 7, 14, 17, 19, 24, 28, 36, 44, 45, 102, 115, 149, 164, 235, 319, 343, 360, 372, 374, 411, 442, 448, 450, 455, 458, 478
folk mental medicine, 203
forming innovative mentality, 419
Forms, 4, 5, 6, 9, 15, 16, 19, 20, 22, 30, 31, 33, 37, 40, 42, 45, 46, 47, 48, 49, 57, 58, 59, 67, 73, 74, 75, 77, 78, 79, 80, 86, 87, 88, 90, 92, 94, 99, 100, 101, 102, 103, 105, 113, 114, 115, 116, 118, 120, 123, 125, 126, 127, 128, 131, 133, 138, 139, 140, 142, 143, 144, 146, 148, 149, 150, 152, 153, 154, 155, 162, 163, 164, 166, 169, 170, 171, 172, 177, 178, 184, 185, 186, 187, 188, 189, 191, 193, 194, 197, 198, 199, 200, 201, 202, 203, 210, 211, 216, 221, 222, 225, 227, 228, 229, 230, 234, 239, 243, 245, 248, 249, 251, 253, 254, 257, 259, 260, 261, 262, 268, 271, 272, 273, 275, 276, 277, 278, 279, 290, 293, 294, 295, 296, 302, 303, 307, 309, 310, 311, 320, 324, 325, 326, 330, 333, 338, 339, 340, 341, 347, 353, 355, 371, 372, 373, 378, 382, 392,

396, 399, 400, 401, 403, 412, 414, 418, 422, 424, 428, 438, 439, 440, 444, 449, 450, 452, 455, 456, 457
forms of mobbing, 234
formula for, 323, 368
forward-looking strategy, 458
four-dimensional space, 30, 34, 37, 94, 279, 281, 372
Fractal trajectory, 30, 226, 378
Freedom for, 28, 295, 296
Freedom for…, 28
frustration tolerance, 209, 210, 237
full-fledged semantic hierarchy, 67
functional, 6, 10, 19, 25, 27, 28, 29, 31, 33, 34, 49, 54, 68, 73, 74, 76, 77, 78, 80, 81, 84, 87, 88, 97, 99, 101, 102, 103, 115, 116, 117, 128, 129, 137, 138, 140, 141, 146, 150, 160, 164, 165, 167, 169, 171, 173, 174, 176, 178, 183, 186, 206, 210, 211, 216, 217, 228, 230, 244, 259, 278, 279, 282, 287, 290, 294, 308, 317, 318, 319, 320, 326, 329, 330, 331, 332, 334, 348, 349, 357, 363, 382, 392, 393, 396, 398, 403, 418, 422, 433, 440, 441, 446, 448, 453, 455, 456, 459, 467, 473, 477
functional disorder, 31, 73, 74, 77, 80, 81, 88, 102, 128, 150, 164, 169, 171, 173, 210, 211, 216, 217, 228, 230, 282, 320, 326, 422
functional disorders, 31, 73, 74, 77, 80, 81, 88, 102, 128, 150, 164, 169, 171, 173, 210, 211, 216, 217, 228, 230, 282, 320, 326, 422
Functional products, 329
functional psychosomatic disorders, 77, 78, 259, 278
functional types of social support, 349
functions of the mental immunity, 442

G

Gambling, 44, 46, 221, 223, 410
game addiction, 222
general practitioners in mental health, 456
General preventology, 421
general satisfaction, 67
Generalized psychological portrait of a terrorist, 249
Global, 4, 14, 17, 21, 22, 35, 37, 38, 41, 47, 51, 63, 67, 72, 236, 244, 248, 254, 256, 257, 261, 265, 266, 267, 268, 269, 270, 273, 275, 276, 280, 281, 300, 357, 364, 375, 376, 378, 390, 394, 399, 411, 412, 413, 415, 416, 441, 442, 449, 451, 452, 459, 460,462
Global Crisis, 4, 21, 22, 38, 236, 357, 390, 411, 460
global dehumanization, 256, 275
global depopulation strategy, 280
goal of mental medicine, 418
golden duet, 433

H

handling, 27, 28, 33, 364
Happiness, 65, 66, 67, 137, 161, 306, 338, 362, 367, 368, 369, 380, 402, 406, 462, 465, 472, 474, 477, 483
hatred, 41, 50, 178, 247, 252, 286
health, 5, 6, 7, 8, 9, 10, 11, 12, 13, 16, 19, 21, 24, 25, 30, 31, 42, 44, 45, 46, 47, 48, 50, 55, 59, 66, 67, 71, 72, 75, 82, 89, 92, 97, 98, 108, 112, 118, 121, 135, 136, 143, 144, 146, 148, 153, 154, 159, 167, 168, 177, 178, 184, 189, 198, 202, 203, 207, 212, 213, 215, 222, 223, 239, 240, 247, 255, 259, 262, 267, 271, 274, 278, 291, 298, 302, 317, 319, 320, 322, 328, 329, 330, 331, 332, 338, 341, 353, 354, 355, 357, 358, 363, 364, 367, 371, 373, 374, 379, 382, 383, 385, 387, 390, 393, 394, 395, 396, 400, 401, 402, 403, 404, 405, 406, 412, 416, 417, 418, 421, 422, 423, 426, 427, 432, 433, 434, 435, 437, 438, 440, 445, 446, 447, 448, 452, 455, 456, 457, 458, 459, 460, 461, 462, 465, 467, 469, 470, 471, 474, 475, 476, 477, 478, 479, 483
Health ecology assessment, 12
Health factors, 9, 10, 25, 458, 479
health promotion and moral purpose of life, 456
health service, 382, 385, 387, 395, 400, 403, 416
Health Service, 143, 382, 385, 387, 395, 400, 403, 416
hereditary loading, 211, 324
hiccups, 191, 194, 195, 196, 197, 198, 199, 200, 201, 202, 203
Hiccups, 191, 194, 195, 196, 197, 198, 199, 200, 201, 202, 203
HIV-infection, 223
human capital, 339, 463
Humanistic strategy, 457
hybrid neurobionic defense systems, 281
hybrid war, 35, 265, 267, 269, 279, 445, 447, 452, 456, 459
hypercompensation attribute legitimating fraudulent, 277
hypercompensatory, 258
hypertogenic diathesis, 85, 87, 90
hypertogenic family, 85, 88, 90
hysterodemonic, 191

I

identities, 39, 361, 407, 450
identity crisis, 54, 444
identity crisis syndrome, 444

illegal participatory consideration of the behavior, 234
immersive virtual reality, 429, 438
immunity, 4, 39, 50, 54, 148, 170, 249, 251, 261, 262, 276, 367, 368, 373, 414, 416, 434, 437, 438, 440, 441, 442, 445, 447, 456, 457, 458
immunodeficiency epidemic, 444
immunomodulation, 288, 319, 382, 452
Incompetence in the sphere of management, 238
independently targetable warheads, 267
Indices of personal mental ecology, 9
Individual mental, 4, 5, 19, 339
information handling, 28
initial, 31, 37, 41, 43, 45, 59, 63, 73, 74, 77, 80, 81, 86, 87, 88, 91, 92, 99, 100, 102, 104, 105, 106, 113, 114, 117, 118, 120, 125, 126, 128, 130, 131, 137, 138, 139, 140, 142, 143, 144, 149, 150, 152, 153, 154, 156, 162, 163, 165, 166, 167, 172, 174, 175, 176, 177, 185, 186, 187, 188, 189, 210, 216, 217, 227, 228, 230, 231, 253, 255, 256, 257, 259, 272, 273, 274, 275, 276, 278, 282, 290, 294, 298, 299, 302, 307, 310, 311, 322, 323, 324, 325, 327, 342, 344, 382, 422, 423, 428, 444, 456, 458, 472
Innovativeness, 339
Institute of Mental Health, 13, 382
integral mission of religion and psychiatry, 380
integrated strategy, 458
integrated treatment and rehabilitation, 381, 383
integrative medicine, 31, 47, 340, 394, 459
integrative psychotherapy, 340, 392, 461
Integrative-synergetic MHS functions, 403
intentional dissemination of false information, 234
intentional failure to provide, 234
interface of the public conscience, 50
Interhemispheric, 28, 29
intermediaries, 371, 375, 451
international neocults' mission, 269
International Scientific Program, 281
inversion, 14, 53, 54, 67, 198, 207, 256, 265, 275, 279, 280, 281, 447, 451

K

Keela, 191, 197

L

lagging or delayed socialization of body functions, 76
late effects, 267
latent, 31, 37, 55, 59, 73, 74, 80, 81, 86, 87, 88, 90, 91, 92, 99, 100, 101, 102, 104, 105, 106, 113, 114, 115, 116, 117, 118, 125, 126, 128, 130, 131, 138, 139, 141, 143, 144, 148, 150, 152, 153, 154, 163, 164, 166, 167, 172, 173, 175, 176, 177, 185, 186, 187,188, 210, 215, 216, 227, 228, 230, 231, 237, 253, 255, 256, 257, 259, 260, 269, 272, 274, 275, 278, 279, 282, 290, 291, 296, 297, 298, 307, 310, 311, 322, 324, 325, 342, 410, 422
Lateral asymmetry, 28, 29
Learnability, 339
Level of activity realization, 28
Level of actuality, 28
Level of information, 28
lishinka, 46, 191, 194
load, 84, 137, 138, 178, 227, 229, 289, 299, 330, 430, 432, 481
logotherapy, 59, 378, 466

M

Macrosocial level, 350, 351, 405
management, 12, 33, 46, 89, 91, 115, 120, 129, 146, 151, 155, 234, 237, 238, 240, 254, 262, 263, 271, 281, 286, 300, 303, 304, 317, 337, 351, 365, 382, 394, 398, 410, 413, 416, 417, 429, 434, 435, 436, 446, 448, 451, 452, 457, 458, 460, 466, 473, 474, 479, 480, 481, 483
mass conscience, 42, 407, 416, 438, 444, 476
mass destruction, 41, 249, 260, 268, 269, 447, 479
mass human, 444
Matrix of mental immunity, 447
mechanism of anonymity, 44
mechanism of autonomy, 45
mechanism of expanded reproduction, 44
mechanism of generalization, 44
mechanism of identity destruction, 45
mechanism of induction, 45
mechanism of polymodal resonanc, 45
mechanism of polymorphic deformation of mind, 45
mechanisms of exposing influence, 251
mechanisms of mental epidemics, 44, 54
medical block, 79, 93, 106, 119, 132, 142, 143, 154, 167, 176, 189, 202, 309, 311
medical ethics with clinical content, 456
Medical-oriented MHS functions, 401
medicine, 1, 4, 5, 6, 7, 13, 14, 15, 17, 19, 20, 21, 22, 23, 24, 25, 27, 30, 31, 33, 35, 47, 49, 56, 71, 72, 74, 107, 111, 146, 151, 203, 206, 207, 208, 225, 231, 233, 236, 271, 279, 287, 293, 297, 298, 302, 303,315, 317, 337, 340, 341, 347, 357, 362, 365, 366, 371, 372, 373, 380, 382, 383, 387, 391, 393, 394, 400, 405, 414, 418, 421, 422, 438, 455, 457, 458, 459, 460, 461, 462, 463, 464, 466, 467, 468,

469, 470, 471, 472, 473, 474, 475, 476, 477, 478, 479, 481, 482, 483
mental and moral, 7, 8, 30, 54, 299
Mental cyber terrorism, 268
Mental ecology, 4, 6, 7, 8, 9, 14, 17, 18, 22, 31, 35, 37, 50, 191, 203, 213, 214, 215, 262, 265, 266, 269, 278, 279, 280, 281, 339, 390, 392, 412, 414, 418, 450, 456, 458, 459, 479
Mental ecology doctrine of national security, 262
mental ecology mission, 7
mental engineering, 50, 407, 408
mental epidemic (ME), 35, 37, 38, 39, 41, 43, 44, 45, 46, 47, 48, 49, 50, 53, 54, 64, 65, 67, 71, 80, 82, 86, 100, 137, 139, 152, 163, 183, 187, 190, 228, 247, 278, 282, 394, 451, 459, 478
mental epidemicity risk, 54
Mental epidemics, 35, 37, 38, 39, 41, 43, 44, 45, 46, 47, 48, 49, 50, 53, 54, 64, 65, 67, 71, 80, 82, 86, 100, 137, 139, 152, 163, 183, 187, 190, 228, 247, 278, 282, 394, 451, 459, 478
Mental epidemics of dependent disorders, 46
Mental epidemics of endoecological disorders, 46
Mental epidemics of induced disorders, 46
Mental epidemics of psychosomatic disorders, 46, 71, 80
Mental epidemics of somatoform disorders, 46
mental epidemiology, 39, 41, 44, 50, 51, 65, 67, 208, 243, 340, 390, 452, 455, 456, 457, 458, 459
Mental Epidemiology, 35, 39, 41, 44, 50, 51, 65, 67, 208, 243, 340, 390, 452, 455, 456, 457, 458, 459
mental health, 4, 5, 6, 7, 8, 9, 10, 11, 13, 15, 17, 19, 20, 23, 24, 25, 30, 31, 33, 40, 42, 44, 47, 48, 50, 54, 56, 59, 65, 66, 79, 81, 82, 93, 119, 142, 146, 178, 189, 196, 203, 213, 217, 231, 246, 247, 259, 262, 263, 266, 267, 271, 277, 279, 288, 302, 308, 309, 311, 313, 331, 332, 337, 338, 339, 350, 356, 357, 358, 359, 362, 365, 371, 372, 376, 378, 381, 382, 388, 389, 390, 391, 392, 394, 395, 396, 397, 398, 399, 400, 401, 403, 404, 405, 406, 408, 409, 411, 412, 416, 417, 418, 422, 423, 424, 427, 431, 433, 434, 435, 436, 438, 440, 447, 448, 451, 452, 455, 456, 458, 459, 460, 461, 463, 467, 468, 469, 470, 478, 479
mental health corporate services, 403
mental health service (MHS), 4, 23, 48, 49, 50, 59, 81, 143, 217, 231, 262, 267, 279, 302, 311, 313, 357, 382, 390, 395, 399, 400, 401, 402, 403, 404, 405, 406, 416, 417, 418, 447, 448, 455, 459, 467, 468, 470, 479
mental health system, 50, 267, 395, 396, 398, 399, 403, 404, 455, 459
mental health system monitoring, 50, 267, 395, 396, 398, 399, 403, 404, 455, 460
mental immunity, 4, 50, 249, 261, 262, 367, 437, 440, 441, 442, 445, 447, 456, 457, 458
Mental Medicine, 1, 6, 7, 13, 17, 18, 19, 20, 21, 22, 24, 25, 27, 29, 31, 32, 33, 34, 35, 37, 41, 44, 45, 47, 48, 49, 50, 51, 54, 58, 67, 73, 74, 79, 90, 94, 95, 109, 121, 133, 142, 146, 151, 155, 158, 165, 168, 175, 176, 186, 191, 203, 212, 229, 243, 260, 262, 265, 271, 278, 279, 280, 281, 287, 297, 302, 303, 304, 309, 315, 317, 337, 338, 339, 341, 347, 348, 349, 350, 356, 357, 358, 359, 363, 371, 372, 374, 377, 378, 379, 380, 382, 383, 387, 388, 391, 393, 394, 401, 405, 406, 408, 409, 411, 412, 413, 414, 416, 417, 418, 422, 433, 435, 437, 444, 446, 447, 452, 455, 459, 460, 469, 478
Mental medicine institute, 405
mental paradigm, 18, 243, 263, 372
mental paradigm of national security, 243, 263, 372
mental peculiarities of terrorists, 250
Mental preventology, 24, 25, 50, 53, 59, 67, 74, 262, 280, 329, 330, 360, 363, 368, 378, 390, 400, 418, 422, 423, 429, 437, 440, 456, 457, 458, 479
mental preventology and recreation therapy, 456
mental preventology as a social institution, 456
mental representation, 58, 170, 174, 254, 256, 257, 261, 266, 273, 275, 293, 368, 418, 452, 456
mental resilience, 42, 49, 50, 82, 125, 262, 424, 425, 426, 427, 429, 430, 432, 433, 436, 437, 445, 447, 456
mental resilience., 50, 82, 125, 430, 432, 436
mental risk, 50
mental safety, 260, 446, 453, 456
mental security of the population, 262
Mental terrorism, 48, 67, 244, 246, 247, 254, 260, 265, 268, 269, 270, 271, 273, 275, 276, 277, 341, 399, 410, 412, 459, 478
mental terrorist war, 268, 270, 273
Mental virology, 41, 42, 50, 268, 279, 280, 281, 437
mental virulence, 50
Mental viruses, 35, 42, 261, 268
mentality, 3, 4, 8, 9, 11, 12, 19, 29, 39, 42, 72, 120, 161, 171, 174, 203, 211, 261, 267, 268, 269, 271, 272, 280, 341, 345, 353, 358, 361, 367, 368, 371, 378, 381, 408, 411, 412, 413, 416, 417, 418, 419, 450, 456, 457, 476
Mentality, 3, 4, 8, 9, 11, 12, 19, 20, 29, 31, 39, 42, 65, 72, 120, 161, 171, 174, 203, 211, 261, 267, 268, 269, 271, 272, 280, 341, 345, 353, 358, 361, 367, 368, 371, 378, 381, 408, 411, 412, 413, 416, 417, 418, 419, 450, 456, 457, 476
mentality as a factor of public, 456
Mentally-psychotherapeutic oriented MHS functions, 402
Mesosocial level, 350, 351, 405

methodological principles of social work, 348
Methodology, 7, 8, 9, 14, 16, 18, 20, 22, 23, 24, 25, 27, 28, 29, 30, 31, 32, 33, 37, 40, 41, 44, 46, 48, 54, 73, 79, 82, 90, 95, 99, 108, 109, 121, 130, 133, 142, 146, 151, 155, 158, 165, 168, 175, 176, 186, 209, 212, 225, 229, 260, 261, 262, 265, 266, 269, 271, 278, 279, 280, 285, 297, 303, 304, 309, 337, 338, 339, 340, 341, 347, 353, 357, 358, 359, 361, 365, 366, 371, 374, 377, 382, 383, 388, 390, 391, 394, 397, 398, 399, 400, 401, 404, 406, 408, 409, 411, 414, 416, 418, 422, 433, 437, 443, 444, 447, 453, 455, 456, 459, 478, 482
Microsocial level, 352
Millisocial level, 350, 352, 405
Mindsight mechanism, 45
Minor biologically active compounds, 330
mirror neurons, 37, 266, 368, 452
mission of mental medicine, 416
mobbing, 44, 46, 48, 55, 82, 90, 143, 158, 178, 203, 206, 233, 234, 235, 236, 237, 238, 239, 240, 246, 247, 251, 253, 256, 258, 259, 261, 277, 311, 313, 357, 410, 457, 458
mobbing family, 253, 256
mobbing-targets, 236, 237
mobilization strategy, 452
mockery and abuse, 234
model of healthy life field, 338
monitoring, 4, 8, 9, 13, 16, 19, 25, 31, 42, 50, 54, 72, 106, 143, 146, 202, 251, 262, 267, 281, 287, 288, 300, 350, 354, 355, 365, 390, 393, 395, 396, 397, 398, 399, 401, 402, 403, 404, 408, 412, 416, 418, 455, 459, 460, 481
moral behavior, 59, 80, 92, 105, 118, 131, 144, 153, 166, 177, 188, 216, 229, 230, 254, 282, 298, 310, 325, 359, 362
moral character, 59, 67, 117, 158, 203, 212, 298, 307, 310, 324, 325, 362, 367
moral condition of Russia, 359
moral development, 51, 56, 67, 82, 90, 91, 95, 158, 179, 363, 378, 464
Moral diagnosis, 54, 364, 365
moral diagnostics, 33, 402
Moral health, 6, 30, 353, 447
moral position, 43, 55, 56, 59, 74, 80, 86, 92, 100, 104, 105, 114, 118, 126, 131, 139, 142, 144, 152, 153, 158, 163, 166, 172, 175, 177, 179, 186, 187, 188, 210, 212, 216, 228, 229, 245, 253, 255, 274, 290, 298, 301, 307, 310, 313, 324, 325, 362, 450
moral resuscitation, 360
moral self-determination of the personality, 53
moral senses, 158, 272, 274, 290, 308, 313, 362, 411
moral sentiments formation, 212, 307, 324
moral socialization, 55, 81, 90, 91, 104, 106, 117, 130, 142, 143, 154, 167, 175, 176, 185, 186, 212, 215, 245, 250, 294, 297, 308, 326, 358, 411, 446
moral standard, 52, 358, 361, 362
Morally and spiritually oriented MHS functions, 402
morally-spiritual feelings, 55
morally-spiritual identity, 55
morally-spiritual position, 56
mother, 16, 75, 76, 77, 99, 108, 125, 127, 162, 289, 290, 291, 292, 293, 297, 298, 306, 322, 324
Multidimensional conscience glassiness strategy, 452
multidisciplinary brigade, 93, 106, 133
multidisciplinary protocol of teamwork, 405
Musical and Vocal Therapy, 430
Myth, 246, 291, 340, 379, 389, 390, 408, 469
mythologization, 387, 388, 390, 408
mythologization of psychiatry, 390

N

national educational ideal, 362
national security., 38, 48, 243, 262, 273, 372, 388, 394, 448, 458
natural mental immunity, 441
negative moral orientation, 367
Neocults, 265, 269, 271, 272, 273, 276
Neuroleptics, 155, 189, 202, 300, 301, 302, 332, 333, 334
Neuro-physiotherapy, 372
neuroplasticity, 47, 303, 429, 431, 433, 436
neurosis, 91, 99, 100, 129, 148, 188, 198, 203, 215, 216, 230, 231, 250, 282, 290, 295, 307, 308, 310, 311, 334, 379, 388
new clinical paradigm of biomedical ethics, 367
none, 72, 78, 270, 334, 375, 376, 413
nones, 270, 375, 376, 461
non-lethal mass destruction weapon, 269
non-lethal weapon, 41, 250, 447, 479
noosphere, 37, 42, 265, 266, 442, 444, 451, 452
noosphere theory, 42
noospheric resilience, 266
Nootropics, 93, 132, 189, 202, 332, 334
normal anomie, 40, 41, 471
normocycle, 52, 53
notion of communication competence, 339
nutritional, 112, 113, 160, 162, 280, 306, 328, 329, 330, 331, 332, 372
Nutritional therapy, 280, 329, 372

O

Object, 4, 24, 27, 28, 41, 52, 53, 72, 137, 226, 235, 297, 369, 396, 405, 422
Objects, 4, 19, 24, 27, 28, 41, 49, 52, 54, 72, 137, 199, 200, 226, 235, 296, 297, 345, 350, 369, 396, 397, 398, 405, 411, 422, 429
occupational burnout syndrome, 205, 207
occupational pathology, 211
occupational risk factors, 208
oncogenic, 149, 152, 153, 158
oncogenic family, 149, 152, 153, 158
Oncological diseases, 147, 153, 480
operational classification of mental epidemics, 46
organization principles for mental health service, 400
orientation, 6, 7, 45, 66, 82, 207, 209, 292, 294, 352, 367, 404, 421, 435, 439, 467, 474
ostentatious refusal, 234
outcome, 31, 37, 59, 73, 74, 79, 80, 81, 86, 88, 89, 90, 92, 93, 94, 99, 100, 101, 103, 104, 105, 106, 108, 113, 114, 116, 117, 118, 119, 125, 126, 129, 130, 131, 132, 139, 140, 141, 142, 143, 144, 149, 150, 151, 152, 153, 154, 161, 163, 166, 171, 172, 174, 175, 176, 177, 185, 187, 188, 189, 210, 211, 212, 216, 217, 227, 228, 230, 245, 254, 255, 256, 257, 259, 273, 274, 275, 276, 277, 278, 282, 290, 295, 296, 298, 307, 310, 319, 320, 322, 323, 324, 325, 326, 410, 422, 425
Overweight, 46, 83, 98, 102, 159, 160, 162, 163, 164, 165, 166, 167, 328, 329, 331, 475, 483
Overweight and obesity, 159, 165, 483

P

pain syndromes, 72, 189
pandemic, 37, 47, 48, 59, 63, 74, 80, 83, 86, 92, 97, 99, 100, 105, 114, 118, 126, 131, 135, 139, 144, 152, 153, 159, 161, 163, 166, 168, 172, 187, 188, 210, 216, 228, 230, 243, 244, 247, 253, 254, 255, 256, 261, 262, 265, 272, 273, 274, 275, 278, 282, 290, 298, 307, 310, 324, 325, 341, 414, 422, 436, 444, 452, 478
pandemic of terrorism, 48, 63, 243, 244, 247, 261, 262, 478
paradigm, 14, 18, 25, 28, 29, 31, 33, 41, 47, 60, 82, 97, 142, 161, 243, 263, 265, 271, 279, 280, 287, 326, 340, 341, 349, 358, 365, 367, 372, 375, 376, 383, 391, 406, 418, 421, 422, 429, 457, 459, 460, 469, 475, 479
paradigmatic, 40, 388
parent demoralization syndrome, 56
parents demoralization, 58
Participativity, 394
patrimonial damnation, 340
paying attention to faked complaints and denunciations, 234
Pedagogic-educational strategy, 457
penetrating information radiation, 267
Peptic ulcer, 111, 112, 113, 114, 115, 118, 480
Permanent self-identification strategy, 450
permissive, 39, 190, 253, 272, 361
permissivity, 44, 249, 263
personal and psychic defects, 211
personal identity, 40, 185, 224, 245, 411, 412, 415, 417, 434, 448, 450
Personality decompensation, 187, 211, 307
Personality disorders, 42, 103, 187, 213, 222, 227, 228, 230, 248, 250, 257, 258, 277, 282, 324, 378, 409, 456
Personality psychopathization, 211
Personalization, 394, 460
Personified (individualized, personalized) medicine, 393
Pharmacotherapy, 16, 80, 92, 105, 118, 131, 144, 153, 166, 177, 188, 216, 282, 310, 311, 312, 332, 333, 335, 387, 401, 456, 483
phenomenon of legitimated recruitment, 271
Philosophy, 14, 17, 19, 20, 22, 33, 289, 358, 365, 366, 372, 378, 462, 465
piblokto, 191, 193, 196, 203
planetary suicide, 248
Political Correctness, 60
political epidemiology, 50
political terrorism, 260
polymodal, 8, 20, 30, 31, 33, 37, 45, 52, 54, 65, 72, 73, 183, 243, 255, 257, 258, 265, 274, 275, 277, 278, 287, 288, 299, 403, 435, 440, 442, 443, 448, 449, 451, 456
Polymodal (cross-, trans-, interactive, etc.) resonance strategy, 451
polymodal mentality, 8, 20, 31, 65
polymodal stress, 73
polymodal trigger, 54
poor, 11, 22, 36, 42, 60, 75, 123, 160, 162, 227, 237, 246, 270, 303, 306, 308, 347, 351, 352, 376, 423, 433, 435
poor faith, 376
population posttraumatic stress, 443
positive affective balance, 67
positive cognitive balance, 67
positive image of the world, 67
positive moral, 367
Possibilities, 4, 5, 18, 24, 28, 31, 43, 48, 68, 108, 145, 174, 211, 265, 301, 302, 338, 348

possibility of, 21, 50, 66, 74, 79, 86, 88, 91, 100, 107, 114, 120, 126, 128, 129, 132, 136, 139, 152, 163, 172, 186, 187, 229, 245, 270, 276, 301, 333, 334, 394, 423, 444, 457
post-Soviet psychosocial stress, 388
prearthritic state, 171, 172, 173, 176, 177
preasthma, 126, 127, 128, 130, 131
pre-cancerous disease, 149
prediabetes, 136, 138, 139, 140, 144
Predictivity, 394
predisposition, 10, 11, 12, 31, 37, 59, 73, 74, 76, 78, 79, 80, 81, 84, 85, 86, 87, 88, 90, 92, 98, 99, 100, 101, 102, 104, 105, 112, 113, 114, 115, 116, 117, 118, 125, 126, 127, 128, 130, 131, 136, 137, 138, 139, 140, 141, 143, 144, 147, 149, 150, 151, 152, 153, 155, 160, 162, 163, 164, 166, 167, 170, 171, 172, 173, 175, 176, 177, 185, 186, 187, 188, 209, 210, 211, 215, 216, 224, 229, 230, 231, 238, 239, 253, 255, 256, 259, 272, 273, 275, 278, 282, 289, 290, 293, 297, 298, 307, 310, 311, 319, 322, 324, 325, 422, 423, 464
pre-hypertension, 87, 88, 91, 467
prevent, 12, 14, 16, 81, 82, 106, 119, 121, 154, 178, 194, 240, 251, 311, 313, 317, 330, 331, 377, 410, 412, 416, 423, 432, 444, 456
Preventivity, 394
primary, 4, 31, 33, 48, 56, 67, 79, 81, 83, 85, 87, 88, 90, 91, 93, 94, 99, 101, 102, 103, 104, 106, 111, 115, 116, 117, 125, 127, 128, 130, 132, 136, 137, 138, 140, 143, 145, 149, 151, 154, 162, 165, 167, 169, 170, 176, 183, 185, 186, 187, 188, 189, 198, 199,200, 215, 225, 227, 231, 245, 247, 250, 254, 257, 267, 272, 275, 292, 299, 300, 301, 305, 306, 307, 308, 310, 311, 317, 318, 322, 323, 350, 360, 374, 387, 422, 423, 437, 455, 456, 457, 458, 466, 471, 477, 481, 483
Primary (physiological) mechanisms of sanogenesis, 317
primary astheno-depressive, 308
Principle of, 18, 19, 28, 347, 355, 365, 369, 380, 415, 428, 438
Priorities, 19, 20, 24, 28, 38, 42, 53, 67, 145, 249, 263, 281, 291, 292, 303, 320, 368, 374, 400, 417, 438, 444, 445, 448, 449
Process, 3, 4, 8, 9, 10, 14, 16, 19, 22, 24, 28, 30, 35, 36, 37, 40, 41, 43, 44, 45, 47, 48, 53, 61, 67, 73, 77, 82, 85, 89, 91, 93, 94, 108, 111, 121, 124, 136, 157, 160, 161, 167, 170, 174, 190, 195, 205, 206, 209, 211, 227, 239, 256, 267, 275, 286, 288, 291, 293, 296, 297, 299, 300, 301, 302, 312, 317, 318, 319, 323, 326, 332, 342, 343, 344, 345, 349, 350, 364, 367, 379, 381, 383, 389, 390, 393, 396, 401, 403, 408, 410, 413, 415, 416, 423, 424, 425, 427, 432, 435, 436, 437, 439, 455, 458, 482
professiogenesis, 11, 24, 43, 46, 81, 82, 90, 91, 143, 154, 158, 175, 178, 179, 186, 203, 205, 206, 207, 208, 209, 210, 212, 215, 216, 217, 231, 235, 236, 238, 239, 241, 262, 263, 277, 296, 308, 311, 313, 357, 364, 381, 400, 401, 402, 403, 404, 405, 406, 418,437, 438, 445, 448, 455, 457, 460, 478
professional and civilization trend, 390
professional deformation, 205, 206, 209, 210, 211, 239
Professional deformation, 205, 206, 209, 210, 211, 239
Program and target-oriented strategy, 457
progressive social deprivation and isolation, 234
Prostitution, 223, 351
provided by a multidisciplinary team, 455
Provision of adaptive professiogenesis, 397, 403, 404
psychiatry, 6, 7, 13, 14, 15, 16, 17, 18, 19, 20, 21, 22, 23, 24, 25, 29, 30, 33, 36, 41, 49, 59, 61, 74, 146, 189, 191, 203, 206, 207, 221, 233, 246, 262, 271, 273, 276, 278, 287, 297, 299, 303, 304, 332, 333, 354, 355, 357,359, 371, 374, 378, 380, 381, 382, 383, 387, 388, 389, 390, 391, 392, 397, 405, 458, 459, 461, 462, 463, 464, 465, 466, 467, 468, 469, 470, 471, 472, 474, 475, 476, 478, 479, 480, 482, 483
Psychic epidemics, 36, 37, 191
psychic health, 5, 7, 30
Psychic health, 5, 7, 30
Psychoemotional stresses, 83, 98
psychogenesis, 8, 9, 22, 30, 31, 33, 37, 42, 46, 68, 74, 79, 86, 88, 93, 100, 102, 114, 116, 126, 128, 139, 140, 142, 150, 152, 163, 164, 165, 172, 173, 174, 176, 187, 199, 210, 211, 213, 226, 227, 228, 239, 255, 256, 272, 274, 275, 279, 290, 291, 292, 294, 295, 296, 307, 309, 320, 324, 326, 372, 409, 418, 434, 442, 444, 446, 447, 449, 469
Psychogenesis of ME, 42
psychoimmunologic dysfunctions, 148
psychological block, 79, 93, 107, 119, 132, 142, 145, 155, 167, 176, 189, 309, 312, 382
psychological diagnosis, 338, 393
psychological diagnostics, 31, 33, 402, 423, 482
psychological theories of schizophrenia, 286
Psychological violence, 57, 58, 233
Psychoprophylaxis, 10, 229, 320, 421, 422, 423
psychosomatic diseases, 71, 72, 73, 78, 79, 81, 124, 151, 202, 213, 227, 229, 278, 282, 432, 434, 468, 473, 475
psychosomatic illness, 44, 206, 211, 255

psychosomatic reaction, 74, 78, 80, 86, 88, 92, 100, 102, 105, 114, 116, 118, 126, 128, 129, 131, 139, 140, 141, 144, 150, 152, 153, 163, 165, 166, 172, 174, 177, 186, 187, 188, 216, 227, 259, 278
psychosomatogenic family, 73, 74, 75, 76, 80, 81, 82
psycho-synergetic teamwork, 337
psychotherapy, 8, 16, 17, 20, 33, 43, 51, 52, 59, 67, 80, 82, 92, 93, 95, 105, 107, 108, 118, 119, 120, 131, 132, 133, 144, 145, 153, 155, 156, 157, 158, 166, 167, 170, 176, 177, 178, 188, 189, 191, 192, 193, 202, 203, 207, 216, 230, 233, 279, 280, 282, 298, 299, 300, 301, 310, 312, 313, 320, 325, 326, 335, 337, 340, 341, 363, 372, 377, 378, 379, 382, 389, 392, 402, 405, 417, 423, 456, 459, 461, 463, 465, 466, 469, 470, 471, 472, 473, 476, 482
psychotraumatic factors, 71
psychovegetative diathesis, 73, 74, 76, 77, 80, 290, 293, 294
public, 4, 5, 6, 7, 8, 9, 11, 13, 14, 17, 23, 31, 35, 36, 37, 38, 41, 42, 43, 44, 46, 47, 48, 49, 50, 53, 54, 58, 63, 64, 65, 67, 71, 72, 81, 82, 94, 142, 143, 161, 198, 201, 243, 244, 247, 248, 249, 251, 254, 255, 259, 262, 265, 266, 267, 268, 269, 270, 271, 273, 274, 276, 277, 278, 280, 281, 290, 311, 312, 339, 351, 354, 355, 356, 357, 358, 360, 361, 364, 367, 372, 373, 374, 381, 382, 387, 394, 395, 396, 398, 399, 402, 403, 405, 406, 407, 408, 409, 411, 412, 413, 414, 415, 416, 418, 421, 422, 424, 431, 440, 443, 444, 445, 446, 447, 448, 449, 450, 451, 452, 455, 456, 457, 458, 459, 460, 466, 472, 476, 478, 481
public conscience, 8, 14, 35, 37, 38, 41, 42, 43, 44, 46, 47, 48, 49, 50, 53, 63, 67, 71, 82, 142, 161, 243, 244, 247, 248, 254, 255, 259, 262, 265, 266, 267, 268, 269, 270, 271, 273, 274, 276, 277, 278, 280, 281, 290, 357, 358, 360, 372, 381, 387, 398, 399, 402, 408, 409, 411, 412, 414, 416, 418, 444, 445, 446, 447, 448, 449, 450, 451, 452, 458, 459, 478, 481
public disorder, 443
Public faculty of mental health, 405
public health, 5, 6, 7, 11, 31, 47, 48, 50, 82, 198, 247, 255, 262, 274, 278, 373, 382, 396, 403, 405, 416, 421, 445, 446, 448, 456, 457, 458, 459
public mental, 5

R

recovery mechanisms, 317, 318
reduction of terms for assignments, 234
regeneration, 112, 119, 318, 319, 323, 326, 382, 436
regress in psychosomatic development, 77
regular physical exercises, 432
regulatory strategy, 459
Relationships, 6, 19, 24, 30, 31, 37, 39, 40, 43, 49, 61, 75, 80, 85, 89, 91, 92, 94, 98, 99, 104, 105, 106, 113, 116, 117, 118, 120, 121, 131, 138, 141, 143, 144, 145, 146, 148, 149, 150, 151, 153, 155, 156, 157, 158, 162, 166, 167, 171, 173, 174, 175, 176, 177, 178, 188, 202, 209, 211, 215, 216, 221, 224, 231, 235, 237, 238, 239, 240, 253, 272, 273, 291, 297, 298, 306, 307, 308, 311, 312, 325, 340, 344, 362, 372, 379, 380, 382, 383, 398, 405, 409, 410, 424, 425, 426, 434, 435, 437, 440, 446, 449, 463, 469, 471, 474
relativity, 30, 94, 372
Religious resource, 371, 372, 374, 377, 381, 382
Religious resource of, 372, 381
Religious resource of animogenesis, 372
Religious resource of mental health, 381
Religious resource of psychogenesis, 372
resilience, 42, 49, 50, 82, 155, 157, 262, 266, 280, 356, 383, 424, 425, 426, 427, 429, 433, 437, 442, 445, 447, 451, 456
Resolved tasks, 28
resonantly-coherent mental illness, 285
restitution, 288, 319, 326, 382
Results, 5, 6, 8, 12, 22, 25, 28, 31, 34, 56, 58, 64, 84, 93, 101, 111, 113, 115, 117, 119, 127, 140, 150, 154, 160, 161, 162, 167, 170, 171, 213, 235, 238, 248, 249, 254, 270, 272, 273, 277, 286, 303, 328, 330, 331, 335, 344, 345, 348, 355, 358, 362, 374, 382, 389, 396, 398, 403, 407, 415, 418, 424, 426, 427, 428, 442, 443, 474, 483
revival of morality, 361
Rheumatoid arthritis, 46, 47, 71, 78, 169, 171, 172, 173, 177, 306, 432, 470, 473, 474, 475, 477, 480, 481
Role of time, 28
Russian mentality, 3, 4, 5, 361, 417

S

Safety Of Living, 446
sanogenetic therapy, 46, 146, 279, 313, 317, 318, 319, 320, 321, 323, 326, 327, 328, 372, 382, 403, 413, 456
sanogenetic therapy for patients in somatic departments, 456
Sanogenetic Therapy of Nicotine Addiction, 320
Satisfaction, 65, 66, 67, 206, 211, 277, 309, 418, 448
scan, 50
schisis, 47, 297, 303, 357
schizogenic family, 290, 291
schizogenic mother, 292
schizoid state, 290

schizophrenia, 46, 47, 49, 62, 63, 170, 203, 213, 285, 286, 287, 288, 289, 290, 291, 294, 295, 296, 297, 298, 299, 300, 301, 302, 303, 304, 354, 381, 434, 463, 466, 467, 469, 470, 472, 479
schizotypical diathesis, 290
Scientology, 265, 269, 270, 271, 272, 273, 276, 277, 278, 280, 462
screening and prediction, 422, 448, 455
secondary child abuse syndrome, 56
secondary mental immunodeficiency syndrome, 281
Secondary sanogenetic mechanisms, 317, 318
self-destructive auto-bullying, 170
Self-development strategy, 449
Semantics, 28, 195, 196, 443
Semiotics, 28, 281
sexaholism, 222
Sexual health, 434, 435
Sexual management, 429, 434, 435, 436, 479
sexual violence, 57, 58, 258
Sexually transmitted, 223
shamanic illness, 191, 192, 193, 196
shamanism, 43, 46, 191, 192, 193, 203
sheva, 46, 191, 194, 195, 196
shopaholism, 222
simulacrum, 260
Sinistrocerebral thinking, 28, 29
Smoking, 9, 10, 11, 36, 83, 84, 87, 91, 94, 98, 101, 102, 106, 112, 115, 149, 154, 169, 222, 223, 224, 320, 322, 323, 324, 325, 409, 410, 427, 462
Social care, 79, 142, 167, 176, 178, 309, 347, 401
social diagnosis, 34, 348, 349
Social epidemics, 3, 43, 47, 48, 64, 215, 225, 243, 245, 247, 248, 249, 251, 253, 257, 259, 261, 262, 267, 268, 276, 277, 278, 279, 280, 358, 376, 388, 412, 414, 430, 438, 447, 449, 456, 458, 478
social health, 7, 10, 30, 259, 390, 447
social identity, 34, 36, 41, 43, 49, 56, 161, 178, 254, 258, 262, 273, 277, 348, 353, 412, 437, 445, 446, 448
social interaction, 121, 312, 335, 361
social organization, 28, 354
social psychiatry, 13, 14, 17, 20
social support, 94, 101, 156, 208, 236, 298, 349, 350, 355, 425, 437, 468, 472
socialization, 38, 55, 73, 74, 76, 80, 81, 86, 89, 90, 91, 92, 100, 104, 105, 106, 114, 116, 117, 118, 126, 129, 130, 131, 138, 139, 141, 142, 143, 144, 150, 152, 153, 154, 162, 163, 166, 167, 172, 174, 175, 176, 177, 185, 186, 187, 188, 189, 205, 206, 209, 210, 211, 212, 215, 216, 236, 239, 245, 250, 255, 256, 274, 275, 282, 294, 297, 298, 307, 308, 310, 311, 322, 323, 324, 325, 326, 328, 350, 351, 358, 360, 411, 416, 446
Socially-oriented MHS functions, 401
society, 4, 5, 6, 8, 10, 11, 13, 14, 15, 16, 17, 18, 22, 36, 38, 39, 40, 41, 43, 44, 48, 49, 54, 55, 58, 61, 62, 64, 65, 67, 89, 90, 93, 95, 99, 135, 159, 161, 184, 197, 198, 203, 206, 211, 221, 222, 244, 246, 247, 248, 249, 251, 254, 255, 257, 261, 262, 263, 265, 267, 269, 271, 273, 274, 287, 292, 298, 299, 302, 312, 321, 340, 348, 349, 351, 353, 354, 355, 357, 358, 359, 360, 361, 367, 371, 373, 376, 382, 389, 392, 395, 397, 400, 407, 411, 414, 416, 417, 418, 421, 437, 438, 439, 441, 442, 443, 445, 446, 447, 448, 449, 456, 459, 460, 462, 464, 466, 470, 476, 484
sociocultural trauma theory, 443
sociogenesis, 8, 9, 22, 30, 31, 33, 37, 38, 46, 68, 74, 79, 86, 89, 90, 93, 100, 104, 114, 116, 117, 126, 129, 130, 139, 141, 142, 150, 152, 163, 165, 172, 174, 175, 178, 186, 187, 199, 209, 210, 211, 213, 226, 228, 238, 255, 256, 272, 273, 274, 279, 289, 290, 292, 294, 296, 307, 309, 320, 324, 326, 349, 350, 352, 353, 372, 410, 418, 434, 442, 444, 445, 447, 449
Sociogenesis of ME, 38
sociogenetic models, 373
Socio-hygienic monitoring, 396
socio-synergetic, 349
somatic health, 6, 30
somatization disorders, 211, 259, 278
somatoform, 42, 44, 46, 47, 74, 77, 78, 86, 87, 88, 92, 100, 103, 105, 114, 116, 126, 129, 131, 139, 141, 144, 150, 152, 153, 163, 165, 166, 172, 174, 177, 181, 183, 184, 185, 186, 187, 188, 189, 206, 210, 213, 216, 227, 228, 230, 248, 255, 259, 274, 278, 282, 307, 310, 324, 325, 334, 461, 465, 471, 477, 480, 482, 483
somatoform diathesis, 185, 187, 188
somatoform disorders, 44, 46, 47, 74, 77, 86, 88, 92, 100, 103, 105, 114, 116, 126, 129, 131, 139, 141, 144, 150, 152, 153, 163, 165, 166, 172, 174, 177, 183, 188, 189, 206, 213, 216, 227, 259, 278, 307, 324, 325, 471, 477, 480, 482
somatoform family, 185, 187, 188
somatoform reactions, 185, 186, 187, 188
Somatogenesis, 8, 9, 22, 31, 37, 44, 46, 68, 74, 79, 86, 88, 93, 100, 102, 114, 115, 116, 126, 128, 138, 139, 140, 142, 149, 150, 152, 163, 164, 172, 173, 176, 187, 210, 211, 213, 226, 227, 228, 239, 255, 259, 272, 274, 278, 279, 289, 290, 291, 295, 296, 307, 309, 324, 326, 331, 372, 411, 418, 442
Somatoneurological complications, 73, 74, 79, 80, 86, 88, 92, 93, 99, 100, 101, 106, 114, 126, 131, 139, 140, 143, 149, 152, 171, 172, 177, 187
Somnology, 429, 433, 434

spiritual and moral, 19, 30, 31, 33, 43, 51, 53, 59, 67, 74, 79, 80, 81, 82, 86, 90, 91, 92, 93, 94, 95, 100, 101, 104, 105, 106, 109, 114, 115, 117, 118, 119, 121, 124, 126, 130, 131, 132, 133, 139, 142, 143, 144, 146, 151, 152, 153, 158, 160, 161, 163, 165, 166, 168, 169, 172, 175, 176, 177, 178, 179, 185, 186, 187, 188, 190, 199, 203, 206, 207, 210, 211, 212, 216, 217, 228, 229, 230, 231, 239, 245, 247, 253, 260, 262, 272, 274, 279, 281, 282, 290, 293, 298, 299, 307, 310, 313, 324, 325, 326, 357, 358, 361, 362, 363, 367, 371, 377, 378, 382, 411, 418, 433, 435, 438, 439, 447, 449, 456, 457, 464, 474, 477, 478, 481, 482, 483
spiritual and moral block, 59, 81, 82, 93, 94, 109, 121, 133, 143, 146, 158, 168, 178, 190, 203, 313
spiritual and moral deficits, 211, 307
spiritual and moral health, 30, 447
spiritual and moral typology, 53
spiritual and religious, 82, 301, 313, 456
spiritual anti-drug immunization, 374
spiritual medicine, 383
spiritually-integrated treatment, 381, 382, 383
state national security, 271
state-civil identity, 448
Strategic Cooperation Approach, 343
strategic mental trap, 267
strategic science, 418
Strategies and target orientation of the mental health service, 404
strategies for mental security, 449
strategies of mental epidemiology, 457
Strategy, 9, 19, 24, 25, 28, 42, 82, 91, 95, 106, 117, 156, 189, 199, 226, 229, 231, 270, 271, 278, 279, 280, 302, 313, 320, 367, 368, 391, 406, 417, 418, 449, 450, 451, 452, 457, 458, 459, 460, 478
strategy of adaptive conscience expansion, 449
structure of happiness, 66
Stylistics, 6, 28, 287, 289
SUNAPCE, 368
syndrome, 17, 46, 54, 55, 56, 57, 58, 59, 64, 72, 77, 78, 81, 82, 87, 90, 98, 102, 104, 106, 117, 128, 130, 137, 140, 142, 143, 145, 148, 154, 155, 156, 158, 161, 164, 174, 175, 176, 179, 186, 205, 206, 207, 208, 212, 213, 221, 224, 225, 226, 227, 228, 229, 231, 233, 235, 240, 243, 245, 246, 251, 253, 254, 256, 259, 272, 273, 275, 277, 278, 281, 289, 290, 294, 296, 300, 301, 306, 308, 309, 313, 323, 324, 333, 334, 358, 360, 393, 410, 411, 412, 415, 419, 441, 444, 445, 452, 472, 482
syndrome of changed reactivity, 259
syndrome of existential despair, 54
syndrome of physical dependence, 259
syndrome of psychic dependence, 259
syndrome of Scientological demoralization, 272, 273
Synergetic Biopsychosociospiritual Methodology, 29, 35, 41, 47, 50, 51, 58, 65, 67, 73, 265, 271, 278, 279, 281, 332, 371, 390, 392, 394, 409, 435, 455, 478
synergetic biopsychosociospiritual Ψ-cluster, 417
Synergetic Functional Diagnosis, 33, 34, 49, 279, 403
synergetic man, 408, 418
synergetic methodology in drug preventology, 374
synergetic person, 31, 455
synergetic personalized model of biopsychosociospiritual care, 455
synergetic psychotherapy, 341
Synergetics, 18, 19, 20, 24, 25, 27, 28, 29, 31, 52, 73, 85, 99, 113, 125, 138, 149, 162, 171, 185, 207, 209, 225, 238, 243, 253, 265, 278, 287, 295, 299, 303, 304, 306, 321, 349, 428, 438, 468, 478, 479
Synergetics of Nicotine Addiction, 321
synergistic functional diagnostics, 455
synergistic person, 372, 378
system, 4, 6, 7, 8, 9, 10, 11, 13, 14, 15, 16, 17, 18, 19, 20, 21, 22, 23, 27, 28, 29, 31, 33, 37, 38, 39, 40, 42, 43, 45, 48, 49, 50, 52, 53, 63, 64, 77, 78, 80, 81, 84, 85, 87, 88, 98, 99, 101, 102, 112, 116, 128, 132,140, 146, 148, 149, 156, 157, 160, 161, 164, 171, 173, 174, 176, 184, 186, 188, 189, 193, 207, 209, 211, 216, 222, 224, 225, 240, 241, 244, 249, 254, 260, 262, 263, 267, 268, 269, 271, 272, 277, 280, 286, 287, 288, 289, 291, 292, 293, 294, 295, 296, 299, 302, 303, 306, 308, 310, 311, 317, 318, 319, 320, 321, 322, 323, 324, 326, 327, 328, 330, 338, 347, 348, 349, 350, 353, 354, 362, 363, 368, 382, 388, 389, 392, 393, 395, 396, 397, 398, 399, 401, 403, 404, 406, 408, 415, 416, 421, 423, 425, 427, 428, 429, 430, 432, 433, 437, 438, 439, 442, 445, 448, 450, 452, 455, 456, 457, 459, 462, 478, 481, 482
System ecological monitoring, 267, 396
system monitoring of, 31, 45, 48, 262, 382, 401, 416, 438, 448, 481
system monitoring of mental health (SMMH), 45, 48, 262, 382, 401, 416, 438, 448
system of action, 211, 348
system of clientele, 348
system of targets, 348
system psychiatric crisis, 23
System synthesis of mental medicine, 19, 20, 478
systemic block-modular protection programs, 71

T

Target levels of mental security, 447
Task(s), 9, 19, 20, 24, 25, 28, 29, 33, 35, 37, 47, 51, 59, 71, 73, 93, 95, 97, 111, 147, 156, 158, 159, 167, 179, 183, 208, 229, 234, 235, 238, 243, 262, 267, 270, 279, 281, 300, 305, 313, 338, 345, 348, 349, 350, 355, 364, 371, 373, 378, 379, 380, 398, 411, 415, 416, 418, 419, 421, 437, 441, 443, 450, 456, 459, 466
Teaching hatred, 252
technological complex of the strategic breakthrough, 418
technological platform of the mental, 394
Technologies, 16, 18, 19, 24, 25, 33, 50, 243, 265, 271, 279, 280, 281, 371, 388, 394, 400, 405, 418, 419, 421, 429, 437, 440, 455, 456, 459
Terrorism, 48, 50, 63, 64, 229, 233, 243, 244, 245, 246, 247, 248, 249, 250, 251, 252, 253, 254, 255, 256, 257, 258, 259, 260, 261, 262, 263, 265, 266, 267, 268, 269, 270, 273, 277, 278, 341, 358, 360, 388, 399, 412, 446, 447, 456, 467, 473, 474, 478, 479, 480, 481, 484
terrorism as a polymodal dependent disorder, 456
terrorist, 17, 48, 54, 234, 236, 238, 239, 240, 243, 244, 245, 246, 247, 248, 249, 250, 251, 252, 253, 254, 256, 257, 259, 260, 261, 262, 268, 269, 270, 273, 276, 280, 388, 410, 484
terrorist attack, 243, 244, 248, 261, 388
terrorist ideology, 280
terrorist war, 252, 261, 268, 270, 273
terrorist world, 262, 273
terroristic community, 258
terroristic world, 256, 260
the happiness level, 65
Theory of Disasters, 427
therapy, 15, 16, 31, 46, 61, 63, 80, 81, 89, 91, 92, 93, 94, 95, 105, 106, 107, 108, 111, 118, 119, 120, 121, 124, 131, 132, 143, 144, 145, 146, 151, 153, 154, 155, 156, 158, 164, 167, 168, 177, 178, 179, 184, 188, 189, 202, 216, 229, 230, 231, 240, 247,279, 280, 282, 298, 300, 301, 302, 304, 310, 311, 312, 313, 317, 318, 319, 320, 321, 323, 325, 326, 327, 328, 329, 335, 340, 353, 371, 372, 373, 377, 382, 389, 401, 402, 403, 406, 413, 424, 429, 430, 431, 432, 456, 461, 464, 465, 466, 468, 470, 474, 475, 479, 481, 483
Time of Troubles, 248
Traditional epidemiology, 35
Tranquilizers, 202, 326, 333, 334
transformation society, 443
traumatic, 155, 170, 171, 173, 184, 199, 202, 206, 225, 257, 259, 267, 276, 277, 306, 319, 345, 410, 423, 424, 425, 427, 431, 435, 443, 447, 465, 482
Trend, 6, 7, 11, 18, 19, 21, 25, 36, 47, 53, 98, 99, 111, 138, 161, 279, 287, 288, 289, 291, 295, 297, 299, 302, 340, 359, 376, 390, 394, 411, 413, 451, 459, 460
Tuberculosis, 124, 223, 306, 396
Types of immunity, 447

U

ulcerogenic diathesis, 113, 114, 115, 116, 118
ulcerogenic family, 113, 114, 117, 118
Unemployment, 22, 57, 99, 223, 256, 263, 275, 351, 424, 447
unexpressed moral orientation, 367
unified multidisciplinary protocol, 279
universal indulgence, 270
unlawful behavior is formed, 212
unwarranted change in wage rate, 234

V

Vector of actions, 28
verbal aggression, 234, 410
Viability, 339
victim, 36, 61, 208, 234, 235, 236, 237, 238, 239, 240, 244, 249, 266, 341, 343, 344, 345, 359, 388, 445
violation of personal, 209
virulent simulacrum, 266

W

Way of object realization, 28
welfare, 10, 57, 66, 347, 418, 449
well-being, 5, 6, 9, 10, 11, 57, 65, 66, 67, 91, 94, 106, 185, 331, 350, 374, 396, 417, 422, 424, 427, 433, 449, 458, 477
workaholism, 46, 205, 206, 209, 210, 211, 221, 227, 410